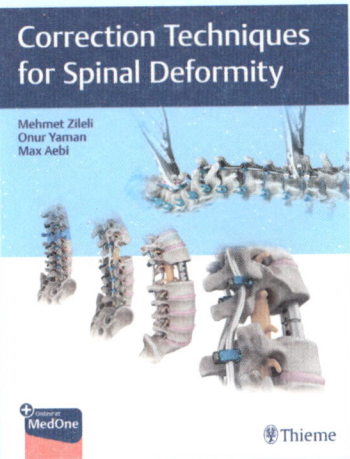

Correction Techniques for Spinal Deformity

Mehmet Zileli
Onur Yaman
Max Aebi

MedOne

Thieme

Access your free e-book now!

With three easy steps, unlock free access to your e-book on MedOne, Thieme's online platform.

1. Note your personal access code below. Once this code is activated, your printed book can no longer be returned.

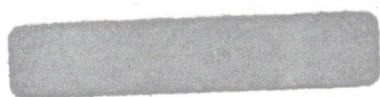

Important Notes

- The personal access code is disabled once the e-book is first activated. Use of this product is restricted to the buyer or, for library copies, authorized users.

- Sharing passwords is not permitted. The publisher has the right to take legal steps for violations.

- Access to online material is solely provided to the buyer for private use. Commercial use is not permitted.

2. Scan this QR code or enter your access code at **medone.thieme.com/code**.

3. Set up a username on MedOne and sign in to activate your e-book on most phones, tablets, or PCs.

Quick Access

After you successfully register and activate your code, you can find your book and additional online media at **medone.thieme.com/9789395390101** or with this QR code.

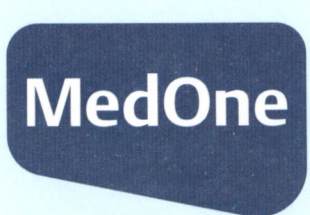

MedOne

Medical information how and when you need it.

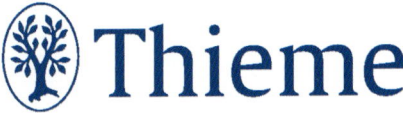

Correction Techniques for Spinal Deformity

Mehmet Zileli, MD
Professor of Neurosurgery
Department of Neurosurgery
Sanko University Hospital
Gaziantep, Türkiye

Onur Yaman, MD
Professor
Department of Neurosurgery
Arel University;
Chief of the Spine Section
Department of Neurosurgery
Memorial Hospital Group Spine Center
Istanbul, Türkiye

Max Aebi, Dr.med. et Dr.h.c.
Senior Consultant
Wirbelsäulenmedizin AG, Salem Spital
Bern, Switzerland;
Professor Emeritus
McGill University
Montreal, Canada;
University of Bern (CH)
Bern, Switzerland;
Member of European Academy of Sciences

Thieme
Delhi • Stuttgart • New York • Rio de Janeiro

Publishing Director: Ritu Sharma
Senior Developement Editor: Dr Nidhi Srivastava
Director-Editorial Services: Rachna Sinha
Project Manager: Nidhi Chopra
National Sales Manager: Bishwajit Kumar Mishra
Managing Director & CEO: Ajit Kohli

Thieme Medical and Scientific Publishers Private Limited.
A - 12, Second Floor, Sector - 2, Noida - 201 301,
Uttar Pradesh, India, +911204556600
Email: customerservice@thieme.in
www.thieme.in

Cover design: © Thieme
Cover image source: © Thieme
Typesetting by RECTO Graphics, India

Printed in India

5 4 3 2 1

DOI: 10.1055/b000000905

ISBN: 978-93-95390-10-1
Also available as an e-book:
eISBN (PDF): 978-93-95390-11-8
eISBN (epub): 978-93-95390-13-2

This book is dedicated to
our patients who have trusted us during their treatment of spinal disorders.

Contents

Contents

Part VI: Special Topics

Henri-Arthur Leroy, MD, PhD
Associate Professor and Neurosurgeon
Neurosurgery
CHU Lille
Lille, France

İdris Avcı, MD
Medical Doctor
Department of Neurosurgery
Memorial Spine Center
Istanbul, Türkiye

İsmail Bozkurt, MD
Consultant
Department of Neurosurgery
Medical Park Ankara Hospital
Batıkent, Ankara, Türkiye

J. Manuel Sarmiento, MD
Clinical Fellow
Spine & Scoliosis Service
Hospital for Special Surgery
New York, NY, USA

Jason W. Savage, MD
Associate Professor
Orthopaedic Surgery
Case Western Reserve University and Cleveland Clinic Lerner
    College of Medicine
Cleveland, Ohio, USA

Jean Charles Le Huec, MD, PhD
Professor
Plyclinique Bordeaux Nord Aquitaine
Spine, Vertebra Department
Bordeaux University
Bordeaux, France

Joao Amorim, MD
Doctor
Department Neurosurgery
UNICEPLAC - Universidade do Planalto
Gama, Distrito Federal, Brazil

John J. Mangan, MD, MHA
Assistant Professor
Department of Orthopaedic Surgery
Thomas Jefferson University Hospital
Philadelphia, Pennsylvania, USA

John Paul Wanner, MD
Assistant Professor
Orthopaedic Surgery
The Medical College of Wisconsin
Milwaukee, Wisconsin, USA

Joseph S. Butler, PhD, FACS, FRCS
Consultant Spine Surgeon
National Spinal Injuries Unit
Mater Misericordiae University Hospital
Mater Private Hospital
Dublin, Ireland

Kazım Yiğitkanlı, MD
Associate Professor
Neurosurgery Department
Konya Medikana Hospital
Konya, Türkiye

Kemal Paksoy, MBBS
Specialist
Neurosurgery
Bahçelievler Memorial Hospital
İstanbul, Türkiye

Leopoldina Pereira, MD
Resident
Neurosurgery
Centro Hospitalar Vila Nova Gaia
Gaia, Portugal

Lisa Boue
Master
Clinical Research Assistant
Clinical Research Department
Polyclinique Bordeaux Nord Aquitaine
Bordeaux, France

Marcos Masini, MD
Professor of Neurosurgery
School of Medicine UNICEPLAC
Department of Neurosurgery, Hospital Lago Sul
Clínica Quéops Millennium
Brasília, Brazil

Margarida Luis Rios Alves, MS
Medical Student
Medical College
Humanitas University
Milano, Italy

Contributors

Max Aebi, Dr.med. et Dr.h.c.
Senior Consultant
Wirbelsäulenmedizin AG, Salem Spital
Bern, Switzerland;
Professor Emeritus
McGill University
Montreal, Canada;
University of Bern (CH)
Bern, Switzerland;
Member of European Academy of Sciences

Mehmet Zileli, MD
Professor of Neurosurgery
Department of Neurosurgery
Sanko University Hospital
Gaziantep, Türkiye

Muhammad Tariq Imtiaz, MD, DABNM, FASNM
Attending/Consultant Physician
National Neurosciences Institute
King Fahad Medical City
Riyadh, Saudi Arabia

Muharrem Yazici, MD
Orthopaedic Surgeon
Orthopedics
Children's Orthopedics and Spine Center
Ankara, Türkiye

Murat Baloğlu, MD
Associate Professor
Department of Neurosurgery
Eskişehir City Hospital
Eskisehir, Türkiye

Nail Özdemir, MD
Professor
Department of Neurosurgery
İstanbul Aydın University School of Medicine
İstanbul, Türkiye

Nevhis Akıntürk, MD
Consultant Neurosurgeon
Department of Neurosurgery
Ege University, Medicine Faculty
İzmir, Türkiye

Nicat Bayram, MD
Professor
Department of Neurosurgery
Memorial Hospital
Istanbul, Türkiye

Nikolay Peev, MD, PhD (Neurosurgery), FRCS (England)
Consultant Neurosurgeon and Spinal Surgeon
Belfast HSC Trust
Belfast, Northern Ireland, UK

Nuri Demirci, MBBS
Medical Student
Medical Faculty
Acibadem Mehmet Ali Aydinlar University
Istanbul, Türkiye

Ömer Akçalı, MD
Professor of Orthopedic Surgery
Department of Orthopedics and Traumatology
Dokuz Eylül University Hospital
Izmir, Türkiye

Onur Yaman, MD
Professor
Department of Neurosurgery
Arel University;
Chief of the Spine Section
Department of Neurosurgery
Memorial Hospital Group Spine Center
Istanbul, Türkiye

Óscar L. Alves, MD
Head
Department of Neurosurgery
Hospital Lusiasas Porto
Porto, Portugal

Özgür Akşan, MD
Specialist
Department of Neurosurgery
Beyin ve sinir
İzmir, Türkiye

Pedro Berjano, MD, PhD
Orthopaedic and Trauma surgeon
Department of G Spine4
IRCCS Ospedale Galeazzi Sant'Ambrogi
Milan, Italy

Pierre Haettel, MD
Neurosurgeon
Service neurochirurgie hôpital Roger Salengro
Université Lille
Lille, France

Preface

Spine surgery is a fast-evolving discipline, and many spine surgeons are opting for subspecializations like spinal deformity surgery.

Spinal deformity correction has its roots in the use of traction techniques and manipulation thousands of years ago; however, surgery for deformity correction gained much interest in the middle of the 20th century. Correction maneuvers used specifically for adolescent idiopathic scoliosis followed by osteotomy techniques and refining them in the current practice have produced many surgical tips and tricks.

Recent trends and progress in geriatric spine surgery, even trying to correct severely degenerated and osteoporotic deformities and applying minimally invasive surgical techniques, have made understanding of this pathology and its treatment even more difficult.

This book, *Correction Techniques for Spinal Deformity*, intends to present and explain all deformity correction maneuvers and different osteotomy types, and tips and tricks behind such surgeries. In addition, it contains numerous illustrations depicting and describing the complex maneuvers to facilitate the readers' understanding.

The book has six main divisions: (1) Techniques for Cervical Spinal Deformity Correction, (2) Techniques for Congenital Spinal Deformity Correction, (3) Spinal Osteotomy Techniques, (4) Sagittal Plane Correction Techniques, (5) Coronal Plane Correction Techniques, and (6) Special Topics. It also covers areas such as neuromonitoring, without which this complex surgery as of today is unthinkable. This book also covers topics like complication avoidance, minimally invasive surgery, lateral access surgery, and dynamic stabilization.

A total of 40 chapters written by world-renowned authors have created this very comprehensive and standard-setting textbook on spinal deformities.

Mehmet Zileli, MD
Onur Yaman, MD
Max Aebi, Dr.med. et Dr.h.c.

Acknowledgments

We acknowledge the great help of Mr. Mehmet Dal, medical illustrator, who has made significant artistic and technical efforts to explain the various details of our surgeries.

Mehmet Zileli, MD
Onur Yaman, MD
Max Aebi, Dr.med. et Dr.h.c.

Contributors

Abhishek Mannem, MS (Ortho), DNB (Ortho), FISS (Spine)
Consultant Spine Surgeon
Spine Surgery
The Bangalore Hospital
Bangalore, Karnataka, India

Adnan Yalçın Demirci, MD
Associate Professor
Department of Neurosurgery
Sağlık Bilimleri University, Bursa Yüksek Ihtisas Education and
    Research Hospital
Bursa, Türkiye

Ahmet Alanay, MD
Professor
Department of Orthopedics and Traumatology
Acibadem University School of Medicine
Istanbul, Türkiye

Ahmet Öğrenci, MD
Associate Professor
Department of Neurosurgery
Medicana Ataşehir Hastanesi
Istanbul, Türkiye

Ali Fahir Özer, MD
Professor of Neurosurgery
Department of Neurosurgery
Koç University School of Medicine
Istanbul, Türkiye

Alice Baroncini, MD, PhD
Spine Fellow
Department of Orthopaedic, Trauma, and Reconstructive Surgery
RWTH Aachen University Hospital
Aachen, Germany

Andrea Redaelli, MD
Orthopedic Spine Surgeon
GSpine4
IRCCS Ospedale Galeazzi - Sant'Ambrogio
Milan, Italy

Areena D'Souza, MS (Ortho)
Facharzt Orthopädie Unfallchirurgie
Consultant Spine Surgeon (Oberärztin)
Department of Pediatric Spine Surgery
Orthopädische Kinderklinik
Aschau i. Chiemgau, Bayern, Germany

Assaker Jordan, MD
Resident
Department of Neurosurgery
Chu Lille
Lille, France

Atul Goel, MD
Consultant
Department of Neurosurgery
Lilavati Hospital & Research Center
Mumbai, Maharashtra, India

Benoit Derre, Master Degree
Engineer
Department of Neurosurgery
Centre Hospitalier Universitaire de Lille
Lille, France

Bronek Boszczyk, Dr. med. habil
Head of Department and Consultant Spine Surgeon
Department of Pediatric Spine Surgery
Orthopädische Kinderklinik
Aschau i. Chiemgau, Bayern, Germany

Çağlar Yılgör, MD
Associate Professor
Pediatric and Adult Spinal Disorders
Comprehensive Spine Center at Acibadem Maslak Hospital
Acibadem University School of Medicine, Department of
    Orthopaedics and Traumatology
Istanbul, Türkiye
Director, Spine Fellowship Program

Çağrı Canbolat, MD
Neurosurgeon
Neurosurgery Clinic
Liv Hospital Vadistanbul
Istanbul, Türkiye

Can Yaldız, MD
Associate Professor
Department of Neurosurgery
Kocaeli Akademi Hospital
Kocaeli, Türkiye

Claudio Lamartina, MD
Orthopedic Spine Surgeon
Chair
GSpine4
IRCCS Ospedale Galeazzi - Sant'Ambrogio
Universita' degli Studi di Milano
Milan, Italy

D. Güçlühan Güçlü, MD
Associate Professor and Head of Neurosurgery
Department of Neurosurgery
University of Health Sciences Bakirkoy Dr. Sadi Konuk Training and
　　Research Hospital
Istanbul, Türkiye

Dileep N. Lobo, MD
Professor of Gastrointestinal Surgery
University of Nottingham; School of Medicine
Queen's Medical Centre
Nottingham, UK

Edward C. Benzel, MD
Emeritus Chair of Neurosurgery
Department of Neurosurgery
Cleveland Clinic
Cleveland, Ohio, USA

Emanuele Quarto, MD
Orthopaedic Surgeon
Department of Orthopaedic Surgery
IRCCS Policlinico San Martino Hospital
Genoa, Italy

Emre Acaroğlu, MD, MAODE
Professor
Orthopedics
Ankara Spine Center
Ankara, Türkiye

Ender Ofluoğlu, MD
Professor
Head of Neurosurgery Department
Arel University School of Medicine
Istanbul, Türkiye

Engin Çetin, MD
Associate Professor
Department of Orthopaedics and Traumatology
Gaziosmanpasa Training and Research Hospital
Istanbul, Türkiye

Faisal R. Jahangiri, MD, CNIM, DABNM, FASNM, FASET
Assistant Professor of Instruction
Neuroscience
University of Texas at Dallas
Richardson, Texas, USA

Ferran Pellisé, MD, PhD
Professor
Orthopedic Surgery and Traumatology
Vall d'Hebron University Hospital
Barcelona, Spain

Filippo Mandelli, MD
Orthopaedic and Trauma surgeon
Department of Spine Surgery
University Hospital Basel
Basel, Switzerland

Francesco Langella, MD
Physician
Spine Surgery
Orthopedic & Traumatology
IRCCS Ospedale Galeazzi - Sant'Ambrogio
Milan, Italy

Frank Schwab, MD
Chairman of Orthopaedic Surgery
Department of Orthopaedic Surgery
Lenox Hill Hospital
New York, NY, USA

Gökhan Gökçe, MD
Assistant Professor
Department of Neurosurgery
Turgut Özal University School of Medicine
Malatya, Türkiye

Göktuğ Akyoldaş, MD
Associate Professor
Department of Neurosurgery
Koç University School of Medicine
Istanbul, Türkiye

Habib Canberk Karakoç, MD
Specialist
Neurosurgery
Reyhanlı State Hospital
Hatay, Türkiye

Richard Assaker, MD
Professor
Department of Neurosurgery
CHRU Lille Hôpital Salengro
Lille, France

Rıza Mert Çetik, MD
Orthopedic Surgeon
Department of Orthopedics and Traumatology
Pursaklar State Hospital
Ankara, Türkiye

Rui Reinas, MD
Resident
Department of Neurosurgery
Centro Hospitalar de vila Nova de Gaia/Espinho
Portugal

Salim Şentürk, MD
Associate Professor
Department of Neurosurgery
Memorial Bahcelievler Hospital
Istanbul, Türkiye

Salman Sharif, MD, FRCS (SN), IFAANS
Chair
WNS Spine Committee;
Professor and Chief
Department of Neurosurgery
Liaquat National Hospital & Medical College
Karachi, Pakistan

Salvatore Petrone, MD
Neurosurgeon
Spine Surgery Unit
Humanitas Gradenigo
Turin, Italy

Sandra O'Malley, BMBS
Registrar
Trauma and Orthoapedics
Mater Misericordiae University Hospital
Dublin, Ireland

Sedat Dalbayrak, MD
Head
Department of Neurosurgery
Medicana International Hospital
Ataşehir, Istanbul, Türkiye

Serkan Şimşek, MD, PhD
Professor of Neurosurgery
Department of Neurosurgery
Lokman Hekim University
Ankara, Türkiye

Shahswar Arif, MD, PG Cert (Surgery)
Senior House Officer (SHO)
Trauma and Orthopaedics
Western Health and Social Care Trust
Londonderry, Northern Ireland

Sleiman Haddad, MD, PhD, FRCS
Associated Coordinator
Spine Unit, Orthopedic Surgery and Traumatology
Vall d'Hebron University Hospital
Barcelona, Catalonia, Spain

Stéphane Bourret, PhD
Clinical Research Assistant
Clinical Research Department
Polyclinique Bordeaux Nord Aquitaine
Bordeaux, France

Susana Núñez-Pereira, MD, PhD
Consultant Spine Surgeon
Spine Unit, Orthopaedics and Traumatology Department
Vall d'Hebron University Hospital
Barcelona, Spain

Turgut Akgül, MD
Professor
Department of Orthopedics and Traumatology
Istanbul University
Istanbul, Türkiye

Ülkün Ünlü Ünsal, MD
Associate Professor
Department of Neurosurgery
Manisa City Hospital
Manisa, Türkiye

Virginie Lafage, PhD
AVP Clinical Research
Department of Orthopaedic Surgery
Lenox Hill Hospital
New York, NY, USA

Contributors

Wendy Thompson, MD
Orthopedic surgeon
Polyclinique Bordeaux Nord Aquitaine
Vertebra Center
DETERCA Center, University Bordeaux
Bordeaux, France

Yahya Güvenç, MD
Associate Professor
Department of Neurosurgery
Marmara University
Istanbul, Türkiye

Yunus Emre Özdemir, MD
Senior Resident
Orthopedics and Traumatology
Acıbadem University School of Medicine
Istanbul, Türkiye

Yurdal Gezercan, MD
Associate Professor of Neurosurgery
Department of Neurosurgery
Adana City Training Research Hospital
Adana, Türkiye

Zarina Brady, MD, PG Cert (Surgery)
Senior House Officer (SHO)
Department of Trauma and Orthopaedics
Western Health and Social Care Trust
Londonderry, Northern Ireland

Part I

Techniques for Cervical Spinal Deformity Correction

1 Cervical Sagittal Balance

Yahya Güvenç, Onur Yaman, and Salman Sharif

Introduction

Humans are characterized by bipedalism, but this is achieved by keeping the body in balance. The spine performs an essential function in maintaining balance. Humans developed cervical curvature, lumbar lordosis, thoracal kyphosis, and horizontal gaze to maintain balance. It is crucial to analyze the matter both statically and dynamically to understand balance. There are differences between the balance people keep while standing and the balance conditions while moving. In addition, the healthy spine and the unhealthy spine show differences in the mechanisms while maintaining balance. To maintain the balance, we need to define the morphological criteria and then analyze the compensation phenomena, physiological or pathological. For this purpose, we should know that we need to evaluate the spine as a whole. Changes in the cervical, thoracic, and lumbar regions affect the global balance of the spine. Therefore, in surgical procedures for any spine region, we need to examine the morphological features. Therefore, cervical measurements should be made for surgical planning before any intervention in the cervical region.

Cervical sagittal balance is an important issue that should be considered in operations.

Some studies show that preoperative cervical kyphosis with sagittal imbalance has worse postoperative outcomes. Kyphotic deformity, one of the types of cervical malalignment, usually occurs after postlaminectomy. Kyphosis causes increased neck pain, intradiskal pressure, degeneration, intraspinal canal pressure, and resulting myelomalacia. Therefore, surgical correction of patients should target cervical lordosis with global spinal balance.[1]

Cervical sagittal balance is an essential part of global spinal sagittal balance. The cervical spine is an effective part for compensating for global sagittal balance to maintain horizontal gaze. Cervical sagittal balance is directly related to health quality of life factors. In cervical fusion, this must be considered when determining the ideal alignment for permanent fixation.

In spinal alignment, the cervical, thoracic, lumbar, and pelvic regions are interconnected. When there is a deterioration in these regions, other areas compensate for this situation. In the degenerative spine with imbalance, compensatory mechanisms work for maintaining the balance. When there is a decrease in the lumbar lordosis of the patients, there will be an anterior malposition; to correct this, there will be an increase in thoracic kyphosis and cervical lordosis due to compensatory mechanisms. When cervical kyphosis occurs, the compensatory mechanism increases lumbar lordosis and decreases thoracic kyphosis. The cervical spine lordosis will change to maintain a horizontal perspective and the position of the head in the vertical plane relative to the body. If there is a severe primary cervical deformity, the lumbar spine and pelvis will be involved in the compensatory mechanism. Therefore, when planning deformity surgery, we need to measure cervical deformation and compensatory changes.

Definitions

There are some cervical spine sagittal alignment parameters. Some are commonly used parameters; others are newly proposed parameters (**Table 1.1**).

There are many values close to each other in the literature regarding "normal" cervical parameters. Therefore, there is no definite value for each angle. However, there is a range of values that can be common for cervical parameters. Many studies in the literature conducted in the asymptomatic population show differences in normal cervical angle result in each study (**Table 1.2**).[2–8] The biggest reason for this is that we are measuring a dynamic spine. Although these measurements vary, the mean values are close to each other. Therefore, these mean values can give us an idea of normal cervical spinal parameters (**Table 1.2**).[2–8]

Table 1.1 Cervical sagittal alignment parameters

Commonly used cervical spine parameters	Newly proposed cervical spine parameters
C0–C2 lordosis	Cranial tilt
C2–C7 lordosis	Neck tilt
C2–C7 SVA	Cervical tilt
CBVA	EAM–C7 sagittal vertical axis
T1 slope	
TIA	

Abbreviations: CBVA, chin brow vertical angle; EAM, external auditory meatus; SVA, sagittal vertical axis; TIA, thoracic inlet angle.

Table 1.2 Cervical parameters of asymptomatic individuals in some studies in the literature

	C0–C2	C1–C2	C2–C7	C0–C7	SVA C0–C7	C7 S	T1 S	T1A	Neck tilt
Hardacker et al[7]		−31.9 ± 7.0°		−40.0 ± 9.7°					
Guo et al[2]	−16.3 ± 7.0° (female) −14.9 ± 6.5° (males)	−28.2 ± 4.0° (females), −26.4 ± 4.6° (males)	−12.7 ± 6.6° (female), −16.3 ± 7.3° (male)						
Lee et al[8]	−22.4 ± 8.5°		−9.9 ± 12.5°		20.7 ± 11.7 mm	19.6 ± 8.8°	25.7 ± 6.4°	69.5 ± 8.6°	43.7 ± 6.1°
Núñez-Pereira et al[3]	−12.7 ± 6.9°	−20.8 ± 7.3°	−15.8 ± 13.2°			−23.4 ± 11.7°			
Iyer et al[4]	−27.4 ± 9.4°		−12.2 ± 13.6°						
Hey et al[5]			−0.6 ± 11.1° (standing), −17.2 ± 12.1° (sitting)	−30.7 ± 13° (standing), −46 ± 12.5° (sitting)			17.4 ± 8.7° (standing), 30.2 ± 7.4° (sitting)		
Chen et al[6]		−26.2 ± 7.2°	−12.1 ± 10.6°		19.6 ± 13.5°		23 ± 7.1°	62.4 ± 8.5°	39.4 ± 8.4°

Cervical Lordosis

There are some ways to measure cervical lordosis. The Cobb method, the Ishihara index method, Harrison's posterior tangent method, and Jackson physiological stress lines are the most known methods.[9–11] The Cobb method (mCM) is most frequently used in practical applications. A study showed C1 to C7 lordosis of −39 ± 9 degrees in adults without neck symptoms.[7] Cervical lordosis is evaluated in two different subgroups because the mobility in the cervical region shows differences between segments. The C1–C2 region where the movement is high is responsible for 77% of the cervical lordosis, and the remaining 23% occurs at C2–C7 level where the movement is less.[10]

The results of some studies have shown that the cervical lordosis (C0–C7) is around 30 degrees.[12–14] Posture and thoracic kyphosis affect cervical lordosis. Therefore, it is recommended to take X-ray images when the patient is standing. As we get older, thoracic kyphosis increases, and lumbar lordosis decreases. Due to this change, compensation mechanisms come into play in cervical lordosis to provide a horizontal view.

- *Cervical lordosis (C0–C2):* This angle is formed by the McGregor's line and the inferior end plate of C2 (**Fig. 1.1**). C0–C2 angle ranges from −12.3 to −27.4 degrees (**Table 1.2**).
- *Cervical lordosis (C2–C7):* This angle is formed by the inferior end plate of C2 and the superior end plate of C7 (**Fig. 1.2**). C2–C7 angle ranges from −12.1 to −16.3 degrees (**Table 1.2**).
- *Cervical lordosis (C0–C7):* The angle is formed by the McGregor's line and the superior end plate of

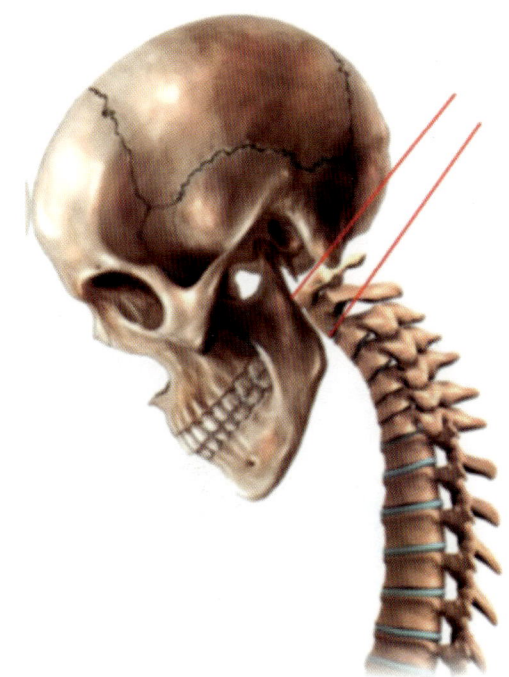

Fig. 1.1 Measurement of C0–C2 lordosis.

C7 (**Fig. 1.3**). C0–C7 angle ranges from −30.0 to −40.3 degrees (**Table 1.2**).

C2–C7 Sagittal Vertical Axis (SVA)

The horizontal distance between a plumb line drawn perpendicularly from the midpoint of the C2 vertebral body and the upper posterior corner of the C7 vertebral body is defined as the SVA (**Fig. 1.4**). C2–C7 SVA measures cervical sagittal alignment, and this angle is correlated with

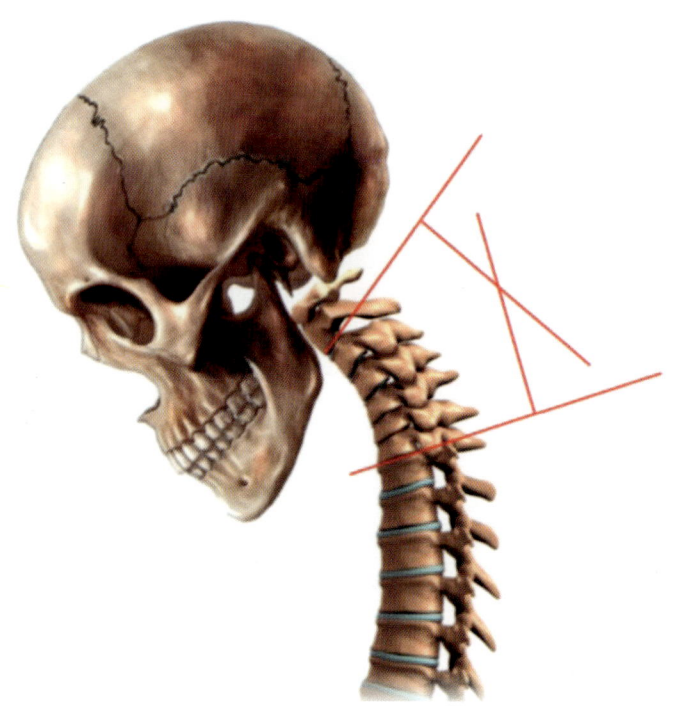

Fig. 1.2 Measurement of cervical lordosis (C2–C7).

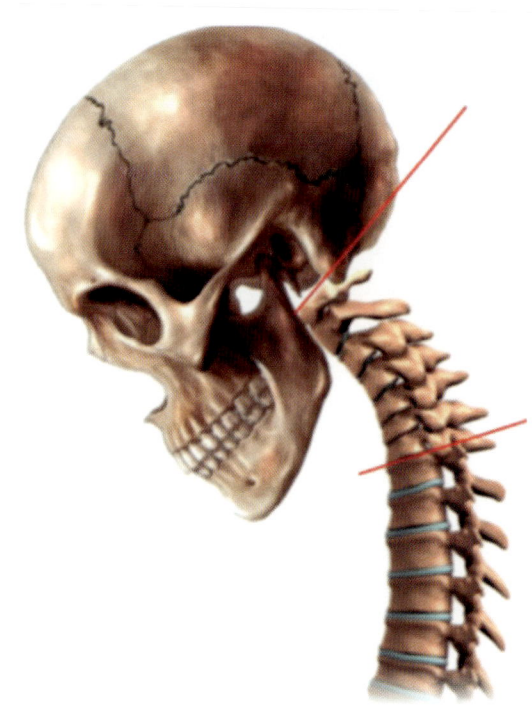

Fig. 1.3 Measurement of cervical lordosis (C0–C7).

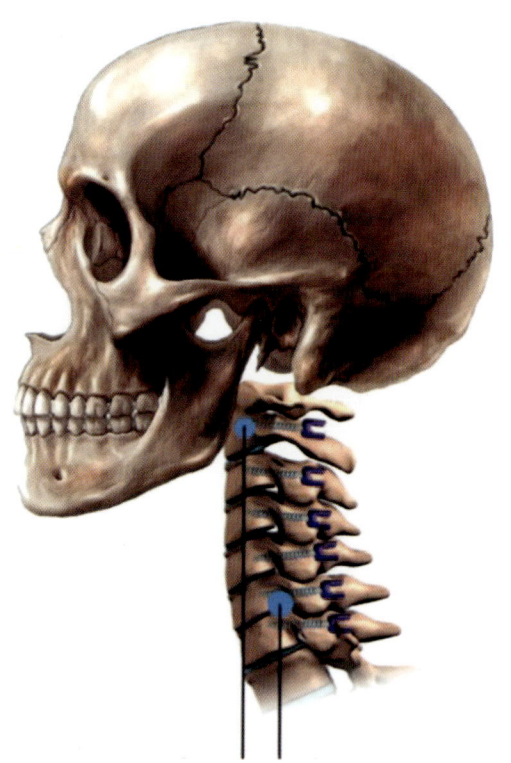

Fig. 1.4 Measurement of C2–C7 sagittal vertical axis (SVA).

health-related quality of life.[15] A study found a mean C2–C7 SVA of 4.74 mm in asymptomatic persons.[16] Iyer et al showed that C2–C7 SVA was 21.3 mm in 120 asymptomatic persons.[4] Tang et al examined the patients who had undergone multilevel posterior cervical fusion surgery and observed that when C2–C7 SVA is >40 mm, there was an increase in the disability.[15]

Chin Brow Vertical Angle (CBVA)

The angle between the line drawn from the chin to the forehead and the vertical is called the chin brow vertical angle (CBVA). This angle is used to determine horizontal gaze (**Fig. 1.5**). CBVA of a patient with ankylosing spondylitis who has been operated on is shown in **Figs. 1.6** and **1.7**. CBVA changes according to head position. For example, CBVA is positive when the head is directed downward; CBVA is negative when the head is directed upwards; when the head is in the neutral position, CBVA is zero. However, in some cervical deformities, the movements of the head are restricted, and CBVA goes outside the normal limits.

Suk et al suggested that CBVA should be within the range of −10 degrees to +10 degrees for providing optimal horizontal gaze when correcting the kyphotic deformity in ankylosing spondylitis.[17]

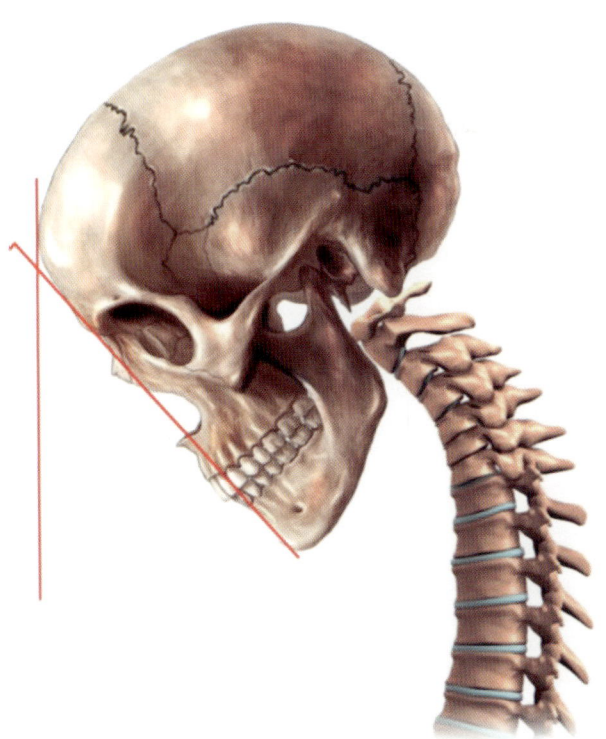

Fig. 1.5 Measurement of chin brow vertical angle.

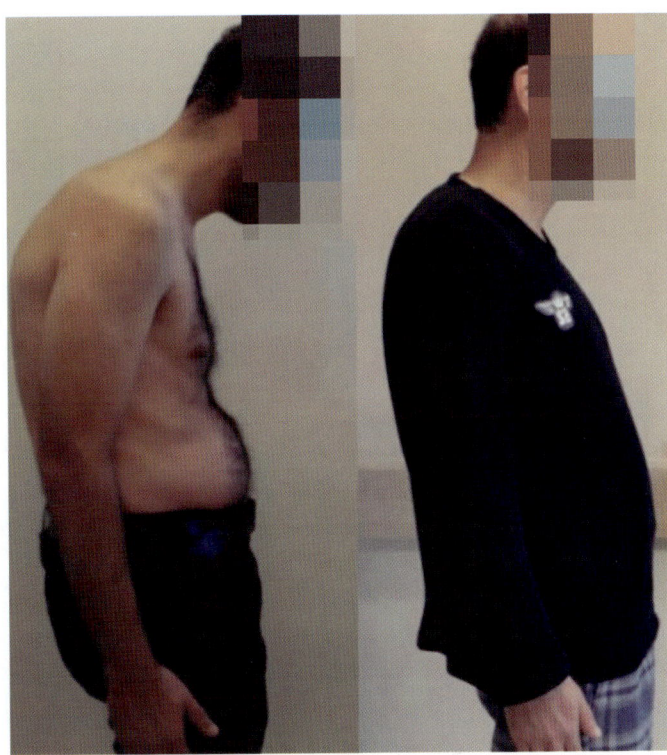

Fig. 1.6 The horizontal gaze of an ankylosing spondylitis case (before and after surgery).

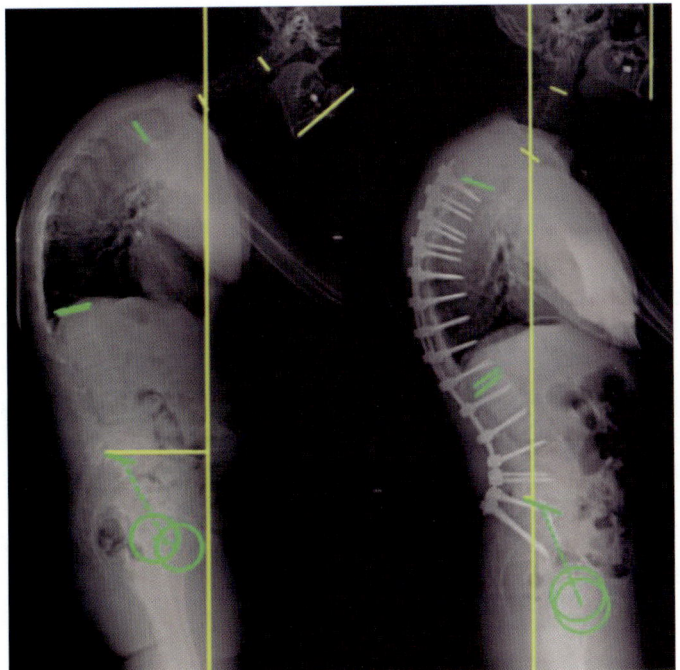

Fig. 1.7 Chin brow vertical angle (CBVA) of 49 degrees was corrected to 0 degree with surgery.

Thoracic Inlet Angle (TIA), T1S, and Neck Tilt

The concepts of T1 slope (T1S) and TIA are similar to the relationship between pelvic tilt, pelvic incidence, and sacral slope in the lumbosacral region. TIA, T1S, and neck tilt used to describe cervical spinal deformities are also used in surgical planning and affect clinical outcomes.

T1 Slope (T1S)

T1S is the angle between the superior end plate of T1 and horizontal (**Fig. 1.8a, b**). T1S is associated with the sagittal alignment of the cervical region. In addition, the T1S reflects the degree of thoracic kyphosis. T1S angle ranges from 17.4 to 25.7 degrees (**Table 1.2**).

Thoracic Inlet Angle (TIA)

The angle between a line perpendicular to the upper end plate of T1 and a line coming from the center of the lower end plate of T1 and the upper end of the sternum is called the

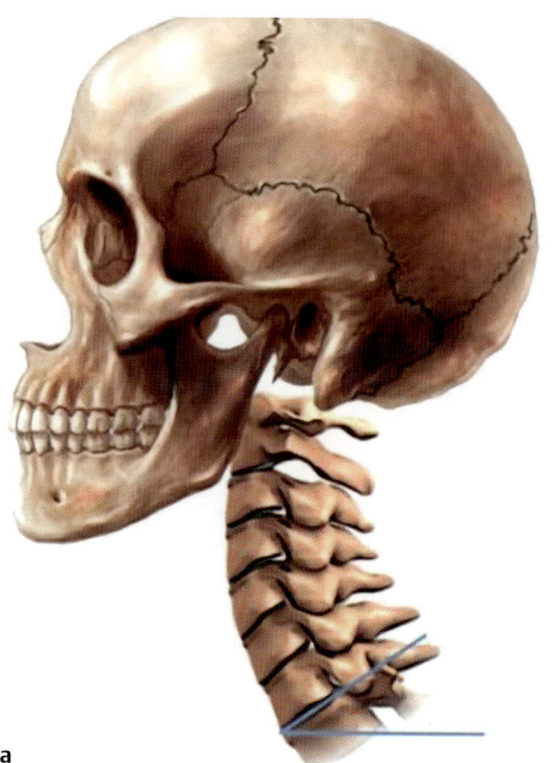

a

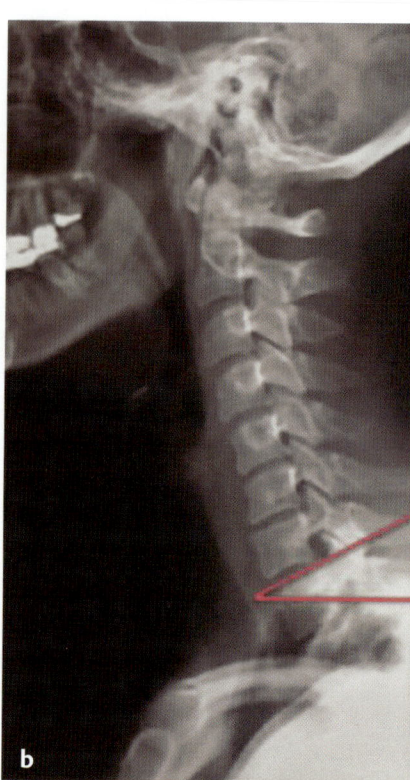

b

Fig. 1.8 (a, b) Measurement of T1 slope.

TIA (**Figs. 1.9a, b,** and **1.10**). TIA determines cervical lordosis. A patient with high TIA has increased cervical lordosis. Lee et al showed that T1S and cervical lordosis are correlated as a compensation mechanism. Their study showed that the horizontal gaze was preserved at around 44 degrees neck tilt by increasing TIA, T1S, and cervical lordosis.[8]

Cervical Tilt

It is the angle between a line at 90 degrees to the T1 superior end plate and a line from the middle of the T1 superior end plate to the tip of the dens (**Fig. 1.11**). The angle between this same line and vertical is called cranial tilt (**Fig. 1.12**). The cranial and cervical tilt angles equal the T1S angle. The cervical tilt angle ranges from 39.4 to 43.7 degrees (**Table 1.2**).

Neck Tilt

Neck tilt is a cervical parameter. It describes the angle between vertical and a line from the middle of the T1 inferior end plate and the upper end of the sternum (**Fig. 1.13**).

Recent studies have defined cervical deformities by using cervical parameters. In these studies, Smith et al defined cervical deformity as C2–C7 kyphosis of >10 degrees and C2–C7 SVA of >4 cm.[18] In addition, Passias et al added other definitions for deformity in their studies. Cervical deformity concepts have been evaluated from many perspectives. According to this study, cervical parameters play a decisive role in defining cervical deformities. For example, when describing cervical kyphosis, it was stated that the C2–C7 Cobb angle should be >10 degrees. In addition, the coronal Cobb angle should be considered when defining cervical scoliosis, and it is indicated in cases where the coronal Cobb angle is >10 degrees. Positive cervical sagittal imbalance is when C2–C7 SVA is >4 cm or T1S–cervical lordosis is >10 degrees. When evaluating the horizontal gaze disorder, we pay attention to cases where the vertical angle of the chin-eyebrow is >25 degrees.[19,20]

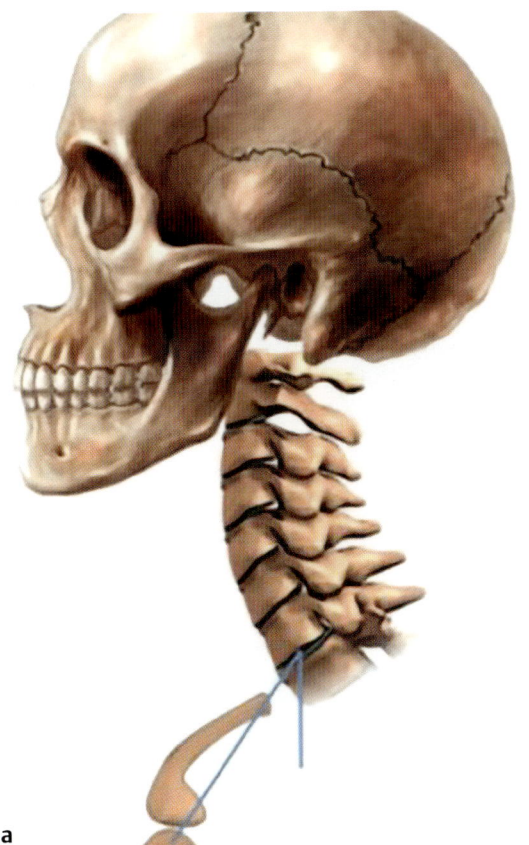

a

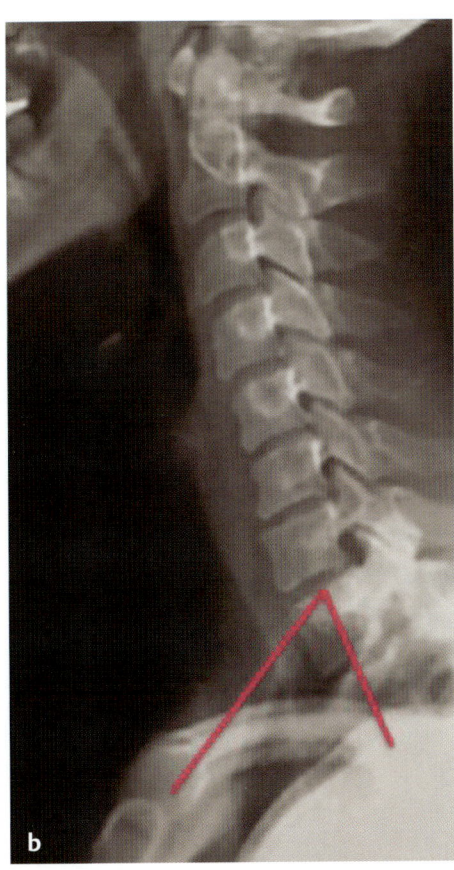

b

Fig. 1.9   (a, b) Measurement of thoracic inlet angle.

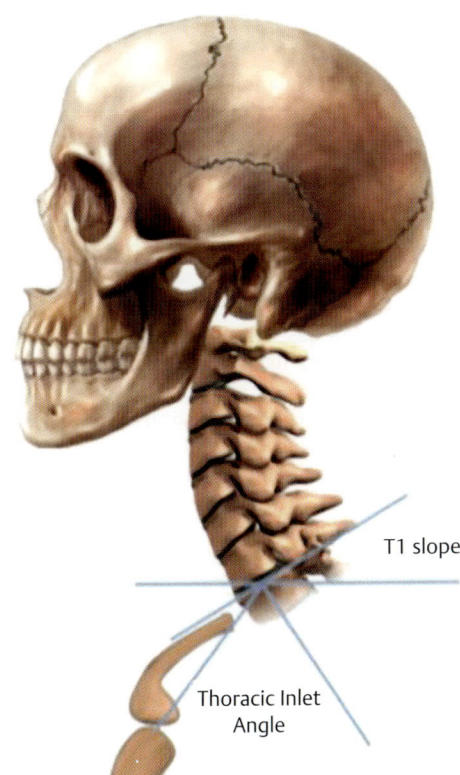

T1 slope

Thoracic Inlet
Angle

Fig. 1.10   Measurement of thoracic inlet angle and T1 slope.

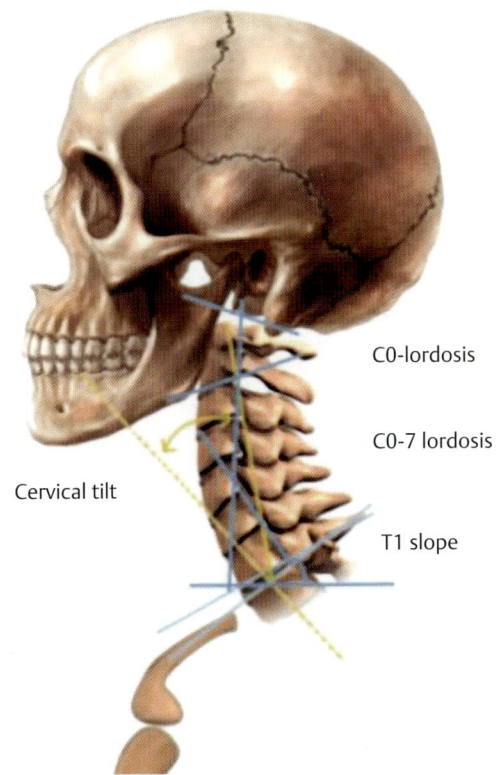

C0-lordosis

C0-7 lordosis

Cervical tilt

T1 slope

Fig. 1.11   Measurement of cervical tilt angle.

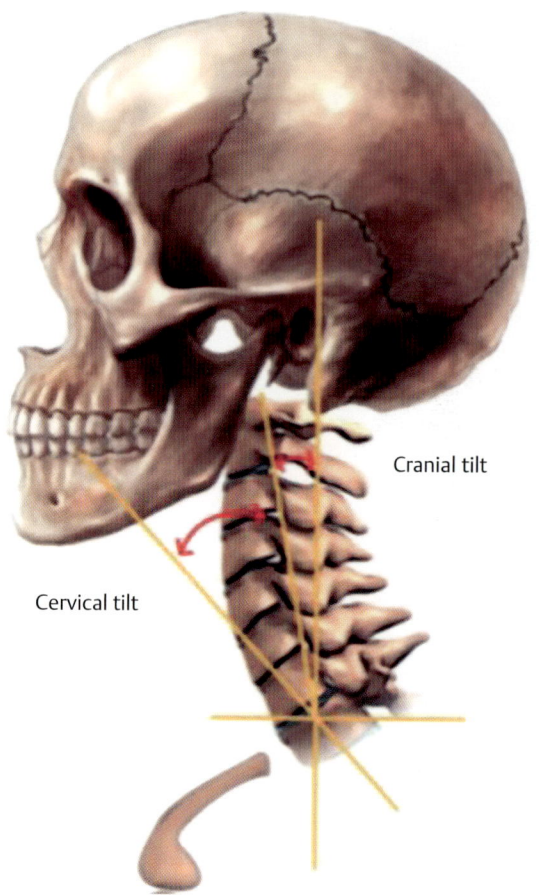

Fig. 1.12 Measurement of cranial tilt angle.

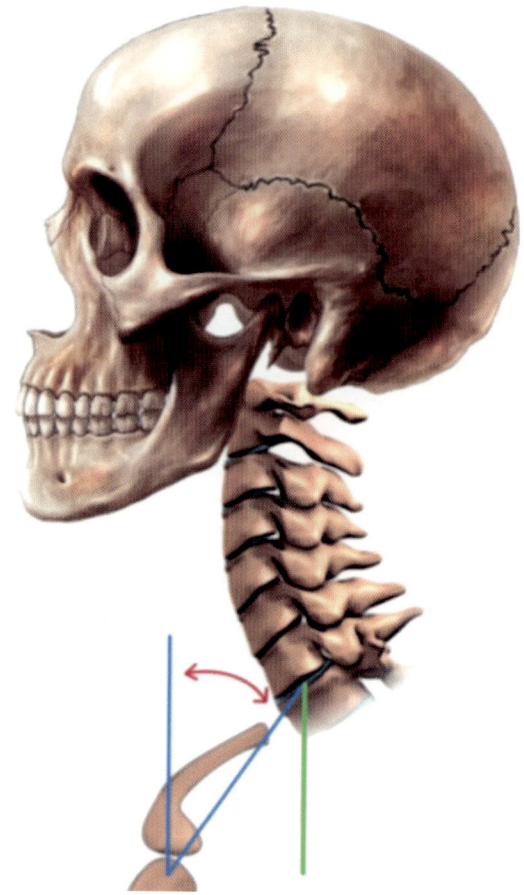

Fig. 1.13 Measurement of neck tilt angle.

Key Points

- Cervical sagittal balance is an essential component of global spinal balance. Therefore, it should be evaluated together with the global spinal balance.

- The cervical spine may change in alignment to maintain a horizontal gaze. It does this with compensation mechanisms.

- Cervical lordosis (C2–C7), T1S, and C2–C7 SVA are the most important considerations during sagittal reconstruction.

- Cervical parameters affect clinical outcomes. Cervical parameters are necessary for surgical planning, and they will help determine the instrument level. Osteotomy planning is done according to cervical parameter results.

References

1. Teo AQA, Thomas AC, Hey HWD. Sagittal alignment of the cervical spine: do we know enough for successful surgery? J Spine Surg 2020;6(1):124–135

2. Guo Q, Ni B, Yang J, et al. Relation between alignments of upper and subaxial cervical spine: a radiological study. Arch Orthop Trauma Surg 2011;131(6):857–862

3. Núñez-Pereira S, Hitzl W, Bullmann V, Meier O, Koller H. Sagittal balance of the cervical spine: an analysis of occipitocervical and spinopelvic interdependence, with C-7 slope as a marker of cervical and spinopelvic alignment. J Neurosurg Spine 2015;23(1):16–23

4. Iyer S, Lenke LG, Nemani VM, et al. Variations in sagittal alignment parameters based on age: a prospective study of asymptomatic volunteers using full-body radiographs. Spine 2016; 41(23):1826–1836

5. Hey HWD, Lau ETC, Wong GC, et al. Cervical alignment variations in different postures and predictors of normal cervical kyphosis: a new understanding. Spine 2017;42(21):1614–1621

6. Chen Y, Luo J, Pan Z, et al. The change of cervical spine alignment along with aging in asymptomatic population: a preliminary analysis. Eur Spine J 2017;26(9):2363–2371

7. Hardacker JW, Shuford RF, Capicotto PN, Pryor PW. Radiographic standing cervical segmental alignment in adult volunteers without neck symptoms. Spine 1997;22(13):1472–1480, discussion 1480

8. Lee SH, Kim KT, Seo EM, Suk KS, Kwack YH, Son ES. The influence of thoracic inlet alignment on the craniocervical sagittal balance in asymptomatic adults. J Spinal Disord Tech 2012;25(2):E41–E47

9. Tan LA, Straus DC, Traynelis VC. Cervical interfacet spacers and maintenance of cervical lordosis. J Neurosurg Spine 2015;22(5):466–469

10. Scheer JK, Tang JA, Smith JS, et al; International Spine Study Group. Cervical spine alignment, sagittal deformity, and clinical implications: a review. J Neurosurg Spine 2013;19(2):141–159

11. Ames CP, Blondel B, Scheer JK, et al. Cervical radiographical alignment: comprehensive assessment techniques and potential importance in cervical myelopathy. Spine 2013;38(22, Suppl 1):S149–S160

12. Kuntz C IV, Levin LS, Ondra SL, Shaffrey CI, Morgan CJ. Neutral upright sagittal spinal alignment from the occiput to the pelvis in asymptomatic adults: a review and resynthesis of the literature. J Neurosurg Spine 2007;6(2): 104–112

13. Abelin-Genevois K, Idjerouidene A, Roussouly P, Vital JM, Garin C. Cervical spine alignment in the pediatric population: a radiographic normative study of 150 asymptomatic patients. Eur Spine J 2014;23(7):1442–1448

14. Yukawa Y, Kato F, Suda K, Yamagata M, Ueta T, Yoshida M. Normative data for parameters of sagittal spinal alignment in healthy subjects: an analysis of gender specific differences and changes with aging in 626 asymptomatic individuals. Eur Spine J 2018;27(2):426–432

15. Tang JA, Scheer JK, Smith JS, et al; ISSG. The impact of standing regional cervical sagittal alignment on outcomes in posterior cervical fusion surgery. Neurosurgery 2012;71(3):662–669, discussion 669

16. Park JH, Cho CB, Song JH, Kim SW, Ha Y, Oh JK. T1 slope and cervical sagittal alignment on cervical CT radiographs of asymptomatic persons. J Korean Neurosurg Soc 2013;53(6): 356–359

17. Suk KS, Kim KT, Lee SH, Kim JM. Significance of chin-brow vertical angle in correction of kyphotic deformity of ankylosing spondylitis patients. Spine 2003;28(17):2001–2005

18. Smith JS, Lafage V, Schwab FJ, et al; International Spine Study Group. Prevalence and type of cervical deformity among 470 adults with thoracolumbar deformity. Spine 2014;39(17):E1001–E1009

19. Passias PG, Jalai CM, Lafage V, et al; International Spine Study Group (Littleton, Colorado). Primary drivers of adult cervical deformity: prevalence, variations in presentation, and effect of surgical treatment strategies on early postoperative alignment. Neurosurgery 2018;83(4):651–659

20. Passias PG, Vasquez-Montes D, Poorman GW, et al; ISSG. Predictive model for distal junctional kyphosis after cervical deformity surgery. Spine J 2018;18(12):2187–2194

Atul Goel

Introduction

Basilar invagination is diagnosed when there is odontoid process migration into the foramen magnum and is confirmed by evaluation based on classical radiological parameters, more popular being those described by Chamberlain and Wackenheim.

Classification of Basilar Invagination

The author classified basilar invagination as Group A and Group B in 2004:

Group A basilar invagination: When there is atlantoaxial instability that is manifested by an abnormal increase in the atlantodental or clivodental interval, it is Group A.[1] In Group A basilar invagination the odontoid process seems to invaginate into foramen magnum, or as von Torklus put it in the year 1972, the spine is migrated or herniated into the brain.[2]

Group B basilar invagination: Basilar invagination is also diagnosed by the parameter described by Chamberlain. In this group, there is no evidence of atlantoaxial instability when assessed by the parameter of abnormal increase in atlantodental or clivodental interval and abnormal transgression of the Wackenheim's clival line by the odontoid tip. In Group B, the entire craniovertebral junctional zone is rostrally positioned.[1]

Group A—Genesis of Nomenclature

Basilar invagination had been classically identified to have "fixed" or "irreducible" atlantoaxial dislocation. As the anomaly was considered fixed, the treatment was decompression. Accordingly, decompression either by transoral route or by foramen magnum was the accepted mode of surgical treatment. In the year 2004, we identified for the first time in the literature that in a specific subgroup of cases with basilar invagination, atlantoaxial joint is not fixed, and is not only mobile but is pathologically "hypermobile" and more importantly is reducible by manual manipulation.[1]

This subgroup of patients was identified as having Group A basilar invagination. There was an abnormal increase in atlantodental or clivodental interval. We identified another subgroup of patients (Group B basilar invagination) where there was basilar invagination when assessed by the classical parameter of Chamberlain's line, but atlantodental or clivodental interval was not abnormally increased. While we recommended atlantoaxial facetal distraction and fixation and craniovertebral junction realignment in cases with Group A basilar invagination, we suggested foramen magnum decompression in Group B cases. This treatment modality was based on the understanding (in the year 2004) that atlantoaxial joint was unstable in Group A cases, and stable or fixed in Group B cases. Group A cases were earlier treated by transoral decompression and Group B cases were treated by foramen magnum decompression.[3] The role of fixation was unclear in both subgroups and was a debated issue.

Revolution in the Understanding and Treatment of Basilar Invagination

As our experience in the subject matured, we have realized that atlantoaxial joint is unstable in both Group A and Group B. Accordingly, based on this understanding atlantoaxial fixation is the treatment. The study concluded that the atlantoaxial joint in patients with Group A basilar invagination is not only not fused or fixed but is excessively or abnormally mobile. More importantly, it was proposed that stabilization of the unstable joint and restoration of craniovertebral alignment can be the optimum surgical treatment for this subgroup of patients. Identification of the fact that atlantoaxial joint was unstable and could be reduced in Group A basilar invagination relegated transoral surgery for decompression into realm of history. Identification of the fact that instability is the nodal point of pathogenesis of Group B basilar invagination and atlantoaxial fixation is the treatment, has the potential of relegating foramen magnum decompression as a form of treatment into historical domain. "Posterior alone" and "fixation alone" method of surgical treatment has currently become the preferred mode of surgical treatment for both Group A and Group B basilar invagination.

Radiological Evaluation of Group A Basilar Invagination

A variety of musculoskeletal and soft tissue alterations are frequent accompaniments of basilar invagination. We recently evaluated our experience with 510 cases having Group A basilar invagination that were treated over a 9-year period.[4] The aim of the study was to assess the musculoskeletal and soft tissue alterations in Group A basilar invagination. We also evaluated if the bone alterations influenced the nature of neo-neural formations that included syringomyelia and Chiari formation. The findings of our study are summarized.

Subclassification of Group A Basilar Invagination Based on Abnormality of CSF Loculations Within or Outside the Spinal Cord[4]

External syringomyelia: We recently identified that excessive amount of cerebrospinal fluid (CSF) was present outside the confines of the spinal cord (or in the extramedullary compartment) in several patients having basilar invagination. The term "external syrinx" was used to refer to the presence of an excessive amount of CSF that occupied the larger space in the widened subarachnoid spaces, and not to loculated tumor-like space occupying collection as seen in arachnoid cysts. Although other terms like "external hydromyelia," "extramedullary hygroma," "spinal cord atrophy," "neural agenesis," and "external hydrocephalus or cyst" were considered to name the presence of excessive amount of CSF outside the spinal cord, the term "external syringomyelia" seemed to best convey the intended meaning and was used in our earlier publications.[4–6] On a parallel note, the term "external syringobulbia" was used to describe the presence of excessive amount of CSF outside the confines of the brainstem and the cerebellar convexity.

This excessive presence of CSF in the extramedullary compartment or "external syrinx" was related to combination of both larger spinal canal and thinner spinal cord girth when compared to normal cohort.

Depending on the type of CSF cavitation/loculation within or outside the spinal cord, the patients were divided into four subgroups (**Table 2.1**). Group A1 (60 cases) included

Table 2.1 Classification of Group A basilar invagination

A1: Internal syringomyelia	60 (12%)
A2: External syringomyelia	354 (69%)
A3: Both internal and external syringomyelia	51 (10%)
A4: No cord abnormality	45 (9%)

Source: Reproduced with permission from Goel et al.[4]

patients having syringomyelia (**Fig. 2.1**). Group A2 (354 cases) included patients who had external syrinx (**Figs. 2.2** and **2.3**). Group A3 (51 cases) had both syringomyelia and external syrinx (**Fig. 2.4**). Group A4 (45 cases) had no abnormality of CSF cavitation in the spinal canal (**Fig. 2.5**). Syringobulbia was identified in 5 patients and external syringobulbia was identified in 401 patients.

The radiological evaluation of Group A basilar invagination was done based on this classification. From the analysis it appeared that the nature of bone malformation in general and angulation of the odontoid process and the extent of basilar invagination directly influenced the presence or absence of external syrinx and syringomyelia.

Radiological Measurements

Radiological measurements were obtained in the four groups individually and analyzed in comparison with the normal cohort. **Table 2.2** summarizes the bone and soft tissue anomalies including presence of Chiari malformation, assimilation of atlas, C2–C3 fusion, bifid arches of atlas, and subaxial bone fusions (Klippel-Feil abnormality).

Some parameters to evaluate basilar invagination and other bone abnormalities are mentioned below.

Cord girth measurements were used not to quantify the volume of the spinal cord, but rather to delineate the thickness of the column of the neural tissue as it relates to the thickness of the column of CSF.

Table 2.2 Radiological parameters

Parameter	Number of patients (%)
Chiari formation	126/510 (24.7)
Syringomyelia	415/510 (91.17)
Types of atlantoaxial instability based on facetal alignment	
Type A atlantoaxial instability	483 (94.7)
Type B atlantoaxial instability	17 (3.3)
Type C atlantoaxial instability	10 (2)
Assimilation of atlas	250/510 (49)
Unilateral	12
Bilateral	238
Bifid arches of atlas	86/510 (16.8)
C2–C3 fusion	234/510 (45.8)
Klippel-Feil syndrome	28/510 (5.5)
Atlantodental/clivodental instability	24/300 (8)
Vertical instability	47/300 (15.6)

Source: Reproduced with permission from Goel et al.[4]

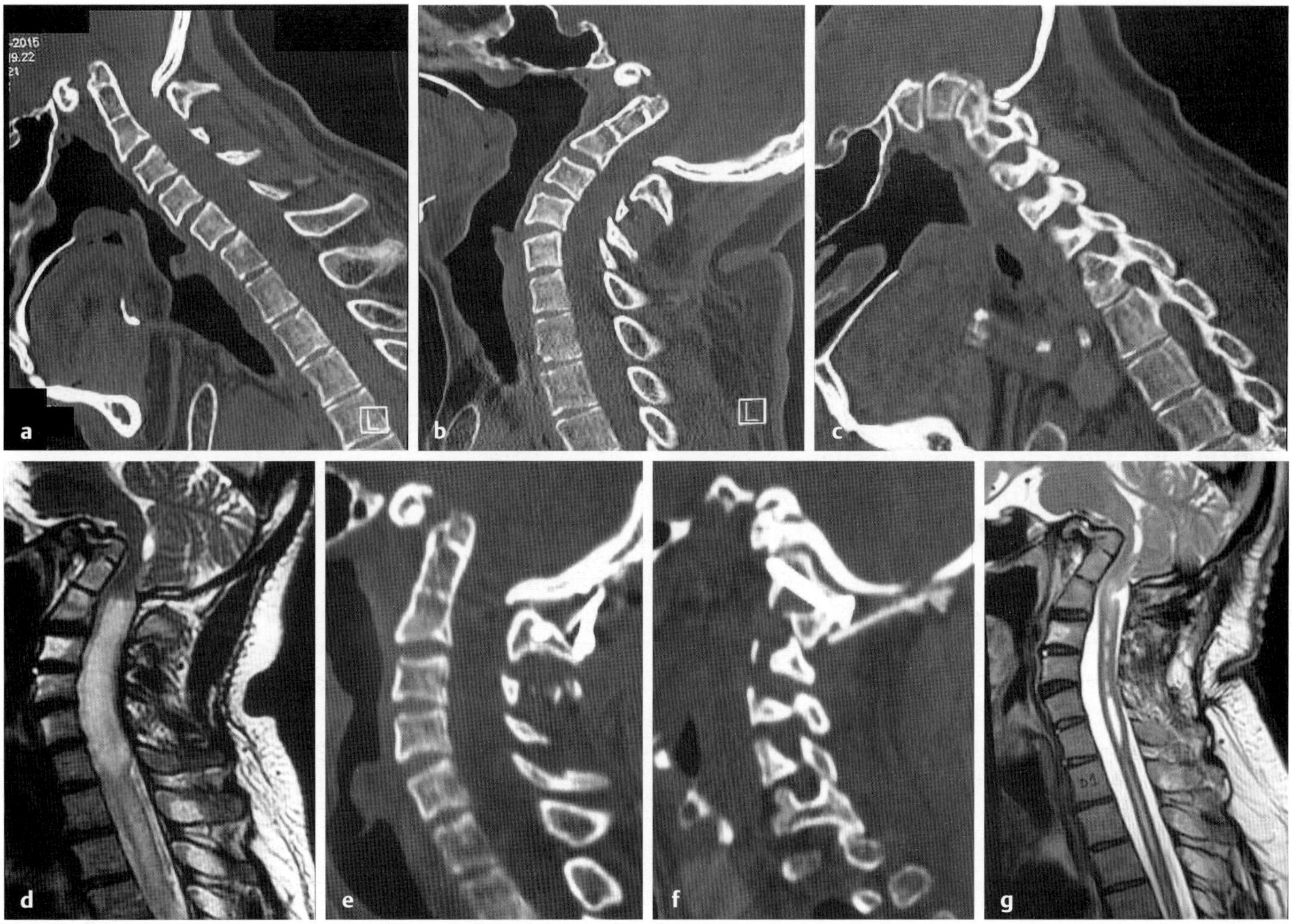

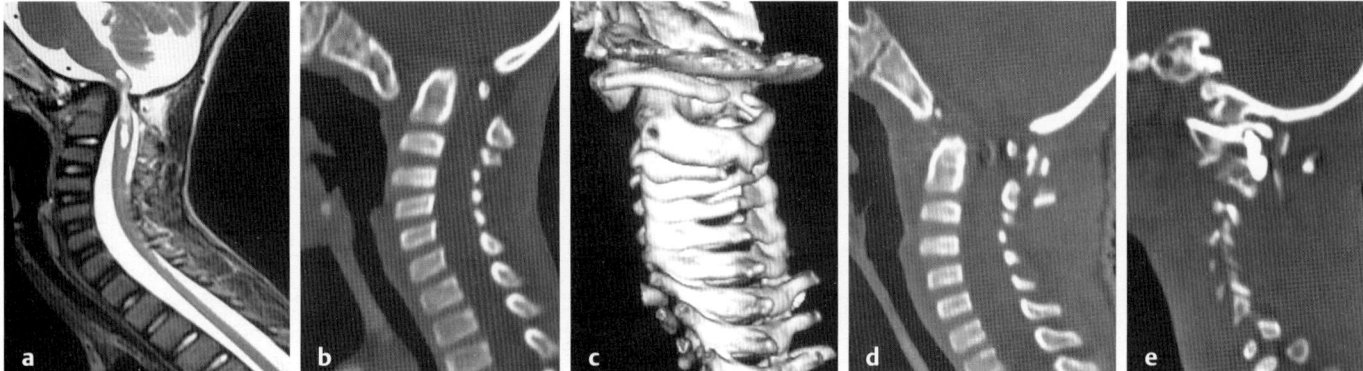

Fig. 2.1 Group A1: Images of a 22-year-old male patient. **(a)** Computed tomography (CT) scan with the head in flexion showing basilar invagination. Assimilation of atlas and C2–C3 fusion can be seen. **(b)** CT scan with the head in extension showing mild reduction in basilar invagination. **(c)** CT scan sagittal image with the cut passing through the facets. Type I atlantoaxial facetal instability can be seen. **(d)** T2-weighted magnetic resonance imaging (MRI) showing syringomyelia and Chiari formation. Note the presence of external syringobulbia. **(e)** Postoperative CT scan showing reduction of atlantoaxial instability and fixation. **(f)** Postoperative CT scan cut through the facets showing the implant. **(g)** Delayed postoperative MRI (9 months after surgery) showing reduction in the size of syrinx.

Fig. 2.2 Group A2: Images of a 7-year-old male child. **(a)** T2-weighted magnetic resonance imaging (MRI) showing Group A2 basilar invagination and cord compression. External syringomyelia and external syringobulbia can be observed. **(b)** Computed tomography (CT) scan showing basilar invagination. **(c)** Three-dimensional CT scan showing type I atlantoaxial facetal instability. Bifid posterior arch of atlas can be observed. **(d)** Postoperative CT scan showing reduction of basilar invagination and fixation. **(e)** Postoperative CT scan with the cut passing through the facets showing the implant.

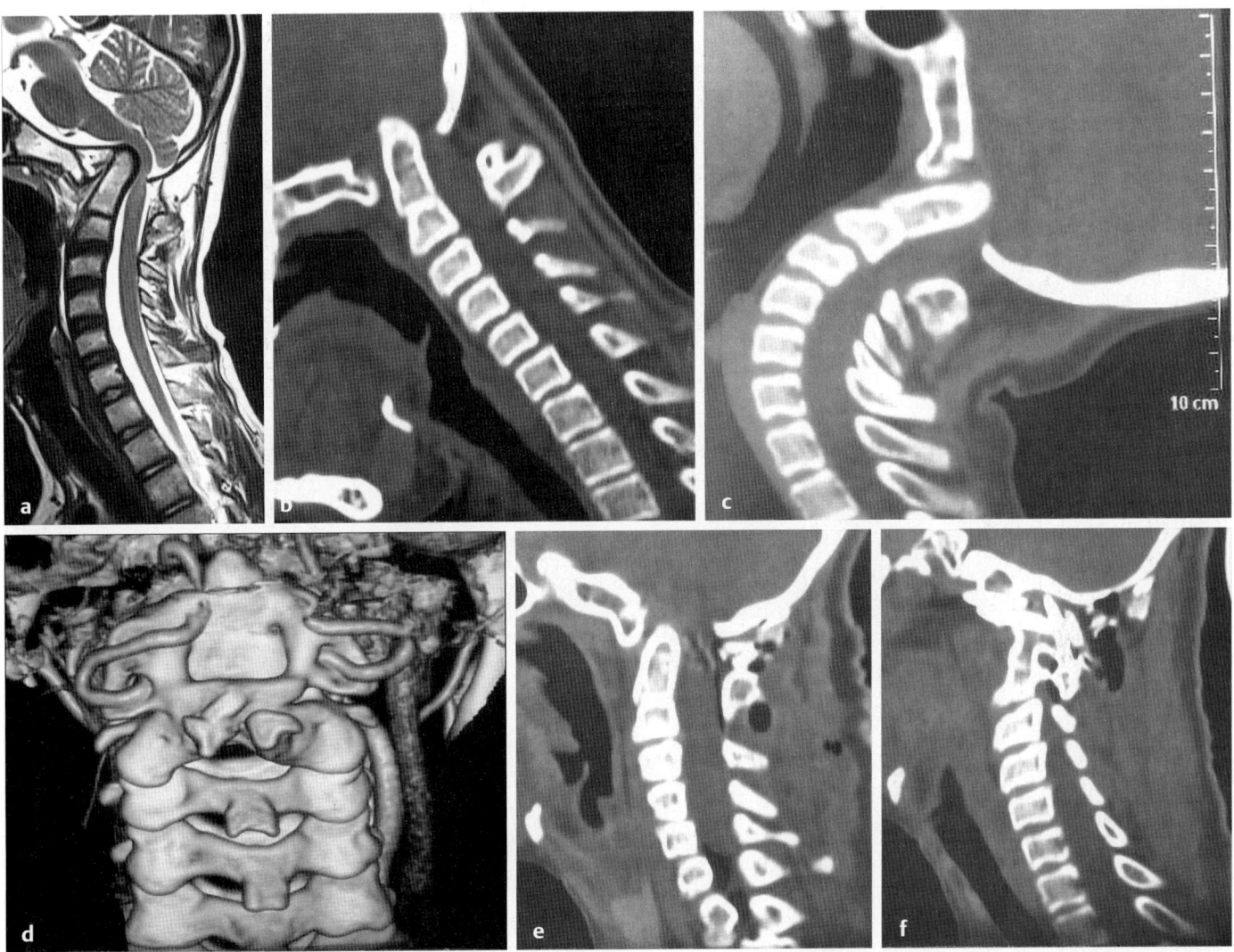

Fig. 2.3 Group A2: Images of a 14-year-old male child. **(a)** T2-weighted magnetic resonance imaging (MRI) showing Group A2 basilar invagination. Assimilation of atlas and C2–C3 fusion can be seen. There is external syrinx and external syringobulbia. **(b)** Computed tomography (CT) scan with the head in flexion showing basilar invagination. **(c)** CT scan with the head in extension showing reduction in vertical atlantoaxial dislocation. **(d)** Three-dimensional CT scan showing the abnormal course of vertebral artery posterior to the facet of atlas. **(e)** Postoperative CT scan showing reduction of basilar invagination. **(f)** Postoperative CT scan showing the fixation construct.

Anteroposterior spinal canal and spinal cord girth measurements were taken at the C6 mid-vertebral body level, mid-D4 vertebral body level, and at mid-L3 vertebral body level on sagittal magnetic resonance imaging (MRI) as the index sites. In cases with syringomyelia, the neural girth was calculated as the sum of measurements of neural tissues both anterior and posterior to the syrinx cavity.

Spinal neural girth, measured in presence or absence of syringomyelia, was reduced and the spinal bony canal was increased in majority of cases when compared to the normal population.

Craniovertebral measurements: With the patient in a neutral head position, a horizontal line (line A) was drawn

connecting the tuberculum sellae to inion. Line B was drawn parallel to line A and coursed over the tip of the odontoid process. Line C was drawn parallel to line B and coursed over the midpoint of the base of the C7 vertebra. Distance between lines A and B was the posterior cranial fossa height and distance between lines B and C was the neck height[7] (**Fig. 2.6**).

Anterior–posterior dimension of the posterior cranial fossa was measured as the distance between the dorsum sellae and the internal occipital protuberance on the mid-sagittal cut of CT scan.

The **length of the clivus** was measured from the tip of the dorsum sellae to the lower edge of the clivus. The clivus

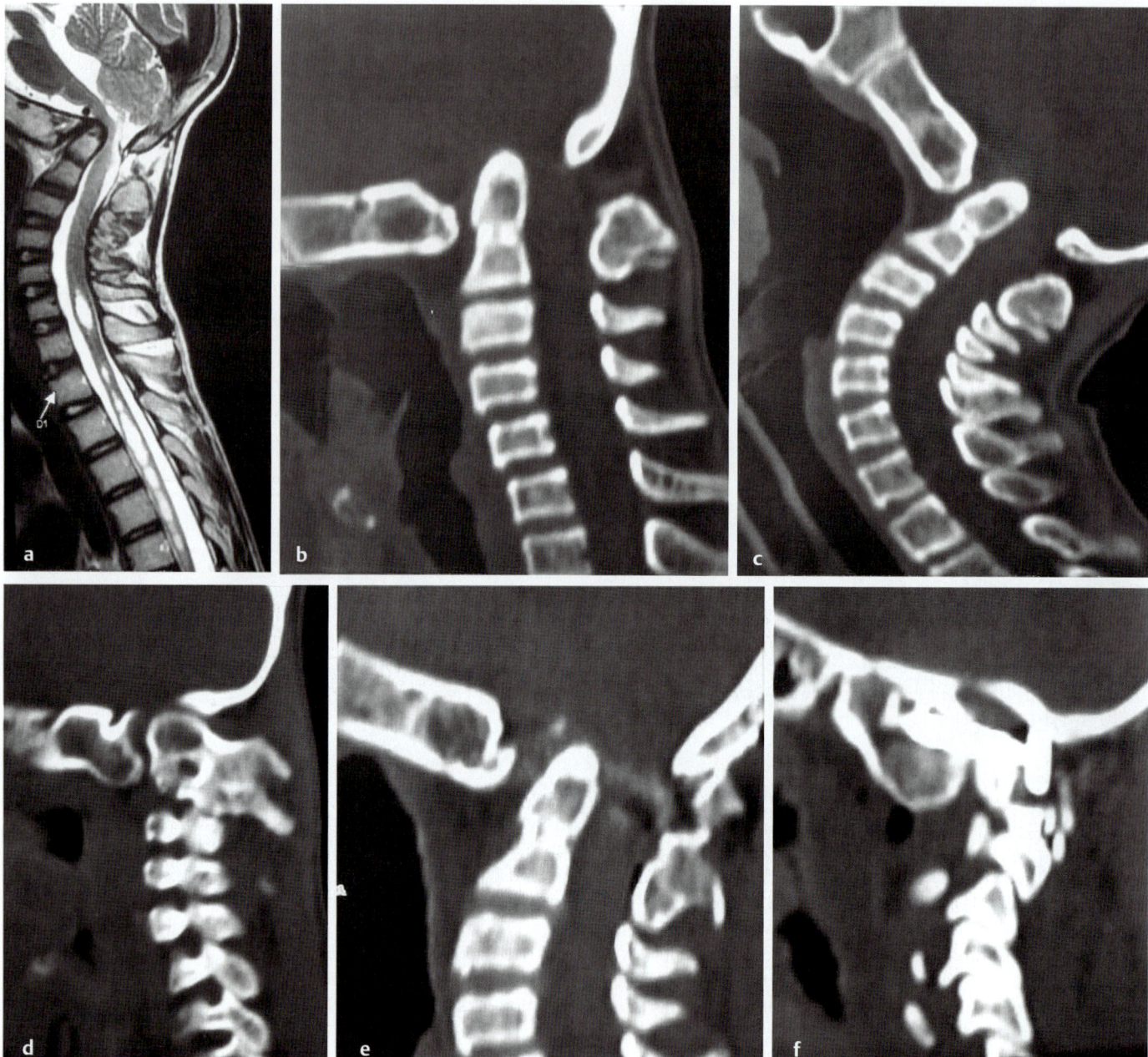

Fig. 2.4 Group A3: Images of a 13-year-old male child. **(a)** T2-weighted magnetic resonance imaging (MRI) showing Group A3 basilar invagination. There is syringomyelia and external syringomyelia. **(b)** Computed tomography (CT) scan with head in flexion showing basilar invagination. There is assimilation of atlas. **(c)** CT scan with the head in extension showing reduction in vertical atlantoaxial dislocation. **(d)** CT scan with the sagittal cut passing through the facets. The facet of atlas is dislocated anterior to the facet of axis (spondyloptosis). **(e)** Postoperative CT scan showing reduction of dislocation and fixation. **(f)** Postoperative CT scan with cuts passing through facets showing the implant.

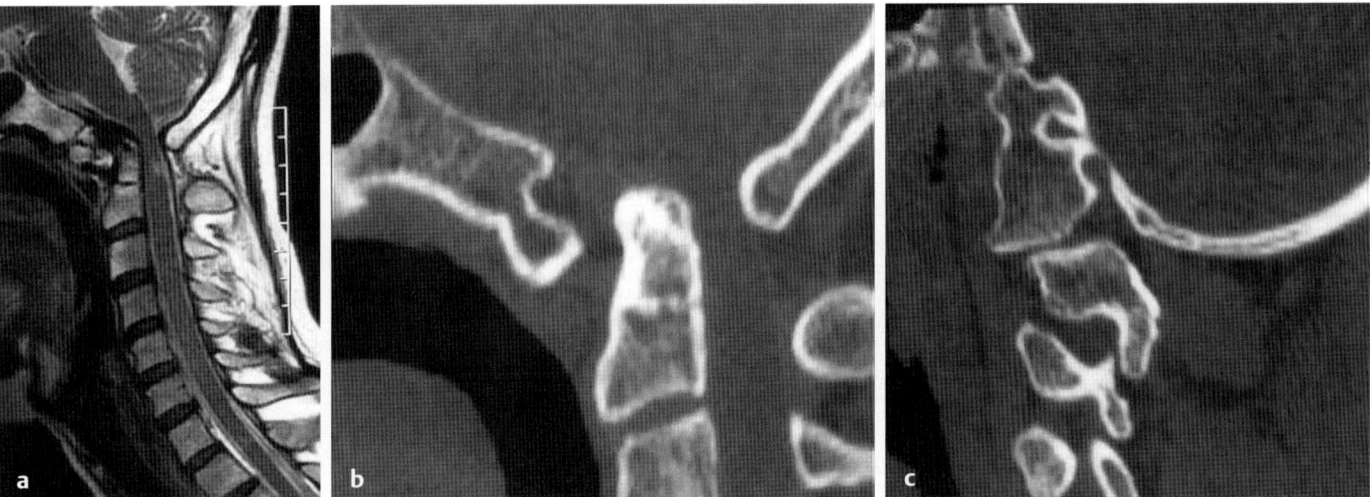

Fig. 2.5 Group A4: Images of a 32-year-old male patient. **(a)** T2-weighted magnetic resonance imaging (MRI) showing Group A4 basilar invagination and cord compression. There is no syringomyelia. **(b)** Computed tomography (CT) scan showing basilar invagination and assimilation of atlas. **(c)** CT scan with cut passing through the facets showing Type 1 atlantoaxial facetal instability.

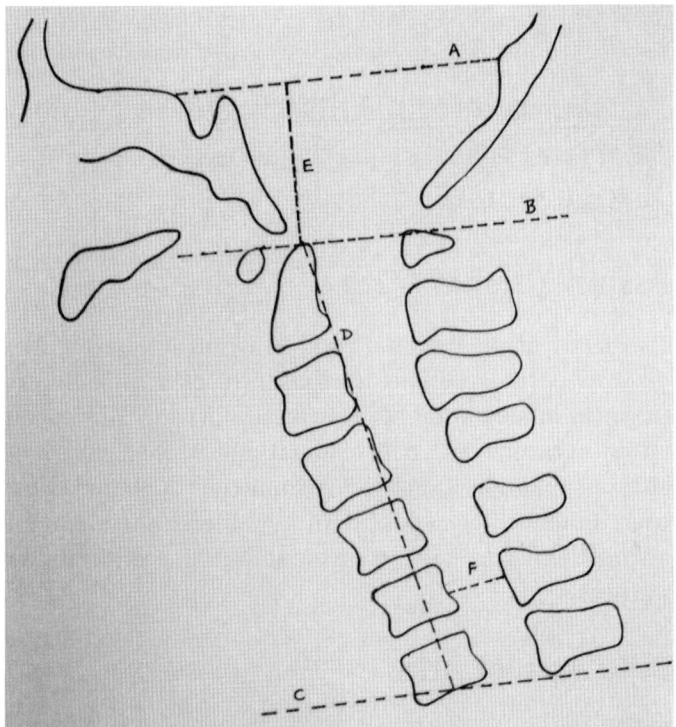

Fig. 2.6 Line drawing used to measure posterior fossa and neck height. With the patient in neutral head position, a horizontal line (line A) is drawn connecting the tuberculum sellae to inion. Line B is drawn parallel to line A and courses over the tip of the odontoid process. Line C is drawn parallel to line B and courses over the midpoint of the base of the C7 vertebra. Distance between line A and B is posterior cranial fossa height and distance between lines B and C is neck height.

length was called as "short" if it was less than 3.5 cm. In the study, 81 patients had short clivus.

The "minimum" **craniocervical neural girth** was measured at the level of tip of the odontoid process.

Wackenheim's clival line was drawn from the tip of the posterior clinoid process and extended along the posterior limit of the clivus.[8]

Platybasia was assessed by measuring the basal angle that was a line drawn from the nasion to the dorsum sellae and the Wackenheim's clival line.

Chamberlain's line was drawn from the posterior tip of the hard palate to the posterior rim of the foramen magnum.[9] Basilar invagination was severe when the tip of the odontoid process was >10 mm above the Chamberlain's line. In the study, 323 patients had severe basilar invagination.

Goel modified omega angle: The degree of neural compression was assessed by the tilt of the odontoid process toward the neural structures and was measured using the modified omega angle.[3] Modified omega angle was measured with the head in neutral position as depicted in the line drawing (**Fig. 2.7**). A line was drawn along the hard palate. As C2–C3 fusion was a frequent observation, line B was drawn parallel to line A and passed through the midpoint or center of the base of C3 (instead of base of C2 as described earlier).[3] Line C was drawn from the midpoint of base of C3 body and extended superiorly along the tip of the odontoid process.

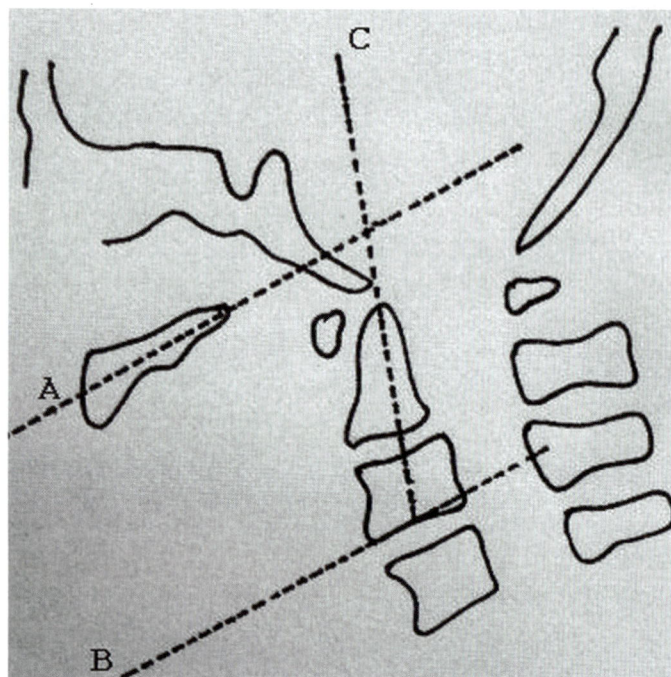

Fig. 2.7 Line drawing showing the Goel modified omega angle. Line A is drawn along the line of had palate. Line B is a line that is drawn parallel to line A. It passes through the midpoint of inferior surface of body of C3 vertebra. Line C is a line drawn from the midpoint of inferior surface of body of C3 vertebra and passes through the tip of the odontoid process. The angle between lines B and C is considered to be the modified omega angle.

Inclination of the odontoid process: The angle subtended between lines B and C was considered to be the inclination of the odontoid process in an anteroposterior perspective.

Inclination of the odontoid process in a transverse perspective: Bimastoid or bidigastric lines were drawn on coronal image of either commuted tomography (CT) scan or MRI. The angle subtended by the line drawn from the midpoint of base of C3 vertebra to tip of odontoid process on either of these lines was the inclination of the odontoid process in a transverse perspective.

Craniovertebral angulation: The angle subtended between Wackenheim's clival line and a line drawn along the odontoid process (line C) was described as craniovertebral angulation.

C1 facetal angle: The C1 facetal angle was measured as the angle between a line drawn along the articular surface of C1 facet and the horizontal in the neutral head position.

C2 facetal angle: The C2 facetal angle was measured as the angle between a line drawn along the articular surface of the C2 facet and the horizontal in the neutral head position.

The author's analysis identified that degree of alteration in the craniovertebral and odontoid process angulation determined the nature of neural abnormalities. The more severe the inclination of the odontoid process (either in the anteroposterior or in the horizontal or transverse perspective) and more acute the craniovertebral angulation, the more frequent was the presence of Group A2 or A3 cord abnormality. Type of facetal instability and the degree of angulation of the inferior surface of the facet of atlas influenced the angulation of the odontoid process and the extent of neural compression. The more severe the inclination of the C1 facet and more severe the cord compression, the higher was the incidence of presence of external syringomyelia.

Epidemiology

In the study cohort, 40% of the patients were younger than 21 years. This age group profile is significantly younger to ages in Group B patients evaluated by us in another series.[5,6] From the age profile evaluation, it appears that the patients in Group A2 were relatively younger than the patients in other groups.

Musculoskeletal Abnormalities Seen in Patients with Group A Basilar Invagination

Assimilation of Atlas

The fusion of the occipital condyle with the facet of atlas determined the presence (or absence) of assimilation of the atlas. Assimilation of atlas was found in 250 patients (49%), of which 238 had bilateral and 12 had unilateral atlas assimilation. Unilateral assimilation of the atlas has been infrequently reported in the literature. Unilateral assimilation was always associated with torticollis of the neck.

Bifid Arch of Atlas

Bifid posterior arch of atlas was observed in 86 (16.8%) patients. Apart from the author's recent report, there is no major case series in the literature that has focused on evaluation of bifid posterior arch of atlas. Although it could not be radiologically demonstrated, the bifid posterior arch probably opens up on flexion of the neck and closes on neck extension in an open–close door format.[10] Such movements of bifid posterior arch of atlas could act as dynamic decompressive laminectomy and probably had a protective function for the critical neural structures in face of abnormal mobility of the odontoid process. As discussed earlier, in cases with bifid posterior arch of atlas, the facets of atlas are laterally displaced in relationship to the facets of axis and are obliquely poised. The lateral displacement of each half of the atlas results in vertical height reduction between the occipital bone and the lamina and spinous process of the axis.[10]

C2–C3 Fusion

C2–C3 fusion was identified in 234 (45.8%) patients. In 201 of these patients there was assimilation of the atlas. Essentially bone fusions were more common above (assimilation of atlas) and below (C2–C3 fusion) the tip of the odontoid process.

Klippel-Feil Abnormalities

Subaxial vertebral bone fusions were identified in 28 (5.5%) cases (**Table 2.2**). Such bone fusions have been named as Klippel-Feil abnormalities.[11]

Os-odontoideum

Os-odontoideum was identified in 9 (1.7%) patients.

Factor of Atlantoaxial Instability

Instability of the atlantoaxial joint was assessed by the classically described parameter of atlantodental or clivodental (in cases with assimilation of atlas) interval.

Mobile and partially reducible atlantoaxial dislocation (24 cases) was assessed by alteration of atlantodental or clivodental interval on dynamic flexion–extension images that were available in 300 patients.

Mobile vertical atlantoaxial instability (47 cases) was diagnosed when the odontoid process moved relative to anterior arch of atlas (or anterior rim of foramen magnum in cases with assimilated atlas) on dynamic flexion–extension images.

In rest of the 229 (76.3%) patients out of the 300 patients in whom dynamic images were available, there was no odontoid process movements or alteration in the atlantodental alignment on dynamic imaging.

Goel's Classification of Atlantoaxial Instability on the Basis of Facetal Alignment

In accordance with recently described classification of atlantoaxial instability based on facetal alignment in neutral head position, atlantoaxial instability was divided into three types: Type I facetal instability (483 cases), when the facet of the atlas was dislocated anterior to the facet of the axis; Type II facetal instability (17 cases), when the facet of the atlas was dislocated posterior to the facet of axis; and Type III (10 cases) facetal instability, when the facets were in alignment and the instability was detected only on direct handling of bones during surgery.[12–14] Type I facetal instability was more frequently associated with Group A2 and A3 cord abnormalities while Type II and Type III atlantoaxial facetal instability was more often associated with Group A1 cord abnormality.[12–14]

Facetal Orientation

Facets of atlas and facets of axis were in an abnormal orientation in all patients. Even though the facetal surfaces were in an abnormal inclination, the joint was functional. This finding was correlated during the operative procedure that involved opening of the joint. The angle of inclination of facet of atlas ranged from 12.1 to 103.6 degrees from the horizontal. Angle of facet of axis from the horizontal ranged from 0 to 103.6 degrees. In 134 (26.2%) cases, the entire articular surface of the facet of atlas was located anterior to the articular surface of facet of axis. We identified such an alignment as spondyloptosis.

Chiari 1 Formation and Syringomyelia

In 126 (24.7%) cases, there was Chiari 1 formation. Our recent studies identify that basilar invagination, Chiari formation, and syringomyelia represent a spectrum of abnormalities wherein the primary etiology is atlantoaxial instability. In five cases there was Chiari formation with tonsillar herniation only on one side, on the side contralateral to the indenting odontoid process in cases presenting with torticollis. Such a form of tonsillar herniation was recorded first by us in the literature.[4]

Bone and Neural Abnormality

The presence of syringomyelia (Group A1), external syringomyelia (Group A2), both syringomyelia and external syringomyelia (Group A3), or absence of any evidence of unusual CSF loculation (Group A4) in the cervical spine could give a clue as to the direction of migration of the odontoid process, degree of basilar invagination, and extent of cord compression. It seems that the pathogenesis of syringomyelia/external syringomyelia is same in cases with Group A and Group B basilar invagination and in cases where there is no bone abnormality at the craniovertebral junction and is related to inclination of the odontoid process and atlantoaxial instability.

It was identified that there was excessive volume of CSF even in the posterior cranial fossa compartment. It was observed that external syringobulbia was associated in all four groups, irrespective of the fact whether CSF was present within the cord (syringomyelia), outside the cord (external syringomyelia), or both within and outside the cord (Group A3). External syringobulbia was present in 35 (77.7% out of 45 cases) cases in Group A4 when there was no significant abnormality of CSF cavitation in the spine. In such cases, the cerebellum was atrophic and more than normal amount of CSF was present around the cerebellum and the brainstem.[4–6]

Short Head, Short Neck, and Short Spine

We labelled shortening of clivus as "shortening of the head." Short neck and short head were simultaneous and proportional. There was an increase in spinal canal and a simultaneous and proportionate increase in anteroposterior dimension of the posterior cranial fossa.[4] There was reduction in the girth or atrophy of the spinal cord. It was identified that there was excessive volume of CSF even in the posterior cranial fossa compartment. It was observed that external syringobulbia was associated in all four groups, irrespective of the fact whether CSF was present within the cord (syringomyelia), outside the cord (external syringomyelia), or both within and outside the cord (Group A3). External syringobulbia was present in 35 (77.7% out of 45 cases) cases in Group A4 when there was no significant abnormality of CSF cavitation in the spine. In such cases, the cerebellum was atrophic and more than normal amount of CSF was present around the cerebellum and the brainstem.

Our observations identify that in Group A basilar invagination the neural structures, both in the posterior fossa and in the cervical spinal cord and both above and below the site of maximum cord compression, were atrophic when compared to the normal cohort population. Additionally, the bone compartments housing these neural structures, both in the spinal canal and in the posterior cranial fossa, were vertically reduced in length resulting in short neck and short head but were anteroposteriorly and transversely increased in their dimensions. Although it could not be confirmed due to absence of adequate number of images, it appears that the length of the entire spine is probably reduced in these patients when compared to the normal cohort. Reduction in the neural girth, decrease in vertical and increase in transverse bone canal dimensions, and an increase in length of neural structures resulted in an outcome that made the neural structures float in excessive volume of CSF that was present either within or outside the neural structures. In this respect the pathogenesis and function of CSF whether it was present within or outside the neural structures appeared to be similar.

Inferences from Radiological Evaluation

Degree of basilar invagination and angulation of the odontoid process are among the key factors that determine presence or absence of syringomyelia or external syrinx formation. Atlantoaxial instability is the primary abnormality in Group A basilar invagination. From the analysis it appeared that the nature of bone malformation directly influenced the presence or absence of external syrinx and syringomyelia.

Evolution of Treatment

Prior to the year 2000, all patients with Group A basilar invagination were treated by transoral decompression.[15] The indication for simultaneous posterior fixation was unclear and was done in approximately 30% cases. In the year 2004, we discussed that atlantoaxial facetal distraction and fixation could result in reduction of basilar invagination and stabilization of the atlantoaxial joint, circumventing the need for any transoral decompression.[1] Our surgical technique involved opening of the atlantoaxial joint, denuding of the articular cartilage, stuffing bone graft pieces and a Goel facet spacer into the articular cavity after manually distracting the facets and subsequent direct atlantoaxial fixation using plates and screws with the technique described by us earlier in 1988.[16,17] Although earlier the intra-articular spacer was introduced into the articular cavity in all cases, after the year 2009, it was identified that opening of the joint, denuding the facets of the articular cartilage, introduction and packing of bone graft within the articular cavity with distracted facets, and subsequent plate and screw fixation of the atlantoaxial joint provided firm stabilization of the region and resulted in reduction of basilar invagination. This change in philosophy was related to our understanding that solid and firm fixation aiming at arthrodesis was the primary aim of surgery. Fixation and fusion were more important surgical goals than realignment and reduction of basilar invagination. In the subsequent cases, the intra-articular spacers were used more as stabilizers than as distractors. Also, intra-articular spacers were used when direct screw insertion into the facets of atlas or axis was not possible due to difficulties in exposure or due to problems related to screw insertion.

Evaluation of Atlantoaxial Instability and Group A Basilar Invagination

Atlantoaxial joint instability is the nodal point of pathogenesis of the entire process. Group A basilar invagination is a result of listhesis of facet of atlas over the facet of axis. Long-term instability results in varying degree of angulation of the facets of atlas and of axis. In majority of cases, there was Goel Type I atlantoaxial facetal instability, meaning thereby that on lateral profile imaging in neutral head position, the facet of atlas was located anterior to the facet of axis. The location of facet of atlas anterior to the facet of axis mimicked the location of vertebral bodies in lumbosacral "spondylolisthesis." In a number of cases, the entire facet of atlas was located anterior to the facet of axis, a radiological situation labelled by us as "spondyloptosis" of atlantoaxial facets. Less frequently, there can be Goel Type II atlantoaxial facetal instability. Infrequently there can be Goel Type III facetal instability. We identify that despite their malalignment, the joints are functional. Such mobility was observed in the form of mobile vertical instability or anteroposterior instability on dynamic imaging. The articular surface of the joint was identified to be larger and extended over wide surface of the joint and over the pedicle. The nature of instability of the atlantoaxial joint determined the clinical symptoms and the secondary musculoskeletal and neural responses.

Surgical Issues

Goel Technique of Atlantoaxial Fixation in Cases with Group A Basilar Invagination

Figs. 2.8 to 2.22 highlight the clinical case scenarios in patients with Group A basilar invagination.

Patient position: The patient is placed in prone position. Cervical traction is applied before the patient is turned prone. The head end of the operation table is elevated to 30 degrees. The head is in a "floating" position, with the headrest providing only minimal support. The traction is applied to keep the head stable and in neutral position during surgery and prevent any excessive or unwanted flexion, extension, or rotation. Distraction of the facets was not the primary aim of surgery, as it was realized that head traction had only marginal effect of the atlantoaxial articulation. Although the traction helps in reducing dislocation in some cases, direct

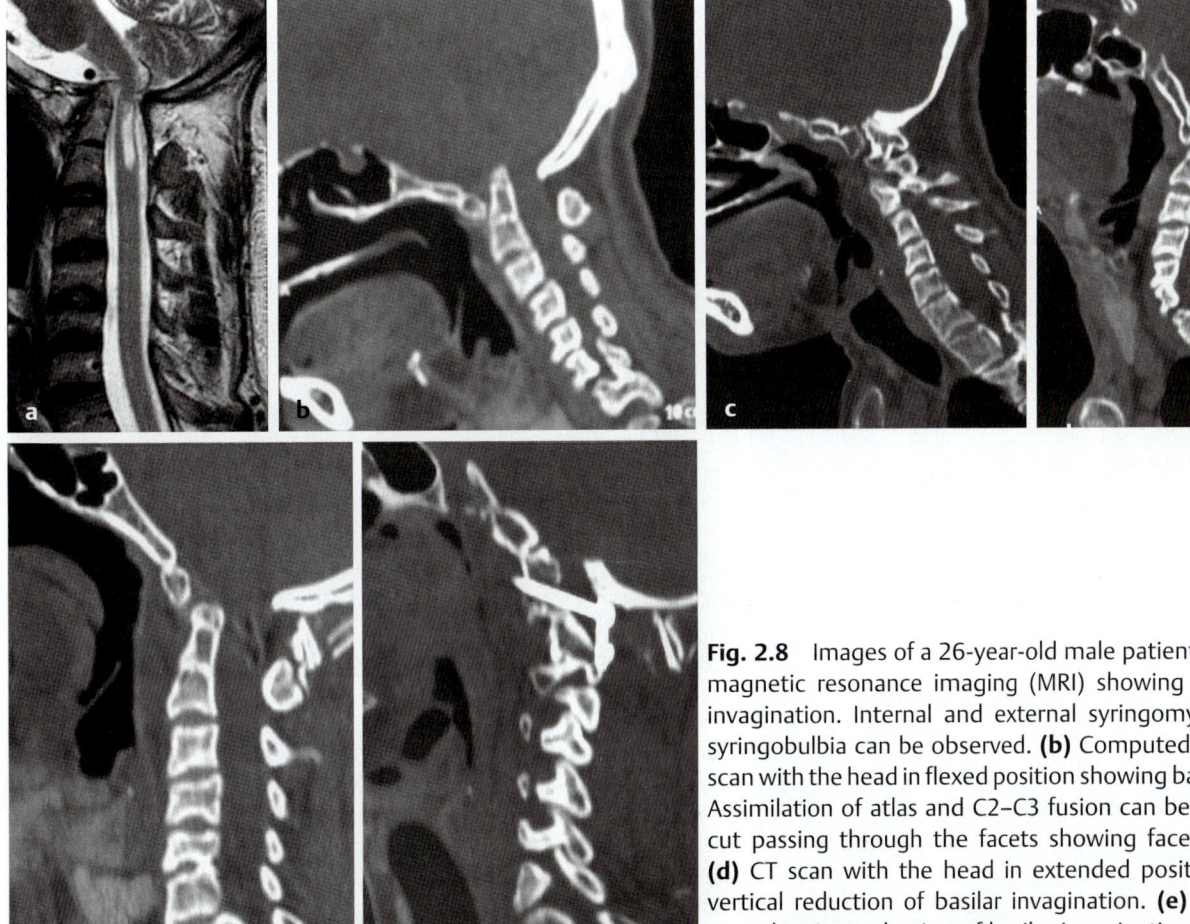

Fig. 2.8 Images of a 26-year-old male patient. **(a)** T2-weighted magnetic resonance imaging (MRI) showing Group A3 basilar invagination. Internal and external syringomyelia and external syringobulbia can be observed. **(b)** Computed tomography (CT) scan with the head in flexed position showing basilar invagination. Assimilation of atlas and C2–C3 fusion can be seen. **(c)** CT scan cut passing through the facets showing facetal malalignment. **(d)** CT scan with the head in extended position showing mild vertical reduction of basilar invagination. **(e)** Postoperative CT scan showing reduction of basilar invagination. **(f)** Postoperative CT scan cut passing through facets showing the implant.

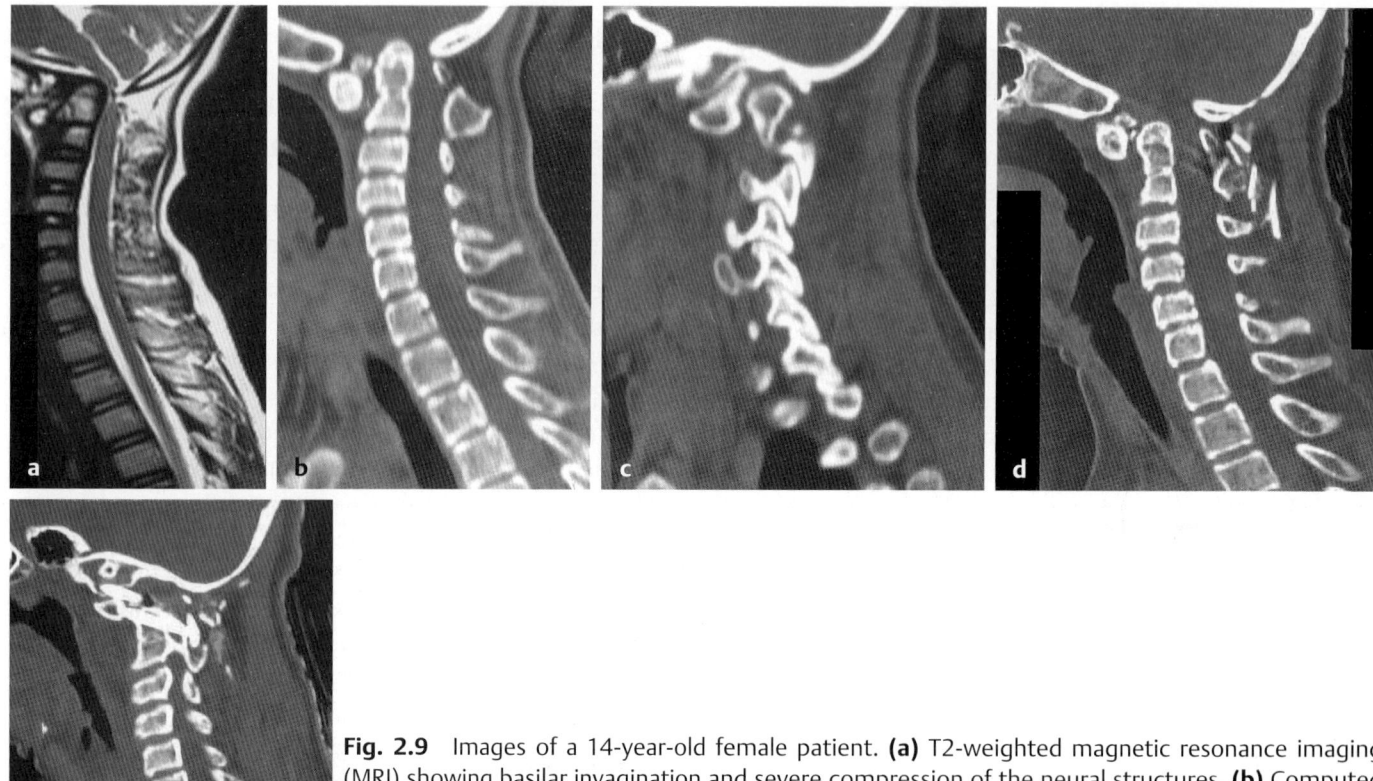

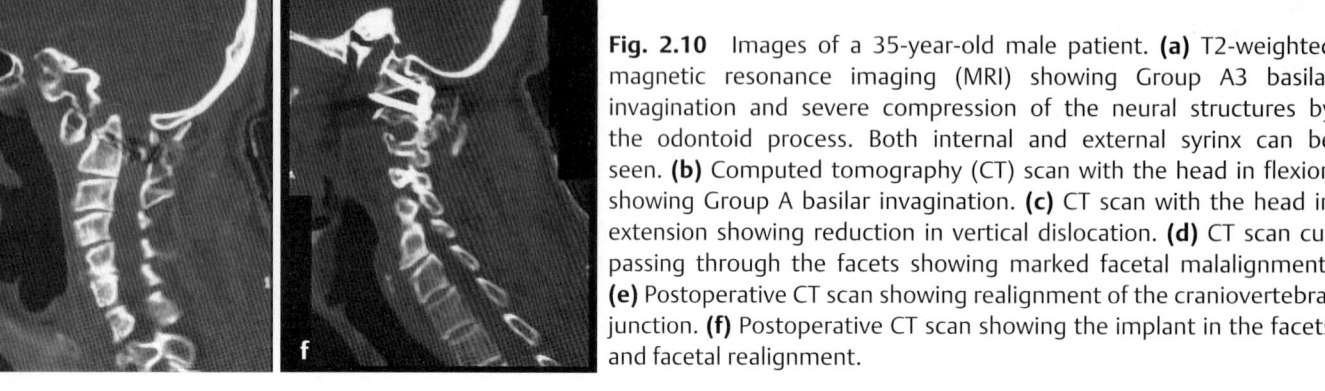

Fig. 2.9 Images of a 14-year-old female patient. **(a)** T2-weighted magnetic resonance imaging (MRI) showing basilar invagination and severe compression of the neural structures. **(b)** Computed tomography (CT) scan showing Group A3 basilar invagination. Os-odontoideum can be observed. **(c)** CT scan cut passing through the facets showing Type 1 facetal instability. **(d)** Postoperative CT scan showing reduction of basilar invagination and atlantoaxial fixation. **(e)** Postoperative CT scan showing the implant.

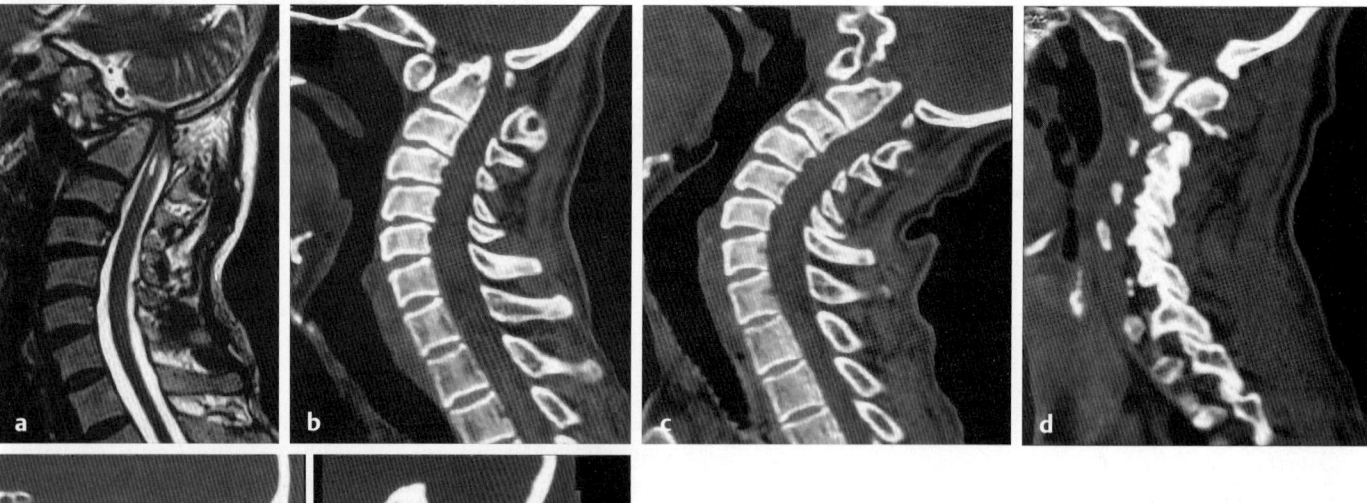

Fig. 2.10 Images of a 35-year-old male patient. **(a)** T2-weighted magnetic resonance imaging (MRI) showing Group A3 basilar invagination and severe compression of the neural structures by the odontoid process. Both internal and external syrinx can be seen. **(b)** Computed tomography (CT) scan with the head in flexion showing Group A basilar invagination. **(c)** CT scan with the head in extension showing reduction in vertical dislocation. **(d)** CT scan cut passing through the facets showing marked facetal malalignment. **(e)** Postoperative CT scan showing realignment of the craniovertebral junction. **(f)** Postoperative CT scan showing the implant in the facets and facetal realignment.

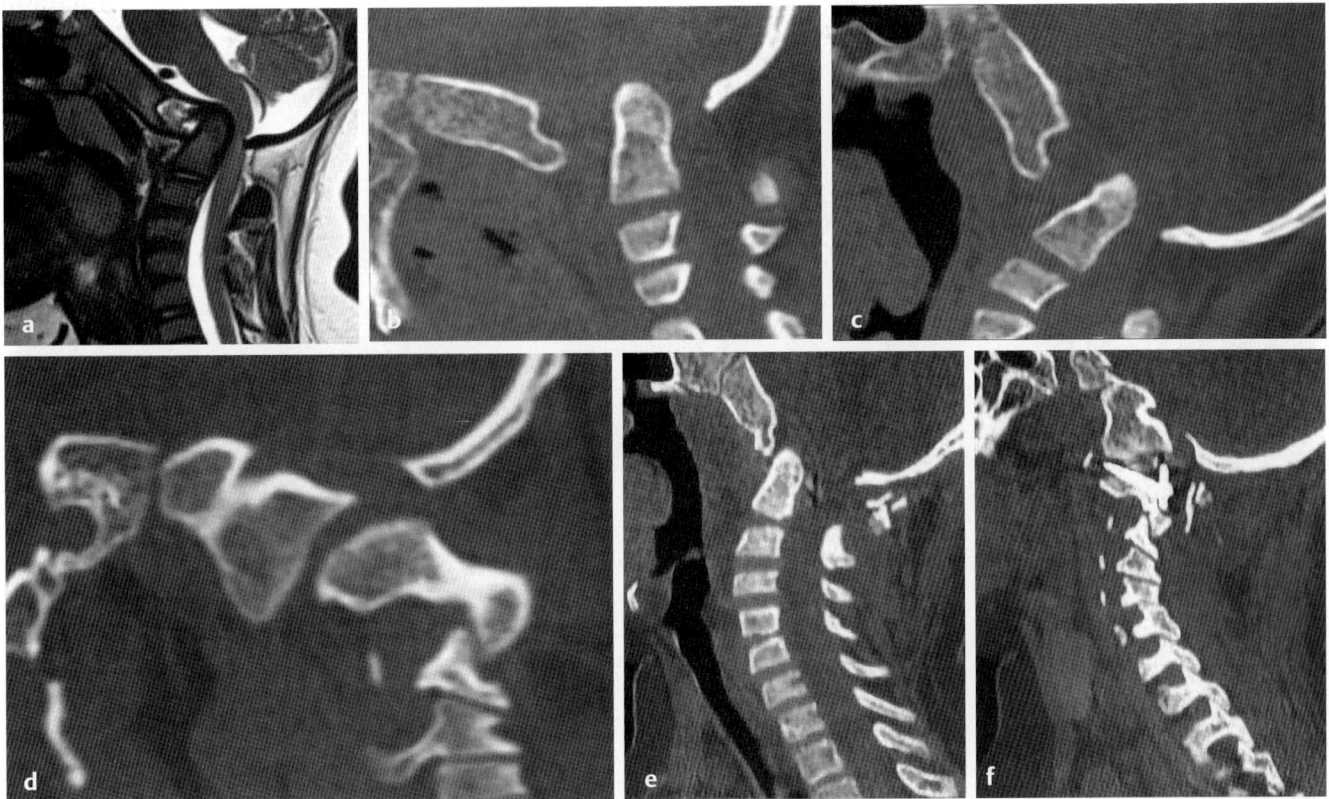

Fig. 2.11 Images of an 8-year-old male child. **(a)** T2-weighted magnetic resonance imaging (MRI) showing Group A2 basilar invagination. External syringomyelia and external syringobulbia can be seen. **(b)** Computed tomography (CT) scan with the head in flexion showing assimilation of atlas and basilar invagination. **(c)** CT scan with the head in extension showing mild reduction of vertical dislocation. **(d)** CT scan with the cuts passing through the facets showing Type 1 atlantoaxial instability. **(e)** Postoperative CT scan showing craniovertebral junction realignment. **(f)** Postoperative CT scan showing the implant.

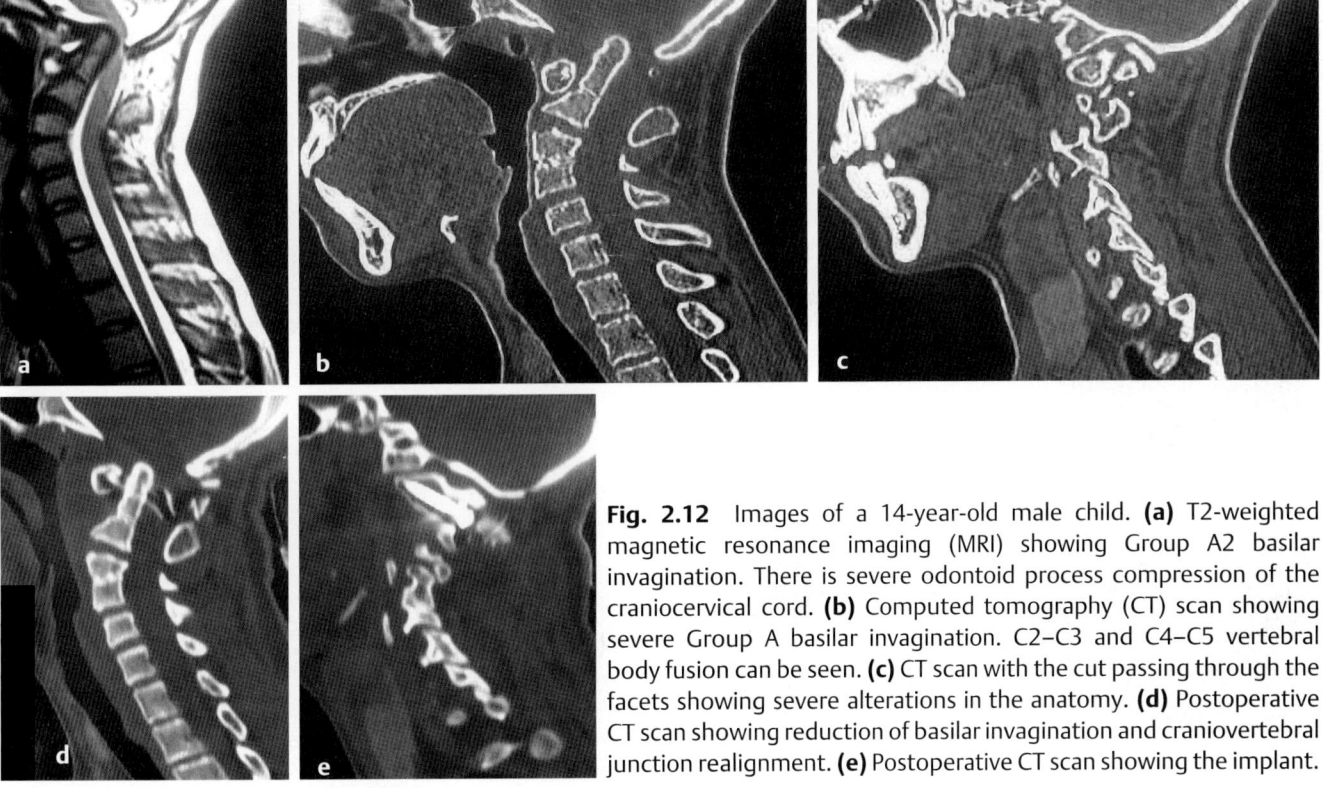

Fig. 2.12 Images of a 14-year-old male child. **(a)** T2-weighted magnetic resonance imaging (MRI) showing Group A2 basilar invagination. There is severe odontoid process compression of the craniocervical cord. **(b)** Computed tomography (CT) scan showing severe Group A basilar invagination. C2–C3 and C4–C5 vertebral body fusion can be seen. **(c)** CT scan with the cut passing through the facets showing severe alterations in the anatomy. **(d)** Postoperative CT scan showing reduction of basilar invagination and craniovertebral junction realignment. **(e)** Postoperative CT scan showing the implant.

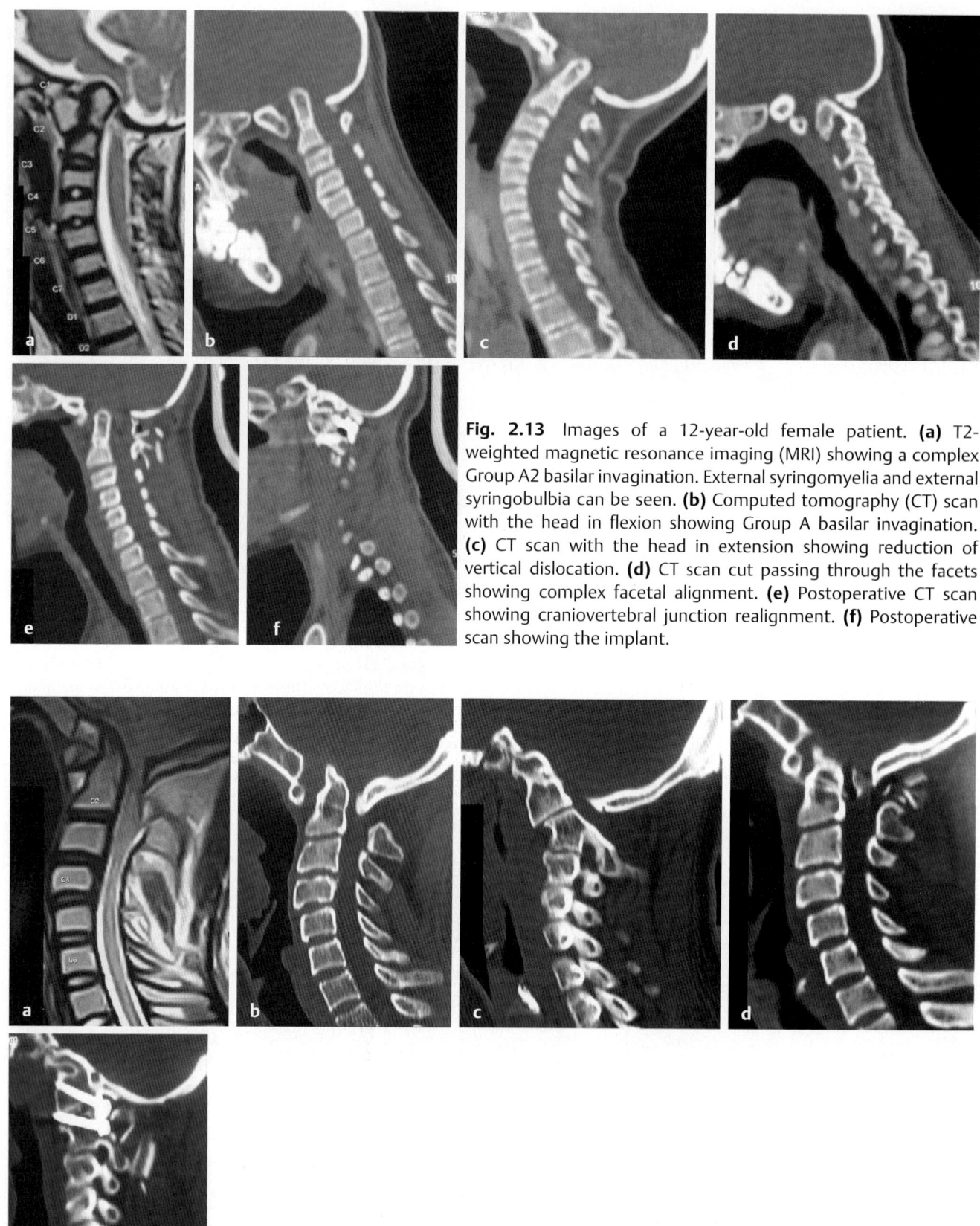

Fig. 2.13 Images of a 12-year-old female patient. **(a)** T2-weighted magnetic resonance imaging (MRI) showing a complex Group A2 basilar invagination. External syringomyelia and external syringobulbia can be seen. **(b)** Computed tomography (CT) scan with the head in flexion showing Group A basilar invagination. **(c)** CT scan with the head in extension showing reduction of vertical dislocation. **(d)** CT scan cut passing through the facets showing complex facetal alignment. **(e)** Postoperative CT scan showing craniovertebral junction realignment. **(f)** Postoperative scan showing the implant.

Fig. 2.14 Images of a 29-year-old male. **(a)** T2-weighted magnetic resonance imaging (MRI) showing Group A3 basilar invagination. Syringomyelia and external syringomyelia can be seen. **(b)** Computed tomography (CT) scan showing Group A basilar invagination. There is assimilation of the atlas. **(c)** CT scan showing Type 1 atlantoaxial facetal malalignment. **(d)** Postoperative CT scan showing craniovertebral junction realignment. **(e)** Postoperative CT scan showing the implant in the facets.

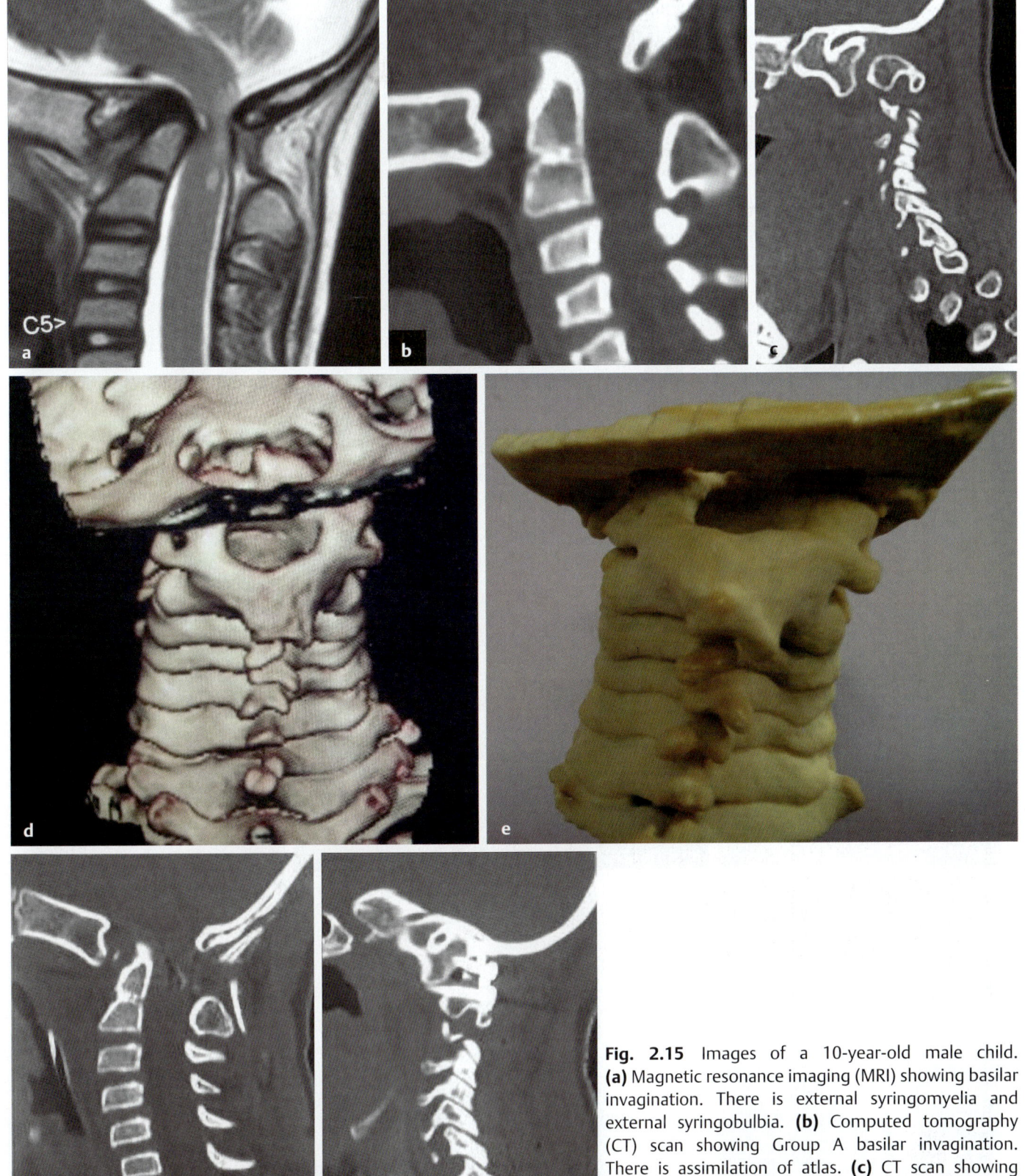

Fig. 2.15 Images of a 10-year-old male child. **(a)** Magnetic resonance imaging (MRI) showing basilar invagination. There is external syringomyelia and external syringobulbia. **(b)** Computed tomography (CT) scan showing Group A basilar invagination. There is assimilation of atlas. **(c)** CT scan showing Type 1 atlantoaxial facetal instability. **(d)** Three-dimensional CT scan showing the craniovertebral junction. **(e)** Three-dimensional model showing the craniovertebral junction. **(f)** Postoperative CT scan showing craniovertebral junction realignment. **(g)** Postoperative CT scan showing the implant.

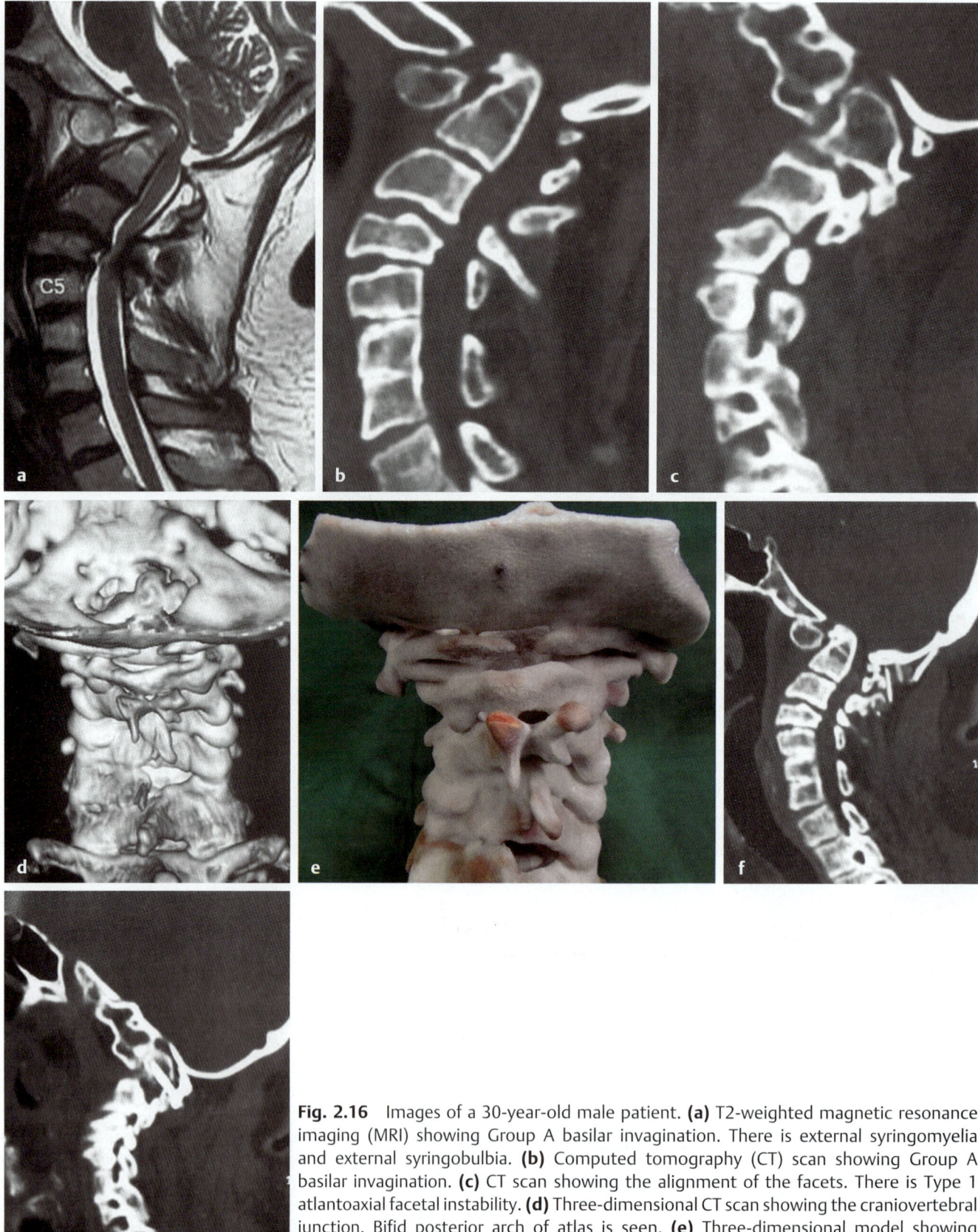

Fig. 2.16 Images of a 30-year-old male patient. **(a)** T2-weighted magnetic resonance imaging (MRI) showing Group A basilar invagination. There is external syringomyelia and external syringobulbia. **(b)** Computed tomography (CT) scan showing Group A basilar invagination. **(c)** CT scan showing the alignment of the facets. There is Type 1 atlantoaxial facetal instability. **(d)** Three-dimensional CT scan showing the craniovertebral junction. Bifid posterior arch of atlas is seen. **(e)** Three-dimensional model showing the craniovertebral junction. The traverse of the vertebral arteries can be appreciated. **(f)** Postoperative scan showing craniovertebral junction realignment. **(g)** Scan showing the implants.

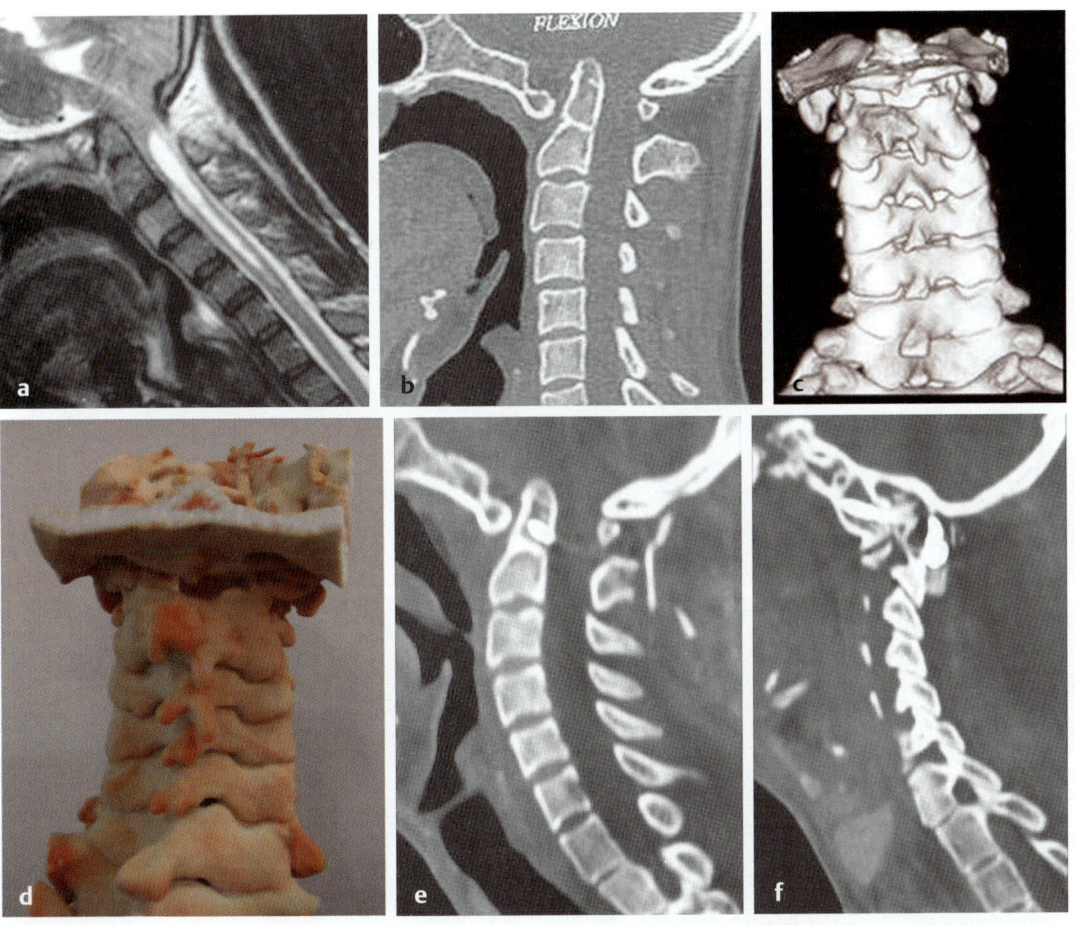

Fig. 2.17 Images of a 25-year-old male patient. **(a)** Magnetic resonance imaging (MRI) showing Group A basilar invagination. There is Chiari formation and syringomyelia. **(b)** Computed tomography (CT) scan showing basilar invagination. **(c)** Three-dimensional CT scan showing craniovertebral junction. Bifid posterior arch of the atlas can be seen. **(d)** Three-dimensional model showing the craniovertebral junction. The location and course of the vertebral artery can be seen. **(e)** Postoperative CT scan showing incomplete but significant craniovertebral junction realignment. **(f)** CT scan showing the facetal implant.

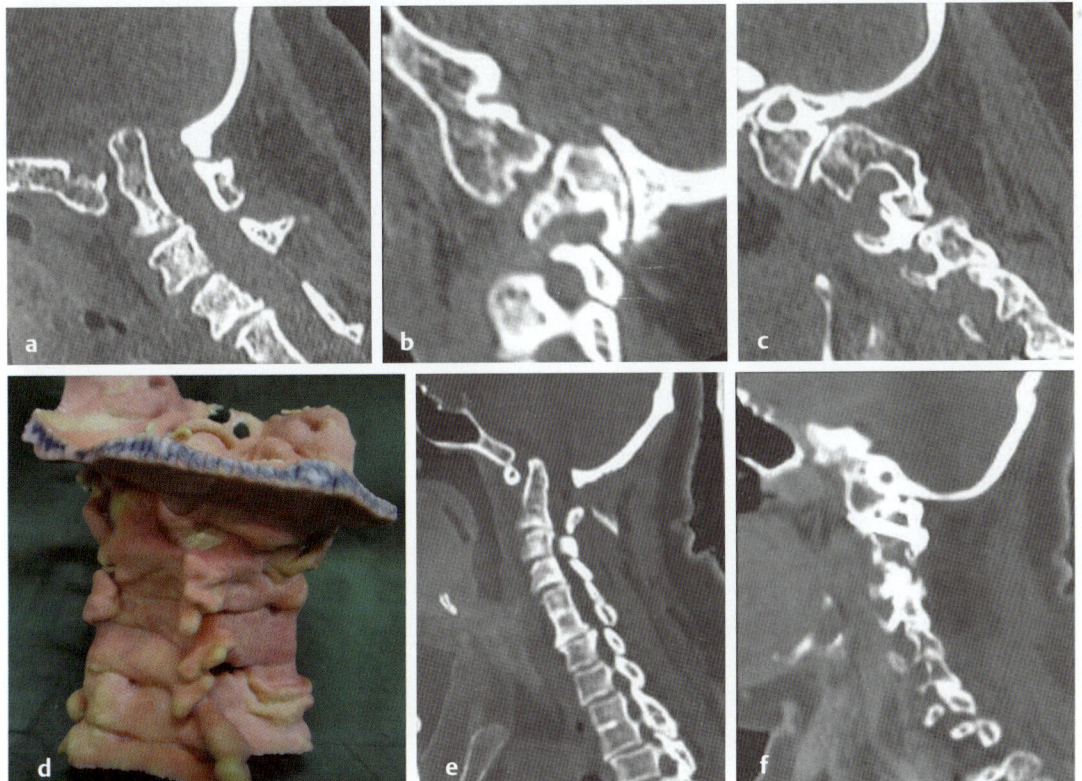

Fig. 2.18 Images of a 48-year-old female patient. **(a)** Computed tomography (CT) scan showing Group A basilar invagination. **(b)** CT scan showing the malalignment of the facets on one side. **(c)** CT scan showing better alignment of the facets of the contralateral side. **(d)** Three-dimensional model of the case showing the malalignment. The location of the vertebral arteries can be seen. **(e)** Postoperative scan showing the craniovertebral junction realignment. **(f)** Scan showing the implant.

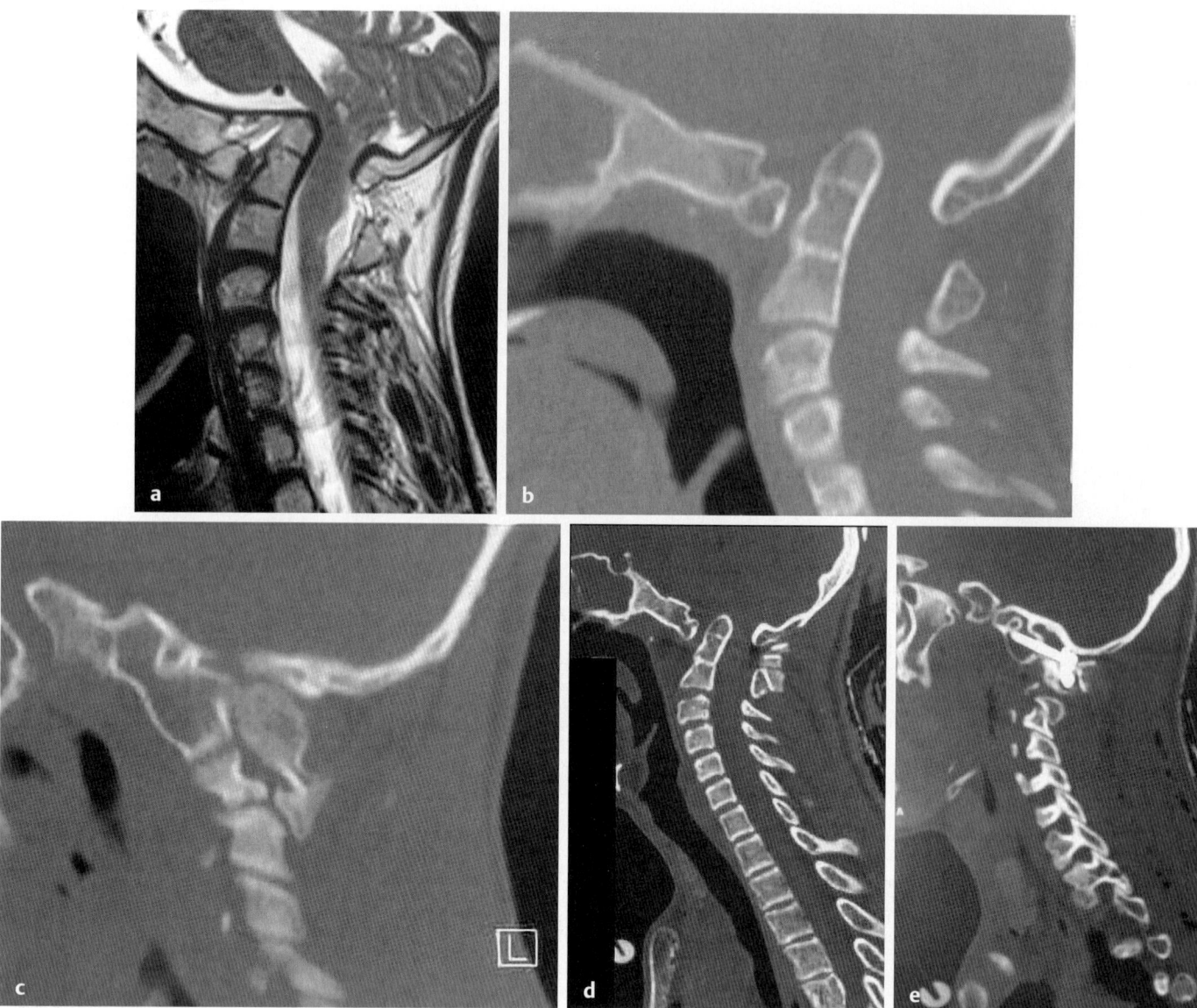

Fig. 2.19 Images of an 18-year-old male patient. **(a)** T2-weighted magnetic resonance imaging (MRI) showing the basilar invagination. External syringomyelia and external syringobulbia can be seen. **(b)** Computed tomography (CT) scan showing basilar invagination. There is assimilation of atlas and C2–C3 fusion. **(c)** CT scan showing severe facetal malalignment. **(d)** Postoperative CT scan showing craniovertebral junction realignment. **(e)** Scan showing the facetal implant.

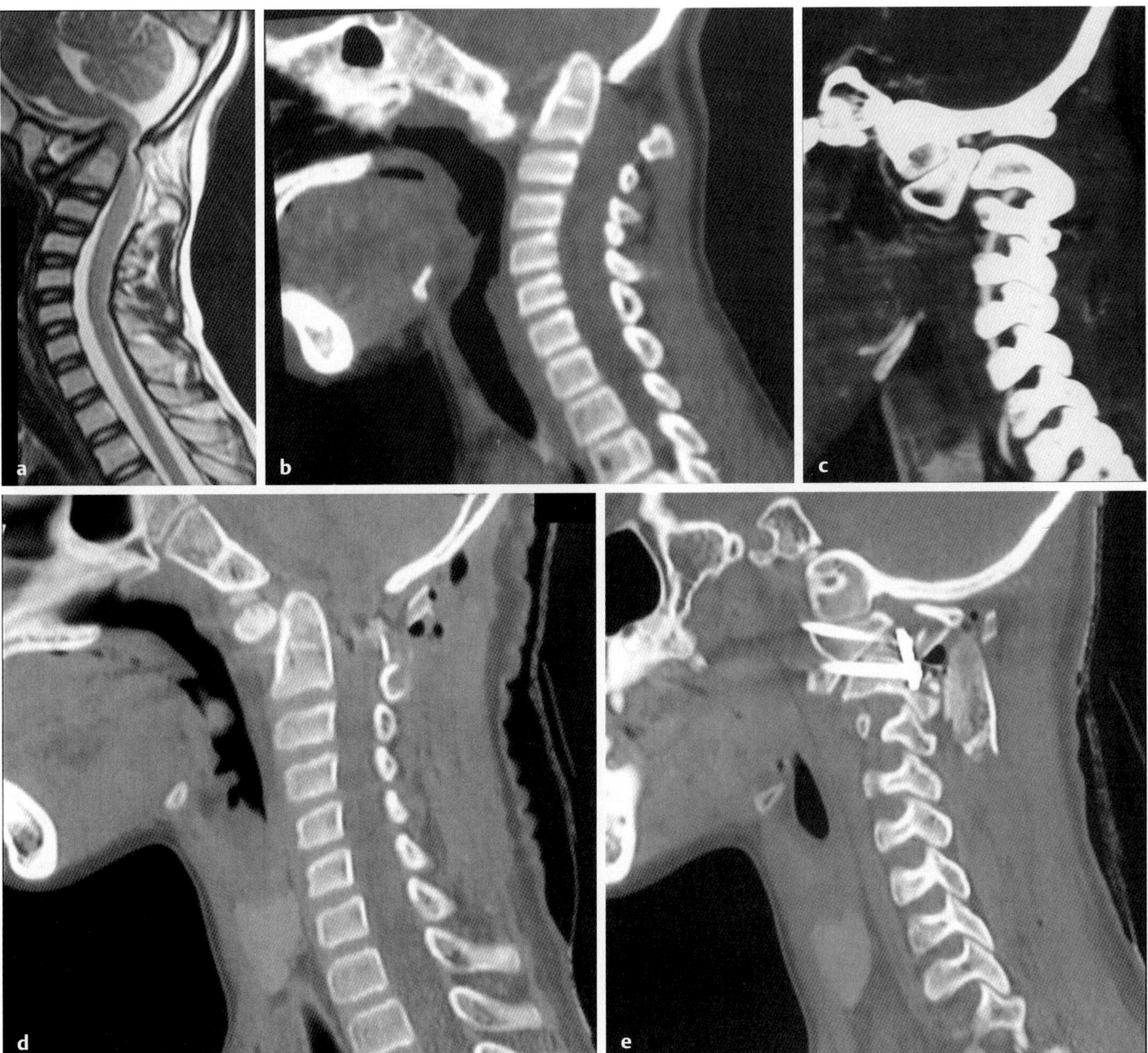

Fig. 2.20 Images of a 12-year-old male child. **(a)** Magnetic resonance imaging (MRI) showing marked basilar invagination and marked neural compression. External syringomyelia and external syringobulbia are seen. **(b)** Computed tomography (CT) scan showing marked basilar invagination. Assimilation of atlas is seen. **(c)** CT scan showing Type I atlantoaxial facetal instability. **(d)** Postoperative CT scan showing craniovertebral realignment. **(e)** CT scan showing the implants.

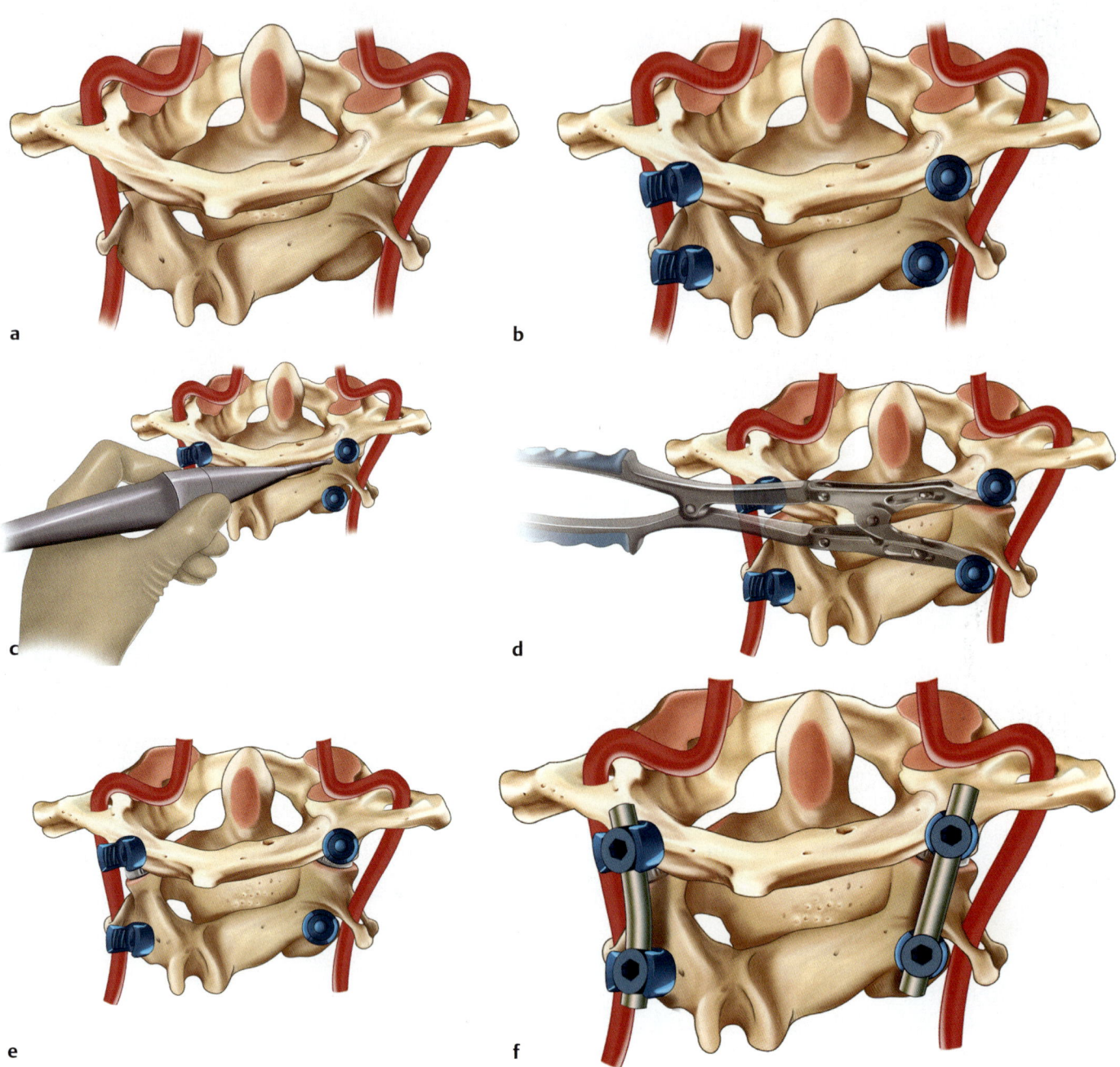

Fig. 2.21 **(a–f)** Illustrations of posterior basilar invagination reduction technique of Goel. Distraction of the atlantoaxial joint can be provided by distraction of C1 and C2 screws **(d)**, and a spacer or a cage or a bone graft is placed into the joint **(e)**, and screws are fixed using a short rod **(f)**.

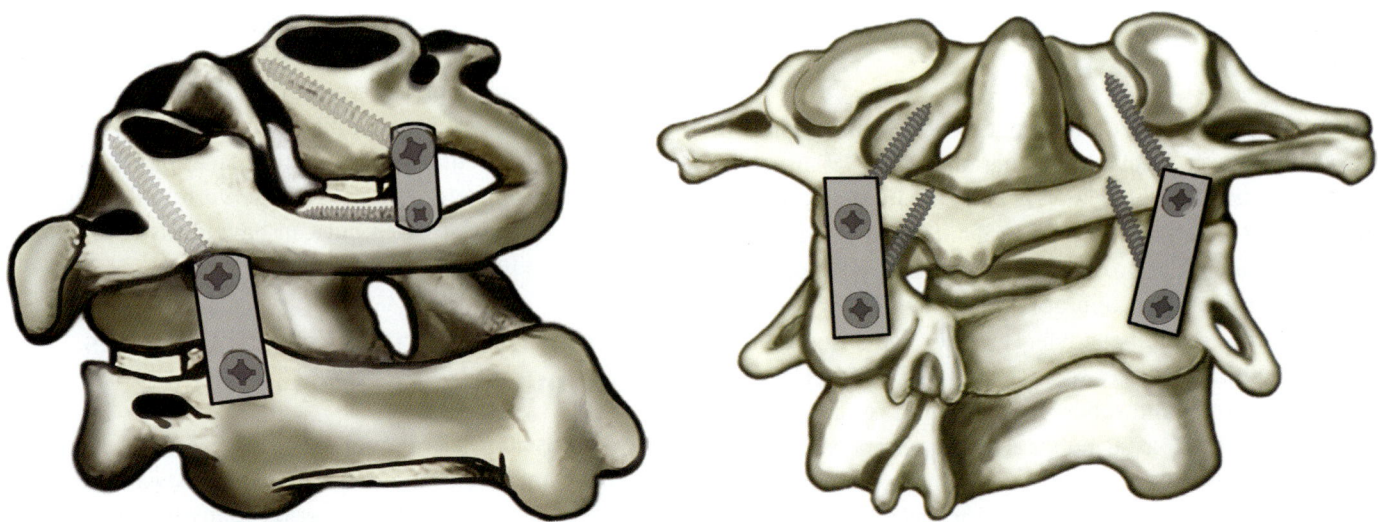

Fig. 2.22   Image showing Goel's technique of distraction and fixation using plate and screws.

and manual facetal handling and distraction resulted in primary reduction. A host of bone abnormalities, fusions, and rotation and an unusual course of the vertebral artery may make the exposure of the joint difficult and unsafe. The rostral location of the joint in some cases and excessive venous pooling of the region can also make the joint exposure difficult. Although C2 ganglion was sectioned in cases treated earlier in the series, the C2 ganglion is elevated in most recent cases to expose the joint. However, wherever the exposure is not satisfactory and screw insertion in atlas and axis is not possible under direct surgical vision, the C2 ganglion is sectioned after its wide exposure. The pedicle of C2 vertebra is the key to joint exposure. It is first exposed widely and then followed with a subperiosteal dissection rostrally toward the atlantoaxial articulation. Manual handling of the bones can depict the unstable nature of the joint. The joint is exposed widely, articular cartilage is denuded, and bone chips harvested from the iliac crest are packed into the joint cavity. Plate/rod and mono/polyaxial screw fixation is subsequently carried out. The muscle attachment to the C2 spinous process and arch of atlas is then sharply and widely cut. The spinous process, lamina, and exposed surface of pars of C2 and posterior arch of atlas are drilled to prepare it as host bone for iliac crest graft. Traction is removed after the patient is turned to supine position.

Parameters of Successful Operation

Symptomatic recovery is the most important parameter of success of the operation. Following a successful operation, immediate postoperative recovery in symptoms is a rule. Improvement in the power and reduction in the stiffness of the limbs and relief from tingling paresthesia are observed as

soon as the patient is completely reversed from anesthesia. The recovery in symptoms continues in the postoperative phase. Careful evaluation will show that there is recovery in all musculoskeletal abnormalities that include torticollis and reduction in neck size. Apart from reduction of basilar invagination or craniovertebral realignment, it is bone fusion of the atlantoaxial region that determines the success of the operation. Any delayed worsening in the neurological condition is a suggestion of persistent atlantoaxial instability. It must be remembered that reduction of basilar invagination or reduction of atlantodental/clivodental interval distance is not the primary aim of surgery. It is firm stabilization and fixation that is the primary aim. In other words, although preferred and most acceptable it is not craniovertebral junction bony realignment that is the aim of surgery, rather firm and solid atlantoaxial fixation is the primary purpose of operation.

Is Inclusion of Occipital Bone in the Fixation Construct Necessary?

Basilar invagination is an outcome of atlantoaxial instability. Atlantoaxial stabilization is treatment. Inclusion of the occipital bone is unnecessary.[13] Moreover, inclusion of the occipital bone in the fixation construct severely restricts neck movements and the strength of the construct is weaker when multiple spinal segments are included in the fixation. In other words, inclusion of the occipital bone in the fixation construct should not be done as it is a harmful surgical procedure. However, in some cases, direct atlantoaxial fixation may not be possible due to technical or anatomical reasons, then in such a case, inclusion of the occipital bone will be the only option, albeit a suboptimal option.

Atlantoaxial Fixation in Cases with Assimilation of Atlas

Assimilation of atlas is a frequent skeletal abnormality in association with basilar invagination. Direct atlantoaxial fixation is technically relatively difficult in such cases as the joint is located rostrally. Several authors feel that in the presence of assimilation of the atlas, inclusion of the occipital bone in the fixation is appropriate as the facet of the atlas is fused with occipital condyle. However, we observed that even in such cases direct screw insertion into facet of atlas provides a strong and robust fixation point for atlantoaxial fixation. The atlantoaxial joint is always open and excessively mobile and never fused in such cases. Wide opening of the atlantoaxial joint, denuding of the articular cartilage, and introduction of the bone graft into the articular cavity are essential components of technique. Long screw can be inserted into the facets of atlas and axis. Direct atlantoaxial facetal fixation is recommended and most optimal even in cases with assimilation of the atlas.

Occipital bone inclusion in the fixation construct is not necessary. Use of long implants and fixation of the occipital bone with screw that measures 2 to 5 mm in length are inherently weak, prone to dislodgment on neck twisting, and severely restrict neck movements.

Inclusion of the Subaxial Spine in the Fixation Construct

Basilar invagination is a long-term outcome of subtle and progressive atlantoaxial instability. Other joints that include occipitoatlantal joint and subaxial joints are unaffected or are not unstable. Atlantoaxial joint segmental stabilization is the aim of treatment. Inclusion of the occipital bone or subaxial bones is not only unnecessary, but also use of long implants and fixing normally functioning spinal segments can make the construct weak and prone to failures.

Protection of the Vertebral Artery

Avoidance of injury to the vertebral artery forms the main surgical issue during surgery. Special care is necessary to preoperatively visualize and determine the course of the vertebral artery in three-dimensional planes. In this respect three-dimensional models can form a useful investigational modality. In any case, the course of the vertebral artery cannot be taken for granted and needs to be adequately studied. Although not used routinely by the author, intraoperative navigation to assess the best and safe passage for the screw that avoids the vertebral artery appears to be essential. Dissection and protection of the supra-axial course of the vertebral artery is particularly important in cases with assimilation of the atlas. The course of the artery is frequently behind the facet of atlas in such cases. Compromise or sacrifice of the vertebral artery can be harmless in most cases but can have disastrous clinical outcome that includes death.

Reversal of Musculoskeletal Changes Following Atlantoaxial Fixation

Several musculoskeletal abnormalities like short neck and torticollis and bone anomalies like platybasia recover in the immediate postoperative period following atlantoaxial stabilization. In our earlier report, we had discussed that there is a potential of bone fusion to un-fuse. Neural abnormalities like Chiari malformation and syringomyelia also have the potential of reduction. It appears that the only abnormality in basilar invagination is atlantoaxial instability, and all other musculoskeletal and neural abnormalities are secondary and have a protective function.

Conclusion

Direct fixation of the facets of atlas and axis and craniovertebral junction realignment are the treatment of Group A basilar invagination.

Key Points

- Group A basilar invagination is a manifestation of atlantoaxial instability.
- Clinical and radiological evidence suggest that the process of atlantoaxial instability is progressive.
- Inclination of the odontoid process and the extent of its superior migration will influence alteration in musculoskeletal and neural malformation.
- The degree and duration of atlantoaxial instability will influence formation of CSF loculations within the spinal cord (syringomyelia) or outside the spinal cord (external syringomyelia) or within the brainstem (syringobulbia) or outside the brainstem (external syringobulbia).
- Opening of the atlantoaxial joint, denuding the articular cartilage, distracting the facets, stuffing bone graft and/or intra-articular spacer within the joint cavity essentially to stabilize the joint and provide space for bone fusion, and

subsequent lateral mass plate/rod and screw fixation are essential elements of surgical treatment.

• Atlantoaxial fixation aimed at segmental arthrodesis is the treatment. Inclusion of the occipital bone or subaxial spine in the fixation construct is not necessary and may be counterproductive.

References

1. Goel A. Treatment of basilar invagination by atlantoaxial joint distraction and direct lateral mass fixation. J Neurosurg Spine 2004;1(3):281–286

2. Von Torklus D, Gehle W. The Upper Cervical Spine: Regional Anatomy, Pathology, and Traumatology. A Systematic Radiological Atlas and Textbook. New York: Grune & Stratton; 1972:1–98

3. Goel A, Bhatjiwale M, Desai K. Basilar invagination: a study based on 190 surgically treated patients. J Neurosurg 1998; 88(6):962–968

4. Goel A, Jain S, Shah A. Radiological evaluation of 510 cases of basilar invagination with evidence of atlantoaxial instability (Group A basilar invagination). World Neurosurg 2018;110:533–543

5. Goel A, Nadkarni T, Shah A, Sathe P, Patil M. Radiologic evaluation of basilar invagination without obvious atlantoaxial instability (Group B basilar invagination): an analysis based on a study of 75 patients. World Neurosurg 2016;95:375–382

6. Goel A, Sathe P, Shah A. Atlantoaxial fixation for basilar invagination without obvious atlantoaxial instability (Group B basilar invagination): outcome analysis of 63 surgically treated cases. World Neurosurg 2017;99:164–170

7. Goel A, Shah A. Reversal of longstanding musculoskeletal changes in basilar invagination after surgical decompression and stabilization. J Neurosurg Spine 2009;10(3):220–227

8. Thiebaut F, Wackenheim A, Vrousos C. [New median sagittal pneumostratigraphical finding concerning the posterior fossa] [in French]. J Radiol Electrol Med Nucl 1961;42:1–7

9. Chamberlain WE. Basilar impression (platybasia): a bizarre developmental anomaly of the occipital bone and upper cervical spine with striking and misleading neurologic manifestations. Yale J Biol Med 1939;11(5):487–496

10. Goel A, Nadkarni T, Shah A, Ramdasi R, Patni N. Bifid anterior and posterior arches of atlas: surgical implication and analysis of 70 cases. Neurosurgery 2015;77(2):296–305, discussion 305–306

11. David KM, Thorogood PV, Stevens JM, Crockard HA. The dysmorphic cervical spine in Klippel-Feil syndrome: interpretations from developmental biology. Neurosurg Focus 1999;6(6):E3

12. Goel A. Goel's classification of atlantoaxial "facetal" dislocation. J Craniovertebr Junction Spine 2014;5(1):3–8

13. Goel A. Occiput, C1 and C2 instrumentation. In: Winn RH, ed. Youmans and Winn Neurological Surgery. Philadelphia, PA; 2017:2643–2655

14. Goel A. Facetal alignment: basis of an alternative Goel's classification of basilar invagination. J Craniovertebr Junction Spine 2014;5(2):59–64

15. Shah A, Serchi E. Management of basilar invagination: a historical perspective. J Craniovertebr Junction Spine 2016; 7(2):96–100

16. Goel A, Laheri VK. Plate and screw fixation for atlanto-axial subluxation. Acta Neurochir (Wien) 1994;129(1-2):47–53

17. Goel A, Desai KI, Muzumdar DP. Atlantoaxial fixation using plate and screw method: a report of 160 treated patients. Neurosurgery 2002;51(6):1351–1356, discussion 1356–1357

3 Ponte Osteotomy for Cervical Spine

Yurdal Gezercan

Introduction

As a natural process of increased life span in our age, we are faced with more cervical deformities in our daily practice. Cervical deformities and malignancies have been the focus of intense attention for spinal surgeons in recent years. Established global and spinopelvic parameters in adult spinal deformities have also been defined for the cervical region and have been widely used in deformities of this region, and pedicle subtraction osteotomy (PSO) (C7–T1 vertebra) has been used in posterior approaches due to the anatomical aspects of the cervical region (vertebral artery). The quality-of-life scores can be increased by obtaining ideal alignments with performance of osteotomies in cervical deformities.[1–4]

In addition to standard plain radiographs, hyperflexion and hyperextension radiographs are also used to evaluate the flexibility of the deformity.

Definition of the Technique

This procedure can be considered as the adaptation of the classical Ponte osteotomy to the cervical region. In his description of the technique for thoracic kyphosis in 1987, Albert Ponte defined osteotomy as wide thoracic facet joint resection, as well as lamina removal and ligamentum flavum excision.[5] This technique, which has been popularized as posterior column shortening osteotomy, corrects closure of thoracic kyphosis osteotomy gaps by significantly shortening the posterior column with segmentally applied and apically

directed compressive forces. This technique, which is applied in the cervical region, can be applied at any cervical region level. After the patient is brought to the operating room, endotracheal intubation is followed by intraoperative neuromonitoring under general anesthesia. The patient is placed in the prone position, the arms are on both sides of the body, and the head is placed in a soft silicon head cap in the modified Concorde position (**Fig. 3.1**). The head is fixed to the table edges with a horizontally placed band from the occiput. The operating table is placed in the reverse Trendelenburg position to prevent venous stasis in the surgical area. Following the suboccipital midline skin incision, the dorsal fascia is passed using the electrocautery and the paravertebral muscles are opened by bilateral subperiosteal dissection from the spinous processes. Wide dissection up to the lateral aspect of the facet joints and complete lateral mass surface exposures are important (**Fig. 3.2**). It should be kept in mind that posterolateral grafting should be done for fusion when closing the osteotomy gap. After placing the retractor, posterior instrumentation (lateral mass or pedicle screw) is applied to the appropriate levels since the pathology and total laminectomy performed are above and below the levels for which osteotomy is planned (kyphosis apex and adjacent levels if necessary; **Fig. 3.3**). The foramen roof is thinned by drilling the upper vertebral inferior facet joint and the lower vertebral superior facet joint under irrigation with saline using a high-speed drill. Then, using a number 1 Kerrison rongeur, foraminotomy is performed by entering from the medial side of the intervertebral foramen. At this point, complete spinal root decompression is achieved by removing the free part of the superior facet joint

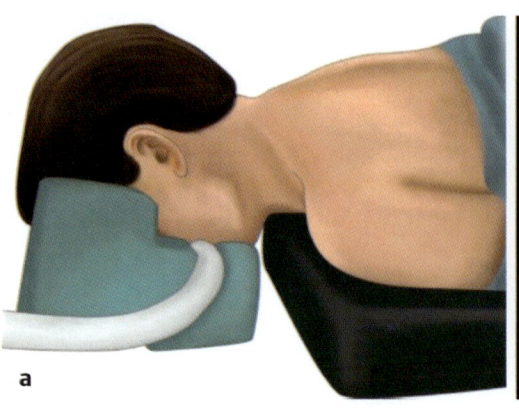
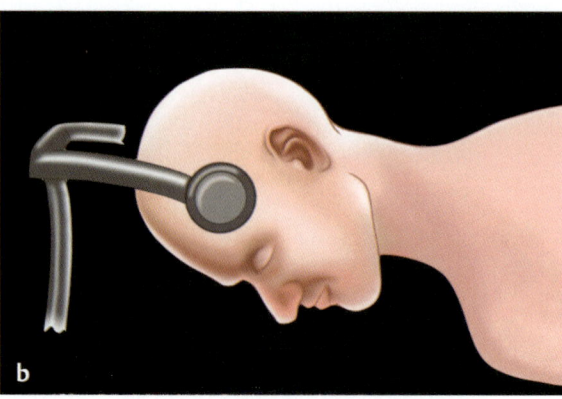

Fig. 3.1 Head position can be attained by using a soft silicone cap **(a)** or by a Mayfield head holder with three pins **(b)**.

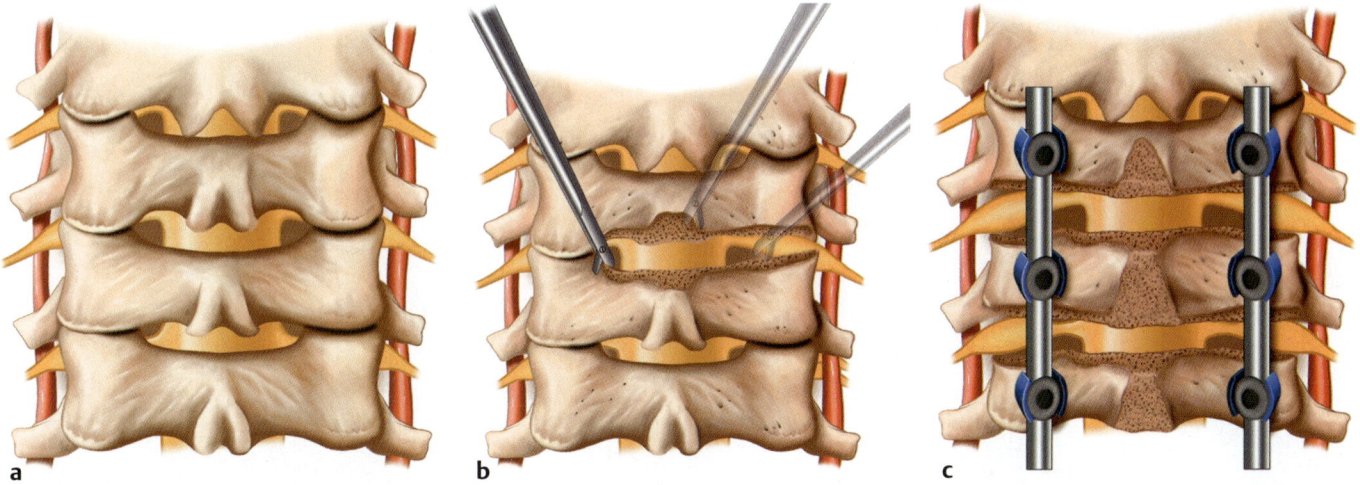

Fig. 3.2 After the surgical field is opened **(a)**, Ponte osteotomies are performed by removing laminar edges and resection facets partially **(b)**. The pedicle screws are inserted **(c)**. The deformity can be corrected by head deflection and compression of the screw heads on the rods. Dura and spinal roots must be observed at this stage.

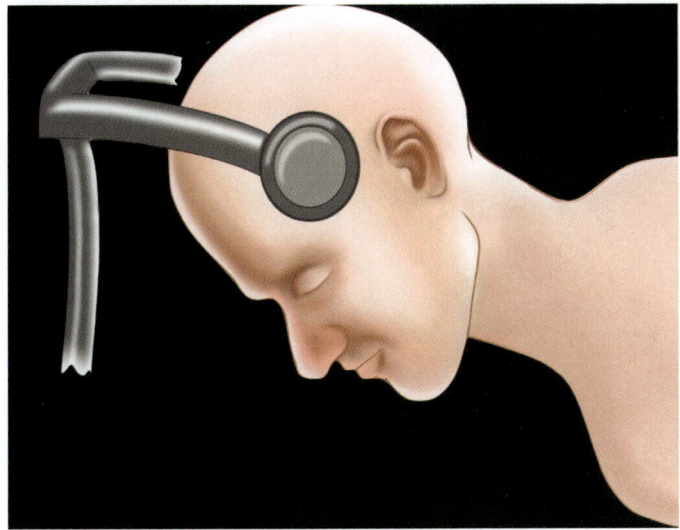

Fig. 3.3 Mayfield head holder is released; the head is moved back in extension to reduce kyphosis and provide lordosis.

after cutting the anatomical ligament from the peduncle as if a tooth was extracted. This bilaterally applied procedure can be safely performed according to the correction needs of the deformity. It gains an average of 5 degrees per level. After the inferior and superior facet joint resection, the osteotomy gap is closed by deflecting the table head, and after the ideal lordotic rod bending is done, the osteotomy line is closed under compressive forces (**Fig. 3.4**). Meanwhile, attention should be paid to possible neural damage by checking the neuromonitoring records. Afterward, posterolateral grafting is performed with autografts obtained from the laminae. A silicone drain is placed in the epidural area, and the anatomical folds are closed in order.

Position

- The patient is placed on the radiolucent surgical table in a Concorde position with silicone head holder (**Fig. 3.1a**) or with Mayfield clamps (**Fig. 3.1b**).
- The patient should be placed on the table so that the anterior–posterior fluoroscopy image can be taken.
- The patient should better have a neuromonitoring.

Surgical Technique

- The area to be operated is determined by fluoroscopy.
- After skin incision, the paravertebral muscles are retracted subperiostally.
- Approximately 5 to 7 degrees corrections are provided for each segment.
- To reduce epidural venous bleeding, the osteotomy site should be closed as quickly as possible.
- With the Ponte osteotomy, the posterior column is closed.
- Partial laminectomy (lamina, ligamentum flavum) is performed on the planned vertebrae with the help of ultrasonic bone cutter (**Fig. 3.2a**).
- A diamond tipped drill or 1- to 2-mm Kerrison rongeur is used to resect the inferior facet of the upper vertebra and the superior facet of the lower vertebral column (**Fig. 3.2b**).
- Facet resection is performed consecutively to the planned vertebrae of the Ponte osteotomy. Roots are thoroughly set free.

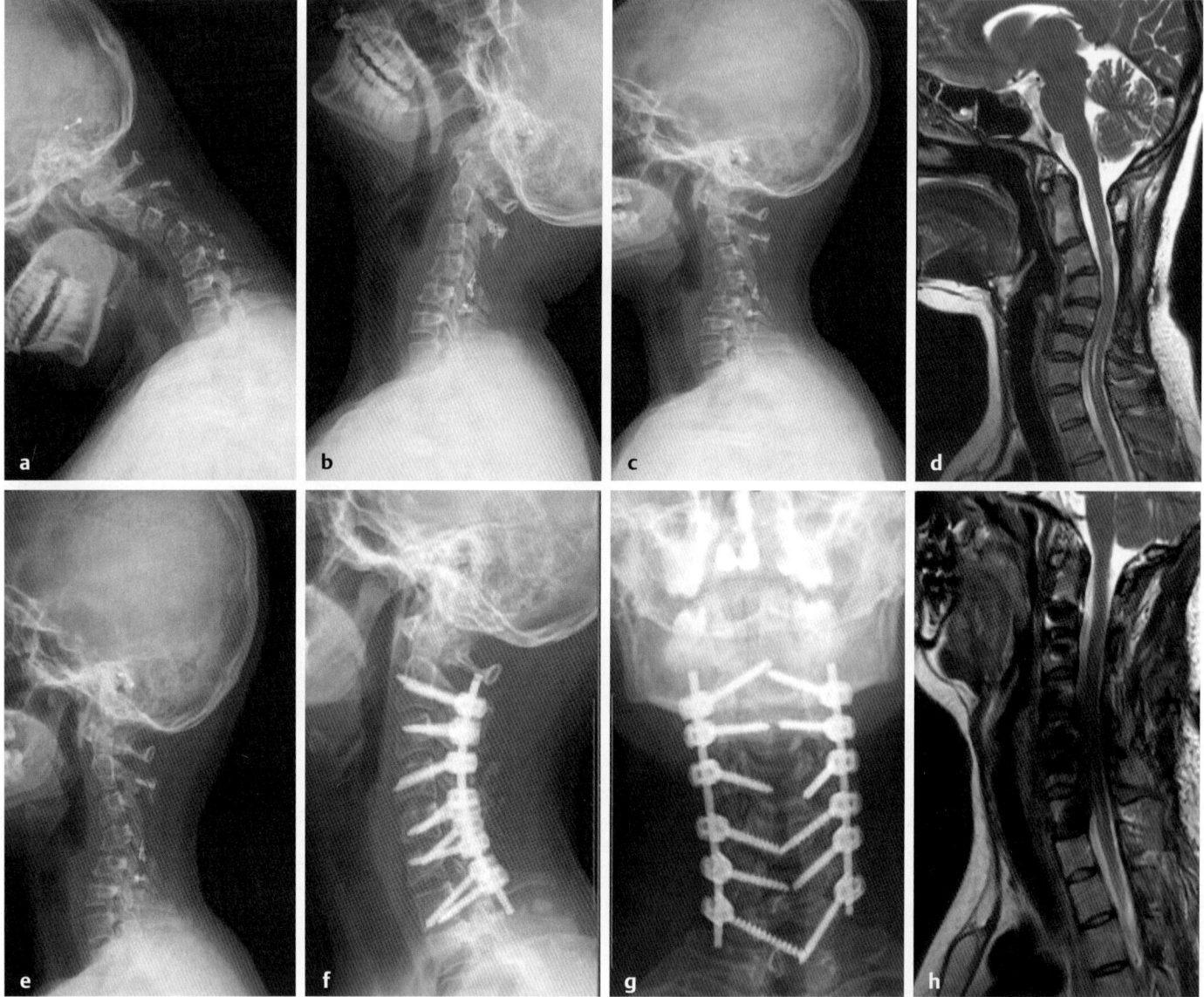

Fig. 3.4   A female patient who developed postlaminectomy kyphosis in 6 months after primary surgery. Preoperative radiographs **(a–c)** showed the flexibility of the neck. A laminoplasty was performed after a dermal sinus excision at the age of 25 years **(d)**. The author considered it as a postlaminectomy kyphosis. A two-level (C4–C5 and C5–C6) Ponte osteotomy and C2–C7 pedicle screw fixation completely corrected the kyphosis **(e–h)**.

- Pre-arranged, pedicular or lateral mass screws are placed with the help of fluoroscopy or neuronavigation (**Fig. 3.2c**).
- An appropriate curve is given to the rod. The Mayfield head holder is released, and the head is manually positioned in the appropriate position (**Fig. 3.3**). Rods are placed in a compressive manner (in the appropriate position). It is checked that the cord and nerve roots are not under compression.
- Neuromonitoring must be used during the closure of the posterior column. During the closure process, changes in the electrophysiologic values should be checked frequently.

- During the closing operation, care must be taken not to fold the dura.
- Autografts from leminectomy are placed on the surgical area.

Indications

Many osteotomy techniques have been described for the management of cervical deformities.[2–4,6–8] Ames et al created a classification by standardizing these osteotomy types, which are defined as anterior, posterior, or both of the spine.[1] Ponte osteotomy is defined as grade 2 complete facet resection in the classification that ranges from grade

1 to 7.[1] Ponte osteotomy, which is one of the three types of flexibility defined by Koller, can be used in semirigid and flexible ones.[9] There should be no ankylosis anterior to the vertebra to correct the deformity in this technique, which is posteriorly applied. Appropriate realignment can be achieved by performing Ponte osteotomy at multiple levels in patients with cervical lordosis loss. Therefore, it can be used in all deformities without solid fusion in the anterior vertebra. Among the indications, it can be used in cervical spondyloses with degenerative sagittal plane deformity; cervical spondylotic myelopathies; postlaminectomy; post-traumatic, postinfectious, post-tumor, and iatrogenic kyphosis; anterior nonunion; and cervical pediatric deformities. It can also be used as an adjunct to anterior osteotomies in combined surgery.

Complication Avoidance

Posterior cervical surgery complications include neurological injury, root damage, C5 palsy, vertebral artery injury, cerebrospinal fluid fistula, hardware failure, pseudoarthrosis, and wound problems (hematoma and infection). Among these, the most frightening is neurological injury.

Cervical Ponte is a surgical method in osteotomy that is performed by excision of the spinous process, lamina, flavum ligamentum, and resection of the superior and inferior facet joint. Particular attention should be paid to continuous neuromonitoring recording during laminectomy and facet joint resection. The superior facet joint must be completely removed for the nerve root to be fully decompressed. Contrarily, while the osteotomy gap is closed, the root may become stuck in the foramen and root damage may occur. Thus, using a diamond tip and complying with microsurgical principles and performing it under a microscope during the foraminotomy stage when using a high-speed drill are recommended.

Tips and Tricks

- The flexibility of preoperative deformity should be well evaluated (**Fig. 3.4**).
- The number of levels and the area for osteotomy under radiological parameters should be carefully determined.
- The final stage of foraminotomy is reached using a diamond-tipped high-speed drill.
- The final stage of foraminotomy is performed with a 1-mm Kerrison rongeur under the microscope and the liberated bone is carefully removed.

- Correction should be done under table deflection and rod compression, seeing that the bone surfaces of the osteotomy space are in absolute contact with each other.
- The osteotomy must be performed under neuromonitoring.

Key Points

- Ponte osteotomy aims to close the posterior column.
- It can create compliance with cervical sagittal parameters.
- Before surgery, assessment of the flexibility of the deformity is necessary.
- Ponte osteotomy is a safe technique for flexible cervical kyphosis.
- Approximately 5 to 7 degrees corrections are provided for each segment.
- To reduce epidural venous bleeding, the osteotomy site should be closed as quickly as possible.

References

1. Ames CP, Smith JS, Scheer JK, et al. A standardized nomenclature for cervical spine soft-tissue release and osteotomy for deformity correction: clinical article. J Neurosurg Spine 2013;19(3):269–278
2. Etame AB, Than KD, Wang AC, La Marca F, Park P. Surgical management of symptomatic cervical or cervicothoracic kyphosis due to ankylosing spondylitis. Spine 2008;33(16):E559–E564
3. Smith JS, Shaffrey CI, Lafage V, et al; International Spine Study Group. Spontaneous improvement of cervical alignment after correction of global sagittal balance following pedicle subtraction osteotomy. J Neurosurg Spine 2012;17(4):300–307
4. Passias PG, Passfall L, Horn SR, et al; International Spine Study Group. Risk-benefit assessment of major versus minor osteotomies for flexible and rigid cervical deformity correction. J Craniovertebr Junction Spine 2021;12(3):263–268
5. Ponte A, Orlando G, Siccardi GL. The true Ponte osteotomy: by the one who developed it. Spine Deform 2018;6(1):2–11
6. Ames CP, Smith JS, Eastlack R, et al; International Spine Study Group. Reliability assessment of a novel cervical spine deformity classification system. J Neurosurg Spine 2015;23(6):673–683
7. Hong JT, Koller H, Abumi K, et al. A new nomenclature system for the surgical treatment of cervical spine deformity, developing, and validation of SOF system. Eur Spine J 2021;30(6):1670–1680
8. Funayama T, Abe T, Noguchi H, et al. Severe, rigid cervical kyphotic deformity associated with SAPHO syndrome successfully treated with three-stage correction surgery combined with C7 vertebral column resection: a technical case report. Spine Deform 2021;9(1):285–292
9. Koller H. Cervical spine profile issues—cervical kyphosis. The XVIII CSRS-ES Cadaveric Instructional Course. Barcelona, Spain March 31–April 1, 2016

4 Pedicle Subtraction Osteotomy for Cervical Spine

Serkan Şimşek and Kazım Yiğitkanlı

Introduction

Rigid cervicothoracic kyphosis cause pain, cervical radiculopathy, and swallowing difficulty, limiting horizontal gaze and upright posture.[1] Surgical correction with cervical pedicle subtraction osteotomy (PSO) with posterior screw fixation is often required for extreme cases. This surgical procedure involves resectioning the posterior column; then, with a transpedicular wedge osteotomy, the posterior and middle columns are shortened.[2] Corrective osteotomy of the cervical spine is one of the most challenging procedures because of catastrophic complications such as irreversible spinal cord injury and possible brain damage from vertebral artery injury. The complication rates in previous papers are between 26.9 and 87.5%; the permanent neurological complication rate is 4.3%, and the mortality rate is 2.6%.[3]

Mason et al[4] first described the cervical PSO; then Urist[5] and Law[6] applied this technique. The osteotomy was done by removing the posterior elements at the T1 level in a wedge shape to obtain extension of the neck.[4] The osteotomy used by Urist,[5] and Law,[6] was similar to the Smith-Petersen osteotomy, which includes removal of the posterior elements at the level requiring correction (spinous process and lamina). Simmons described controlled fracture (osteoclasis) at the C7 level in patients with ankylosing spondylitis.[7] Simmons et al performed a C7 laminectomy and C6–C7 and C7–T1 wide facetectomies to decompress C7–C8 nerve roots bilaterally. Under halo-traction with local anesthesia, manually extending the cervical spinal cord resulted in osteoclastic fractures through the anterior column of the spine.[7] Halo immobilization was kept until fusion occurred, and the procedure had a 4% mortality rate.[7] The Smith-Petersen osteotomy has been the standard to restore sagittal balance and horizontal gaze at the cervicothoracic junction. In ankylosing spondylitis cases, controlled fractures are better suited to accomplish the goal than in patients with normal bone.[8]

Mehdian et al[9] recognized the need for a controlled extension after the osteotomy to limit the possibility of sagittal translation of the posterior segments into the spinal canal. A temporary fixation rod would prevent sudden translation of the vertebral bodies during the correction maneuver. The translational rod also helps the contralateral titanium rod to be placed, locked at the degree of extension.

Here we discuss technical modifications of this procedure, permitting maximum safe resection of cervical bone and performing extension osteotomy with extension maneuvers.

Etiology

Postlaminectomy kyphosis is the most common cause of iatrogenic kyphosis, followed by ankylosing spondylitis. Trauma, infection, neoplasm, and congenital anomalies also cause rigid cervical kyphosis.[10]

Postlaminectomy kyphosis develops with disruption of the posterior tension band, increasing compressive force on the anterior spinal elements and resulting in the shifted head with the increased anterior axial load leading to further kyphosis. The incidence of postoperative kyphosis after multiple-level laminectomy is 21% in grown-ups[11] and 37 to 100% in children.[11–14]

Ankylosing spondylitis is a seronegative spondylo-arthropathy associated with the major histocompatibility complex antigen HLA-B27.[15] The typical deformity is a forward shift of the head due to a combination of thoracic hyperkyphosis and loss of lumbar lordosis, resulting in fixed sagittal imbalance. The cervical spine typically shows cervical and cervicothoracic junction kyphosis, leading to difficulty in horizontal gaze, swallowing, and lying flat, with limited activities of daily life. The spine in ankylosing spondylitis loses its flexibility, and it acts like a long bone, becoming susceptible to significant injury even with minor forces.[16,17] These patients also tend to have osteoporosis due to stress shielding with ankylosing spondylitis.[18] Even minor trauma may result in the development of an acute cervical kyphotic deformity and neurological deficit.

Surgical Technique

Correction of kyphotic deformity with spinal stabilization and decompression of the neural elements are the goals of the surgery.

Surgical Planning

Factors affecting the surgical plan are:

- Symptoms.
- Neurological examination, degree of neural compression.
- Etiology.
- Deformity characteristics like location and flexibility, presence of ankylosis, and fusion levels.
- Proximal and distal degenerative changes.
- Medical comorbidities.
- Surgical anatomy of the vertebral artery.
- Bone quality.

The amount of correction should be considered by using the radiographic parameters. T1 slope (T1S) minus C2–C7 lordosis <15 degrees, C2–C7 sagittal vertical axes (SVA) <40 mm, and chin-brow vertical angle (CBVA) between –10 degrees and +20 degrees are generally acceptable ranges.[19–22]

The most important goal is to know how much correction may be acquired. On average, single-level PSO yields 35 degrees of lordosis correction.

Preoperative Evaluation

All patients planned for a cervical PSO require a detailed medical evaluation before surgery, including diabetes, smoking, and previous spinal infection. In addition, surgeons should analyze baseline functional levels of the respiratory and gastrointestinal systems.

Plain radiographs, flexion–extension, and lateral bending views are valuable to assess the rigidity of the deformity, and evaluate both sagittal and coronal plane deformities. Preoperative computed tomography (CT) scans and magnetic resonance imaging (MRI) scans are also necessary. When planning deformity correction, it is critical to maintain and restore the patients' ability to see the front of their body. Modification at a slightly flexed position, usually up to 20 degrees, is required when the patient has complete ankylosis of the cervical spine. A slightly flexed position is less critical when the patient has preserved motion from the occiput to C2. Aligning the posterior vertebral line of C2 as close to the anterior vertebral line of C7 is fundamental to achieving a balanced cervical posture.

Surgery

Awake nasotracheal intubation may be a safer way to anesthetize the patients. Document somatosensory-evoked potentials (SSEP) and motor-evoked potentials (MEP) as a baseline before positioning. Once the patient is intubated,

sterile Gardner-Wells tongs are carefully arranged and placed.

The patient is then placed in the prone position on the operating room table with gel rolls on the sides. Arms are kept on both sides. In the beginning, the head of the bed is flexed, and the bed is positioned in approximately 30 degrees of reverse Trendelenburg to decrease bleeding (**Fig. 4.1**). Following positioning, SSEP/MEPs are recorded furthermore. Next, the traction force is applied to the Gardner-Wells tongs with a sterile rope with controlled SSEP/MEP.[23]

Standard posterior midline cervicothoracic exposure is accomplished. The rear cervical facet joints are exposed. Using intraoperative pedicle visualization and palpation, particularly the medial boundaries of the pedicles, helps in safer screw fixation of upper thoracic pedicles. Biplanar fluoroscopy may be utilized to ascertain the optimal position of the screws. Bilateral C2 pedicle and C3 to C6 lateral mass screws are placed. Bilateral T1-2-3 pedicle screws are also inserted (**Fig. 4.2**). A unilateral temporary fixation rod is inserted into one side before the osteotomy is started. This prevents sudden translation of the vertebral bodies and decreases the stretching force on the spinal cord and nerve roots (**Fig. 4.3**).

A C7 laminectomy is accomplished with a high-speed, diamond-tipped burr or rongeur. The inferior third of the C6 laminae and the superior third of the T1 laminae are removed with Kerrison rongeur. Wide laminectomy prevents compression of the dura and C7/C8 nerve roots while closing the osteotomy sites (**Fig. 4.3**).

Preparation of the pedicles and exposure of the exiting nerve roots are crucial, laminoforaminotomies are performed through the exiting C7–C8 nerve roots bilaterally. The pedicles of C6, C7, and T1 are palpated with a dissector while performing the laminoforaminotomies. An internal

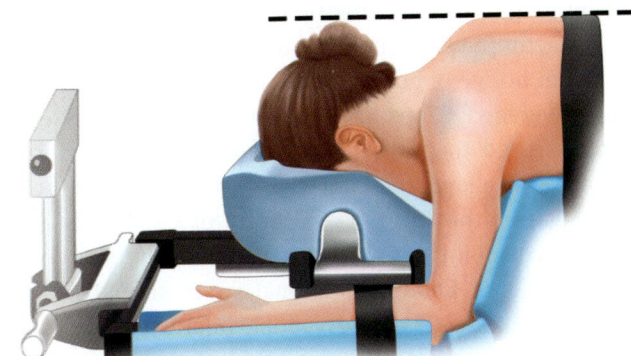

Fig. 4.1 Prone position of the patient in preparation of the surgical field. The entire head is included in the sterile field. Sterile rope may be placed and connected to traction through Gardner-Wells tongs.

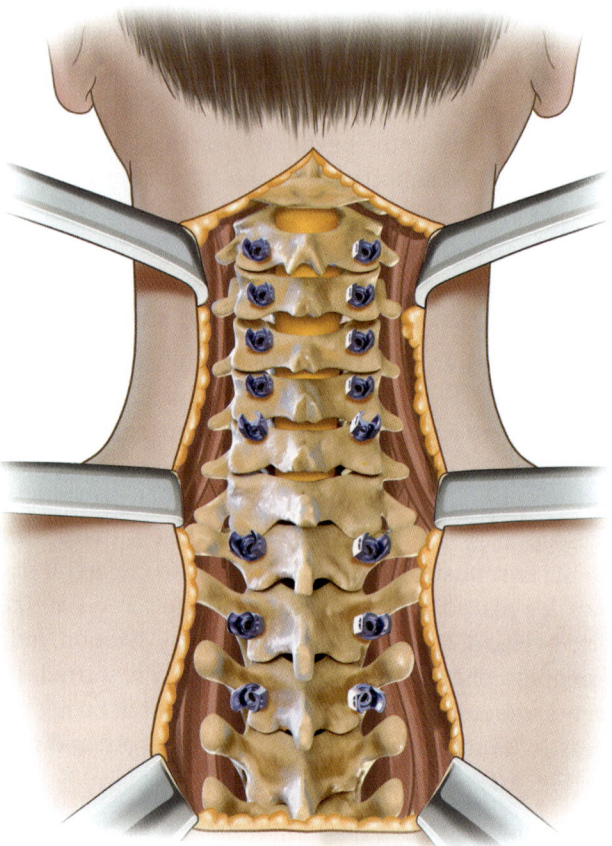

Fig. 4.2 A posterior cervical incision is performed through C2 to T4. The heads of the C2 pedicle, C3, C4, C5, and C6 lateral mass, and T1, T2, and T3 pedicle screws are depicted.

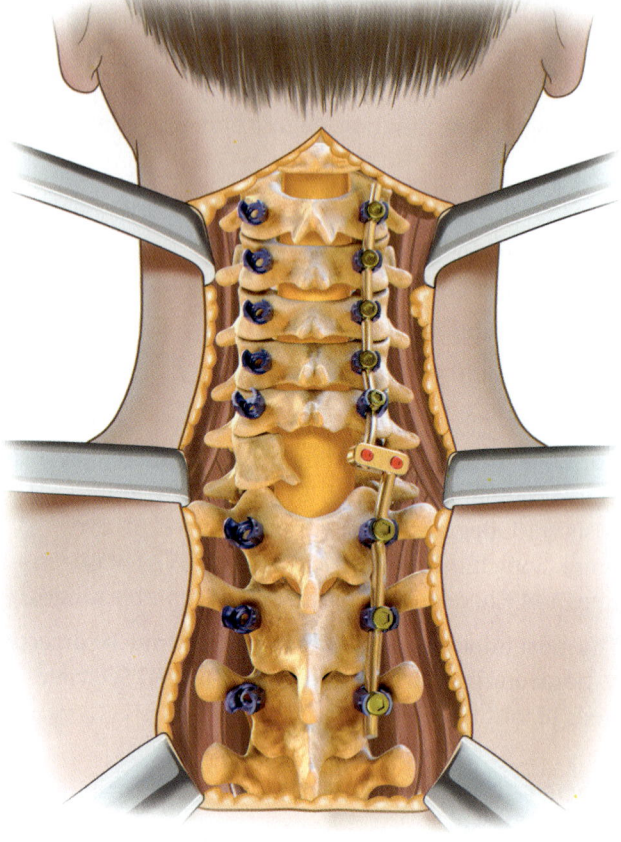

Fig. 4.3 Illustrative image of the wide laminectomy and unilateral facetectomy at C7 level. Before contralateral facetectomy and osteotomy, unilateral temporary cervicothoracic rods (cervical rod 3 mm and thoracic rod 6 mm diameter) with an off-set connector are placed.

pediculectomy of the C7 pedicle is accomplished so that the exiting C7 and C8 nerve roots are inspected entirely. A high-speed burr may also be employed during this phase. A probe is passed from the hollow pedicles bilaterally into the C7 body. At this level, the ventral C7 body and the attached posterior longitudinal ligament remain completely intact. A dural retractor may be employed to protect the spinal cord. Once a thin bridge of bone remains between the hollowed-out and widened C7 pedicles, a curved micro curette or elevator is used to push the posterior cortex in a dorsal direction. This allows the cancellous bone to be indirectly packed against the front of the body of C7, forming an anterior pivot point onto which the osteotomy site could close posteriorly. Enough foraminal space should be left available for exiting C7–C8 nerve roots bilaterally (**Fig. 4.4**).

Four-rod technique with extension correction maneuvers is utilized during the closure of the osteotomy.

After completing a bilateral pediculectomy, the cervicothoracic rod with an off-set connector is contoured in place and fixed loosely to the other side of the temporary

fixation rod (**Fig. 4.5**). The operator holds the Gardner-Well tongs with one hand, and the other assistant releases the traction force of the sterile rope. Intraoperative manual extension reduction is performed. During this phase, monitoring impingement of the spinal dura and nerve root is of the utmost importance. This method may be repeated multiple times to obtain the desired correction angle. During manual extension, the operator may not continuously monitor the surgical field, so observing the surgical area by the other assistant is vital.[23] Close visual observation of the osteotomy gap is done, with the support of the caudal part of the osteotomy with the surgeon's other hand. A controlled and gentle reduction is performed; the surgeon extends the head so that the patient's eyes are perpendicular to the floor. Surgeons should take care not to hyperextend the head (**Fig. 4.6**).

Osteotomy closure, cervical spinal cord, and C7/C8 nerve roots should be monitored continuously. Finally, rods are contoured and locked (**Fig. 4.7**). The osteotomy site and exiting nerve roots are reinspected. Local laminectomy

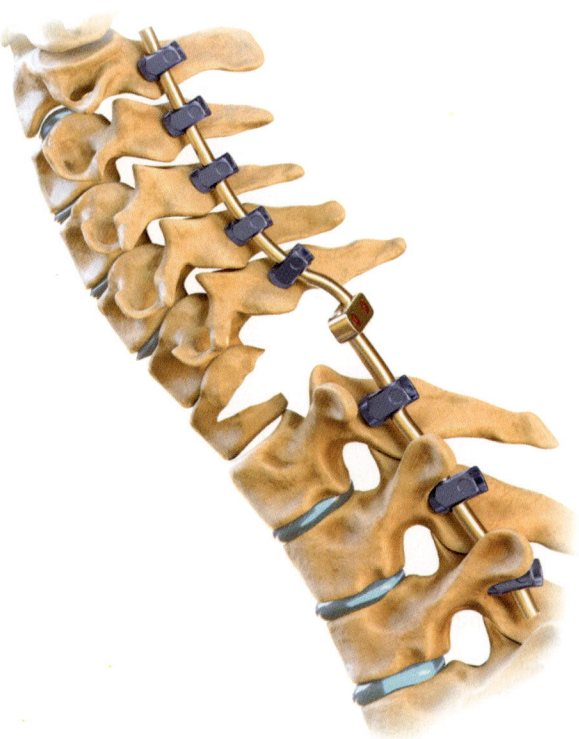

Fig. 4.4 Illustrative sagittal image of C7 pedicle subtraction osteotomy.

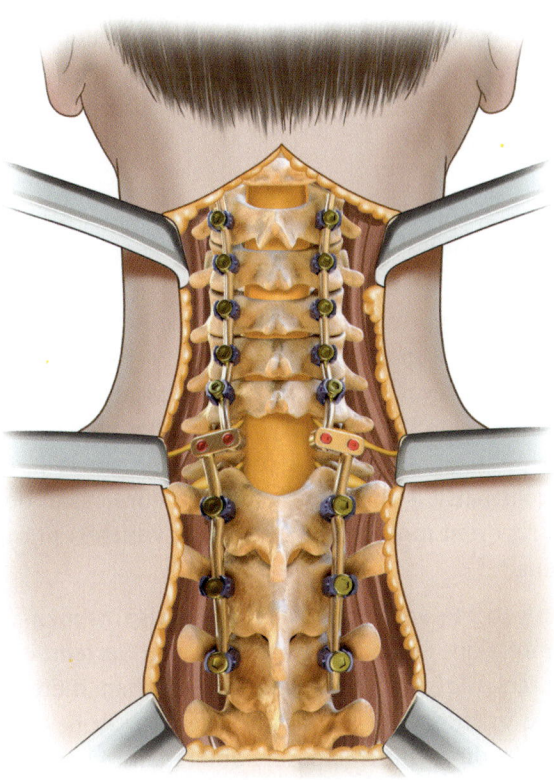

Fig. 4.5 After completing bilateral pediculectomy, double cervicothoracic rods with two off-set connectors are contoured in place and fixed loosely. Note bilateral C7 and C8 nerve roots, and C7 and T1 pedicles.

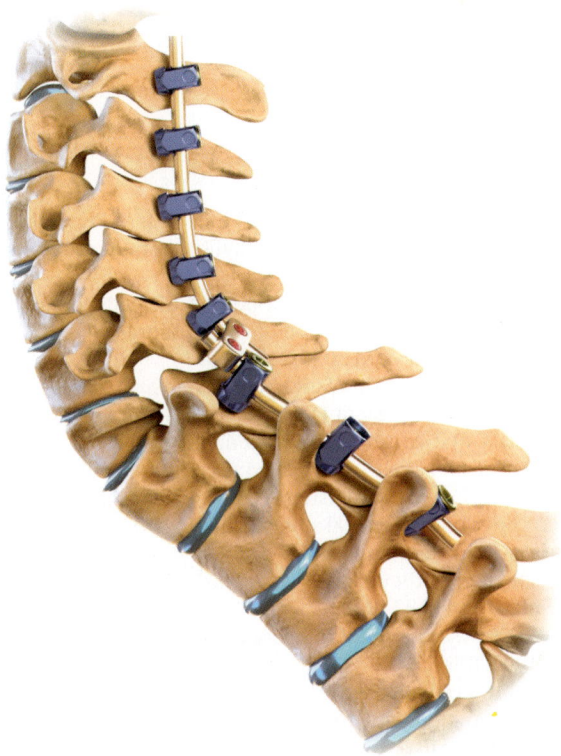

Fig. 4.6 Sagittal illustrative view after the closure of the osteotomy site with extension maneuver.

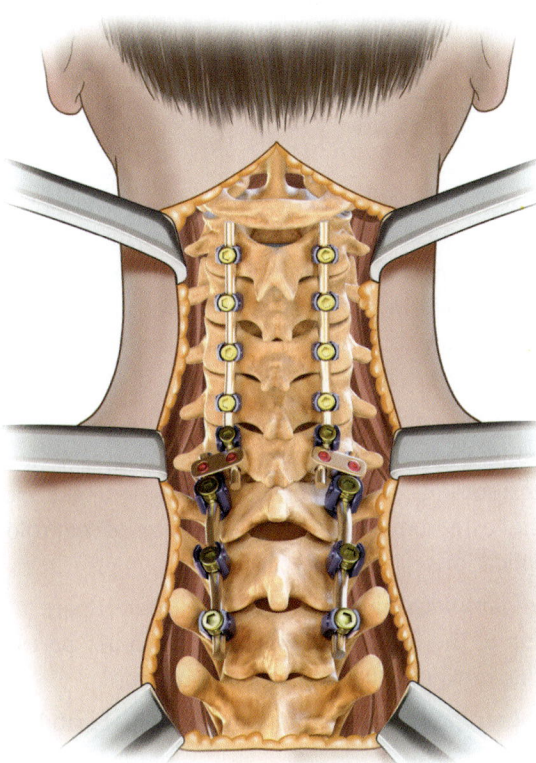

Fig. 4.7 Posterior illustrative view after the closure of the osteotomy site with extension maneuver.

autografts are packed into the osteotomy site, a subfascial drain is placed, and the layers are closed. Postoperatively, once the airway is suitable for extubation, the patient is waked up, and extubated. A rigid collar is placed for comfort for up to 6 weeks.

Complications

Smith et al reported 9.2% mortality following surgery.[24] Other studies reported 2.3% mortality rate, and 3.3% significant medical and 13.5% neurological complication rates.[25] The neurological injury rate is approximately 23%, and the permanent neurologic complication rate is 4.3%.[3] C8 nerve root palsy is the most common neurological deficit, with a reported incidence of 19 to 38%, which is primarily transient.[26,27]

Injury to the vertebral artery could also happen when decompression extends laterally to the vertebral body and enters the transverse foramen or when there is an anomaly in the path. Hemostatic agents may be used to control bleeding. Direct exposure and repair may be tried if possible or interventional radiology can stent or embolize the vertebral artery.

Treatment of severe kyphoscoliosis with osteotomies is associated with significant blood loss. Therefore, preoperative and intraoperative blood loss monitoring is mandatory.

Tips and Tricks

- Profuse bleeding from the epidural space can occur during removal of the ligamentum flavum. Do not start a flavectomy before completing all necessary bone removal. Gelatin sponges help hemostasis (Carefully packing does not cause spinal cord compression). Maintaining a hemoglobin level > 10 g/dl is essential.

- Strict adherence to the osteotomy technique, using intraoperative neuromonitoring and a closed look to the osteotomy site, especially throughout the closure of the osteotomy, decreases the rate of neurological complications.

- Wide laminectomy, including the lower part of the lamina of the upper vertebra and the upper part of the lamina, prevents buckling of the spinal cord.

- Temporary rod helps to maintain the spinal stability.

Conclusion

Kyphotic cervical deformity is rare and troublesome, requiring significant spinal surgical reconstructive techniques to restore sagittal deformity. However, cervical PSO can provide excellent sagittal correction in extreme deformity cases.

Key Points

- Controlled reduction of deformity is a critical step for successful reduction of the deformity.

- Maximal amount of bone removal at the osteotomy site increases the safety.

- Head extension reduction maneuver is an effective method to provide reduction after corrective osteotomies of the cervical spine.

- The status of the dura should be reviewed and the exiting C7/C8 nerve roots should be evaluated carefully after fixation of the rods.

Acknowledgment

The authors thank Arda Yigitkanli, Georgia Tech Biomedical Engineering Student, US, for kindly editing the manuscript's grammar.

References

1. Kubiak EN, Moskovich R, Errico TJ, Di Cesare PE. Orthopaedic management of ankylosing spondylitis. J Am Acad Orthop Surg 2005;13(4):267–278

2. Meng Y, Ma J, Shu L, et al. Modified C7 pedicle subtraction osteotomy for the correction of cervicothoracic kyphosis. BMC Musculoskelet Disord 2020;21(1):28

3. Etame AB, Than KD, Wang AC, La Marca F, Park P. Surgical management of symptomatic cervical or cervicothoracic kyphosis due to ankylosing spondylitis. Spine 2008;33(16): E559–E564

4. Mason C, Cozen L, Adelstein L. Surgical correction of flexion deformity of the cervical spine. Calif Med 1953;79(3):244–246

5. Urist MR. Osteotomy of the cervical spine; report of a case of ankylosing rheumatoid spondylitis. J Bone Joint Surg Am 1958;40-A(4):833–843

6. Law WA. Osteotomy of the cervical spine. J Bone Joint Surg Br 1959;41-B:640–641

7. Simmons EH. The surgical correction of flexion deformity of the cervical spine in ankylosing spondylitis. Clin Orthop Relat Res 1972;86(86):132–143

8. Deviren V, Scheer JK, Ames CP. Technique of cervicothoracic junction pedicle subtraction osteotomy for cervical sagittal imbalance: report of 11 cases. J Neurosurg Spine 2011; 15(2):174–181

9. Mehdian SM, Freeman BJ, Licina P. Cervical osteotomy for ankylosing spondylitis: an innovative variation on an existing technique. Eur Spine J 1999;8(6):505–509

10. Ogura Y, Dimar JR, Djurasovic M, Carreon LY. Etiology and treatment of cervical kyphosis: state of the art review-a narrative review. J Spine Surg 2021;7(3):422–433

11. Kaptain GJ, Simmons NE, Replogle RE, Pobereskin L. Incidence and outcome of kyphotic deformity following laminectomy for cervical spondylotic myelopathy. J Neurosurg 2000;93(2, Suppl):199–204

12. Bell DF, Walker JL, O'Connor G, Tibshirani R. Spinal deformity after multiple-level cervical laminectomy in children. Spine 1994;19(4):406–411

13. Cattell HS, Clark GL Jr. Cervical kyphosis and instability following multiple laminectomies in children. J Bone Joint Surg Am 1967;49(4):713–720

14. Yasuoka S, Peterson HA, Laws ER Jr, MacCarty CS. Pathogenesis and prophylaxis of postlaminectomy deformity of the spine after multiple level laminectomy: difference between children and adults. Neurosurgery 1981;9(2):145–152

15. Wells LJ, Edwards JH, Webley M, et al. Ankylosing spondylitis, HLA, and BF. Lancet 1979;1(8107):104–105

16. Detwiler KN, Loftus CM, Godersky JC, Menezes AH. Management of cervical spine injuries in patients with ankylosing spondylitis. J Neurosurg 1990;72(2):210–215

17. Kanter AS, Wang MY, Mummaneni PV. A treatment algorithm for the management of cervical spine fractures and deformity in patients with ankylosing spondylitis. Neurosurg Focus 2008;24(1):E11

18. Bronson WD, Walker SE, Hillman LS, Keisler D, Hoyt T, Allen SH. Bone mineral density and biochemical markers of bone metabolism in ankylosing spondylitis. J Rheumatol 1998;25(5):929–935

19. Iyer S, Lenke LG, Nemani VM, et al. Variations in occipitocervical and cervicothoracic alignment parameters based on age: a prospective study of asymptomatic volunteers using full-body radiographs. Spine 2016;41(23):1837–1844

20. Suk KS, Kim KT, Lee SH, Kim JM. Significance of chin-brow vertical angle in correction of kyphotic deformity of ankylosing spondylitis patients. Spine 2003;28(17):2001–2005

21. Song K, Su X, Zhang Y, et al. Optimal chin-brow vertical angle for sagittal visual fields in ankylosing spondylitis kyphosis. Eur Spine J 2016;25(8):2596–2604

22. Ames CP, Smith JS, Eastlack R, et al; International Spine Study Group. Reliability assessment of a novel cervical spine deformity classification system. J Neurosurg Spine 2015;23(6):673–683

23. Lee SH, Kim KT, Suk KS, Kim MH, Park DH, Kim KJ. A sterile-freehand reduction technique for corrective osteotomy of fixed cervical kyphosis. Spine 2012;37(26):2145–2150

24. Smith JS, Shaffrey CI, Kim HJ, et al; International Spine Study Group. Prospective multicenter assessment of all-cause mortality following surgery for adult cervical deformity. Neurosurgery 2018;83(6):1277–1285

25. Etame AB, Wang AC, Than KD, La Marca F, Park P. Outcomes after surgery for cervical spine deformity: review of the literature. Neurosurg Focus 2010;28(3):E14

26. Tokala DP, Lam KS, Freeman BJ, Webb JK. C7 decancellisation closing wedge osteotomy for the correction of fixed cervico-thoracic kyphosis. Eur Spine J 2007;16(9):1471–1478

27. Langeloo DD, Journee HL, Pavlov PW, de Kleuver M. Cervical osteotomy in ankylosing spondylitis: evaluation of new developments. Eur Spine J 2006;15(4):493–500

5 Anterior Cervical Osteotomy

Gökhan Gökçe and Onur Yaman

Introduction

Cervical spine deformities can be rigid or flexible. These deformities cause severe neck pain, decrease in quality of life, and disability. Surgical correction of cervical deformities can be done anteriorly or posteriorly. As a result of these surgical corrections, horizontal gaze, chest–jaw, and shoulder–ear deformities have improved in most patients, while clinically significant improvements have been made in neck pain and quality of life. Most patients have high satisfaction rates.

Flexible cervical spine deformities can often be corrected with multiple-level anterior cervical diskectomy and fusion (ACDF), total or partial corpectomies, and posterior instrumentation, while rigid cervical deformities require osteotomy (anterior or posterior).[1] ACDFs have limited correction rates. They provide approximately 6 degrees of correction per level when multiple levels are corrected.[2] With the combined effect, an effective correction rate can be achieved. Total or partial corpectomy can provide sagittal correction by opening the spinal canal when there is anterior compression behind the vertebral body. Considering the morbidity of multiple level corpectomies, hybrid surgeries, namely, diskectomy–corpectomy, may be preferred.

Rigid cervical deformities should be evaluated separately. They often require anterior cervical osteotomy. Anterior cervical osteotomy with bilateral complete uncinectomy is effective in correcting rigid kyphosis and is particularly beneficial in the midcervical spine. However, most of the time, combined intervention, that is, anterior–posterior surgery, is required for the correction of these rigid deformities.[3–5]

Objectives of cervical deformity surgery include instrumentation–arthrodesis for a sound stabilization to provide neural decompression, correction of deformity, horizontal parallel view, and surgical correction.

When the literature is examined, posterior surgeries have been shown to be preferred in the correction of cervical deformities. These surgeries are wedge opening osteotomies, such as pedicle subtraction osteotomy (PSO) and Ponte osteotomy. However, these surgeries have some limitations; for example, PSO is usually limited to the lower cervical region (C7–T1). Again, during the closure of these osteotomies, the cervical nerve roots may be damaged, and the vertebral artery may be injured.[2] In comparison, wound infections, postoperative neurological deficits, proximal junction kyphosis (PJK), and additional cardiorespiratory complications may be more common in posterior cervical surgeries.[6]

These complication rates can be as high as 56%. In order to avoid these complications and difficulties, anterior cervical osteotomies have become popular in the last decades. With this surgical technique, both sagittal and coronal deformities can be effectively corrected.[2]

Patients scheduled for anterior cervical osteotomy should be carefully selected preoperatively. Careful preoperative preparation and evaluation process are necessary.[4] Surgical tricks should be done step by step, and the surgeon must be able to foresee possible risks at all stages. Bilateral complete unsinectomy performed after cervical diskectomy in anterior cervical osteotomy should extend to the transverse foramen. And at these stages, the vertebral arteries in close proximity should be carefully protected. An osteotomy performed in this way can effectively and powerfully correct the deformity in two planes.[3]

Cervical spine deformities have only received the necessary attention in the last decades compared to other parts of the spine. The development of knowledge in the literature in this field and the introduction of new surgical techniques (such as anterior Riew osteotomy) have resulted in new advances in this field.[3] A holistic view of the cervical spine, new measurements, classifications, and algorithms have given a new impetus to cervical deformity surgery. A defect in another part of the spine, such as a pathology in the thoracic region, can cause a dynamic result in cervical deformity, so imaging of the entire spine is often necessary.

In the literature review, Ames et al have described seven different types of posterior osteotomies ranging from partial facet resection to vertebral column resection (VCR).[8] Again, Tan et al defined algorithms for anterior and posterior surgical techniques for planning surgical interventions used in the correction of cervical deformities.[7] Thanks to these algorithms, it has become easier to decide on the type of surgical intervention. However, like all algorithms, they have limitations.[8,9]

Anterior cervical surgery is a more well-known technique with relatively fewer complications. This has allowed the development of anterior osteotomy techniques for the correction of cervical deformities.[10] For example, anterior Riew osteotomy is a powerful correction technique that can be applied to the entire cervical spine. This osteotomy includes an effective sagittal and coronal correction by cleaning the anterior cervical disc distance and extending to the bilateral uncovertebral joint border and applying a force from above to the forehead.

Indications

Indications include rigid cervical deformities with no motion on flexion and extension radiographs, the presence of anterior cervical osteophytes, decreased C2–C7 lordosis angle and marked kyphotic angulation, and increased C2–C7 sagittal vertical axis (SVA). Ear–shoulder and jaw–chest deformities in which the horizontal gaze is impaired are the most appropriate indications for anterior cervical osteotomy.

Preoperative Planning

Patients who are planned for anterior cervical osteotomy should be examined in detail preoperatively. It is important to evaluate whether the deformity is rigid or flexible. Efforts of cervical anterior or posterior fusion should be looked for (anterior osteophyte bridges, posterior fusion patterns). Detailed patient history should be taken; detailed clinical examination and full radiological examination should be performed. All cervical X-rays (anteroposterior [AP]/lateral, dynamic flexion/extension X-ray, scoliosis film, computed tomography [CT] and magnetic resonance imaging [MRI]) should be done. Scoliosis X-ray is important especially for the evaluation of thoracic and even lumbar pathologies that may affect the cervical deformity. The apex of the cervical deformity, the foraminal stenosis areas, the neighborhood of the vertebral artery, and the relationship of the bone structure should be determined. Cervical balance measurements (cervical C2–C7 SVA, cervical lordosis angle, T1 slope, chin–eyebrow vertical angle) should be performed on direct radiographs.

Preoperative CT is performed to evaluate the condition of the facets, the condition of the foramen, posterior and anterior fusion masses, and disc distances. MRI is performed to evaluate spinal cord compression, myelopathic hypersignal, and nerve root compressions.

Clinical and imaging studies may be incompatible in some cases. In these cases, additional etiological investigations are necessary. For example, additional electromyography (EMG) for nerve entrapment syndromes, additional somatosensory evoked potentials (SEP), motor evoked potentials (MEP), or different imaging studies may be needed for possible amyotrophic lateral sclerosis (ALS) disease.

Prior cervical surgery requires careful consideration in some conditions. For example, the condition of vocal cords after previous surgery should be documented by ENT consultation. If vocal cord dysfunction has occurred in previous surgery, ipsilateral surgery should be planned to prevent bilateral injury. Considering the long course of the recurrent laryngeal nerve, the left-sided approach should be preferred in patients with normal vocal cord function. The anatomy of the deformity is also important in the surgical approach. In patients with significant coronal deformity, the convex side approach is preferred.

The course and localization of the vertebral artery are critical for patients scheduled for anterior cervical osteotomy. Preoperative CT and CT angiography can provide information about the course and condition of the vertebral artery.

Preoperative comorbid pathologies (diabetes mellitus [DM], advanced age, osteoporosis, short neck, obesity, immunodeficiency, etc.) should be considered in the preoperative planning.

Surgical Technique

Awake fiber-optic intubation of the patient who is scheduled for anterior cervical osteotomy is important for safe surgical initiation. The surgeon and anesthesia team should take this into account, especially in patients with severe spinal cord compression and instability. Excessive neck extension should be prevented and the risks that may occur in the first positioning should be minimized. Patients with rigid cervical deformity are at high risk of neurological loss during correction. Therefore, these operations must be performed under neuromonitoring. Spinal cord perfusion is critical throughout the surgical phase, so mean arterial pressure (MAP) should be maintained at around 80 mmHg.[2,3] In the surgical positioning of the neck, support pads should be placed under the neck, and support pads should be carefully placed under the chest so that the neck remains in the air.[2,3]

The Gardner-Wells device should be placed at a traction force of 15 lb for comfortable manipulation of the head and neck. With the help of this device, the desired coronal and rotational alignment can be achieved. When the osteotomy is completed with the correct positioning, the anesthetist removes these pillows one by one under the neck in a controlled manner, and the surgeon presses them on the forehead and provides adequate reduction of the kyphosis.[3] This maneuver will cause osteoclasis of the posterior fusion mass and the head will lean toward the operating table after the deformity is corrected. The higher the correction desired here, the higher the head should be from the table. The surgeon's full dominance of the surgical field is important at this stage.[2]

At the beginning of the operation, after the final positioning is completed, the neck is prepared and covered in a sterile way. An operating microscope is used throughout the surgery. Using the Smith-Robinson approach, which is the standard for anterior surgery, anatomical folds are crossed with blunt and sharp dissections, and the anterior cervical line and kyphosis apex are exposed. Fluoroscopy is used for level verification. The apex of the kyphosis must be exposed, which can sometimes be difficult, unlike a degenerative spine.[2,3,11]

After the anterior cervical fascia is done with blunt scraping, the longus colli is stripped with the help of bipolar cautery, leaving a cuff where retractors can be easily inserted. In the meantime, maximum care should be taken to protect the sympathetic chain that runs close to the longus colli. Cutting the longus colli muscles is often required because of their contribution to neck flexion.

It is beneficial to use fixed retractors placed under the table-mounted longus colli. Anterior cervical osteophytes are removed with the help of a lexel ronguer and cervical diskectomy is completed up to the posterior longitudinal ligament with the help of a disc ronguer.

The disc space is thoroughly cleaned (**Fig. 5.1**). Correct placement of the Caspar retractor and pins is an important step in anterior cervical osteotomy (**Fig. 5.2**). The pins of the Caspar retractor should be placed perpendicular to the

vertebral body, but sometimes in an osteoporotic spine, due to insufficient bone strength, a double set of pins should be preferred instead of a single set of pins.[3]

Upright positioning of the pins may cause different pegging, but the distraction maneuver to these pins will help to give the appropriate cervical lordosis after the osteotomy is completed.[2,3]

In anterior cervical osteotomy, 2.5-mm burr tip of high-speed drill is used when working deep. To achieve symmetrical resection in the coronal plane, the bone resection should be perpendicular to the spine in the same plane as the disc space (**Fig. 5.2**). In patients with mixed coronal and kyphotic deformities, bone resection may be asymmetrical to restore alignment in the coronal and sagittal planes. Although an osteotomy in the same plane with the disc distance is required to achieve a symmetrical resection in the coronal plane, this osteotomy can be performed asymmetrically in patients with mixed type coronal and sagittal plane deformities.

The osteotomy should extend across the disc space lateral to the uncovertebral joint and beyond the posterior longitudinal ligament (PLL). At this stage, attention should be paid to the localization and possible injury of the vertebral artery. At the lateral margin, the osteotomy should extend to the uncinate processes. Curettes and dissectors are used to thin the uncinate process (**Fig. 5.1b**).

It is beneficial to place a dissector lateral to the uncinate process to prevent vertebral artery injury. In this way, the lateral extent can be determined. In order to protect the vertebral body, the lateral edge of the uncinate is thinned

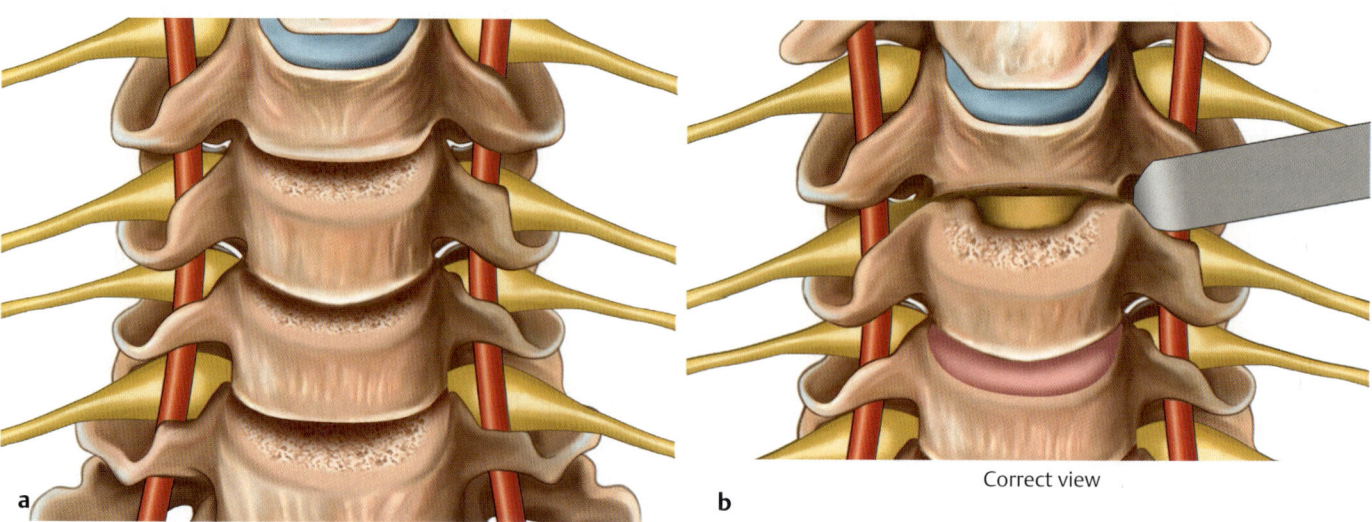

a   b   Correct view

Fig. 5.1 Anterior cervical osteotomy. Disc space is thoroughly cleaned (**a**). The vertebral artery is protected using a dissector during resection of the uncinates (**b**).

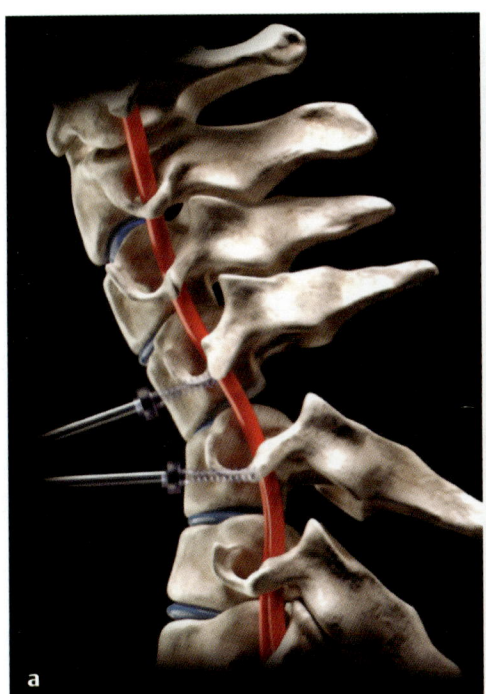
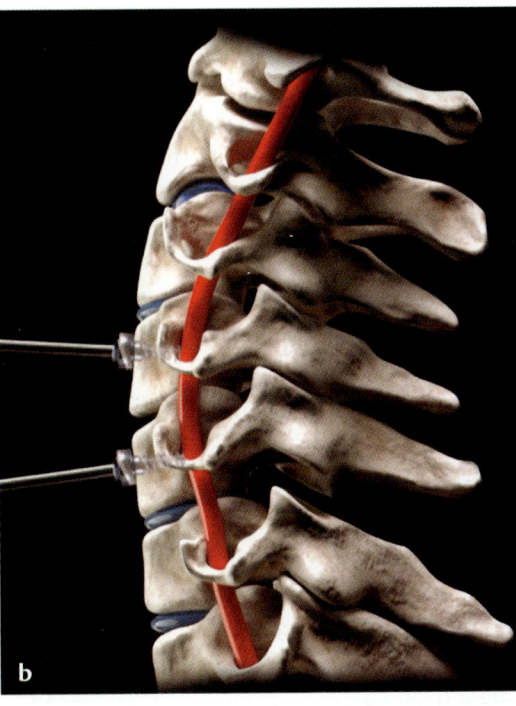

Fig. 5.2 Placement of Caspar pins for anterior osteotomy. The pins of the Caspar retractor should be placed perpendicular to the vertebral body. Kyphotic angulation before correction **(a)**, and after correction by providing a lordotic angulation **(b)**.

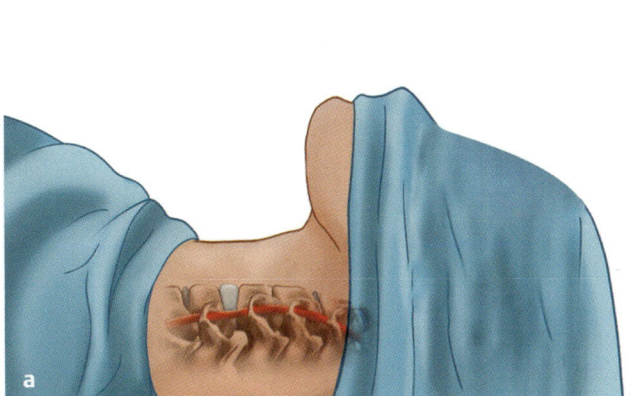
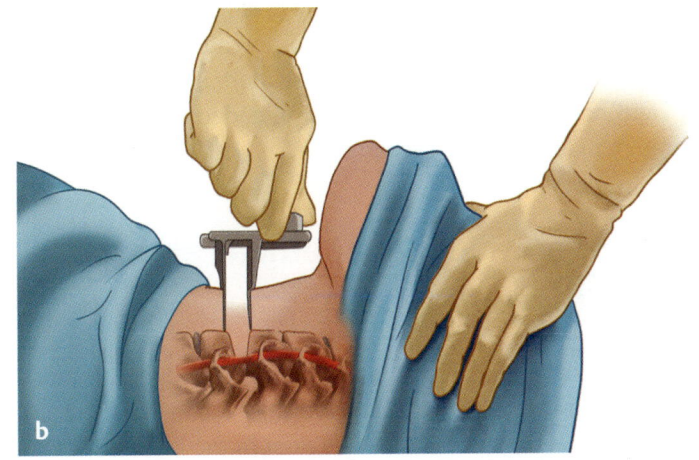

Fig. 5.3 Distraction pins are perpendicular to the anterior surface of the spine and distracted to maximize lordosis across the osteotomy site **(a)**. Correction of cervical deformity after completion of anterior osteotomy. Gentle downward force is applied to take advantage of the large moment provided by the long lever arm, while simultaneously distracting across the osteotomy using the Caspar pins **(b)**. (Modified from Safaee MM, Tan LA, Riew KD. Anterior osteotomy for rigid cervical deformity correction. J Spine Surg. 2020 Mar;6(1):210–216.)

and broken with the help of a curette and carefully removed (**Fig. 5.1b**).

Now that the nerve root tracing is at a detectable stage, the foraminotomy is completed with the aid of a curette to allow nerve root decompression and completion of the osteotomy.[2,3]

After making sure that the osteotomy extends beyond the bilateral neural foramen, the stage of correction of the deformity is started. The surgeon begins the correction of the deformity by pressing the forehead in a controlled manner,

while the anesthetist gradually removes the pillows under the patient's neck (**Fig. 5.3**). This powerful lever arm may pose a risk for vertebral body fracture, while distraction with Caspar pins slowly corrects the deformity (**Fig. 5.3b**). In addition to the Caspar pins, we use larger disc space sizers in sequence, starting at 5-mm high, an independent cervical cage. After each disc sizer is placed in the disc space, it is swung slightly in the head and caudal direction while pressing down on the forehead. The Caspar distractor is enlarged to continue the correction. By the time the back of the head reaches the operating table, the anterior portion of the kyphosis correction is usually complete[12] (**Fig. 5.2b**). If additional lordosis is needed during the scope control, the anesthesia team may place a folded pillow under the patient's shoulder, thereby pushing the head further back. Additional weight (up to 25 lb) can be added to the Gardner-Wells device at this point to maintain the desired correction. It is important that the bone graft to be placed in the distracted osteotomy area is of the right height; generally the highest bone graft should be used considering the possibility of graft collapse. After adequate correction is achieved, the anterior cervical plate is placed.[2–4,11,13]

However, if posterior oscillations are required to achieve the desired correction, we recommend using a trapezoidal bone graft that only contacts the anterior osteotomy site to obtain additional lordosis. In these cases, we usually use a self-contained cage secured with a single screw, but an interference screw or support plate can be used to prevent graft removal at the posterior stage.[14] After meticulous hemostasis is completed in the surgical field, the wound is meticulously closed without leaving a dead space. In order to not leave a hematoma behind, it is recommended to use penrose drains, which are less likely to clog, instead of high-suction drains. Generally, it is recommended to complete the posterior fixation in the same session, if not the use of a rigid neck collar or halo is recommended until the final surgery planned in the second stage.

Postoperative Management and Complications

If the retraction in the cervical region is less than 3 hours, the patient is extubated after the operation. However, if this period is long, the patient is taken to the intensive care unit in intubated condition for possible airway problems and followed up with hourly neurological examinations throughout the night.[3] In the absence of neurological deficit, blood pressure can be switched to normotension. The Penrose drain is held for 8 consecutive hours, usually on the 1st or 2nd postoperative day, until the dressing dries. A rigid collar is used if posterior fixation has been added or if there is concern about the strength of the soft bone.

Complications of anterior cervical osteotomy are similar to classical anterior surgery. Dysphagia, vocal cord paralysis, trecheal/esophagial injury, vertebral artery injury, spinal cord and nerve root injuries, cerebrospinal fluid (CSF) leak, wound infection, instrument failure, graft collapse, and pseudoarthrosis can be seen. Among these, dysphagia is often transient and responds to steroid therapy. Psodorarthrosis can be reduced with posterior fusion added to anterior surgery. Wound infections are relatively rare in those who have only anterior surgery, but their incidence increases in cases where posterior surgery is also added. The addition of vancomycin powder to the wound site and meticulous surgery can reduce the frequency of hemostasis and complete closure. The overall medical complication rate is between 3.1 and 44.4%. Neurological loss rate is approximately 13.5%; mortality rate varies between 3.1 and 6.7%.[3] In general, patient satisfaction rate is high after anterior cervical osteotomy and correction.

Anterior Riew osteotomy is a powerful technique to correct rigid cervical deformity. Patients with chest–jaw and shoulder–ear deformities can be treated safely and effectively. Some studies have shown that PSO combined with anterior cervical osteotomy provides equal or better corrections than isolated PSOs with equal working times and less intraoperative blood loss. So combined interventions may be associated with better outcomes. Correct patient selection, good preoperative planning, and technique contribute to the success of the operation. Anterior cervical osteotomy is a powerful but underused tool for deformity correction. Spinal surgeons should become more familiar with this technique because it can provide effective correction and eliminate the need for cervical PSO.[3,4,15]

Tips and Tricks

The most critical decision for anterior cervical osteotomy is to determine that the deformity is rigid. Flexible deformities can be corrected with conventional ACDF, partial/total corpectomies, wedge osteotomies, or posterior techniques. Anterior cervical osteotomy (Riew anterior cervical osteotomy) offers an important alternative for rigid cervical deformities. Important limitations of posterior techniques (PSO being limited to C7–T1, nerve root injury that may occur during correction closure, risks of injury to the vertebral artery, relative increase in neurological deficits, etc.) may make this technique more reliable and effective. This is a significant advantage for spinal surgeons who are more accustomed to anterior cervical surgery. In this respect, it is possible that it will be used more frequently and will become popular.

Key Points

- Correct patient selection and preoperative planning are important in anterior cervical osteotomy.

- The entire stage of surgery should be performed under neuromonitoring.

- The surgical positioning of the patient is important. Cervical support pillows are placed according to the deformity, and the anesthetist gradually removes the pillows from under the patient's neck during the correction of the deformity.

- It is a critical step to perform an unsinectomy by preserving the vertebral artery area with a dissector when the uncinate prominence is reached after complete and effective cleaning of the cervical disc space with disc punches.

- One of the trick points of anterior cervical osteotomy is that the surgeon pushes the forehead down by distracting the Caspar pins and gradually corrects the deformity.

References

1. Quadros DG, Guiroy A, Fontes RBV. Total subaxial reconstruction. J Spine Surg 2020;6(1):280–289

2. Tan LA, Riew KD. Anterior cervical osteotomy: operative technique. Eur Spine J 2018;27(Suppl 1):39–47

3. Safaee MM, Tan LA, Riew KD. Anterior osteotomy for rigid cervical deformity correction. J Spine Surg 2020;6(1):210–216

4. Tan LA, Riew KD, Traynelis VC. Cervical spine deformity—part 2: management algorithm and anterior techniques. Neurosurgery 2017;81(4):561–567

5. Zuckerman SL, Goldberg JL, Riew KD. Multilevel anterior cervical osteotomies with uncinatectomies to correct a fixed kyphotic deformity associated with ankylosing spondylitis: technical note and operative video. Neurosurg Focus 2021;51(4):E11

6. Tan LA, Riew KD, Traynelis VC. Cervical spine deformity—part 3: posterior techniques, clinical outcome, and complications. Neurosurgery 2017;81(6):893–898

7. Tan LA, Riew KD, Traynelis VC. Cervical spine deformity—part 1: biomechanics, radiographic parameters, and classification. Neurosurgery 2017;81(2):197–203

8. Ames CP, Smith JS, Eastlack R, et al; International Spine Study Group. Reliability assessment of a novel cervical spine deformity classification system. J Neurosurg Spine 2015;23(6):673–683

9. Safaee MM, Tan LA, Ames CP. Posterior osteotomy techniques for rigid cervical deformity correction. J Spine Surg 2020;6(1):274–279

10. Echt M, Mikhail C, Girdler SJ, Cho SK. Anterior reconstruction techniques for cervical spine deformity. Neurospine 2020;17(3):534–542

11. Kim HJ, Nemani VM, Daniel Riew K. Cervical osteotomies for neurological deformities. Eur Spine J 2015;24(Suppl 1): S16–S22

12. Protopsaltis TS, Stekas N, Smith JS, et al. Surgical outcomes in rigid versus flexible cervical deformities. J Neurosurg Spine 2021:1–9 (Epub ahead of print)

13. Kim HJ, Piyaskulkaew C, Riew KD. Comparison of Smith-Petersen osteotomy versus pedicle subtraction osteotomy versus anterior-posterior osteotomy types for the correction of cervical spine deformities. Spine 2015;40(3):143–146

14. Yoshihara H, Abumi K, Ito M, Kotani Y, Sudo H, Takahata M. Severe fixed cervical kyphosis treated with circumferential osteotomy and pedicle screw fixation using an anterior-posterior-anterior surgical sequence. World Neurosurg 2013; 80(5):654.e17–654.e21

15. Kim HJ, Piyaskulkaew C, Riew KD. Anterior cervical osteotomy for fixed cervical deformities. Spine 2014;39(21):1751–1757

6 Surgery for Cervical Spondylosis and Deformity

John J. Mangan, John Paul Wanner, Edward C. Benzel, and Jason W. Savage

Introduction

The cervical spine is a highly complex structure with unique articulations that ultimately function to support the head, maintain horizontal gaze, protect the neurovascular elements, and allow for the greatest range of motion of any of the spinal segments. The complexity of the bony and neurovascular anatomy, as well as any pathological or congenital variation, must be fully understood prior to surgical intervention. Age-related degenerative changes, inflammatory conditions, and previous surgical intervention can cause neurologic manifestations including radiculopathy, myelopathy, or myeloradiculopathy. The main objectives of cervical deformity surgery include restoration of horizontal gaze, decompression of neural elements, and reestablishment of balanced spinal alignment.

The presence of cervical deformity has been shown to significantly impact overall function and lead to significant pain as well as decreased health-related quality of life (HRQOL).[1] In order to properly treat these patients, the provider must have a thorough understanding of the clinical and radiographic evaluation necessary for appropriate preoperative planning. The surgeon must understand radiographic parameters used to define the extent of the cervical deformity and help determine if it is a primary deformity or compensatory deformity due to a thoracolumbar derangement.

The purpose of this chapter is to review the necessary elements of the clinical evaluation as well as the various radiographic parameters used to define and understand any co-existing deformity. The authors then provide an overview and rationale for the various surgical options available to address the deformity and any neurologic compromise. Finally, we discuss the outcomes of patients with neurologic compromise in the setting of cervical deformity.

Clinical Evaluation

The clinical presentation of patients with cervical deformity can vary greatly with complaints of neck fatigue and pain, difficulty in maintaining a horizontal gaze, neurologic deterioration, and even difficulty in swallowing and/or breathing. Thus, it is crucial that the provider perform a complete neurologic history and physical examination to understand the patient's problems and develop a comprehensive surgical plan. The physical examination should include an assessment of the patient's alignment in both the seated and supine positions as well as standing with the hips and knees extended (to limit compensatory mechanisms).[2] The seated position is crucial in understanding the origin of the deformity as it removes the effect of a lumbar and/or pelvic deformity.[2] The supine position gives an indication of the rigidity of the cervical deformity as gravity will help to passively correct the deformity (this may take 5 or more minutes). A severely rigid cervical deformity will not correct but if the primary deformity is thoracic or lumbar, the compensatory cervical deformity will usually correct in the supine position.

Neck fatigue and pain are common presenting symptoms. Degenerative cervical spondylosis results in degeneration and height loss of the discs, which ultimately leads to kyphosis and increased stress on the posterior elements and cervical musculature. In an attempt to correct the mechanical imbalance, the cervical musculature over-compensates resulting in fatigue, increased energy expenditure, and muscle strain. Coupled with the concurrent disc and facet degeneration, patients with cervical deformity can have intractable neck pain.

Cervical deformity is often associated with neurologic deterioration and myelopathy. Increasing cervical kyphosis is associated with cord flattening which ultimately leads to increased pressures and decreased blood flow which can cause demyelination and neuronal loss.[3,4,5,6,7,8] It is also important to realize that decompression alone may not relieve pressure on the spinal cord. With a kyphotic cervical deformity, the ventral cord becomes draped over the posterior aspects of the vertebral bodies and only deformity correction will provide sufficient relief. A comprehensive neurologic examination is needed to understand the patient's preoperative neurologic state and aid in discussions of postoperative expectations. Without surgery, many of these changes are progressive but even with surgery the changes may be irreversible.

Radiographic Evaluation

In case of cervical deformity, developing the correct surgical plan begins with obtaining the correct images. Evaluation should start with anteroposterior (AP) and lateral static radiographs. Most radiographic measures that will be discussed below can be obtained from these images. However, it is tremendously important to understand the rigidity of any deformity. Along with the physical examination, dynamic images such as flexion and extension radiographs can aid in this determination. Additionally, it is essential that the treating physician understand if the cervical deformity is the primary deformity or is a compensatory deformity due to a concomitant thoracolumbar deformity. This can be determined by routinely obtaining AP and lateral, 36-inch standing scoliosis radiographs. The surgeon can then define the spinopelvic parameters and begin to understand the etiology, and ultimately, treat the cervical deformity.

Computed tomography (CT) of the cervical spine is required during the workup and preoperative planning of cervical deformity surgery. The complex bony architecture, especially at the occiput–C1 and C1–C2 articulations, needs to be evaluated carefully to understand the deformity and plan for surgical decompression and fixation. If the deformity is contributed by cervical spondylosis, the CT scan can help to determine which levels have undergone auto-fusion. In the same manner, if the deformity has an iatrogenic component, it is crucial to determine if pseudarthrosis is present so that it may be addressed during any future operation.

Magnetic resonance imaging (MRI) should also be a component of the initial workup as many of these patients present with neurologic deficits. MRI allows the surgeon to understand the location and extent of stenosis that may require direct decompression. MRI also allows for a greater understanding of vertebral artery anatomy which is crucial for planning surgical approach and fixation technique. The presence of myelomalacia may also help to inform a preoperative discussion of postoperative recovery.

Cervical Alignment Measurements

The primary load distribution of the cervical spine is in the posterior two columns (composed of the two facet joints) which bears 64% of the total weight. The anterior column (disc and vertebral body) bears the remaining 36%.[9] An essential component of this physiologic load distribution is the lordotic curvature of the cervical spine. There are three primary methods to quantify cervical lordosis: Cobb angles,[10] Jackson physiological stress lines,[11] and the Harrison posterior tangent line method.[10] All the three methods utilize upright lateral radiographs of the cervical spine. The Cobb angle is generally measured from C1–C7 or C2–C7. It is a four-line method in which the first line is drawn parallel to the inferior end plate of C2 and the second line parallel to the inferior end plate of C7. Two lines perpendicular to the first two lines are then drawn and the angle between the crossing perpendicular lines is the Cobb angle (**Fig. 6.1a**).[10] The Jackson physiological stress line method uses two lines. Both lines are drawn parallel to the posterior bodies of C2

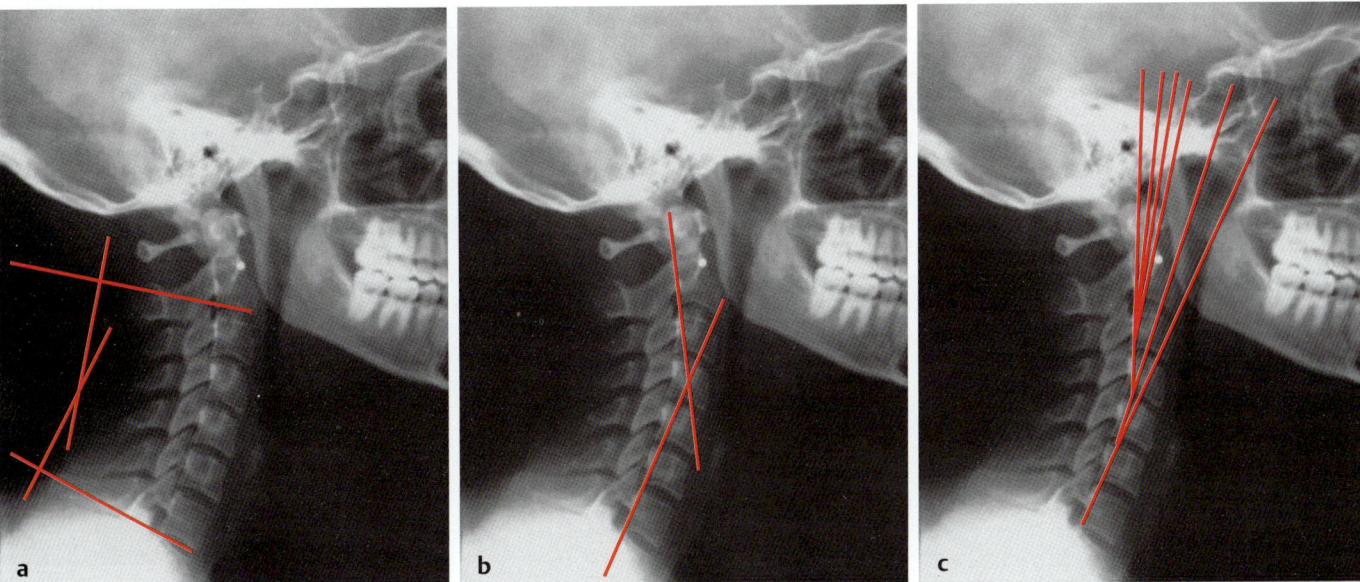

Fig. 6.1 Lateral cervical spine radiographs demonstrating three primary methods of quantifying lordosis: Cobb angle **(a)**, Jackson physiologic stress lines **(b)**, and Harrison posterior tangent lines **(c)**.

and C7 and the angle created by their intersection is used (**Fig. 6.1b**).[11] Finally, the Harrison posterior tangent line method involves drawing lines parallel to the posterior vertebral body spanning from C2 to C7. The segmental angles are then summed to achieve an overall lordosis angle (**Fig. 6.1c**). Although it has been demonstrated that the Harrison method may provide the best estimate of lordosis,[10] the Cobb angle is more commonly used due to its ease of use and high intra- and interrater reliability.[12] It is important that segmental lordosis be distinguished from overall lordosis as only about 6 degrees (15%) of cervical lordosis occurs at the lowest three levels of the subaxial spine (C3–C7) and the occiput–C1 segment is generally kyphotic.[13] Thus, the majority of cervical lordosis is found at the C1–C2 articulation (**Table 6.1**).

Cervical C2–C7 sagittal vertical axis (SVA) is a common measurement derived from upright lateral radiographs to help measure sagittal translation of the cervical spine. This is an important measurement as prior studies have shown that increasing C2–C7 SVA values is associated with poorer HRQOL.[1] C2–C7 SVA is obtained by dropping a plumb line from the centroid of the C2 vertebral body and then measuring the distance between that line and the posterior, superior aspect of the superior end plate of C7 (**Fig. 6.2**). Normal distances for C2–C7 SVA range from 15 to 17 ± 11.2 mm.[13]

Three additional measurements have been defined by Lee et al[14] in hopes of contextualizing cervical deformity and drawing analogies to the spinopelvic relationships in the lumbar spine. These include the thoracic inlet angle, neck tilt, and T1 slope. The thoracic inlet angle is analogous to pelvic incidence (PI) in the lumbar spine and is defined as the angle between a line from the center of and perpendicular to the T1 superior end plate and a line from the center of the T1 end plate and the upper end of the sternum (**Fig. 6.3**). Neck tilt is the angle obtained by drawing a line from the center

of the T1 superior end plate to the top of the sternum and a second vertical line drawn from the top of the sternum. Neck tilt is similar to the more familiar pelvic tilt which defines retroversion of the pelvis in the lumbar spine. T1 slope is defined as the angle between a line drawn parallel to the superior end plate of T1 and a horizontal line (sacral slope in lumbar spine). A relationship exists such that thoracic inlet angle equals T1 slope plus neck tilt (analogous to pelvic incidence equals sacral slope plus pelvic tilt).

When evaluating patients with cervical deformity, it is necessary to evaluate the cervical spine as it relates to the entire spine. Regional cervical alignment as well as global sagittal balance of the cervical and thoracolumbar spine must be examined. Global sagittal balance can be determined through the C7 SVA. This measurement uses a plumb line from the centroid of the C7 vertebral body, and the distance between this line and the posterior, superior aspect of the S1 end plate is measured. Pelvic incidence correlates with lumbar lordosis (LL), lumbar lordosis correlates with thoracic kyphosis, and thoracic kyphosis correlates with cervical lordosis. Thus, high pelvic incidence (a static measurement)

Table 6.1 Average segmental lordosis in asymptomatic cases

Level	Angle (°)
Occiput–C1	2.1 ± 5.0
C1–C2	−32.2 ± 7.0
C2–C3	−1.9 ± 5.2
C3–C4	−1.5 ± 5.0
C4–C5	−0.6 ± 4.4
C5–C6	−1.1 ± 5.1
C6–C7	−4.5 ± 4.3
C2–C7	−9.6
C1–C7	−41.8

Source: Table recreated with data from Hardacker et al.[13]

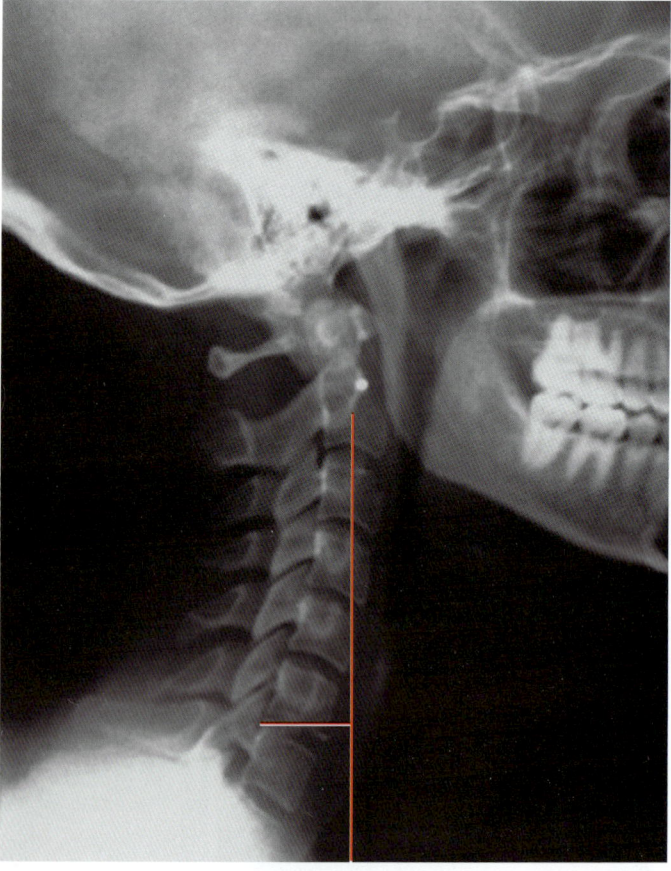

Fig. 6.2 C2–C7 sagittal vertical axis (SVA) measurement with plumb line dropped from centroid of C2 and distance measured between C2 plumb line and the posterior, superior aspect of C7 superior end plate.

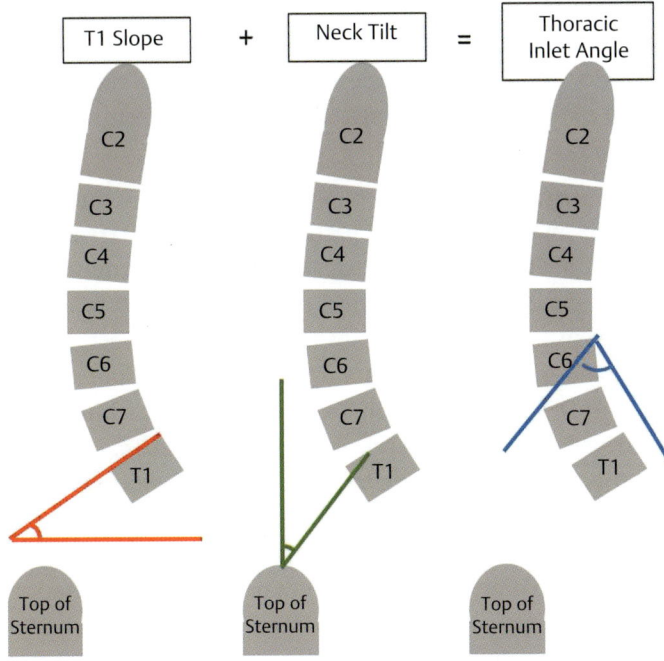

Fig. 6.3 Illustration demonstrating measurements of T1 slope, neck tilt, and thoracic inlet angle. These are analogous to sacral slope, pelvic tilt, and pelvic incidence, respectively.

will correlate with increased amounts of lumbar lordosis, thoracic kyphosis, and cervical lordosis in order to maintain horizontal gaze and reduce energy expenditure.[15,16] This complex relationship must be understood when attempting to understand if a deformity is the primary deformity or a compensatory deformity. For example, patients with a lumbar deformity (pelvic incidence-lumbar lordosis [PI-LL] mismatch) will compensate through pelvic retroversion (increased pelvic tilt) and compensatory changes in their thoracic (decreased kyphosis) and cervical (increased lordosis) spine. Similarly, a primary cervical deformity will compensate by increasing its pelvic tilt and lumbar lordosis. An accurate evaluation of spinopelvic parameters should also be made as it has been well established that a patient's LL is within 9 degrees of PI.[16] If a significant PI–LL mismatch exists, the primary deformity is most commonly caused by loss of lordosis in the lumbar spine.

Although not a radiographic measurement, the chin-brow vertical angle (CBVA) is an important aspect of evaluating patients with cervical deformities. It is the angle subtended between a line drawn between the patient's chin and brow and a vertical line. In order to obtain the measurement, a clinical photograph must be taken with the patient standing with hips and knees extended and cervical spine in a neutral (or fixed deformity) position. This angle has been found to have a significant impact on quality of life and should be restored to near neutral. Over- or

undercorrection will prevent the patient from maintaining horizontal gaze without requiring an inordinate amount of energy expenditure.[17]

Preoperative Planning

Preoperative planning starts with first understanding the "goals of the operation" which requires a thorough understanding of the patient's overall deformity and what functional or neurologic issues need to be addressed. A detailed history, physical examination, and radiographic assessment are paramount to being able to appropriately treat patients with spinal deformity.

As part of the planning process, examining the patient in the standing, seated, and supine positions will help to further understand the characteristics of each deformity. By evaluating the patients in these various positions, the flexibility of their deformity can be identified as well as any global sagittal imbalance derangement. Assessing the patients while standing and walking allows for evaluation of the thoracolumbar posture and identification of any functional abnormalities that may be contributing to their symptoms. Evaluation in seating position will prevent lumbopelvic pathology from interfering in the cervical examination.

It is important to recognize and understand the relationships between the craniocervical, subaxial, and thoracolumbar spine.[18] For instance, patients with subaxial cervical hyper- kyphosis will have hyperextension at the craniocervical junction while patients with positive sagittal balance that is driven by a thoracolumbar deformity may also present with hyperextension of the craniocervical junction due to compensatory subaxial cervical hyper-lordosis. It is important to understand and identify the driving pathology causing each patient's deformity.

A complete imaging assessment including X-ray, CT, and MRI scans will allow for areas of neurologic compromise to be identified as well as any congenital or degenerative bony abnormalities that may be contributing to the patient's derangement. X-ray evaluation including cervical AP, lateral, flexion, and extension radiographs can help define the deformity as well as the rigidity or flexibility of the cervical spine. In addition to cervical spine radiographs, full-length standing scoliosis films are helpful to identify any thoracolumbar pathology that may be contributing to the cervical deformity. CT scans are helpful to identify areas of ankyloses, spondylosis, or other pathologies, such as ossification of the posterior longitudinal ligament, that may be contributing to the deformity or neurologic symptoms that need to be addressed during surgical correction. An MRI should also be obtained to identify areas of neural compression or flattening of the spinal cord due to kyphosis as well as identify areas of myelomalacia that may be present.

In the end, the goals of surgery are to restore sagittal balance and decompress the neural elements. The magnitude of correction is typically the result of the flexibility of the spine. Through physical examination and imaging modalities a surgical plan can be derived to ensure safe and adequate correction of the cervical spinal deformity.

Surgical Treatment Options

Surgical planning for correction of a cervical spinal deformity begins with a thorough physical examination and radiographic evaluation. Patients are indicated for surgery due to either compromised neurologic status including radiculopathy or more commonly myelopathy as well as intractable pain or functional decline due to cervical malalignment. Radiographic evaluation aids in the surgical decision-making by identifying areas of listhesis, kyphosis, and stenosis. It is also important to note any areas of congenital or degenerative ankylosis as this may affect surgical decision-making. It is also paramount to identify if the patient has undergone previous procedures which may alter the surgical plan. In addition to obtaining imaging of the cervical spine, full-length standing scoliosis films may aid with understanding of the patient's pathology by evaluating the global coronal and sagittal alignment.

Cervical deformities are often categorized as either rigid or flexible. A flexible deformity or kyphosis will be passively correctable while a rigid deformity will not. One way to identify the flexibility of the cervical spine is to lie the patients down during the physical examination to identify to what degree they are able to passively extend or correct their kyphosis. Flexion and extension radiographs may also be helpful in categorizing the deformity. Surgical treatment options vary based on the type of cervical deformity, either flexible or rigid. Flexible deformities are often more amenable to smaller procedures and do not typically require an osteotomy to realign the spine. Rigid deformities are typically more complex and may require an osteotomy to correct the spine's alignment or in some scenarios a combined anterior and posterior operation. For example, the patient shown in **Fig. 6.4** developed a proximal kyphosis above the previous thoracolumbar fusion and below the previous multilevel anterior cervical diskectomy and fusion (ACDF). Standing 36-inch scoliosis films show this problem

is driven by an upper thoracic deformity, and the CT scan demonstrates that this a relatively fixed kyphosis. An all-posterior approach was undertaken, which shows reduction in the patient's positive sagittal balance and restoration of horizontal gaze.

The magnitude of correction needed and obtainable is dictated by the patient's pathology. Anterior treatment options include ACDF, anterior cervical corpectomy with fusion, and an anterior cervical opening wedge osteotomy. ACDF typically allows for 3 to 5 degrees of correction per level, and multilevel ACDFs are more effective than single-level ACDFs particularly in fixed deformities.[19] Kim et al described the anterior cervical osteotomy in 2014.[21] In their experience they were able to generate 1.3 cm of translation with an isolated anterior column osteotomy and 23 degrees of correction compared to 3.7 cm of translation and 32 degrees for patients who underwent posterior augmentation after the anterior osteotomy. Posterior based correctional procedures include Smith-Peterson osteotomies (SPOs) and pedicle subtraction osteotomies (PSOs). SPOs can contribute approximately 10 degrees of lordosis or correction per level and a PSO may provide approximately 35 degrees of correction.[19] Furthermore PSOs can provide 2.2 to 4.3 cm of cervical sagittal vertical axis (cSVA) reduction.[22] Anterior and posterior approaches can be performed in conjunction with one another, which can allow for a significant amount of deformity correction. **Fig. 6.5** demonstrates a patient with an iatrogenic deformity secondary to a multilevel cervical decompression for a previous epidural abscess. The patient developed a kyphosis of the proximal cervical spine with subsequent loss of horizontal gaze. This patient underwent an anterior based approach in the form of a multilevel ACDF and a posterior based posterior cervical osteotomies (PCOs) which successfully restored sagittal alignment. Etame et al evaluated the degree of correction of cervical kyphosis that was achieved with different corrective procedures. They identified that ACDF provided the least amount of correction while anterior/posterior procedure provided similar correction to PSO.[19]

PSOs can be performed classically at C7, T1, or T2.[23] However, due to the inability to sacrifice the lower cervical nerves, C8 and T1, C7 and T1 PSOs have fallen out of favor for some. In addition to concerns regarding the exiting nerve roots, some patients will have an anomalous vertebral artery that runs through C7, which makes preoperative planning and proper imaging crucial if performing a C7 PSO. We prefer to perform three-column osteotomies at T2, which allows us to apply compression across T1 and T3 pedicle screws and avoid the risk of postoperative hand dysfunction.

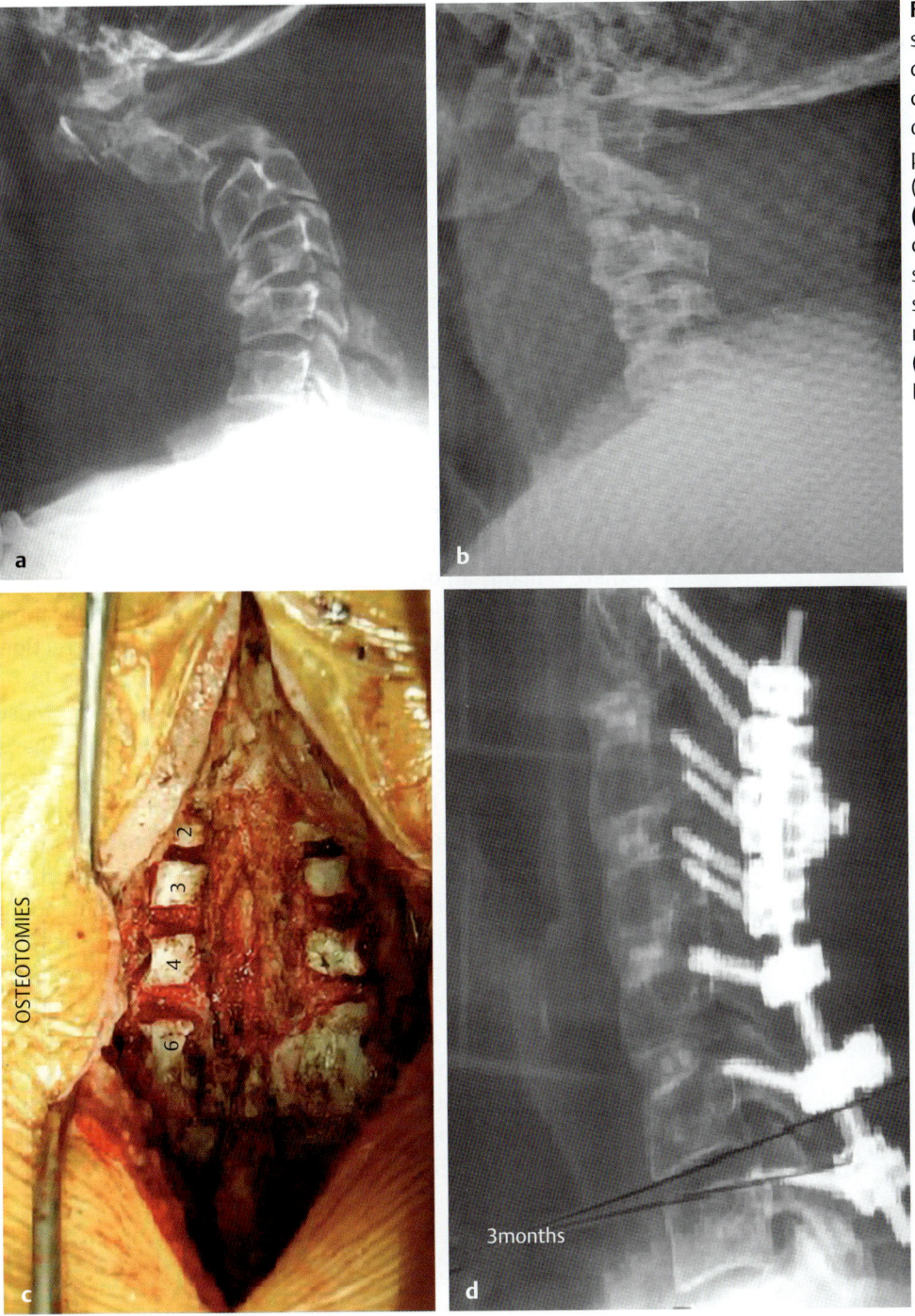

Fig. 6.4 Iatrogenic cervical kyphosis secondary to previous multilevel cervical laminectomy **(a)**. Radiographs demonstrating corrective ability of anterior based procedure once posterior cervical osteotomies (PCOs) are performed posteriorly **(b)**. Demonstration of posterior column osteotomies of the cervical spine **(c)**. Postoperative radiographs show neutral cervical alignment with restoration of horizontal gaze **(d)**. (Photos courtesy of Thomas Mroz, MD.)

Outcomes

Commonly, cervical spinal deformity has a negative impact on a patient's quality of life and frequently leads to disability.[1] Surgical correction of these deformities can result in significant improvements for patients. Radiographic measures have been correlated to outcome, specifically cSVA and CBVA.[17] cSVA has demonstrated worse outcomes if greater than 40 mm. CBVA is associated with forward gaze and should be kept to around 10 degrees.[17] Improvement in both of these measurements has been associated with improvements in activities of daily living and HRQOL scores. Cervical deformity can also contribute to a positive sagittal alignment and play a role in a patient's overall spinal misalignment. It has been well established that a positive sagittal balance of more than 50 mm is associated with worse disability and patient-reported outcome measures.[15,16]

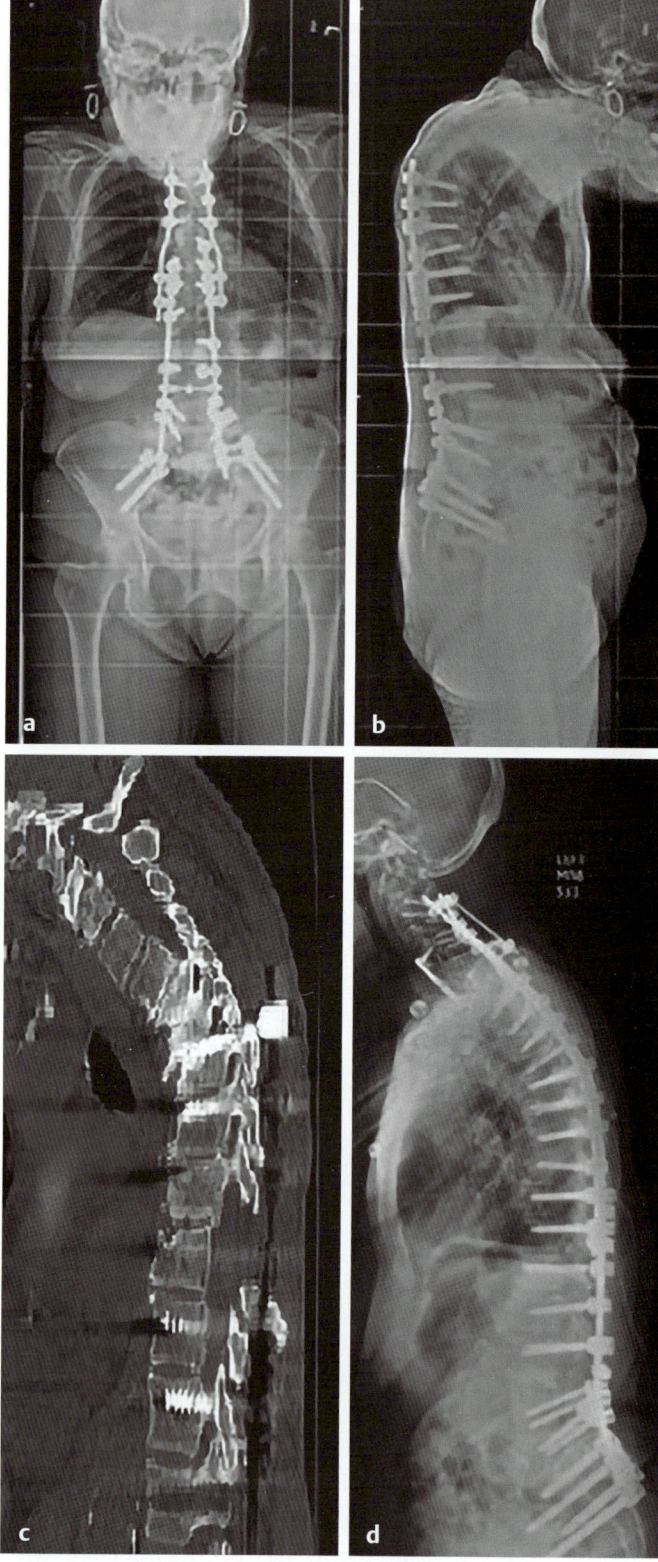

Fig. 6.5 Preoperative radiographs showing positive sagittal balance secondary to proximal thoracic kyphosis **(a, b)**. Preoperative computed tomography (CT) scan of the cervicothoracic junction shows this is fixed or rigid deformity **(c)**. Postoperative radiographs demonstrating an all-posterior approach through multilevel posterior column osteotomies **(d)**.

While cervical kyphosis has been well demonstrated to be associated with lower HRQOL, cervical lordosis is less correlated with patient outcomes. This is likely due to the large variability in cervical lordosis in the general population. However, the correction of focal cervical kyphosis has been demonstrated to result in improved neurologic outcomes.[20] Cervical kyphosis leads to cord flattening and neuronal loss resulting in severe myelopathic symptoms and worse patient-reported outcome scores.[6,23,24]

Complications

The recognition and treatment of cervical deformity have evolved over recent years but our knowledge still lags behind that of thoracolumbar deformity. Despite the improvement in treatment strategies, techniques, and instrumentation, there remains an overall high complication rate. Smith et al published a prospective study evaluating the complication rates of patients undergoing cervical deformity correction across 13 sites in North America.[25] They found that 74 of 132 patients (55.4%) had at least one complication. Most complications occurred during the early postoperative phase but up to 20% of complications occurred at the time of last follow-up, which in this study was 18 months on average. The most common complication was dysphagia, which occurred in 11.3% of patients, followed by distal junctional kyphosis, which occurred in 9% of patients. Nerve root motor deficits occurred in 5.3% of patients and new sensory deficits in 4.5%. There were two mortalities from cardiopulmonary complications. Furthermore, of the 133 patients, 23 underwent high-grade osteotomies in which 18 complications occurred. Numerous other studies report the high rates of complications that occur with surgical correction of cervical deformity. Appropriate perioperative patient optimization is critical in minimizing these complications.

Key Points

- The cervical spine is a complex structure which may have a wide variety of anatomic variations.

- The treatment of patients with a cervical spinal deformity requires a thorough understanding of each patient's anatomy and pathology.

- Radiographic parameters should include the cSVA and T1 slope in addition to evaluation of the patient's global sagittal alignment.

- Identifying the rigidity or flexibility will help decision-making in the surgical planning process.

- ACDF provides the least amount of angular correction, while PSO provides significant correction.

- Each patient's surgical plan should be devised based on individual pathology.

References

1. Tang JA, Scheer JK, Smith JS, et al; ISSG. The impact of standing regional cervical sagittal alignment on outcomes in posterior cervical fusion surgery. Neurosurgery 2012;71(3):662–669, discussion 669

2. Scheer JK, Ames CP, Deviren V. Assessment and treatment of cervical deformity. Neurosurg Clin N Am 2013;24(2):249–274

3. Ames CP, Blondel B, Scheer JK, et al. Cervical radiographical alignment: comprehensive assessment techniques and potential importance in cervical myelopathy. Spine 2013;38(22, Suppl 1):S149–S160

4. Chavanne A, Pettigrew DB, Holtz JR, Dollin N, Kuntz C IV. Spinal cord intramedullary pressure in cervical kyphotic deformity: a cadaveric study. Spine 2011;36(20):1619–1626

5. Iida H, Tachibana S. Spinal cord intramedullary pressure: direct cord traction test. Neurol Med Chir (Tokyo) 1995;35(2):75–77

6. Jarzem PF, Quance DR, Doyle DJ, Begin LR, Kostuik JP. Spinal cord tissue pressure during spinal cord distraction in dogs. Spine 1992; 17(8, Suppl):S227–S234

7. Kitahara Y, Iida H, Tachibana S. Effect of spinal cord stretching due to head flexion on intramedullary pressure. Neurol Med Chir (Tokyo) 1995;35(5):285–288

8. Shimizu K, Nakamura M, Nishikawa Y, Hijikata S, Chiba K, Toyama Y. Spinal kyphosis causes demyelination and neuronal loss in the spinal cord: a new model of kyphotic deformity using juvenile Japanese small game fowls. Spine 2005;30(21): 2388–2392

9. Pal GP, Sherk HH. The vertical stability of the cervical spine. Spine 1988;13(5):447–449

10. Harrison DE, Harrison DD, Cailliet R, Troyanovich SJ, Janik TJ, Holland B. Cobb method or Harrison posterior tangent method: which to choose for lateral cervical radiographic analysis. Spine 2000;25(16):2072–2078

11. Jackson RP, McManus AC. Radiographic analysis of sagittal plane alignment and balance in standing volunteers and patients with low back pain matched for age, sex, and size. A prospective controlled clinical study. Spine 1994;19(14): 1611–1618

12. Polly DW Jr, Kilkelly FX, McHale KA, Asplund LM, Mulligan M, Chang AS. Measurement of lumbar lordosis. Evaluation of intraobserver, interobserver, and technique variability. Spine 1996;21(13):1530–1535, discussion 1535–1536

13. Hardacker JW, Shuford RF, Capicotto PN, Pryor PW. Radiographic standing cervical segmental alignment in adult volunteers without neck symptoms. Spine 1997;22(13): 1472–1480, discussion 1480

14. Lee SH, Kim KT, Seo EM, Suk KS, Kwack YH, Son ES. The influence of thoracic inlet alignment on the craniocervical sagittal balance in asymptomatic adults. J Spinal Disord Tech 2012;25(2):E41–E47

15. Schwab F, Lafage V, Boyce R, Skalli W, Farcy JP. Gravity line analysis in adult volunteers: age-related correlation with spinal parameters, pelvic parameters, and foot position. Spine 2006;31(25):E959–E967

16. Schwab F, Patel A, Ungar B, Farcy JP, Lafage V. Adult spinal deformity-postoperative standing imbalance: how much can you tolerate? An overview of key parameters in assessing alignment and planning corrective surgery. Spine 2010;35(25):2224–2231

17. Suk KS, Kim KT, Lee SH, Kim JM. Significance of chin-brow vertical angle in correction of kyphotic deformity of ankylosing spondylitis patients. Spine 2003;28(17):2001–2005

18. Hann S, Chalouhi N, Madineni R, et al. An algorithmic strategy for selecting a surgical approach in cervical deformity correction. Neurosurg Focus 2014;36(5):E5

19. Etame AB, Wang AC, Than KD, La Marca F, Park P. Outcomes after surgery for cervical spine deformity: review of the literature. Neurosurg Focus 2010;28(3):E14

20. Grosso MJ, Hwang R, Mroz T, Benzel E, Steinmetz MP. Relationship between degree of focal kyphosis correction and neurological outcomes for patients undergoing cervical deformity correction surgery. J Neurosurg Spine 2013;18(6):537–544

21. Kim HJ, Piyaskulkaew C, Riew KD. Anterior cervical osteotomy for fixed cervical deformities. Spine 2014;39(21):1751–1757

22. Lau D, Ames CP. Three-column osteotomy for the treatment of rigid cervical deformity. Neurospine 2020;17(3):525–533

23. Deviren V, Scheer JK, Ames CP. Technique of cervicothoracic junction pedicle subtraction osteotomy for cervical sagittal imbalance: report of 11 cases. J Neurosurg Spine 2011;15(2): 174–181

24. Iida H, Tachibana S. Spinal cord intramedullary pressure: direct cord traction test. Neurol Med Chir (Tokyo) 1995; 35(2):75–77

25. Smith JS, Buell TJ, Shaffrey CI, et al. Prospective multicenter assessment of complication rates associated with adult cervical deformity surgery in 133 patients with minimum 1-year follow-up. J Neurosurg Spine 2020:1–13. doi: 10.3171/2020.4.SPINE20213. Online ahead of print

Part II

Techniques for Congenital Spinal Deformity Correction

7 Kyphectomy in Newborns

Nail Özdemir and Özgür Akşan

Introduction

Severe kyphosis is observed in 15% of newborns with meningomyelocele (MMC) in the lumbar and thoracolumbar regions.[1-3] It is associated with a high prevalence of hydrocephalus and serious neurological problems that lead to poor quality of life in newborns with MMC. Also, severe kyphotic deformity causes chronic epidermal ulceration, osteomyelitis, decreased abdominal and functional capacity, and sitting problems.[1] The degree of the kyphotic curve is usually large initially and increases by 4 and 12 degrees per year.[4] Progression is usually seen from the time the child sits down. Thoracic lordosis is frequently observed in older children and is often fixed in this period. It is absent in newborns and increases by about 2.5 degrees per year.[1]

In MMC, kyphectomy performed simultaneously with closure of the dural sac is a safe surgery that provides effective correction. Primary surgical wound healing is earlier and better in newborns who have undergone kyphectomy. Even if recurrent deformity occurs, it is better tolerated, and revision surgery is easier than in older child.[1]

The authors in this chapter aim to explain the technique, its indications, methods of prevention from complications, and convey their clinical experience to the readers.

Description of the Technique

The newborn is placed on chest rolls in the prone position. The MMC pouch is removed by turning around the borders. The dura is carefully exposed. The transverse processes are dissected from fascia and muscles. Kyphotic deformity called gibbus is revealed by dissecting with bipolar cautery to reveal the lateral corpus. Working from lateral to medial, the right and left sides are dissected separately. It is important not to injure the retroperitoneal structures and the iliopsoas. Therefore, dissection should be done bluntly with sponges and cottonoids. The dural layer is very thin and often attached to the posterior longitudinal ligament. To avoid cerebrospinal fluid leakage, it is safer to separate the dural layer from the ligament than to separate it from the bone. The dural layer is carefully separated from the transverse processes. The apical vertebra and usually three or four nerve roots coming out of it are observed. Transverse processes and abnormal pedicles

are excised. Nerve roots are completely shown on all points from the spinal cord to the point where they enter the psoas muscle from the front and are protected by a blunt dissector. After the transverse processes are removed and lateral corpus is dissected, the kyphotic deformity is fully revealed. The posterior longitudinal ligament is separated anteriorly from the vascular structures (inferior vena cava, aorta) with blunt dissection. Then, the dural sac is carefully retracted. No binding is applied to access the vertebral body (**Fig. 7.1a–e**). After the deformity is revealed, the apex vertebra is excised starting from disc areas. The vertebrectomy procedure is initiated and created by removing the posterior surface of the caudal segment and the posterior dorsal portion of the lower surface of the cranial segment as a wedge. One and a half vertebrae may need to be removed to create the lordosis after kyphectomy. A high-speed drill (8-mm cutting burr) is used for vertebrectomy. The procedure is carried out by carefully working through the roots above and below the level of the spine. A #1 large needle silk suture is passed through the upper and lower vertebrae of the resected kyphosis. Usually up to four to six silk sutures throughout the disc space are essential to obtain the strongest uptake in the vertebral bodies. An assistant should gently press and hold the vertebral body with finger to close the gap. Bones from vertebrectomy should be placed anteriorly (**Fig. 7.1f**). After repair of the dura, the surgical floors should be closed properly (**Fig. 7.1g, h**). After the operation, the treatment should be continued in the prone position in the incubator. The orthosis makes it difficult for the newborn to breathe. For this reason, it is not necessary to use it (**Fig. 7.1i**).

In authors' series, there were six female and two male newborns who underwent kyphectomy. The average birth weight of the newborns was 2,780 g. The average age at the time of operation was 5.6 days. All newborns had lumbar S-shaped type of kyphotic deformity. Partial vertebrectomy (vertebral body decancellation) was performed in four newborns, while total vertebrectomy was performed in four newborns. The mean operating time was 116 minutes. No patient received transfusion for blood. No serious complications were experienced in any of the patients and wounds of each newborn were closed successfully. The average follow-up period was 4 years and 3 months (from 3 to 61 months). A patient who died 1 week after discharge was excluded from the follow-up period. The average

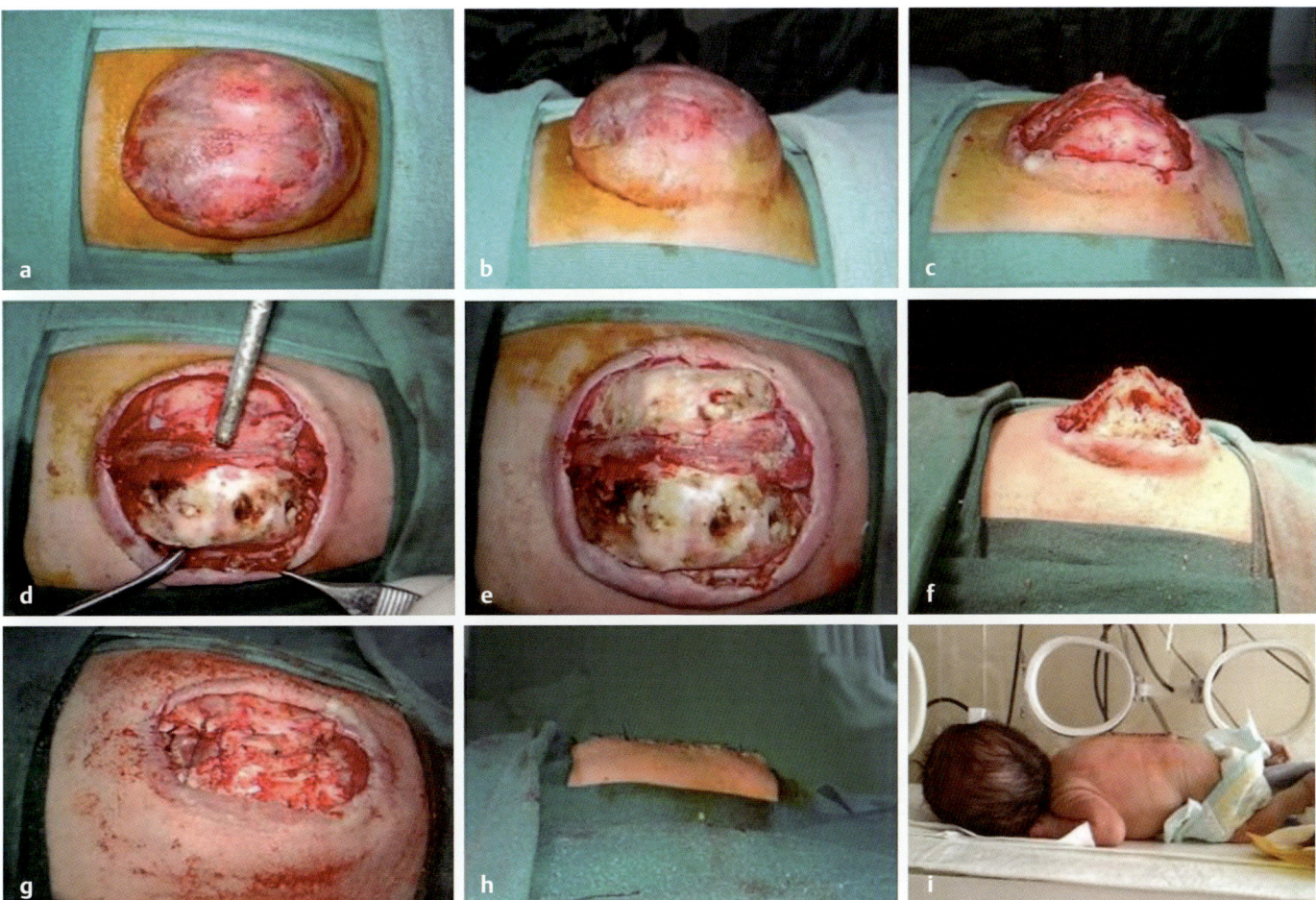

Fig. 7.1 **(a)** Anterior picture of meningomyelocele (MMC). **(b)** Lateral picture of MMC. **(c)** The dura is carefully exposed. The transverse processes are dissected from fascia and muscles. **(d, e)** Kyphotic deformity is revealed by dissecting with bipolar cautery to reveal the lateral corpus. Working from lateral to medial, the right and left sides are dissected separately. **(f)** An 8-mm cutting drill is used for vertebrectomy. **(g, h)** After repair of the dura, the surgical floors should be closed properly. **(i)** After the operation, the treatment should be continued in the prone position in the incubator until the skin is fully healed.

preoperative kyphosis angle of 75.6 degrees (from 50 to 90 degrees) had improved to 35 degrees (from 15 to 55 degrees) at the last follow-up. All patients underwent surgery because of hydrocephalus (ventriculoperitoneal shunt in seven patients, third ventriculostomy in one patient). In addition, decompression surgery was performed in three patients with Chiari type II malformation. The newborns stayed in the hospital for an average 27.7 days (**Table 7.1**).[1]

Indications

Such newborns with a preoperative kyphosis angle greater than 50 degrees should undergo kyphectomy.

Kyphosis in MMC can significantly reduce quality of life. The kyphectomy procedure is effective in preventing progression and improving the quality of life in these patients. In addition to its benefits in terms of correcting surgical sitting balance and chronic skin problems, it also provides benefits such as increasing respiratory capacity, relieving the abdominal cavity, and stopping deformity progression.

It is controversial whether kyphectomy should be performed in the neonatal period or in childhood. During childhood, a fixed compensatory lordosis develops in thoracic region as well as hardening of the deformity takes place. In newborns with MMC, kyphectomy provides effective correction in the early period. Also, contrary to popular belief, it is a reliable operation. Even if kyphosis recurs, it is easier to revise. Surgery in older children is more difficult, is prone to complications, and often requires instrumentation.[1]

Table 7.1 Reported eight cases for neonatal kyphectomy with MMC

No.	Gestational age, sex	Birth weight (gram)	Time of surgery (days)	Surgical technique	Length of surgery (minutes)	Need of blood transfusion	Preoperative kyphosis angle	Postoperative kyphosis angle (1st week)	Postoperative kyphosis angle (1st year)	Postoperative kyphosis angle (2nd year)	Additional surgery and surgical time	Hospital stay (days)	Follow-up (months)
1	38 weeks, female	2,700	10	L3 total vertebrectomy	90	No	90°	50°	50°	45°	VP shunt (12th day)	24	61
2	38 weeks, female	2,780	3	L3–L4 total vertebrectomies	120	No	85°	45°	45°	30°	VP shunt (9th day)	17	59
3	35 weeks, male	1,950	4	L3 total vertebrectomy	90	No	80°	35°	50°	65°	VP shunt (18th day), SOC + CL + DP (28th day)	34	59
4	38 weeks, female	2,440	3	L2–L3 partial vertebrectomies	180	No	50°	15°	25°	25°	VP shunt (13th day)	18	59
5	38 weeks, female	3,400	11	L2–L3 partial vertebrectomies	120	No	60°	25°	35°	45°	VP shunt (27th day)	31	44
6	38 weeks, male	3,510	2	L2–L3–L4 partial vertebrectomies	120	No	70°	35°	45°	70°	VP shunt (13th day), SOC + CL + DP (26th day)	40	41
7	38 weeks, female	3,000	6	L2–L3 partial vertebrectomies	120	No	80°	65°	65°	75°	Third ventriculostomy (90th day)	15	36
8	35 weeks, female	2,470	6	L3 total vertebrectomy	90	No	90°	50°	-	-	VP shunt (25th day), SOC + CL + DP (34th day)	43	Death (1st week after the discharge)

Abbreviations: MMC, meningomyelocele; SOC + CL + DP, suboccipital craniectomy, cervical laminectomy, and duraplasty; VP, ventriculoperitoneal.

Complication Avoidance

Total and partial vertebrectomy are two approaches for kyphectomy. Lindseth[5] described kyphotic deformity as C- and S-shaped. S-shaped type is more rigid, and total vertebrectomy is usually required. Lindseth and Stelzer[6] showed better results for lordosis if added to the vertebrectomy in the cephalic spine along with the apical vertebra. In C-shaped type, partial vertebrectomy may be sufficient. Lindseth advocated vertebrectomy by evacuating the lower and upper parts of the apex vertebra.[5] Theoretically, partial vertebrectomy procedure allows the growth centers of the vertebral body to grow continuously. In addition, kyphectomy should be performed if it is thought that skin will not close when the MMC sac is closed. Kyhpectomy should be performed during dural sac excision. Compared with total vertebrectomy, partial vertebrectomy better preserves minor neurologic functions if present. It has additional benefit that it does not reach the anterior column and therefore does not damage the vessels. Surgery in the neonatal period results in less blood loss compared to childhood. Although complications have been reported for S-shaped type deformity in newborns in previous series in the literature, this procedure is quite safe.

Tips and Tricks

The procedure is carried out by carefully working through the roots above and below the level of the spine. It is important to put #1 silk sutures from the top to bottom to close the gap formed after kyphectomy. For correction, it is sufficient for the assistant to apply gentle pressure to the lower vertebrae. Usually up to four to six silk sutures throughout disc space are essential to obtain the strongest uptake in the vertebral bodies. Bone chips obtained during vertebrectomy should be placed in the gap for fusion purposes. Afterwards, silk sutures should be tied, and kyphosis should be corrected.

Key Points

- Kyphectomy in the newborn with MMC is a safe method that provides an effective correction in the early period.

- Kyphotic deformity one of the most problem in meningomyelocele.Because this problem causes chronic epidermal ulceration, osteomyelitis, decreased abdominal and functional capacity, and sitting problems.

- Kyphectomy in the newborn with MMC is a safe method that provides an effective correction in the early period.

- Primary surgical wound healing is earlier and better in newborns who have undergone kyphectomy. Even if recurrent deformity occurs, it is better tolerated, and revision surgery is easier than in older child.

References

1. Özdemir N, Özdemir SA, Özer EA. Kyphectomy in neonates with meningomyelocele. Childs Nerv Syst 2019;35(4):673–681
2. Crawford AH, Strub WM, Lewis R, et al. Neonatal kyphectomy in the patient with myelomeningocele. Spine 2003;28(3):260–266
3. de Amoreira Gepp R, Quiroga MRS, Gomes CR, de Araújo HJ. Kyphectomy in meningomyelocele children: surgical technique, risk analysis, and improvement of kyphosis. Childs Nerv Syst 2013;29(7):1137–1141
4. Karlin LI. Kyphectomy for myelodysplasia. Neurosurg Clin N Am 2007;18(2):357–364
5. Lindseth RE. Spine deformity in myelomeningocele. Instr Course Lect 1991;40:273–279
6. Lindseth RE, Stelzer L Jr. Vertebral excision for kyphosis in children with myelomeningocele. J Bone Joint Surg Am 1979;61(5):699–704

8 Surgery for Diastematomyelia

Adnan Yalçın Demirci and Óscar L. Alves

Introduction

Spinal cord dysraphism is a term which is used to describe various spinal cord malformations. Diastematomyelia (DM) (also called diplomyelia, pseudo diplomyelia, and split spinal cord syndrome) is one of these malformations. It is an anomaly that divides the cord into two symmetrical or unsymmetrical parts along the midline of the cord, forming two neural tubes.[1,2] The anomaly was first described by Ollivier in 1837.[3] There are two subtypes of DM: DM is classified as Type 1, if there is a separate dural sac covering each hemicord and an extradural bony septum separating these two hemicords, and as Type 2, if there is only one dural sac covering both hemicords without a compact bony septum between them (**Fig. 8.1**). A soft fibrous septum is seen between the two spinal cords in Type 2.[1,4] The septum is mostly seen in the lumbar vertebrae (70%) and the thoracolumbar junction, and it is very rare in the cervical region and sacral vertebrae.[5]

The anomaly is frequently seen in children and rarely in adults and its incidence is higher in girls than boys.[6,7] Neurological findings vary based on the age and the presence of other comorbid spinal malformations.[1] Although there may be cutaneous anomalies alone, orthopedic syndromes related to the spine and lower extremities and varying degrees of neurological findings may also accompany the cutaneous anomaly.[8] Cutaneous anomalies are seen in 69% of cases. Hypertrichosis is one of the most common cutaneous anomalies, followed by naevus and capillary hemangiomas.[8,9] Symptoms due to stretching of the spinal cord occur as the patient gets older.[4] Pain in the lower extremity, which is prominent in adults, is less common in children. Leg cramps and pain associated with physical activity are typical. Weakness in the lower extremity, loss of sensation, decreased deep tendon reflexes and/or anal reflexes, sphincter dysfunction, and loss of sensation in the perineal region may be seen in the clinical examination.[1,7,10]

There are several theories regarding DM. Herren's theory of neurulation disorder states that DM is an exaggerated folding of the neural plate. This theory further argues that DM is always associated with a spinal anomaly.[11] Dryden used X-rays as a teratogenic agent in chick embryos and showed the folding of neural folds, as Herren suggested, but failed to show the splitting.[12] Gardner's hypothesis states that two neural tubes are formed as a result of rupture of the neural tube with hydromyelic distension from both ventral and dorsal directions and then this space is filled by fibrous or bone tissue.[13] However, this hypothesis was rejected by Mann on the grounds that cerebrospinal fluid (CSF) that is produced from the choroid plexuses does not yet have an effect.[14] Bremer suggested that DM emerges as an accessory neuroenteric canal. The neuroenteric canal is the only midline structure capable of dividing the neural epithelium during embryogenesis.[15,16] Pang et al supported the theory that DM is caused by a fundamental ontogenetic error that occurred during closure of the primitive neuroenteric canal.[1] Dias and Walker argued that DM emerges as a result of abnormal formation during gastrulation of paired notochordal and paired neuroepithelial cells that remain separated before neurulation because the neural plate becomes a single layer after the completion of gastrulation.[17]

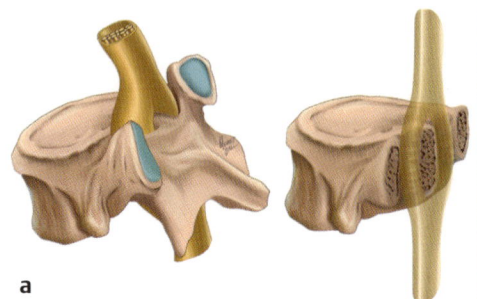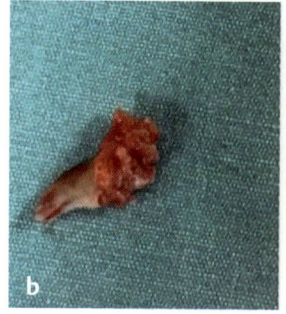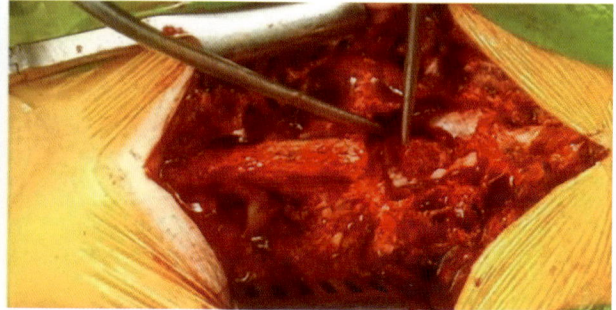

Fig. 8.1 **(a, b)** Extradural bony septum separating two hemicords.

Surgical Technique

The surgery is performed in the prone position with general anesthesia. The genu-pectoral position, which is mostly used in disc surgery, is not recommended as it may cause redundant stretching.[7,18] Pillows should be used to prevent abdominal compression. Neurophysiological monitoring has not been used universally in studies on DM, but today it is highly advisable to perform surgery accompanied by neurophysiological monitoring. Once the target area is cleaned and covered, the distance is determined by fluoroscopy. Afterwards, the skin, subcutaneous tissue, and fascia are incised. Paravertebral muscle dissection is performed bilaterally. It should be kept in mind that there may be large lamina defects during muscle dissection with cautery; therefore, care must be taken not to cause dural damage. The pathological vertebrae and the laminae of the upper and lower vertebrae should be clearly identified. In Type 1 DM, a laminectomy should be performed to expose the median bone septum by means of an ultrasonic bone cutter (**Fig. 8.2**). The median dural cleft and the cranial and caudal single dural sheath should be clearly visible. The dural cleft region is rich in vascular structures. The median bone septum should be carefully excised under the microscope to avoid opening the dura. Bone cutters can also be used during this procedure, and care should be taken not to traumatize the neural tissues. Often there is an artery in the middle of the septum and may bleed due to excision of the septum.[1] Bleeding should be brought under control with the help of bipolar cautery and bone wax. After removal of the bone septum, the dura should be opened with a scalpel no. 15 around the dural cleft under the microscope, and afterwards, the dural piece surrounding the bone septum should be removed by cutting it into an ellipse using microscissors (**Fig. 8.3** and **8.4**). The part of this piece adhering to the base of the dura should also be cut with microscissors without damaging the integrity of the dura, and if bleeding occurs, it should be stopped with bipolar cautery. The dural bands, if present, that anchor the spinal cord extending from the dorsal or ventral aspects of both halves of the spinal cord to the septum dura are cut and released. After that, the dura opened from the dorsum is sutured.

Since the bony septum is absent in Type 2 DM and the dural sheath is single, the dura is opened under the microscope after laminectomy with an ultrasonic bone cutter. In order to prevent deformation of the spine in pediatric patients, laminoplasty is to be preferred instead of laminectomy. In the next step, the spinal cords are released by cutting the connections between the dura and the fibrous septum, which is located between the half spinal cords and fixes them to the dorsal or ventral dura. The dorsal dura is sutured in a CSF-leakage-proofed manner.

Frequently, tethered cord is seen in DM.[19] When a tethered cord is present in the preoperative radiological examinations, laminectomy should be performed at the relevant level and the thick filum should be explored, even if it is not in the area of operation, and it should be cut after checking with the neuromonitoring probe.

Surgical Indications

Traditionally, surgical indications of DM are considered to be rapid deterioration in neurological, urological, or orthopedic functions. A rapid recovery is seen in these patients after surgery.[7] However, Matson et al argued that the purpose of DM surgery is primarily prophylactic rather than curative.[20] Prophylactic surgery should be discussed in terms of preventing future aggravation with minimal morbidity or no morbidity.[7] Mathieu et al believe that asymptomatic children will eventually develop neurological symptoms and therefore argues that performing prophylactic surgery is necessary.[18] More recent articles recommend prophylactic treatment of DM as well.[5,6,21] Conversely, Zuccaro noted that the majority of unoperated asymptomatic patients remained asymptomatic for an average of 7 years.[22,23]

Most orthopedists recommend performing surgery for intraspinal pathology prior to scoliosis surgery for patients with scoliosis related to DM.[24] Since performing laminectomy and removing bone spur in a scoliotic spine will increase spinal deformation, it is recommended that these patients

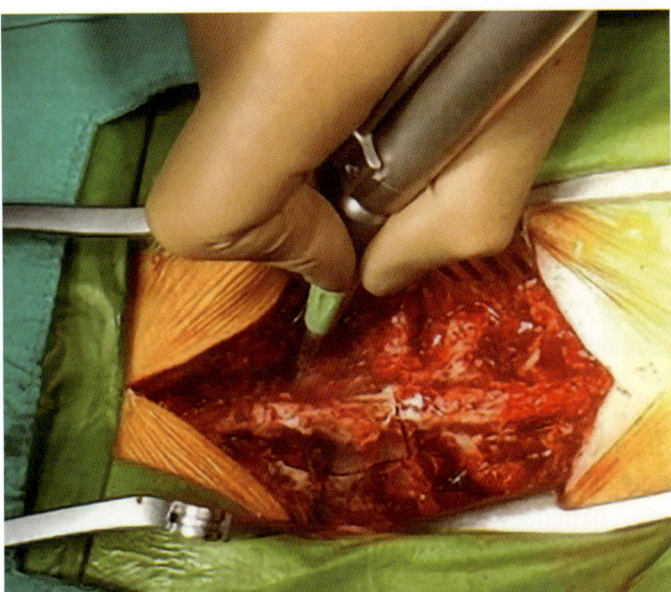

Fig. 8.2 Laminectomy should better be performed with an ultrasonic bone cutter.

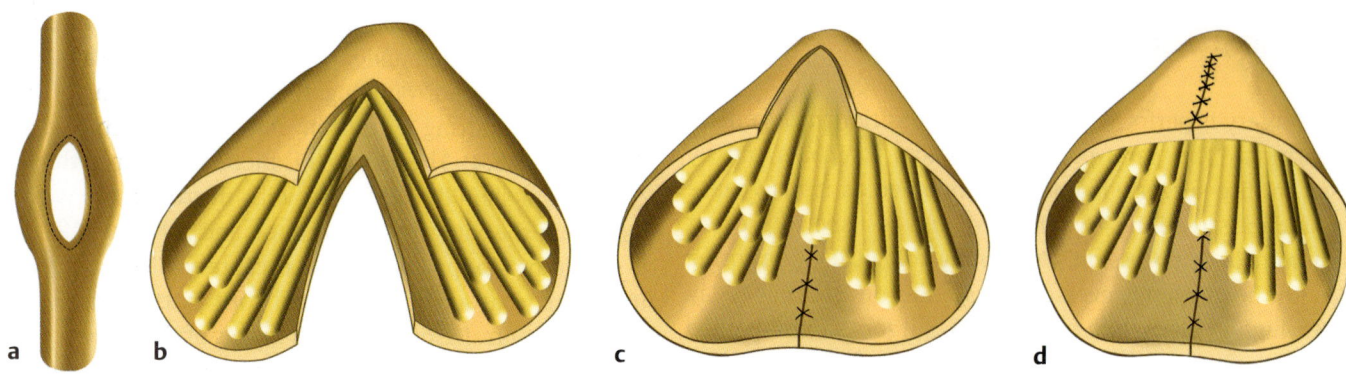

Fig. 8.3 **(a–d)** The dura should be opened around the dural cleft. Then anterior dura is repaired followed by posterior dura repair.

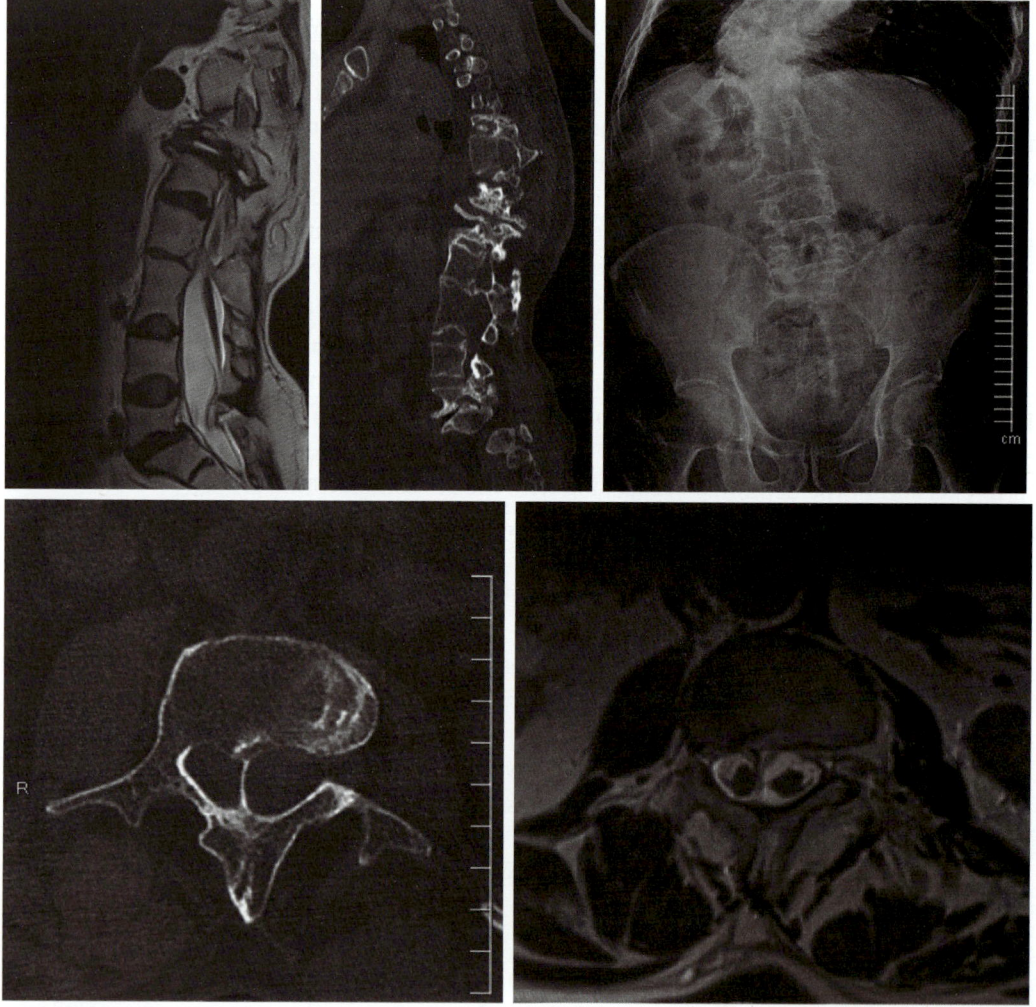

Fig. 8.4 A 61-year-old male patient with scoliosis had weakness and numbness of both legs that increased with walking. Magnetic resonance (MR), computed tomography (CT), and direct radiograms showed a diastematomyelia at T12 level.

be fixed by stabilization. This can be performed in the same or in a different session.[25]

Guthkelch divided 22 patients with stable deficits into two groups. In the conservatively followed group, 8 out of 10 patients required surgery due to the aggravation of a pre-existing condition. In the other group, 12 patients with stable deficits who were operated immediately after diagnosis did not have an increase in neurodegenerative deficits. Therefore, they concluded that surgery is indicated in all patients with stable neurological deficit.[26]

Patients admitted mainly due to worsening of their sphincter functions are candidates for emergency surgery. Meyrat et al recommend systematic use of urodynamic and anorectal manometry.[27] As they are the most sensitive parameters for patients' deterioration, even if these patients are otherwise asymptomatic and their surgeons should be encouraged to perform operation.[27]

Adult DM patients rarely complain of sexual disturbances. Chehrazi and Haldeman reported on a patient with sphincter and erectile dysfunction who was persuaded for insertion of a penile prosthesis.[28] Although another case with improved sphincter function and sexual disturbances has been reported after removal of the fibrous septum, this result is rather exceptional. In fact, sphincter disturbances reported in the adult tethered cord rarely show such remarkable improvement.[29]

DM surgery can cause improvement or regression of trophic ulcers, despite the chronic course of trophic lesions in extremities.[6,30]

In addition, the indication for surgery is certain in the presence of DM and other diseases such as dermal sinus, dermoid tumor, neuroenteric cyst, or teratoma.[7]

Complication Avoidance

In general, the morbidity and mortality rate of DM surgery is very low. While perioperative complications are mostly related to hemostasis, postoperative complications result from insufficient watertight closure of the dura.[7]

It is necessary to obtain prior information about bone defects with CT scan before surgery. If there are lamina defects, cautery should not be used during paravertebral muscle dissection to avoid dural and neural damage.

Instead, ultrasonic bone cutter should be used during laminectomy and median bone septum should be removed to avoid traumatizing dural and neural tissues. Bleeding caused by removal of the bone septum can be controlled with bipolar cautery and bone wax.

Careful removal of the median bone septum and the surrounding dura under the microscope is important in order to prevent damage to neural tissues.

These surgeries should not be performed without neurophysiological monitoring, especially when considering cutting the thick filum.

Finally, extreme care should be taken when closing the dura; it should be sutured in a waterproof manner to prevent CSF leakage.

Tips and Tricks

- The genu-pectoral position, which is generally used in disc surgeries, is not recommended.

- Neurophysiological monitoring should be applied during the surgery.

- It should be remembered that there may be large lamina defects during paravertebral muscle dissection.

- Ultrasonic bone cutter should be utilized during laminectomy.

- A microscope should be used in the stages after the laminectomy procedure.

- The dural bands extending from the dorsal or ventral surfaces of the spinal cord and anchoring the spinal cord should be cut and released.

- The thick filum should be explored and cut.

- Dorsal dura should be sutured in a manner to prevent CSF leakage.

Key Points

- Surgery is indicated in all patients with stable deficits.

- Surgery of intraspinal pathology is recommended before scoliosis surgery for patients with scoliosis and associated DM.

- There is usually an artery in the middle of the septum that may bleed due to excision of the septum.

- While perioperative complications are mostly related to hemostasis, postoperative complications result from insufficient closure of the dura in terms of watertightness.

References

1. Pang D, Dias MS, Ahab-Barmada M. Split cord malformation: Part I: A unified theory of embryogenesis for double spinal cord malformations. Neurosurgery 1992;31(3):451–480

2. Naidich TP, Zimmerman RA, Mclone DG, Raybaud C. Congenital anomalies of the distal spine and spinal cord: embryology and malformations. Riv Neuroradiol. 1995;8(Suppl 1):13–23

3. Ollivier d'Angers CP. Traité des maladies de la moelle e'pinière, 3rd edn. Me'quignon-Marve's: Paris, 1837:1160

4. Alnefaie N, Alharbi A, Alamer OB, et al. Split cord malformation: presentation, management, and surgical outcome. World Neurosurg 2020;136: e601–e607

5. Erşahin Y, Mutluer S, Kocaman S, Demirtaş E. Split spinal cord malformations in children. J Neurosurg 1998;88(1):57–65

6. Mahapatra AK, Gupta DK. Split cord malformations: a clinical study of 254 patients and a proposal for a new clinical-imaging classification. J Neurosurg 2005; 103(6, Suppl): 531–536

7. Rilliet B. Diastematomyelia. In: Özek MM, Cinalli G, Maixner WJ, eds. The Spina Bifida Management and Outcome. Italia, PA: Springer; 2008:487–513

8. Choux M, Lena G, Genitori L, Foroutan M. The surgery of occult spinal dysraphism. Adv Tech Stand Neurosurg 1994;21: 183–238

9. Wendelin DS, Pope DN, Mallory SB. Hypertrichosis. J Am Acad Dermatol 2003; 48(2):161–179, quiz 180–181

10. Akay KM, Erşahin Y, Cakir Y. Tethered cord syndrome in adults. Acta Neurochir (Wien) 2000;142(10):1111–1115

11. Pickles W. Duplication of the Spinal Cord (Diplomyelia). Journal of Neurosurgery 1949; 6(4): 324–331

12. Dryden RJ. Spina bifida in chick embryos: ultrastructure of open neural defects in the transitional region between primary and secondary modes of neural tube formation. In: Persaud TVN, eds. Advances in the Study of Birth Defects. Neural and Behavioural Teratology. Vol. 4. Lancaster: MTP Press Limited; 1980: 75–100

13. Gardner WJ. The Dysraphic States. Amsterdam: Excerpta Medica; 1973

14. Mann RA, Persaud TVN. Experimental open defects in the early chick embryo. In: Persaud TVN, ed. Advances in the Study of Birth Defects. Vol. 4. Neural and Behavioural Teratology. Lancaster: MTP Press Limited; 1980:63–74

15. Bremer JL. Dorsal intestinal fistula; accessory neurenteric canal; diastematomyelia. AMA Arch Pathol 1952;54(2): 132–138

16. Emura T, Asashima M, Hashizume K. An experimental animal model of split cord malformation. Pediatr Neurosurg 2000; 33(6):283–292

17. Dias MS, Walker ML. The embryogenesis of complex dysraphic malformations: a disorder of gastrulation? Pediatr Neurosurg 1992;18(5-6):229–253

18. Mathieu JP, Decarie M, Dube J, Marton D. Diastematomyelia. Study of 69 cases (author's transl) Chir Pediatr 1982; 23(1): 29–35

19. Pang D. Split cord malformation: Part II: Clinical syndrome. Neurosurgery 1992;31(3):481–500

20. Matson DD, Woods RP, Campbell JB, Ingraham FD. Diastematomyelia (congenital clefts of the spinal cord); diagnosis and surgical treatment. Pediatrics 1950;6(1):98–112

21. Gan YC, Sgouros S, Walsh AR, Hockley AD. Diastematomyelia in children: treatment outcome and natural history of associated syringomyelia. Childs Nerv Syst 2007;23(5): 515–519

22. Zuccaro G. Split spinal cord malformation. Childs Nerv Syst 2003;19(2):104–105

23. Schijman E. Split spinal cord malformations: report of 22 cases and review of the literature. Childs Nerv Syst 2003; 19(2):96–103

24. McMaster MJ. Occult intraspinal anomalies and congenital scoliosis. J Bone Joint Surg Am 1984;66(4):588–601

25. Leung YL, Buxton N. Combined diastematomyelia and hemivertebra: a review of the management at a single centre. J Bone Joint Surg Br 2005;87(10):1380–1384

26. Guthkelch AN. Diastematomyelia with median septum. Brain 1974;97(4):729–742

27. Meyrat BJ, Tercier S, Lutz N, Rilliet B, Forcada-Guex M, Vernet O. Introduction of a urodynamic score to detect pre- and postoperative neurological deficits in children with a primary tethered cord. Childs Nerv Syst 2003;19(10-11): 716–721

28. Chehrazi B, Haldeman S. Adult onset of tethered spinal cord syndrome due to fibrous diastematomyelia: case report. Neurosurgery 1985;16(5):681–685

29. Pang D, Wilberger JEJ Jr. Tethered cord syndrome in adults. J Neurosurg 1982;57(1):32–47

30. 'Serratrice G, Gastaut JL, Pouget J. Mutilating ulcerative acropathy in diastematomyelia. Rev Neurol (Paris) 1990; 146(11): 702–704

9 Resection of Congenital Hemivertebra for Thoracic and Lumbar Spine

Alice Baroncini, Francesco Langella, Max Aebi, and Claudio Lamartina

Introduction

Congenital scoliosis is a rare deformity caused by a failure in the segmentation or formation of the vertebrae during the 4th to 6th gestational weeks. Hemivertebra represents the most frequent cause of congenital scoliosis and is defined as a complete failure of the formation of a vertebral body.[1] The development of three-dimensional computed tomography (CT) scans allowed a more detailed analysis of the posterior elements of the hemivertebrae, allowing for a further classification based on the level of formation of the pedicles and laminae[2] (**Fig. 9.1**). As bracing proved ineffective for correcting the deformity,[3] surgical therapy is required. Royle described the first case of hemivertebra resection in 1928, but over time other options such as hemiepiphisiodesis or local fusion without resection have been proposed. The latter two possibilities showed, however, unpredictable results. Currently, the most common technique for correcting the deformity is represented by posterior resection and fusion, as described by Ruf and Harms in 2002.[4]

In this chapter, the authors aim to describe the surgical technique and offer some insight into the possible complications and their prevention and management.

Definition and Steps of the Technique

Surgery is performed with the patient in prone position without pressure on the abdominal structures. A radiolucent operating table is required. The use of neuromonitoring (somatosensory and motor-evoked) is highly recommended, along with a cell-salvage device.

- Perform a standard midline incision to expose the hemivertebra and the adjacent cranial and caudal vertebrae and expose the pedicles and transverse processes of the adjacent vertebrae enough to allow placement of pedicle screws. For thoracic hemivertebrae, 2 to 3 cm of the attached rib must also be exposed.

- Inferior facetectomies of the hemivertebra and the cranial vertebra can be performed to increase flexibility.

- Insert pedicle screws. Particular attention should be paid when placing the screws on the concave side, as the scoliotic curve pushes the spinal cord toward this side. Place a temporary rod between the screws on the convex side to ensure stability while the resection is performed.

- Begin the resection of the hemivertebra.

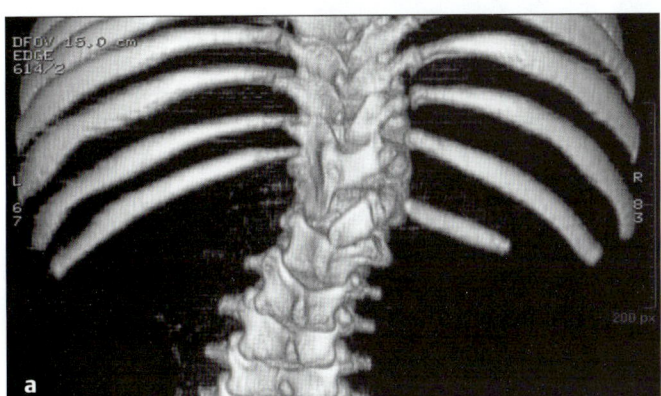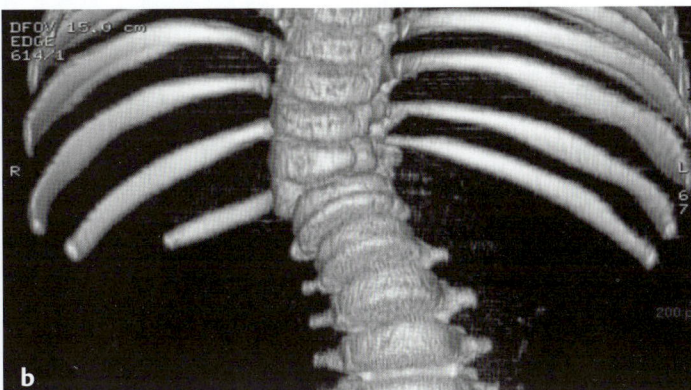

Fig. 9.1 **(a, b)** Computed tomography (CT) scan of an 18-month-old baby diagnosed with hemivertebra at the thoracolumbar junction.

First, the posterior elements should be resected (spinous process, hemilamina, inferior facet, transverse process, 2–3 cm of the attached rib in the thoracic spine). Removing the facet and transverse process will open the cranial and caudal foramina, and the nerve roots will be exposed after removing the pedicle. Epidural bleeding is to be expected at this stage. It can be controlled by bipolar vessel cautery or hemostatic agents, while bony bleeding can be controlled using bone wax.

Once the lateral side of the hemivertebra is exposed, piecemeal resection can be performed. Different instruments can be used at this stage, such as Kerrison rongeur/punch osteotomes, curettes, or drills. The dural sac and the nerve roots need to be visible during the entire resection and can be protected with nerve retractors. As the dural sac is usually pushed toward the convex side of the curve, the neural structure usually does not represent an obstacle when resecting the hemivertebra.

After removal of the bony structures, the cranial and caudal intervertebral discs and any remaining cartilaginous structures need to be resected. Careful end plate preparation is crucial to obtaining anterior fusion.

- After the removal of the temporary rod, pre-bent titanium or cobalt-chrome rods can be inserted for the final correction. The correction should be performed by compression over the screw heads until the end plates of the now adjacent vertebrae are touching. Correction by distraction over the screws on the convex side should be avoided or limited to a minimum to prevent damage to the neural structures. Small gaps can be filled with grafts obtained from the resected bone. Cages should be used to fill more significant gaps or when anterior support is required.

A nerve hook can be used to check that the nerve roots on the concave side do not impinge after compression. The correction should be checked under fluoroscopic guidance: when the correction is sufficient, the rods can be locked in the screw heads.

- To enhance posterior fusion, decortication of the posterior elements of the instrumented vertebrae is performed. The autologous, morselized bone graft obtained by the resection must be placed on the prepared posterior elements and between the transverse processes in the lumbar spine.

- After inspecting the site for bleeding and placing subfascial drainage, wound closure can be performed.

A case example is shown in **Fig. 9.2**.

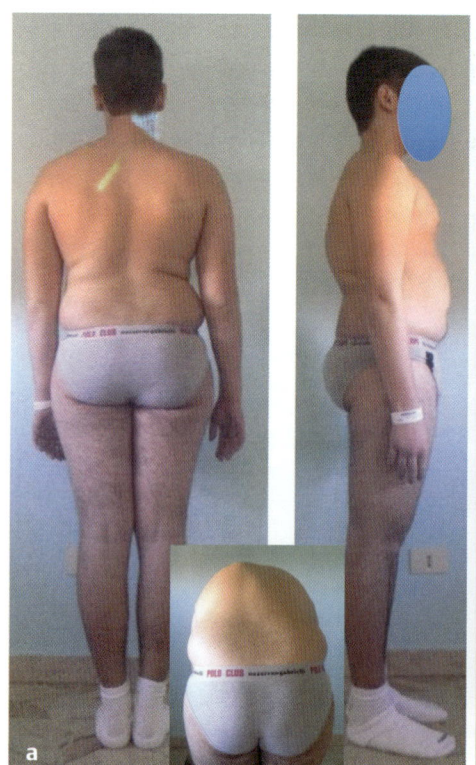 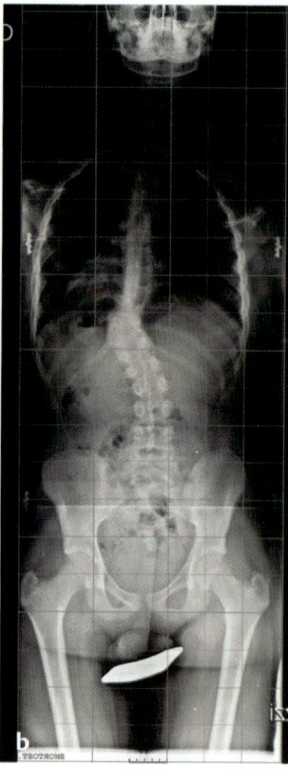 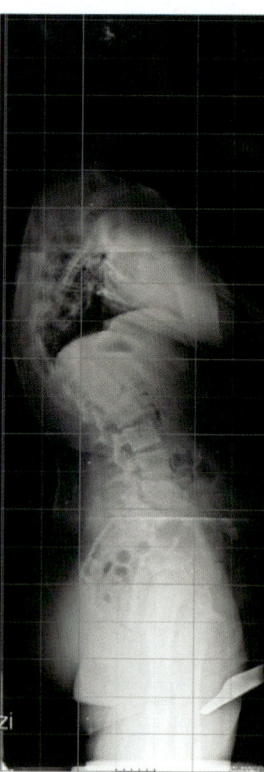

Fig. 9.2 Clinical presentation **(a)** and X-rays **(b)** of a 15-year-old boy diagnosed with T11 hemivertebra. (*Continued*)

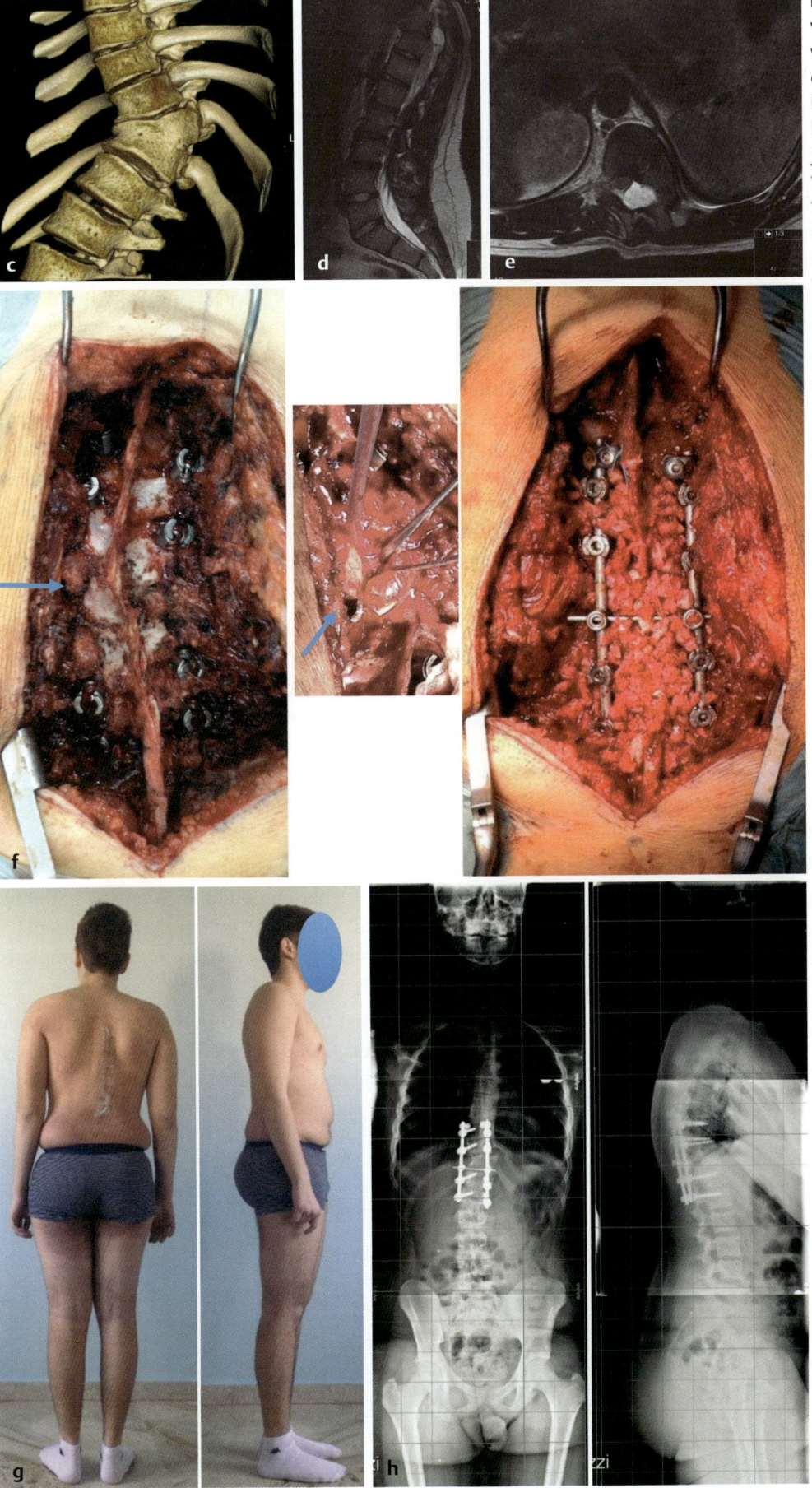

Fig. 9.2 (*Continued*) T11 hemivertebra (**c**). An arachnoid cyst was also evident at the level of the deformity (**d**). Due to hyperkyphosis and location of the hemivertebra at the thoracolumbar junction, a bisegmental fusion would not have been sufficient to warrant correction, and a longer construct was required. After exposure of the vertebrae that would be instrumented and placement of the pedicle screws (**e**), the hemivertebra was exposed while protecting the dural sac with nerve retractors (**f**) and was resected. The pre-bent rods were inserted, and the correction was performed. The autograft obtained with the resected hemivertebra was placed over the decorticated posterior aspects of the instrumented vertebrae (**g**). After surgery, the coronal and sagittal alignment was restored (**h**). This is also shown by the now symmetrical appearance of the patient's back.

Indications

Treating congenital scoliosis caused by hemivertebrae is always surgical, as conservative treatment with a brace has proved to be ineffective. Surgery aims to obtain a straight spine with a physiological sagittal alignment while keeping fusion as short as possible. However, the timing of surgery in congenital scoliosis is still debated.

As nonincarcerated hemivertebrae have a growth potential similar to that of fully formed vertebrae, the deformity is bound to progress over time.[5] In the case of a single, fully segmented hemivertebra, the rate of curve progression is 1 to 3 degrees per year. This rate increases to 2 to 5 degrees per year in the case of two fully segmented hemivertebrae. The location of the hemivertebra also represents a critical factor in determining the progression of the deformity.[6] Hemivertebrae in the thoracolumbar or lumbosacral junction typically leads to a significant trunk shift (and kyphosis in the thoracic spine).

Similarly, the upper thoracic spine hemivertebrae will present with an evident shoulder imbalance. The fastest progression rate is seen in the hemivertebrae of the thoracolumbar junction. Low thoracic or lumbar curves generally show a milder course. Three-dimensional characterization of the hemivertebra also predicts the progression rate, with fully segmented, unison hemivertebrae (a hemivertebra with exactly corresponding anterior and posterior components) showing the highest rate of progression in early childhood.[7]

These factors should be taken into account when planning the timing of surgery. As a general rule, early treatment is advisable. Observation can be prolonged in the case of curves with a slow progression or limited trunk shift (e.g., middle to low thoracic curves, lumbar curves). Conversely, early or prophylactic treatment is required in transitional areas. It is paramount to perform surgery to keep the fusion as short as possible and limit the intraoperative risks. At the same time, the curve is still somewhat flexible before secondary curves become structural.

Complication Avoidance

It is known that hemivertebrae is associated with other spine anomalies or anomalies of the central nervous system, including meningocele.[5] Thus, a preoperative magnetic resonance imaging (MRI) and intraoperative neuromonitoring are essential to perform surgery safely.

When performing the incision and the preparation of the hemivertebra and the adjacent vertebrae, it is fundamental to limit the exposure to the area that will be fused. This is because excessive exposure may lead to an unwanted junctional spontaneous fusion.

Although this will sound obvious to the experienced reader, sharp tools or hammers should not be employed when preparing the placement for the screw. In particular, on the concave side, where the dural sac is pushed against the pedicle, excellent three-dimensional knowledge of the patient's anatomy and the use of blunt tools with careful and controlled movements are required to avoid damage to the neural structures.

Once the posterior elements of the vertebra have been removed, the anterior structures, particularly the blood vessels, can be protected with a spatula or a sheet of surgicel. Starting from the exposition of the lateral aspect of the hemivertebra, the spatula can be carefully pushed anteriorly without losing bone contact. This will create a separation plane between the hemivertebra and the surrounding soft tissues, allowing the safe use of sharp tools.

Although fusion should be kept as short as possible, the construction must be long enough to ensure stability. Proximal and distal junction failure can represent a complication of hemivertebra resection. A case example is shown in **Fig. 9.3**.

Finally, fusion must be achieved in the spine's posterior and anterior aspects. A 360-degree fusion limits the risk of the crankshaft phenomenon. This is relevant in patients with large curves or subjects with open triradiate cartilages, as these present the highest risk of developing this complication.

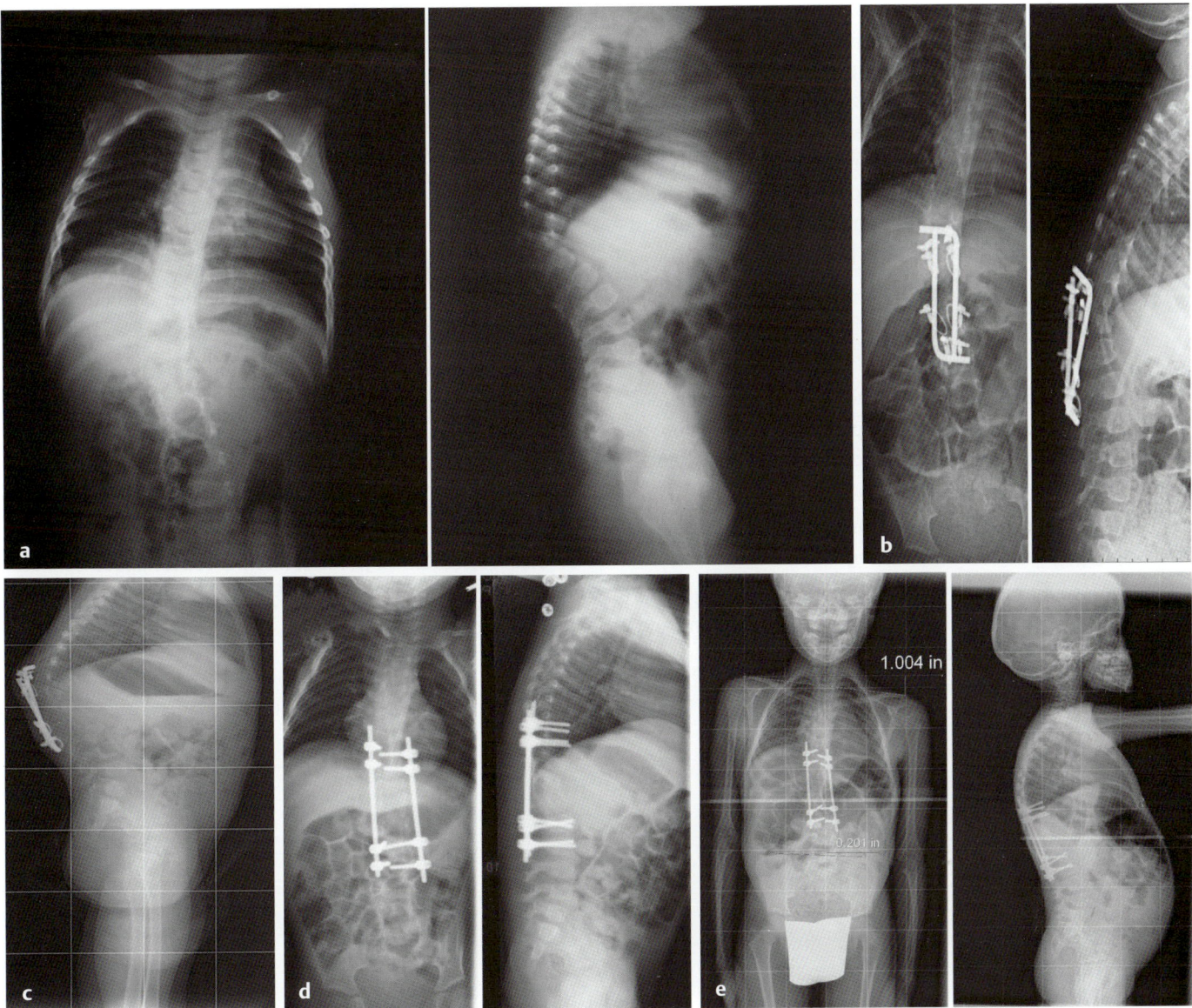

Fig. 9.3 An 18-month-old patient (same subject as in **Fig. 9.1**) underwent hemivertebra resection. The fusion was performed with a Luque construct **(a, b)**. After 4 months, a proximal failure was diagnosed **(c)**, fortunately without neurological symptoms, and a revision with pedicle screws and proximal extension was performed **(d)**. At the 5-year follow-up, the patient presented a correct coronal and sagittal alignment, even though shoulder imbalance was still present **(e)**.

Tips and Tricks

Although the pedicles of the vertebrae above and below the hemivertebra are usually fully formed, they may still be too weak in case of correction of significant deformities. In the worst case, this may lead to a fracture of the pedicle and the vertebral body. Different techniques can be employed to avoid this complication or salvage once a fracture has occurred.

- Although a hemilaminectomy of the cranial and caudal vertebra may allow for better exposure of the neural structures, a resection should be avoided or kept to a minimum to allow for a strong anchorage in case sublaminar hooks be required.

- After exposure of the posterior elements, the upper border of the cranial lamina and the lower edge of the caudal lamina can be prepared to lodge laminar hooks. The preparation takes very little time but can be helpful in quick insertion of laminar hooks in case of fracture.

- When a considerable amount of correction is expected, a three-rod technique can be performed as described by Hedequist et al.[8] After placing the pedicle screws, two hooks are placed on the convex side—one supralaminar hook facing downwards on the cranial vertebra and one intralaminar hook facing upwards on the caudal vertebra. Once the resection is performed and the two rods have been placed between the pedicle screws, a third rod can be placed between the hooks. In this way, the compressive forces on the convex side can be shared between the spine's posterior and mid/anterior elements to safeguard the integrity of the pedicles.

Key Points

- Congenital scoliosis due to hemivertebra formation requires surgical therapy. It is essential to perform surgery before the deformity becomes too rigid and before secondary curves become structural.

- The posterior resection of a hemivertebra can be safely and feasibly performed to correct congenital scoliosis.

- Fusion should be kept as short as possible; the goals are to achieve a straight alignment on the coronal plane and a physiological sagittal balance.

References

1. McMaster MJ, Ohtsuka K. The natural history of congenital scoliosis. A study of two hundred and fifty-one patients. J Bone Joint Surg Am 1982;64(8):1128–1147
2. Nakajima A, Kawakami N, Imagama S, Tsuji T, Goto M, Ohara T. Three-dimensional analysis of formation failure in congenital scoliosis. Spine 2007;32(5):562–567
3. Winter RB. Congenital kyphosis. Clin Orthop Relat Res 1977; (128):26–32
4. Ruf M, Harms J. Hemivertebra resection by a posterior approach: innovative operative technique and first results. Spine 2002;27(10):1116–1123
5. Ruf M, Harms J. Posterior hemivertebra resection with transpedicular instrumentation: early correction in children aged 1 to 6 years. Spine 2003;28(18):2132–2138
6. Hedequist D, Emans J. Congenital scoliosis. J Am Acad Orthop Surg 2004;12(4):266–275
7. Chang SY, Nam Y, Lee J, et al. Predicting the natural course of hemivertebra in early childhood: clinical significance of anteroposterior discordance based on three-dimensional analysis. Spine 2019;44(23):E1362–E1368
8. Hedequist D, Emans J, Proctor M. Three rod technique facilitates hemivertebra wedge excision in young children through a posterior only approach. Spine 2009;34(6):E225–E229

10 Vertical Expandable Prosthetic Titanium Rib (VEPTR) Procedure for Early-Onset Scoliosis

Ömer Akçalı

Introduction

Robert Campbell first performed thoracic expansion surgery in 1987 on an 8-month-old baby who was connected to a ventilator due to a costal developmental anomaly and advanced scoliosis and had no chance of treatment.[1] The implants used in the first procedure were in the form of vertical extension nails modified from Steinmann pins. Shortly after the procedure, the baby was disconnected from the device, started to breathe freely, and then mobilized as the baby grew up. With this development, the idea of relieving breathing by stretching the thorax in individuals with rib and spine anomalies that cause severe respiratory distress has found widespread support. The implant system used for this purpose has also changed over time and has gained an up-to-date and modern appearance thanks to the support of the users.

Child spine growth involves two distinct peak periods.[2] The first is the period from birth to 5 years of age. After this period, there is a slowdown in the growth rate of the spine. The second growth peak starts with puberty; after the closure of the triradiate cartilage, the growth rate increases with the onset of secondary sex signs. Around 2 years after puberty, growth slows down again and stops at the end of adolescence. These are when congenital anomalies impacting the spine show the fastest progression potential.

On the other hand, the thorax grows slightly differently compared to the growth of the spine. While the thoracic cavity has reached 30% of the adult volume in a child who has reached the age of 5, this rate reaches 50% at the age of 10 and 100% at the age of 15.[2] Thus, if chest wall growth is impaired in a child before the age of 10, it can be considered that almost half of the thoracic cavity volume may be impacted. If the child is under the age of 5, the impact on the thorax volume will be higher. Hence, congenital rib and spine anomalies that would adversely affect the growth of the thorax could cause severe restrictive respiratory failure.

Congenital spinal anomalies can cause severe thoracic deformities from a young age. Congenital absence of ribs or fusion abnormalities accompanying spinal deformities may also lead to increased spine curvature. Both spine and rib anomalies can reduce the capacity of the rib cage.

This manifestation, called thoracic insufficiency syndrome, may sometimes reach life-threatening levels.[3] The working area of the lungs may be limited due to the narrowing of the thorax caused by bone anomalies. Besides, anomalies or location disorders of the ribs in the lower thoracic region may cause diaphragmatic insufficiency as they change the diaphragm's insertion point. As a result, severe oxygenation deficiencies may occur if diaphragmatic respiration is impaired on a narrower rib cage floor. These children may become dependent on ventilators at a very young age. The expected lifespan may shorten remarkably as well. In addition to congenital spine and rib anomalies, progressive muscle diseases such as muscular dystrophy and demyelinating spinal cord injuries may also cause a similar manifestation. Campbell divided the abnormalities that narrow the thoracic cavity into three main types.[1] Type I deformities have congenital scoliosis with chest wall rib deficiencies, Type II deformities have congenital scoliosis with rib fusions, and Type III deformities have a hypoplastic thorax. He also divided thoracic hypoplasia into two groups: shortened-foreshortened (Type IIIa) and narrowed-narrowed (Type IIIb). This distinction is crucial in surgical techniques.

The vertical expandable prosthetic titanium rib (VEPTR) system aims to increase thoracic volume by expanding between the ribs, between the ribs and the pelvis, or between the ribs and the distal segments of the spine. In addition to that, the forces applied to the ribs are indirectly transmitted to the spine, helping to decrease the curvature of the spine. As the child grows, the statically locked system becomes relatively short after some time. If extending is not performed regularly, the VEPTR system can act as a tension band and increase curvature.

Indications

The only definitive indication for VEPTR is thoracic insufficiency syndrome. This is the only indication that was also reported to have been approved by the inventor of the system.[3] It has been recommended for patients who must live dependent on the device for a long time after its first use, with significant respiratory failure caused by congenital scoliosis accompanied by costal anomalies or advanced chest wall anomalies. With the introduction of implants modified from Steinman nails used in the beginning, hooks that develop over time and grip the ribs all around, and spine-pelvic fixation elements, the indications have started to expand. Successful outcomes have been reported with its use in hypoplastic thorax syndromes (such as Jarcho-Levin syndrome and Jeune syndrome).[1,4] Its prevalence, especially in European countries, has been reported to be used at an early age in other early-onset scoliosis types and congenital scoliosis without rib anomaly and neuromuscular scoliosis.[5–9]

Scoliosis that begins under 10 years of age is classically known as early-onset scoliosis and falls under the risky group for progression. In general terms, early-onset scoliosis is categorized into five groups: idiopathic, congenital, neuromuscular, thoracogenic, and syndromic.[4] In early-onset scoliosis, treatment can sometimes be very challenging, and the curvature's progression cannot be controlled. In untreated early-onset scoliosis, the patient's trunk may be short reducing thoracic capacity. Severe lung insufficiency may occur, especially since the development of lung alveoli will continue until the age of 10. Respiratory failure and death rates are higher in these patients than in treated patients.[10] Since fusion surgeries at young ages will lead to morbid effects in both spine and thorax growth, conservative approaches or approaches that allow growth are preferred. Growing rod systems or growth-regulating systems can be used in early-onset scoliosis. VEPTR is one of the systems that will enable spine and trunk growth.

The indication for VEPTR use may vary depending on the causes of early-onset scoliosis. When VEPTR application outcomes were compared in terms of etiological factors, it was revealed that the best correction outcomes in the early stages were in the idiopathic and neuromuscular patient groups, and the least correction was in the congenital group.[6] Moreover, in the same study, complications of VEPTR were as high as 45%. Complication rates are much lower in other systems that allow growth. Besides controlling curvatures and regulating growth can also be more controlled. Hence, VEPTR should not be considered as the first-treatment option in all early-onset scoliosis. VEPTR can be performed if other growth-assisting techniques cannot be used or if chest wall and rib deformities are remarkable. Considering trunk development, VEPTR is suitable for early-onset scoliosis in children under 5 to enable the growth of the rib cage, because in young children, the vertebrae may not always have reached sufficient maturation for implantation. In such cases, curvatures can be controlled by distraction from the ribs.

Description of the Technique

After the first application, significant changes have been experienced in both implants and application techniques. This chapter discusses the author's clinical experience.

Preoperative preparation is of great importance. Congenital pathologies that may be present in the canal and neural structures should be investigated via preoperative magnetic resonance imaging (MRI). Since the VEPTR system is mainly a stretch-based correction technique, neurological problems may develop in congenital anomalies such as tethered cord or diastematomyelia. Lung capacities and respiratory functions of patients should be assessed. The risk of general anesthesia and the necessity of postoperative intensive care should be considered, and necessary measures should be taken.

Implantation levels should be determined before the patient is taken to the operating room. VEPTR can be performed between the ribs and the ribs, between the ribs and the spine, or between the ribs and the pelvis. There can be more than one lateral combined application and bilateral application. For example, if the patient has congenital scoliosis accompanied by extensive costal insufficiency, it would be more appropriate to expand the thorax volume between the ribs. In these patients, if necessary, trunk balance can be achieved by distraction between the ribs and spine on the same side. However, in idiopathic, syndromic, or neuromuscular scoliosis without spinal anomalies, bilateral VEPTR application may give better results in achieving trunk balance.

The patient is placed on the operating table in the prone position. The two sides of the body are supported with pillows, and the abdomen is freed. It is vital to ensure the continuation of abdominal breathing as these children may have respiratory failure.

Neuromonitoring is appropriate since the spine, and thus the spinal cord, would need to be stretched. Since children are tiny, they can easily slide off the side supports on the operating table. It should be ensured that the anterior part of the abdomen is empty and that the fluoroscopy image can be obtained before starting the surgery.

Before starting the incision, marking the skin following the surgical plan made in the preoperative period creates convenience in terms of adaptation (**Fig. 10.1**). The attachment point on the caudal side should be between the second and fifth ribs. However, the second and third or second and fourth ribs may be preferred, depending on the thickness of the child's ribs. It is entered through a

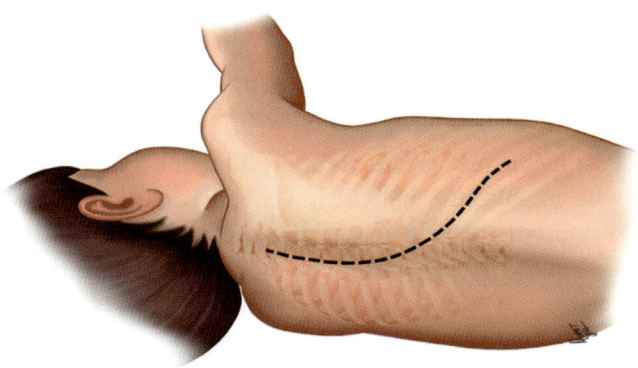

Fig. 10.1 Incision line used for vertical expandable prosthetic titanium rib (VEPTR) procedure.

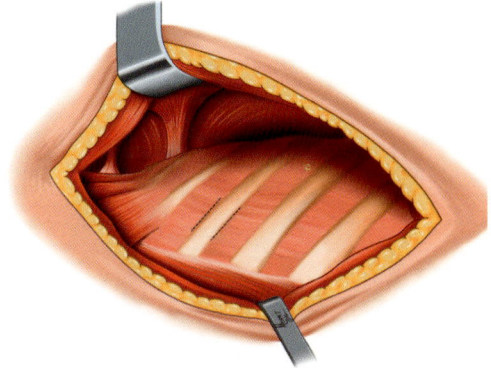

Fig. 10.2 Exposing the rib to fix.

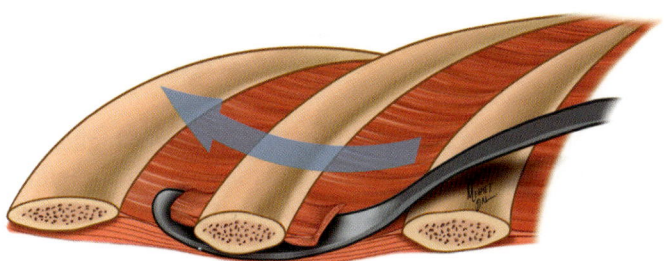

Fig. 10.3 Passing underneath the rib.

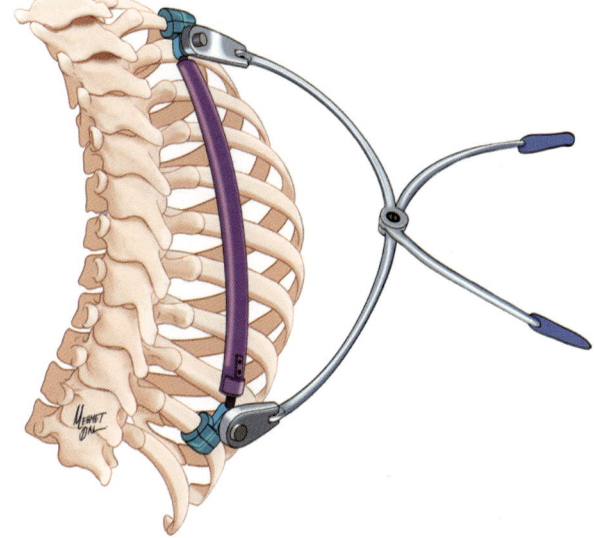

Fig. 10.4 Distraction between the upper and lower ribs.

short longitudinal incision 2 to 3 cm lateral to the midline. After the dorsal fascia is opened, the chest wall is reached by moving laterally under the trapezius muscle, which separates from the midline and between the erector spinal muscle. The rib area for attachment is just lateral to the junction with the transverse process (**Fig. 10.2**). This area is the thickest and most robust area of the ribs. It better transmits the distraction force to the spine. Care should be taken not to injure the costovertebral ligaments during the opening. Otherwise, costovertebral dislocations may occur when distraction is performed. After the pleura is carefully stripped from the parietal regions of the upper and lower ribs, it is entered under the ribs with the help of an elevator(**Figs. 10.3** and **10.4**). All-round and extensive stripping of the costal periosteum may lead to malnutrition in the bone and cause fractures.

For this reason, the periosteum should be preserved as much as possible. The cranial locking hook of the VEPTR system is placed on the superior edge of the rib mentioned above (T2). The inferior hook is also placed on the caudal edge of the lower rib (preferably T4 or T5). Meanwhile, the rod-bearing part of the lower hook extending distally is stretched caudally under the dorsal fascia. When the two hooks are brought closer to each other and locked with the compression device in the set, the proximal ribs are caught (**Fig. 10.5**).

If the distal attachment point is determined as the rib, the same procedure is applied to T11 and T12 levels (**Fig. 10.4**). Next, the ring element of the sliding piece between the distal and proximal hooks is placed. After it is distracted under the control of the scope, it is locked, and the process is finished (**Fig. 10.5**).

If the distal attachment point is chosen as the spine, a hook is generally preferred to reduce the risk of loosening. Sometimes, supralaminar hooks are used if the pedicles are thick and strong, though sometimes screws are also preferred. The rod that will enter the distal hook is first placed into the proximal distraction plate. Considering the distraction processes to be made in the future, the length of the rod should be chosen as long as possible; the lamina of the predetermined stable lumbar spine is exposed. The ligamentum flavum at the upper edge of the lamina is stripped, and the laminar hook is inserted from cranial to caudal through this gap. The appropriate size rod is placed from

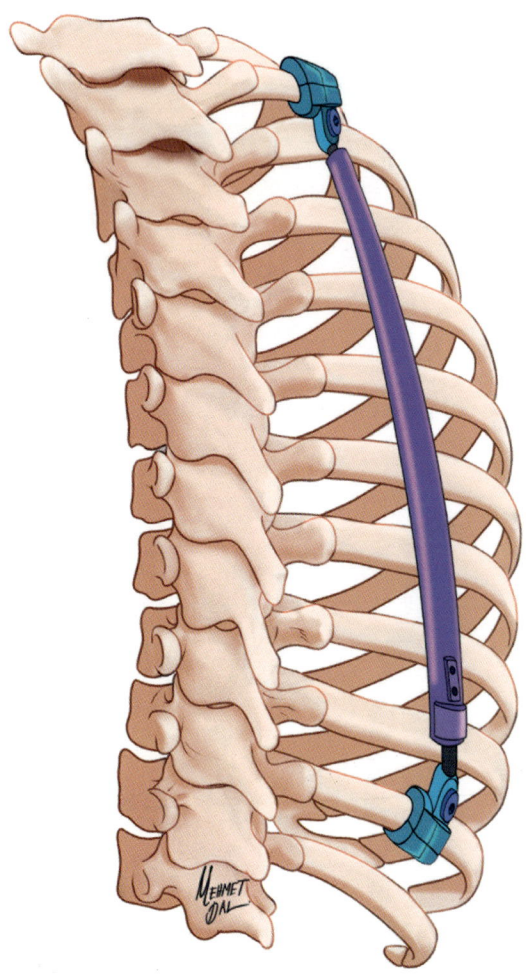

Fig. 10.5 Final position of the vertical expandable prosthetic titanium rib (VEBTR) system.

distal to proximal with the help of a chest tube or directly subcutaneously. The subcutaneous rod is inserted into the lamina hook and fixed by tightening the locking screw. The required amount of distraction is made in the scope control, the lock ring is placed, and the system is locked.

If it is decided to descend into the pelvis distally, the iliac apophysis is reached by entering just lateral to the posterior superior iliac process. The gluteal muscle fibers are stripped, and the apophysis is exposed. The iliac hook is placed close to the mid-k-point of the rear iliac wing. During this process, care must be taken not to injure the cortical bone of the iliac wing. Otherwise, hook dislocation or distal migration may occur. Following the placement of the hook, the rod, which is shaped by lordosis, is placed from distal to proximal. The two components are connected via a small incision made over the proximal VEPTR plate. The pelvic hook and rod connection are interlocked with a connector. Subsequently, an adequate amount of distraction is made to the VEPTR plate and the distal rod junction in the middle section,

and a lock ring is attached and fixed. Pelvic fixations carry a high risk of implant failure in mobilized children. Hence, patients who undergo pelvic fixation are more likely to have neuromuscular scoliosis with lower walking potential.

Postoperative corset use is often not required. The patient can be mobilized when their general condition is good. It is appropriate to make a lengthening with an interval of 6-month periods. Lengthening should be performed under general anesthesia, fluoroscopy control, and without excessive tension on the system. Extreme extensions may cause implant dislocations. During lengthening procedures, it should be noted that the primary goal of using the system is to protect the spine and rib cage and to prevent excessive thoracic collapse.

Complications and Precautions

The complication rate of the VEPTR system is higher than other growth-friendly systems. Thus, it should not be chosen as the first choice in patients for whom alternative methods can be applied. In general, the incidence of complications is reported to be remarkably high, between 45 and 80%.[1,4,5,11–13]

The most common complication is implant failure. Pelvic hooks may become dislocated or migrated at high rates, particularly in children who are beginning to mobilize. Hence, spine fixation should be preferred over pelvic fixation in children with mobilization ability. Laminar hooks may be dislocated. If attention is not paid, lamina fractures and hook dislocations may occur during distraction. Implant fractures or joint release may occur at the rod and VEPTR plate junction. In addition, proximal attachment hooks may come off the ribs. To reduce implant failures, fixation sites must be chosen meticulously, and the fasteners holding the bones must be fixed with adequate but not excessive rigidity. Implant dislocations are more common, especially in patients with thoracic kyphosis. Despite all precautions, the VEPTR system is a fixation technique with a high incidence of implant failure.

In children who have undergone VEPTR, a lengthening procedure should be performed every 6 months. If the lengthening process is prolonged due to another reason or due to the carelessness of the family, the length of the system may be short with the growth of the child. While waiting for a correction, the VEPTR system may create a tension band, bending the spine in the opposite direction.

The implants in the VEPTR system, particularly the proximal plate, are not very low profile. Therefore, pain problems or skin problems because of implant swelling and pressure on the skin are not rare.

Respiratory problems and thus immune deficiencies are common among children with costal anomalies. In addition, deep or superficial infections may occur in syndromic or neuromuscular scoliosis. It may even be necessary to remove the implants in deep infections that cannot be controlled with debridement and antibiotherapy.

Key Points

- The VEPTR system should be considered a reserve for patients who will not use other growth-friendly systems with better outcomes. It can be used as a last resort in cases where other systems cannot be performed or in case of their complications. VEPTR should not be the first choice if more straightforward and trouble-free alternatives are available.

- The upper connection point should be between T2 and T5, and if the ribs are not too thick, both ribs should be clung. The periosteum of the ribs should not be stripped too expansively and devitalized. Otherwise, rib fractures may occur more easily.

- For walking children, the spine should be chosen if the distal endpoint is possible. Hooks should be preferred as fixation material. As some movement between the hooks and the lamina can be tolerated, distal implant failures may occur less than screw fixation. In children with intact pedicle cortex, transpedicular screws can be used as well.

- It will be easier to pass the rod toward the cranial side in a child placed in prone position. Hence, the distal rod should be advanced from the bottom-up.

- It should be ensured that the ring and locking mechanism at the connection point of the proximal VEPTR plate and the rod are extended from the distal face dorsally. Thus, the procedure can be performed without excessive soft tissue injury during extensions.

- More substantial than all these surgical recommendations is assessing the patient and family. The family needs to be communicative and caring people. This system can do more injury if they cannot be counted on to come for an extension on time. For this reason, the cruciality of extension and timing should be explained.

References

1. Campbell RM Jr. VEPTR: past experience and the future of VEPTR principles. Eur Spine J 2013;22(Suppl 2):S106–S117
2. Dimeglio A, Canavese F, Bonnel F. Normal growth of the spine and thorax. In: Akbarnia BA, Yazici M, Thompson GH, eds. The Growing Spine. Berlin Heidelberg: Springer; 2015:47–82
3. Campbell RM Jr, Smith MD, Mayes TC, et al. The characteristics of thoracic insufficiency syndrome associated with fused ribs and congenital scoliosis. J Bone Joint Surg Am 2003;85(3):399–408
4. Smith JT. Bilateral rib-to-pelvis technique for managing early-onset scoliosis. Clin Orthop Relat Res 2011;469(5):1349–1355
5. Danielewicz A, Wójciak M, Sawicki J, Dresler S, Sowa I, Latalski M. Comparison of different surgical systems for treatment of early-onset scoliosis in the context of release of titanium ions. Spine 2021;46(10):E594–E601
6. Almajali A, Obeidat M, Bashmaf O, Wagokh R, Harahsheh B, Alzaben R. Early childhood scoliosis management by vertical expandable prosthetic titanium rib (VEPTR): experience of Royal Medical Services (RMS). Med Arh 2020;74(6):433–438
7. Hasler CC, Mehrkens A, Hefti F. Efficacy and safety of VEPTR instrumentation for progressive spine deformities in young children without rib fusions. Eur Spine J 2010;19(3):400–408
8. Studer D, Hasler CC. Long term outcome of vertical expandable prosthetic titanium rib treatment in children with early onset scoliosis. Ann Transl Med 2020;8(2):25
9. Konieczny MR, Ehrlich AK, Krauspe R. Vertical expandable prosthetic titanium ribs (VEPTR) in early-onset scoliosis: impact on thoracic compliance and sagittal balance. J Child Orthop 2017;11(1):42–48
10. Bachabi M, McClung A, Pawelek JB, et al; Children's Spine Study Group, Growing Spine Study Group. Idiopathic early-onset scoliosis: growing rods versus vertically expandable prosthetic titanium ribs at 5-year follow-up. J Pediatr Orthop 2020;40(3):142–148
11. Bin Majid O, Al-Zayed ZS, Alsultan AM, Altalhy A, Alsadoun NF, Al-Mohrej OA. Radiological outcomes and complications of vertical expandable titanium rib instrumentation in congenital scoliosis with or without rib fusion: a retrospective study. Cureus 2021;13(3):e14167
12. Fletcher ND, Bruce RW. Early onset scoliosis: current concepts and controversies. Curr Rev Musculoskelet Med 2012;5(2):102–110
13. Matsumoto M, Watanabe K, Hosogane N, Toyama Y. Updates on surgical treatments for pediatric scoliosis. J Orthop Sci 2014;19(1):6–14

11 Growing Rod Technique for Early-Onset Scoliosis

Rıza Mert Çetik and Muharrem Yazıcı

Introduction

Early-onset scoliosis (EOS) in children presents one of the most challenging situations in modern spine surgery. Progressive deformity of the spine in the early age group compromises pulmonary development,[1] which in turn causes thoracic insufficiency, cardiac problems, and possible early mortality.[2] With a growing amount of knowledge and experience in this subject and introduction of new treatment methods, remarkable progress has been made in the treatment of this disorder. However, treating a growing spine affects the body as a whole and presents unique challenges.

When treating EOS, the aim must be to control the deformity while preserving the potential for spinal growth and optimizing pulmonary function. Nonsurgical methods can be used with success, including different methods of serial casting[3,4] and bracing.[5] Curves that cannot be controlled by conservative methods may require surgical intervention. Early surgical fusion can control the deformity better than most techniques, but it is no longer preferred due to serious disadvantages such as decreased pulmonary capacity and trunk shortening.[1]

With early fusion out of the picture, the so-called growth-friendly techniques are mostly preferred, which can be divided into three categories: distraction based, compression based, and growth-guidance procedures.[6] The first example of distraction based systems was introduced by Moe et al which consisted of a single rod.[7] Later, development of the dual growing rod technique brought new enthusiasm into this field, and with the good initial results reported by Akbarnia et al,[8] dual growing rods have become the main surgical method for the treatment of EOS.

More recently, magnetically controlled growing rods (MCGRs) have been developed as a new distraction-based device for use in the treatment of EOS. MCGRs do not need the repetitive surgeries for lengthening, and allow outpatient noninvasive lengthenings. These devices aimed to reduce the surgical and psychosocial burdens of repeated surgeries that come with traditional growing rods (TGRs). Their superiority over TGRs may have been questioned,[9,10] but these new devices are being used increasingly every day.

In this chapter, we will focus on the surgical techniques of applying dual growing rods, both traditional and magnetically controlled.

Definition of the Technique

Preoperative Planning

Before the application of dual growing rods, proper preoperative planning is of utmost importance. The deformity should be carefully analyzed on standing anteroposterior and lateral radiographs. In our practice, traction radiographs under general anesthesia (TRUGA) are also an integral part of this treatment plan.

Proximal and distal anchor levels are chosen according to Harrington's principles, as dual growing rods are fundamentally similar to the Harrington rods, both being distraction-based systems.[11] However, just like adolescent deformities, saving motion segments with shorter instrumentations is an important focus for early-onset deformities too. Using TRUGA to choose the fusion levels has been shown to achieve this in adolescent idiopathic scoliosis.[12] In a similar effort, the "stable-to-be vertebra (StbV)" concept has been defined by Dede et al as the most proximal vertebra distal to the main curve that was most closely bisected by the central sacral vertical line (CSVL)[13]: using the StbV as the lower instrumented vertebra helps save motion segments. The surgeon must select the anchor levels on a case-by-case basis.

Surgical Technique—Traditional Dual Growing Rods

When the preoperative planning is complete, the patient is brought into the operating room and general anesthesia is induced. The patient is placed prone on the operating table. A Jackson type operating table or a Relton-Hall frame can be used for larger patients, and small patients can be placed on appropriately sized chest rolls. Proper positioning must be ensured with special attention on the sagittal alignment. Multimodal intraoperative neuromonitoring must be used. Prophylactic antibiotics are administered. Based on surgeon's preference, one or two midline incisions can be used for this procedure (**Fig. 11.1**). We will proceed with the description of the single incision technique.

A midline longitudinal incision is made. The dissection is carried down to the submuscular level, which means that the fascia is incised and the muscle is thinned throughout the incision, but subperiosteal exposure is done only on the anchor sites to prevent autofusion at the intervening segments. Careful preparation of the anchor sites is extremely important. Only the facet joints between two anchor levels, proximally and distally, should be excised—the supra- and interspinous ligaments and the facet joint capsules of the adjacent segments must be preserved. This technique limits the fusion to the anchor sites, and helps prevent inadvertent fusion and junctional problems.

Both hooks and screws can be used for the anchor sites, with at least four anchors each in proximal and distal foundation sites (**Figs. 11.1** and **11.2**). More than two segments of fixation can be preferred in patients with severe and/or kyphotic deformities and weak bone disease. In our practice, we use pedicle screws whenever possible. In their biomechanical study, Mahar et al demonstrated that screw–screw constructs had significantly higher pull-out failure load when compared to screw–hook and hook–hook constructs.[14] They also noted that adding a cross-link to the screw–screw construct did not enhance the strength. When the anatomy of the patient does not allow the use of pedicle screws, hook constructs can be used with the addition of a cross-connector as the upper foundation. When hooks are used, the so-called "claw" constructs have been used frequently on the upper foundation, with an over-the-top

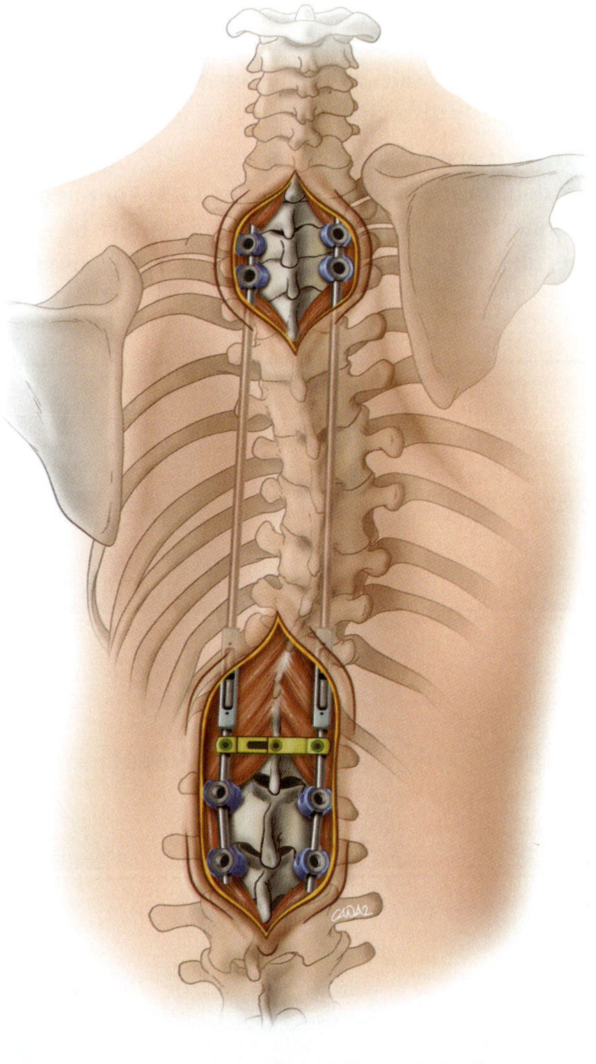

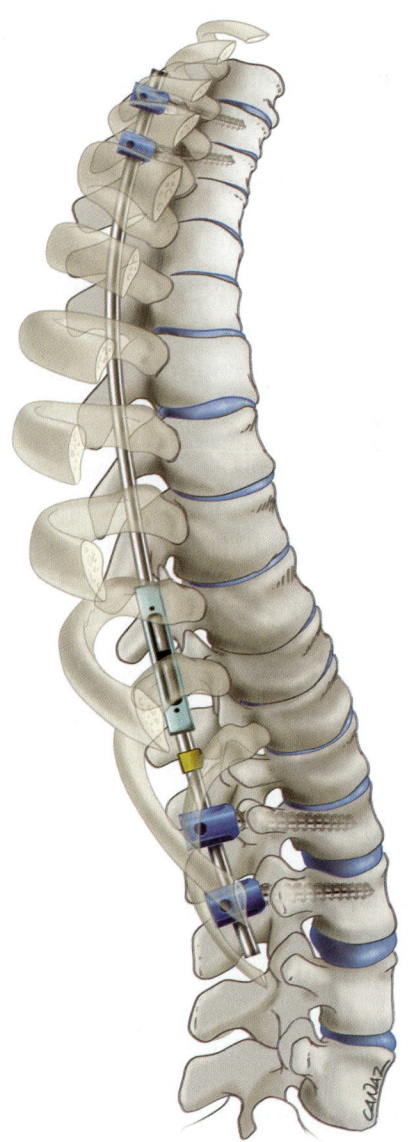

Fig. 11.1 Application of the traditional dual growing rod (GR) by the dual incision technique. The patient is viewed from posterior. Levels of instrumentation chosen are as T2–T3 proximally and L2–L3 distally.

Fig. 11.2 Sagittal view of the patient from **Fig. 11.1**.

laminar hook cranially and a sublaminar hook caudally. Rib anchors are also a viable option. Akbarnia et al showed that rib hook–hook constructs are biomechanically similar to screw–screw constructs by means of ultimate load to failure, and both were stronger that lamina hook–hook and transverse process to lamina hook–hook constructs.[15] Distal foundations are almost always instrumented with pedicle screws. When pelvic obliquity is present, as in the case of neuromuscular scoliosis, a lower distal foundation including sacrum or iliac wings may be chosen by the surgeon. Multimodal neuromonitoring should be used at the index procedure.

When implantation of the anchors with low-profile pediatric implants is done, two 4.5 mm rods are cut (either titanium or stainless steel) and contoured appropriately in the coronal and sagittal planes (**Fig. 11.2**). Larger rods (5.0 or 5.5 mm) can be used in older children, or in revision cases. The rods are then cut in the region where the connectors are going to be placed. If tandem connectors are going to be used, they must be located on the thoracolumbar junction if possible. The connectors and the parts of the rods entering them should not be contoured, and the anatomically straight thoracolumbar region of the spine makes placement easier. Another option is side-to-side connectors, which can be placed on other regions of the spine and the rods on that segment can be contoured. This approach would be more practical for kyphotic deformities.

Once the rods are ready, they are placed in a submuscular fashion, within the thinned paravertebral muscular layer. After proper correction maneuvers and the initial lengthening, the rods are secured to the anchors. The surgeon must take care not to over-correct the deformity or over-distract the rods, to avoid implant failures or immediate neurologic complications. As previously mentioned, cross-connectors can be placed if hooks are used at the proximal anchor sites, just before reducing the rods on the distal anchor sites.[16] Before closure, bone graft or substitutes are placed at the anchor sites to augment the fusion.

The two-incision technique can be used in patients where the deformity is not very rigid, the subcutaneous tissue is of sufficient thickness, and there is no severe sagittal alignment problem. In this case, the proximal and distal anchors can be joined by by-passing the rod through a tunnel created between the incisions with the help of a chest tube.

Closure of the wound is an important step of the procedure and must be done carefully. A drain may be used if deemed necessary by the surgeon. After that, paravertebral muscles and the fascia are tightly closed over the rods with number 1 Vicryl. We prefer to close the subcutaneous layer with 2-0 Vicryl, and the final layer with a 3-0 absorbable suture in a subcuticular fashion.

A thoracolumbosacral orthosis (TLSO) is used during the first 6 months after the index procedure. After solid fusion is achieved at the anchor sites, the brace can be discontinued.

Lengthenings—Traditional Dual Growing Rods (TGR)

The rods must be periodically lengthened, usually once in every 6 to 9 months. This period may change with the patient's age, comorbidities, or surgeon's preference. These procedures can be done on an outpatient basis, but it is not uncommon that even intensive care may be needed due to associated comorbidities of this patient population. Multimodal neuromonitoring is not necessary during the lengthenings if there was no neuromonitoring problem in index surgery.

The connectors are located under fluoroscopy, and a short midline incision is made. Dissection is performed to the submuscular level, and a single thick layer of tissue is created on each side, without separating the anatomical layers. Then, by dissecting laterally, connectors are reached.

If there is enough gap between the rods, the lengthening can be done inside the connector (**Fig. 11.3**). For this purpose, the connector and the upper set screws must be exposed. Connectors on both sides must be properly exposed before

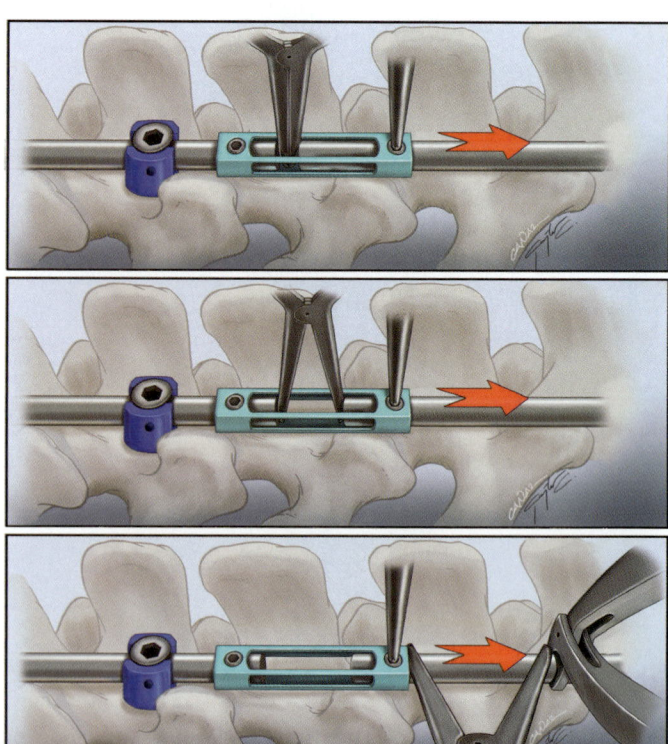

Fig. 11.3 Lengthening of the traditional dual growing rod (GR) by inserting a distractor within the connector.

the lengthening is performed. Generally, the concave side is lengthened first. Place a distractor in the distance between the rods, and firmly open it. Then slowly loosen the upper set screw and use the distractor to gently lengthen the gap by 5 to 10 mm. When the desired lengthening is achieved, tighten the screw again. If the distal rods are going to be used for lengthening, the same process is applied with the difference of loosening and tightening the lower set screws instead of the upper ones. The surgeon must be careful not to over-distract the rods. The spine will be quite flexible especially during the first few lengthenings.

Lengthening can also be done outside the tandem connectors. For this purpose, a rod holder is placed outside the connector, paying attention to leave enough gap that will accommodate a distractor. Then a distractor is placed and firmly opened between the rod holder and the connector. Then slowly loosen the set screw on the side that is going to be lengthened, and gently open the distractor 5 to 10 mm. When the lengthening is done, tighten the set screw again.

Serial lengthenings are continued until skeletal maturity is reached. Sankar et al reported that with each repeated lengthening, the T1–S1 height gain tends to decrease and called this the "law of diminishing returns."[17] The increasing rigidity of the spine can be felt by the surgeon as well, and after a certain amount of lengthening procedures, it may not be possible to distract 5 to 10 mm as planned. If there is no distraction happening at all, then the surgeon might consider finalizing dual growing rod treatment.

Surgical Technique—Magnetically Controlled Growing Rods (MCGR)

Currently, the only available MCGR device in Europe and North America is the MAGEC® (MAGnetic Expansion Control; NuVasive, San Diego, USA). This system basically consists of an implantable rod with an actuator in the middle, which is the part that includes the magnet. This actuator is activated by an external controller device, and by this mechanism distraction is performed.

Implantation of the MCGR is similar to the TGR. One or two midline incisions can be used for this procedure. Preparation of the proximal and distal foundations, and seating the rods are similar to the previously described technique of TGR implantation (see the section Surgical Technique—Traditional Dual Growing Rods). In this section, we are going to focus on the special considerations of MCGR implantation technique.

Two different actuator sizes are offered by the manufacturer: 70 and 90 mm. Based on the fact that the actuator on the rod cannot be contoured, treating surgeon must choose the best option for each patient. The 90 mm

actuator allows 48 mm of distraction while the 70 mm actuator allows 28 mm. MCGRs also have different sizes: 4.5, 5.5, and 6 mm. As in TGR surgery, 4.5 mm is mostly preferred for younger children and index surgery, while larger rods can be used in the revision setting, or in older children.

When the anchors are prepared, the concave rod is generally placed first. A temporary rod on the convex side may help with an initial reduction and easier placement of the MCGR. While contouring the rod, be careful not to bend the actuator or within 1 cm of it. Overbending the remaining proximal part to fit the rod may increase the risk of proximal junctional kyphosis (PJK), and recent literature suggests that it also negatively affects the distractive capacity as well.[18] In patients with an increased thoracic kyphosis, the surgeon may seek other alternative treatment strategies (e.g., preoperative halo gravity traction), or choose the 70 mm actuator. The surgeon must make sure that the actuators work properly before implantation.

In dual growing rod treatment with MCGRs, most surgeons prefer to use one standard (distraction toward caudal direction)/one offset (distraction toward cranial direction) rod orientation. In this setting, the rods must be lengthened separately by the external controller device, which also allows the surgeon to make adjustments on the coronal balance. Standard/standard orientation is also possible and allows lengthening both rods simultaneously, while creating higher distractive forces.[19] With either orientation, for the construct to function best, the actuators must be placed at the same level, preferably on the thoracolumbar junction.

When both anchors are ready, the rods must first be seated on and attached to the proximal anchors. Cross-connectors can be used especially if hooks are used. Then, after appropriate correction maneuvers, the rods are attached to the distal foundation and tightened. First lengthening is done before closure. Bone graft or substitutes are placed at the anchor sites to augment the fusion, and the wound is closed in an anatomic fashion. A drain may be used.

A TLSO brace is advised during the first 6 months after the index procedure, similar to TGR application.

Lengthenings—Magnetically Controlled Dual Growing Rods

Lengthening is a noninvasive procedure in MCGRs and can be performed safely in the clinic (**Fig. 11.4**). Another advantage is that the rods can be lengthened more frequently than TGRs, therefore mimicking physiological growth more closely. Most surgeons prefer lengthening the rods every 2 to 3 months, and there is no consensus in the literature about the ideal interval.

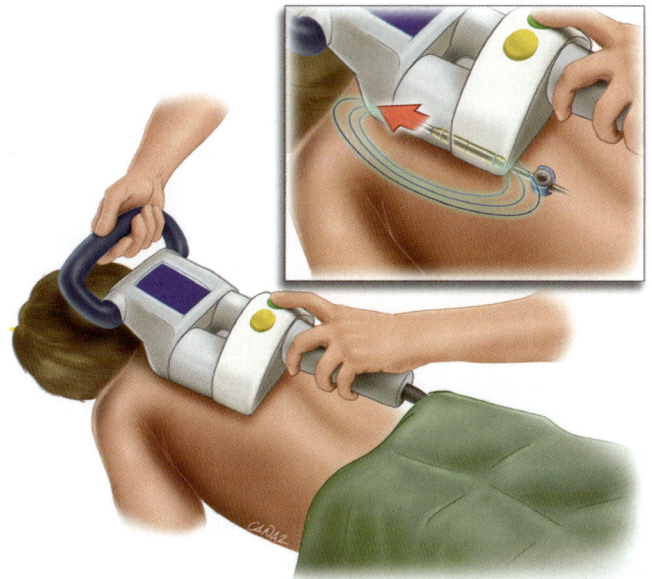

Fig. 11.4 Office lengthening of the magnetically controlled dual growing rod (GR). Please note that the handheld lengthening device is located directly above the actuators.

There are two different strategies for MCGR lengthening. The predetermined distraction length can be entered into the external controller device, and the device stops after reaching that amount. The length of distraction can be set to a standard (e.g., 2 mm for every month), or chosen according to the "tail-gate" principle. Growth charts are used to estimate the expected growth of the children, and the device is set to a distraction length that will catch up.[20] The other one is the "distraction-to-stall" strategy in which the external controller device is set to the continuous mode, and the lengthening is continued until the actuator "clunks," which indicates that the maximum force is generated and the rod can no longer lengthen. The achieved lengthening has not been shown to differ between these two techniques.[21]

To perform the lengthening, the patient is placed prone on the examination table. By using the external magnet locator device provided by the manufacturer, actuators are located and marked on the skin. Then the external controller device is placed directly over the actuators, so that the marking on the skin should be seen inside the window on the device. The controller device must be oriented parallel to the rod, which can be ensured by pointing the device toward the patient's head. Lastly, the device is turned on and the lengthening is performed, according to one of the previously described methods.

MCGR lengthening can also be performed with the patient in a sitting position. In patients with an early clunk sound during lengthening, it is recommended to repeat the magnetic lengthening attempt under light traction to be applied from the head and neck.

Indications

Indications for dual growing rod treatment should be considered together with the general treatment principles guiding EOS management. Generally, curves with a major scoliosis angle less than 25 degrees can be observed with radiographs every 4 to 6 months. Curves that are >25 degrees that show progression of >10 degrees or with a rib–vertebra angle difference (RVAD) of >20 degrees should be actively treated. When nonoperative treatment is considered, serial casting is the most frequently applied method, especially for younger children.[3,4] Bracing can also be effective in a certain group of patients with idiopathic EOS.[5] Rib head phase is also another radiographic variable that is used in estimating curve progression,[22] and a phase 2 rib head warrants treatment.

If the curve progresses over 45 degrees, operative treatment can be considered. Scoliosis angle is not the only criteria: patients with failure or inability to cooperate with cast/brace treatment and patients who show progression despite nonsurgical treatment are also candidates for surgery. Once the decision is made for surgical treatment, the surgeon must choose the most suitable method for that patient. Currently, dual growing rods, either traditional or magnetically controlled, are the mainstay of surgical treatment. Treatment with a single growing rod should only be used when the patient-specific factors do not allow the use of dual rods: previous reports showed clear advantages of dual rods in coronal plane deformity correction and lengthening when compared to single rods.[23,24]

MCGRs are taking the place of TGRs in many centers due to the previously mentioned surgical and psychosocial advantages. It is true that for most patients, indications allow the use of both devices with similar success. However, certain conditions should prompt the use of TGRs instead of MCGRs, including: (1) requirement of repeated magnetic resonance imaging (MRI) scans for the medical follow-up, (2) presence of history of metal hypersensitivity, (3) presence of implanted electronic devices (e.g., pacemaker), (4) under 2 years of age or 25 lb of weight, (5) hyperkyphosis, (6) patient with a short stature that does not allow enough space between the anchors to fit the actuators.[25] Again, in patients with obesity, the distance of the actuator from the magnet makes it difficult to transmit magnetic signals to the rod, making nonsurgical distraction impossible. This situation should also be considered a relative contraindication. Another possible concern is the revision setting. Keskinen et al reported that MCGRs do not achieve the same amount of lengthening when implanted after conversion from TGRs.[26]

Other alternatives for the treatment of EOS include vertical expandable prosthetic titanium rib devices (VEPTR) and growth guidance systems such as the Shilla and Luque-Trolley. The VEPTR system (DePuy Synthes, West Chester, PA, USA) is a titanium longitudinal rib distraction device, which is indicated for patients with primary thoracic insufficiency syndrome (TIS) or certain conditions that put the patient at risk for secondary TIS. In other words, VEPTR can be used when the primary concern is with the thoracic cage, not the spine: congenital scoliosis with rib fusions is an example.[27] Growth guidance techniques direct the spine into a more physiologic alignment, and do not need routine distractions.[28] Their use can be considered when better apical control is required.

Complication Avoidance

Treatment of EOS with dual growing rods is long term, and unfortunately not without complications. Bess et al reported the results of 140 patients who were treated with growing rods, among whom 69 had dual growing rods: 38 (55%) of these patients had at least one complication.[29] Complication rate per surgical procedure was 18%, and mean number of complications per patient was 1.2. High complication rates have also been reported with MCGRs. Lebel et al reported an overall complication rate of 66%, with 45% of the patients experiencing an unplanned return to the operating theater.[30]

The effort to avoid complications starts even before the surgery. General medical condition of the patients should be improved as much as possible prior to surgery. Certain disorders such as cerebral palsy and urinary/bowel incontinence may increase the risk of postoperative complications, and the patients/caregivers must be properly counselled.[31] Patient's age is another very important factor. Younger age at initial surgery means more operations, which in turn means more complications. Delaying the surgery by 1 year was shown to reduce the complication rate by 12%,[29] so the surgeon may consider trying nonoperative measures (e.g., casting, bracing) as long as possible.

Implant-related complications are one of the most important issues with this treatment method. Among 69 patients with dual growing rods, Bess et al reported 42 implant-related complications in 29 (42%) patients.[29] As the most frequent implant-related complication, rod fractures were seen on 22 occasions. Using the dual growing rod technique instead of a single rod may be the most important factor in reducing implant-related complications. Yang et al studied the risk factors of rod fracture in 327 patients with growing rods and reported that single rods had a significantly higher fracture rate when compared to dual rods (36% vs.

11%, $p < 0.001$).[32] This protective effect of dual rod constructs may be because of the reduced mechanical strain on a single rod. Another advantage is that unlike single rod constructs, when one of the rods break, as long as the other rod is intact, the revision can be postponed until the next lengthening. But if a single rod breaks, the revision surgery should be undertaken urgently. Another factor influencing the rate of rod fractures is rod diameter[32]: increasing the rod diameter by 1 mm decreased odds ratio by a factor of 0.6 (95% confidence interval [CI]: 0.44–0.86, $p = 0.025$). Especially after a fracture is encountered, the surgeon may consider replacing the rods with thicker ones in order to prevent further fracturing. We also recommend replacing both rods when one of them is broken. Using pedicle screws instead of hooks whenever possible is another strategy to prevent implant-related complications. Myung et al compared the complications of hooks and anchors in 159 patients with growing rods: rate of complications directly related to screws was 3.7% while for hooks it was 7.3% ($p = 0.02$).[33]

Surgical site infection is another serious complication, with rates ranging between 1.7 and 25%.[28] Bess et al reported 21 wound-related complications in 15 patients, among 69 treated with dual growing rods.[29] They also found that submuscular placement of the rods protects against wound problems, when compared to subcutaneous placing ($p < 0.05$). Other important surgical factors that increase the risk of wound infections in pediatric spine surgery are implant prominence and stainless steel implants.[31] Implant prominence may be an issue especially in smaller children, and the surgeon must be extra careful when selecting and properly contouring the implants. Good general surgical practice must never be underestimated in this population: meticulous surgical technique and good handling of the tissues is always extremely important for preventing complications in pediatric spine surgery, as in every other area of surgery.

Prevention of PJK starts at first dissection. As previously mentioned, when preparing the proximal anchor, the surgeon must be extremely careful not to harm the facet joint capsules and ligamentous structures of the adjacent segments. Other factors also increase the risk of this condition. Watanabe et al studied the risk factors of PJK and identified a lower instrumented vertebra at or cranial to L3, a proximal thoracic scoliosis of 40 degrees or more, and a main thoracic kyphosis of 60 degrees or more to increase the risk significantly.[34] Proper contouring of the rods is also very important. The surgeon must be aware that mismatch between the proximal thoracic sagittal alignment and rod contouring was identified as a risk factor for PJK in adult deformities.[35]

Despite the possible advantage of avoiding repetitive surgeries, MCGRs are not free of complications. In a systematic review of 15 studies, a mean complication rate of 44.5% and an unplanned revision rate of 33% was found.[36] In the study by Lebel et al, in addition to a 66% overall complication rate and 45% rate of unplanned return to the operating room, it was also reported that unplanned surgeries were significantly correlated with thoracic kyphosis greater than 40 degrees (Odds ratio: 5.42, 95% CI: 1.3–23).[30] Due to avoiding planned distraction surgeries, the rate of surgical site infections drops significantly with these implants. However, the ability of avoiding repeated operations has been questioned.[37] The technical considerations for preventing complications in TGRs must be followed in MCGRs as well, since these two different implants share the same biomechanical principles. Clunking is a problem that comes with the complicated design of MCGRs. Increased body habitus, older age, increased spinal heights, and less distance between the actuators (due to cross-talk) have been found to increase the risk of this mechanical issue in the early period.[38] Increased tissue thickness above the rods is another patient-related factor that might result in suboptimal distractions. The decrease in lengthening was found to be 2.1% for each millimeter of increased tissue thickness.[39] When treating patients with a large body habitus, these considerations must be kept in mind by the surgeon. Metallosis has been observed by surgeons during revisions or graduations of MCGRs, which is concentrated around the actuators and rod–anchor junctions. Serum levels of certain ions were found to be elevated in these patients, but the clinical implications of this phenomenon is not yet clear.[40] It is advised not to leave these devices in the tissue longer than necessary, and when growing rod treatment is over, they should be replaced with other instruments.

Outcomes

Current evidence proves that treatment of EOS with traditional dual growing rod allows efficient lengthening of the spine, and while doing so can also control the deformity.[8,23,41] Nearly 50% of the height gain achieved by dual growing rod treatment is provided by the index surgery.[8] On 13 patients treated with TGRs, Akbarnia et al reported that the T1–S1 height gain between post-index surgery and post-final fusion was 1.46 cm/year.[41] In the same study, the mean scoliosis angle decreased from 81 to 35.8 degrees after the index surgery. During lengthenings, the deformity increased to 39.5 degrees, which decreased to 27.7 degrees after the final fusion procedure.

The "true" spinal growth is the height gain that is measured between the index and final fusion procedures, which accurately reflects the effect of serial lengthenings of the dual growing rods. In a systematic review, results from four studies with a total of 176 patients revealed a true T1–S1 growth of 0.6 cm/year.[42] Dimeglio's data suggests that between 5 and 10 years of age, the expected T1–S1 growth is 1 cm/year,[43] which indicates that even with the gold standard treatment method, improvements are required to reach a physiologic level of spinal growth.

Studies on MCGR have reported results that are comparable with TGRs. In a systematic review, an average T1–S1 height gain of 0.9 cm/year was reported from the pooled analysis of 187 patients.[44] It should be kept in mind that for MCGR studies, the follow-up duration may be shorter than ideally expected. The "law of diminishing returns" is a well-known concept for TGR lengthenings,[17] and a similar reduction in lengthening efficiency has also been observed in MCGRs.[45,46] In their multicenter retrospective study on 47 patients with a mean 50 months of follow-up, Lebel et al reported that the mean scoliosis angle of the cohort increased from 40 to 52.8 degrees during lengthenings.[30] As evident by these results, MCGRs are comparable to TGRs by means of deformity control. Avoidance of surgical lengthenings raises the expectancy of a more comfortable treatment period for the children and family, but this presumed positive psychosocial effect on health-related quality of life has been questioned by Bekmez et al.[47] Nevertheless, MCGRs are being preferred over TGRs at an increased rate each year.

Tips and Tricks

Treatment of EOS is a race against time. Proper patient selection and timely interventions are extremely important for successful outcomes.

The surgeon must establish an effective communication with the patient and caregivers, and counsel them before the surgery. Both the patient and the caregivers must be aware of the long treatment period that lies ahead, and the high possibility of encountering complications.

A considerable portion of patients with EOS have serious comorbidities. These fragile children must be managed with extreme care, and in order to avoid complications, their medical conditions must be properly managed before the surgery.

Meticulous surgical technique is the key to preventing a problematic treatment duration. Unlike fusion procedures, dual growing rod constructs are dynamic, which makes them more vulnerable to mechanical failure. The surgeon can significantly lower the risk of failure by careful application. Traditional dual growing rods represent the golden standard for many patients with EOS, even in its most severe form.

Development of MCGRs has caused a lot of excitement among pediatric spine surgeons, and their use has been increasing especially in the developed world. Although not perfect, it is a significant improvement in the treatment of EOS. No single technique is perfect for every patient: the choice is not only between TGRs and MCGRs; there are many other surgical methods (growth guidance systems, VEPTR etc.), which all have their specific indications.

Key Points

- Dual growing rods are the mainstay of surgical treatment of EOS.

- MCGR is the most recent innovation in this field, which has been developed with the expectation of avoiding periodic surgical lengthenings and lowering complication rates.

- Correct application of the dual growing rods requires a detailed preoperative planning combined with careful surgical implantation. A successful index procedure is the key to avoiding many of the possible complications throughout the lengthening period.

- TGRs and MCGRs both share the same principle of distraction-based growth preservation; therefore, the surgical implantation techniques are similar.

- Operative treatment is generally considered in EOS when the scoliosis angle of the major curve exceeds 45 degrees. It must be kept in mind that the scoliosis angle is not the only criteria in decision-making.

- Indications for TGRs and MCGRs are mostly overlapping; however, the surgeon must be aware of certain conditions that will cause to prefer one over the other.

- Treatment of EOS with dual growing rod is a very long process, and complications may be seen in more than half of the patients. Proper counseling of the patient and the family is of utmost importance.

- MCGRs may be helpful in avoiding routine surgical lengthenings, but they are not free of complications or unplanned surgeries.

References

1. Goldberg CJ, Gillic I, Connaughton O, et al. Respiratory function and cosmesis at maturity in infantile-onset scoliosis. Spine 2003;28(20):2397–2406

2. Karol LA. The natural history of early-onset scoliosis. J Pediatr Orthop 2019;39(6, Suppl 1):S38–S43

3. Mehta MH. Growth as a corrective force in the early treatment of progressive infantile scoliosis. J Bone Joint Surg Br 2005; 87(9):1237–1247

4. Waldron SR, Poe-Kochert C, Son-Hing JP, Thompson GH. Early onset scoliosis: the value of serial Risser casts. J Pediatr Orthop 2013;33(8):775–780

5. Li Y, Swallow J, Gagnier J, et al; Pediatric Spine Study Group. A report of two conservative approaches to early onset scoliosis: serial casting and bracing. Spine Deform 2021;9(2):595–602

6. Akbarnia BAYM, Thompson GH. The Growing Spine: Management of Spinal Disorders in Young Children. 2nd ed. Springer; 2016

7. Moe JH, Kharrat K, Winter RB, Cummine JL. Harrington instrumentation without fusion plus external orthotic support for the treatment of difficult curvature problems in young children. Clin Orthop Relat Res 1984;(185):35–45

8. Akbarnia BA, Marks DS, Boachie-Adjei O, Thompson AG, Asher MA. Dual growing rod technique for the treatment of progressive early-onset scoliosis: a multicenter study. Spine 2005;30(17, Suppl):S46–S57

9. Aslan C, Olgun ZD, Ayik G, et al. Does decreased surgical stress really improve the psychosocial health of early-onset scoliosis patients?: A comparison of traditional growing rods and magnetically-controlled growing rods patients reveals disappointing results. Spine 2019;44(11):E656–E663

10. Tognini M, Hothi H, Dal Gal E, et al. Understanding the implant performance of magnetically controlled growing spine rods: a review article. Eur Spine J 2021;30(7):1799–1812

11. Yazici M, Olgun ZD. Growing rod concepts: state of the art. Eur Spine J 2013;22(Suppl 2):S118–S130

12. Hamzaoglu A, Ozturk C, Enercan M, Alanay A. Traction X-ray under general anesthesia helps to save motion segment in treatment of Lenke type 3C and 6C curves. Spine J 2013; 13(8):845–852

13. Dede O, Demirkiran G, Bekmez S, Sturm PF, Yazici M. Utilizing the "stable-to-be vertebra" saves motion segments in growing rods treatment for early-onset scoliosis. J Pediatr Orthop 2016;36(4):336–342

14. Mahar AT, Bagheri R, Oka R, Kostial P, Akbarnia BA. Biomechanical comparison of different anchors (foundations) for the pediatric dual growing rod technique. Spine J 2008; 8(6):933–939

15. Akbarnia BA, Yaszay B, Yazici M, et al; Complex Spine Study Group. Biomechanical evaluation of 4 different foundation constructs commonly used in growing spine surgery: are rib anchors comparable to spine anchors? Spine Deform 2014;2(6):437–443

16. Mundis GM, Kabirian N, Akbarnia BA. Dual growing rods for the treatment of early-onset scoliosis. JBJS Essential Surg Tech 2013;3(1):e6

17. Sankar WN, Skaggs DL, Yazici M, et al. Lengthening of dual growing rods and the law of diminishing returns. Spine 2011;36(10):806–809

18. Pasha S, Sturm PF. Contouring the magnetically controlled growing rods: impact on expansion capacity and proximal junctional kyphosis. Eur J Orthop Surg Traumatol 2021; 31(1):79–84

19. Helenius IJ. Standard and magnetically controlled growing rods for the treatment of early onset scoliosis. Ann Transl Med 2020;8(2):26

20. Mardare M, Kieser DC, Ahmad A, et al. Targeted distraction: spinal growth in children with early-onset scoliosis treated with a tail-gating technique for magnetically controlled growing rods. Spine 2018;43(20):E1225–E1231

21. Dragsted C, Fruergaard S, Jain MJ, et al; Texas Children's Hospital Spine Study Group. Distraction-to-stall versus targeted distraction in magnetically controlled growing rods. J Pediatr Orthop 2020;40(9):e811–e817

22. Mehta MH. The rib-vertebra angle in the early diagnosis between resolving and progressive infantile scoliosis. J Bone Joint Surg Br 1972;54(2):230–243

23. Thompson GH, Akbarnia BA, Kostial P, et al. Comparison of single and dual growing rod techniques followed through definitive surgery: a preliminary study. Spine 2005;30(18):2039–2044

24. Xu GJ, Fu X, Tian P, Ma JX, Ma XL. Comparison of single and dual growing rods in the treatment of early onset scoliosis: a meta-analysis. J Orthop Surg Res 2016;11(1):80

25. Varley ES, Pawelek JB, Mundis GM, Jr., et al. The role of traditional growing rods in the era of magnetically controlled growing rods for the treatment of early-onset scoliosis. Spine Deform. 2021 Sep;9(5):1465–72

26. Keskinen H, Helenius I, Nnadi C, et al. Preliminary comparison of primary and conversion surgery with magnetically controlled growing rods in children with early onset scoliosis. Eur Spine J 2016;25(10):3294–3300

27. Yazici M, Emans J. Fusionless instrumentation systems for congenital scoliosis: expandable spinal rods and vertical expandable prosthetic titanium rib in the management of congenital spine deformities in the growing child. Spine 2009;34(17):1800–1807

28. Hardesty CK, Huang RP, El-Hawary R, et al; Growing Spine Committee of the Scoliosis Research Society. Early-onset scoliosis: updated treatment techniques and results. Spine Deform 2018;6(4):467–472

29. Bess S, Akbarnia BA, Thompson GH, et al. Complications of growing-rod treatment for early-onset scoliosis: analysis of one hundred and forty patients. J Bone Joint Surg Am 2010;92(15):2533–2543

30. Lebel DE, Rocos B, Helenius I, et al. Magnetically controlled growing rods graduation: deformity control with high complication rate. Spine 2021;46(20):E1105–E1112

31. Glotzbecker MP, Riedel MD, Vitale MG, et al. What's the evidence? Systematic literature review of risk factors and preventive strategies for surgical site infection following pediatric spine surgery. J Pediatr Orthop 2013;33(5):479–487

32. Yang JS, Sponseller PD, Thompson GH, et al; Growing Spine Study Group. Growing rod fractures: risk factors and opportunities for prevention. Spine 2011;36(20):1639–1644

33. Myung KS, Skaggs DL, Johnston CE, et al. The Use of Pedicle Screws in Children 10 Years of Age and Younger With Growing Rods. Spine Deform. 2014 Nov;2(6):471–4

34. Watanabe K, Uno K, Suzuki T, et al. Risk Factors for Proximal Junctional Kyphosis Associated With Dual-rod Growing-rod Surgery for Early-onset Scoliosis. Clin Spine Surg. 2016 Oct;29(8):E428–33

35. Yan P, Bao H, Qiu Y, et al. Mismatch between proximal rod contouring and proximal junctional angle: a predisposed risk factor for proximal junctional kyphosis in degenerative scoliosis. Spine 2017;42(5):E280–E287

36. Thakar C, Kieser DC, Mardare M, Haleem S, Fairbank J, Nnadi C. Systematic review of the complications associated with magnetically controlled growing rods for the treatment of early onset scoliosis. Eur Spine J 2018;27(9):2062–2071

37. Teoh KH, Winson DM, James SH, et al. Do magnetic growing rods have lower complication rates compared with conventional growing rods? Spine J 2016;16(4, Suppl):S40–S44

38. Cheung JPY, Yiu KKL, Samartzis D, Kwan K, Tan BB, Cheung KMC. Rod lengthening with the magnetically controlled growing rod: factors influencing rod slippage and reduced gains during distractions. Spine 2018;43(7):E399–E405

39. Gilday SE, Schwartz MS, Bylski-Austrow DI, et al. Observed length increases of magnetically controlled growing rods are lower than programmed. J Pediatr Orthop 2018;38(3):e133–e137

40. Cheung JPY, Cheung KM. Current status of the magnetically controlled growing rod in treatment of early-onset scoliosis: what we know after a decade of experience. J Orthop Surg (Hong Kong) 2019;27(3):2309499019886945

41. Akbarnia BA, Breakwell LM, Marks DS, et al; Growing Spine Study Group. Dual growing rod technique followed for three to eleven years until final fusion: the effect of frequency of lengthening. Spine 2008;33(9):984–990

42. Wijdicks SPJ, Tromp IN, Yazici M, Kempen DHR, Castelein RM, Kruyt MC. A comparison of growth among growth-friendly systems for scoliosis: a systematic review. Spine J 2019;19(5):789–799

43. Dimeglio A, Canavese F. The growing spine: how spinal deformities influence normal spine and thoracic cage growth. Eur Spine J 2012;21(1):64–70

44. Guan D, Zhang Y, Xu J. Clinical Outcome of Magnetically Controlled Growing Rod in Early-onset Scoliosis: A Systematic Review. Clin Spine Surg. 2020 May;33(4):150–5

45. Ahmad A, Subramanian T, Panteliadis P, Wilson-Macdonald J, Rothenfluh DA, Nnadi C. Quantifying the "law of diminishing returns" in magnetically controlled growing rods. Bone Joint J 2017;99-B(12):1658–1664

46. Lebon J, Batailler C, Wargny M, et al. Magnetically controlled growing rod in early onset scoliosis: a 30-case multicenter study. Eur Spine J 2017;26(6):1567–1576

47. Bekmez S, Afandiyev A, Dede O, Karaismailoğlu E, Demirkiran HG, Yazici M. Is magnetically controlled growing rod the game changer in early-onset scoliosis? A preliminary report. J Pediatr Orthop 2019;39(3):e195–e200

Part III

Spinal Osteotomy Techniques

12 Posterior Column Osteotomy

Can Yaldız, Yahya Güvenç, and Onur Yaman

Introduction

Posterior column osteotomy (PCO) is a surgical method that is used to correct spinal deformities. It is also called as Smith-Petersen osteotomy (SPO) or Ponte osteotomy.[1-5] Smith-Petersen first defined this procedure in 1945. In 1984, Ponte described a very similar technique in cases of Scheuermann's kyphosis.

There are several PCO techniques described in the literature. Although some of the related procedures in scientific publications are similar, they are named differently. For example, SPO, opening wedge osteotomy, Chevron osteotomy, and extension osteotomy are identical. Ponte osteotomy, Briggs osteotomy, and polysegmental osteotomy are similar to each other too. For this reason, osteotomy classifications have been developed in recent years. Despite the classifications, many spine surgeons still apply the most commonly known osteotomy techniques in their surgeries and describe them with known names. In this chapter, the authors will discuss the PCO.

Pedicle subtraction osteotomy and Ponte osteotomy have been developed to shorten and straighten the posterior column significantly. While Ponte osteotomy is more commonly used for the thoracic region, SPO is described for the lumbar area. However, it has been stated that it can be used both in the lumbar and thoracic regions. It has been described for biomechanically the same purpose as an shortening posterior column. However, the location of the inferior and superior articular processes is different in the lumbar and thoracic regions. Therefore, adapting the SPO osteotomy described for the lumbar region in the thoracic region is not sufficient to obtain the desired correction.

For this reason, shortening osteotomy in the thoracic region should be different from the lumbar area. When we look at its historical development, it is seen that SPO was described in 1945, and Ponte osteotomy was described in 1984.[1,2] However, using these widely used osteotomy techniques interchangeably in the literature has led to conceptual confusion.[6,7] For this reason, the Ponte technique was re-described in an article published by Ponte in 2018.[8]

Difference Between Smith-Petersen and Ponte Osteotomies

SPO and Ponte osteotomy are release of posterior spinal articulations in the presence of a mobile disc to increase the flexibility of spinal deformities. SPO is used for flexion-type deformity correction with fused disc spaces. Fracture is created along the fused discs. Ponte osteotomy is a method applied with posterior compression along the unfused disc spaces of the kyphotic deformity.

PCO is used for the following indications[5]:

- It enables correcting the spinal deformity in the coronal and lordosis planes.
- PCO is a less invasive and less morbid method than other procedures.
- It may be applied at more than one level by loosening spinal segments.
- It is not three-column osteotomy; it is helpful for minor and single-plane deformities. In addition, operating time is shorter and causes less morbidity.
- It is easier for less experienced surgeons.
- It is used for symmetric shortening of the posterior column.
- Sagittal corrections obtained per level are:
  - 10 to 15 degrees per level
  - 1 degree/mm of bone resected

PCO provides approximately 10 degrees of correction for each spinal level. Therefore, around 1 mm of resection would result in 1 degree of correction (**Fig. 12.1**).[1-4,9]

Surgical Technique

Preoperative Planning

Preoperative evaluation is one of the essential steps in osteotomy. It should be done in detail to reduce perioperative and postoperative complications. A detailed neurological examination of the patient is required. If the patient has neurological deficit, the source of the neurological deficit

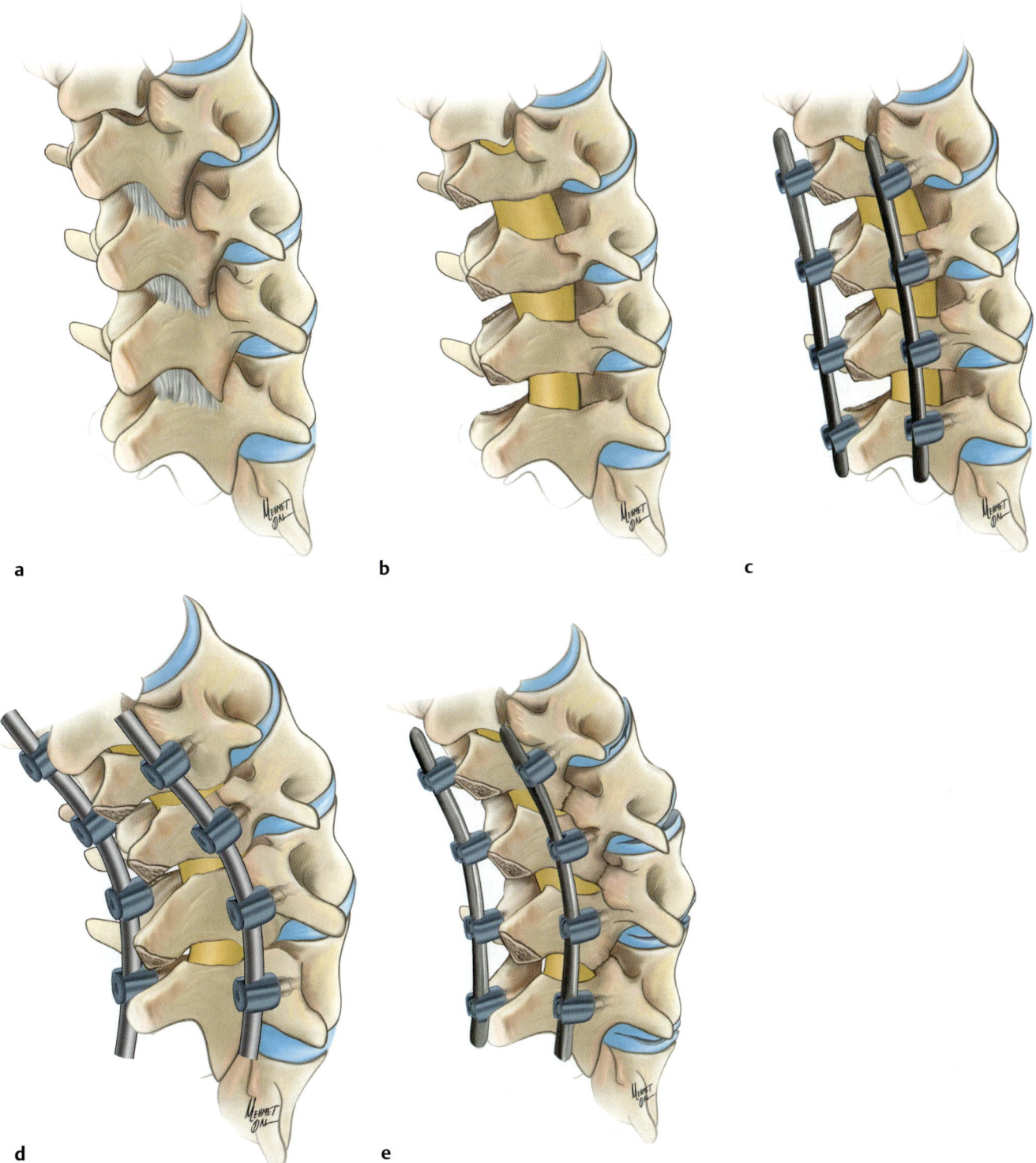

a   b   c

d   e

Fig. 12.1 Posterior column osteotomy is done by removal of inferior and superior articular processes, interspinous and supraspinous ligaments, and a part of the laminae in different degrees **(a, b)**. After placing pedicle screws and rods **(c)**, posterior compressive forces are applied to shorten the posterior column and approximate the remaining articular processes **(d)**. This approach is more like Ponte osteotomy. In case the anterior longitudinal ligaments are opened and anterior disc heights are increased **(e)**, this osteotomy can be called as Smith-Petersen osteotomy.

should be investigated. Preoperative radiological imaging, such as X-ray and computed tomography (CT) and sometimes magnetic resonance imaging (MRI), is required.

The osteotomy levels should be determined before the operation if the neurological deficit is secondary to the deformity. For example, in a patient with thoracic or lumbar kyphotic deformity, the angle of the kyphotic deformity affects the level of osteotomy that will be performed. An insufficient number of Ponte osteotomy levels may cause an insufficient correction in advanced kyphotic angulation. In addition, it may cause an increase in the load on the instrument made in the posterior. This may cause complications such as instrumentation failure, fracture, and screw pull-out. In addition, the existing neurological deformity also affects the width of the decompression area. Therefore, if a posterior closure osteotomy is to be performed in the presence of a neurological deficit in the patient, it should be Ponte osteotomy instead of SPO.

Choosing the right osteotomy and applying the right and adequate level of osteotomy are required. We need sagittal and pelvic parameters when making these choices. Preoperative global balance, sagittal and coronal balance, and cervical, thoracic, and lumbar Cobb angles of the patient should be evaluated as a whole (**Fig. 12.2**). The targeted measurements after surgery should be determined based on these measurements. It will be revealed which osteotomy is needed to achieve the targeted measurements. In addition, with the help of these measurements, the level of osteotomy will be determined.

Classic protractors can be used to make these measurements. In addition, many radiological examinations are evaluated in a digital environment with developing technology. Many spinal angle measurement applications are available to make measurements in a digital environment. Measurements can be made using these applications (**Fig. 12.2**). Before the patient enters the operating room, the level of instrumentation, the type, and the number of osteotomies to be performed should be determined preoperatively.

In addition, neuromonitoring should be used during surgery. First, there should be quality neuromonitoring, including transcranial motor evoked potential (tcMEP) and somatosensory evoked potential (SSEP).

Definition of the Technique

Position

- The patient is placed on the operating table in prone position.

- The abdominal region should stay empty to prevent venous hemorrhages during surgery.

Surgical Technique

SPO consists of resection between the lumbar facet joints and separation of the ligamentum flavum from the lower edge of the lamina and where it attaches to the joint. Lamina resection is not performed in SPO.

For Ponte osteotomy, resection is performed between the facet joints, but this resection is wider than the resection performed in SPO. In addition, wide laminectomy and complete resection of ligamentum flavum are performed in Ponte osteotomy (**Fig. 12.1**).

Compression maneuver to the posterior area is performed in the Ponte region where the implant is placed. This technique provides posterior shortening, and anterior lengthening occurs in the posterior and the anterior (**Fig. 12.1**).

The steps of the surgical procedure are as follows:
- The surgical level is determined with fluoroscopy.
- Following skin incision, paravertebral muscles are skimmed subperiosteally.
- Spinous processes of the level, bilateral laminae, and facets are revealed (**Fig. 12.1**).
- The inferior part of the spinous process and the following interspinous ligament are removed through a rongeur.
- Ligamentum flavum is separated from the attached points at the inferior and superior laminae.
- It is completely excised with the aid of Kerrison rongeur. It is essential not to hurt the dura during this excision (**Fig. 12.1**).
- Hemorrhages in epidural venous structures, if present, are stopped with the aid of bipolar coagulation Surgicel or Spongostan.
- After the dura is revealed, facet joints are partially removed with Kerrison rongeur or high-speed drill (**Fig. 12.1**).
- Transpedicular screws are placed at osteotomy segments (**Fig. 12.1**).
- The posterior column is closed with the aid of a compressor or hyperextension of the operating table (**Fig. 12.1**).

Complication Avoidance

- *Epidural hemorrhage* is usually seen during flavectomy and facetectomy, particularly when the upper part of the

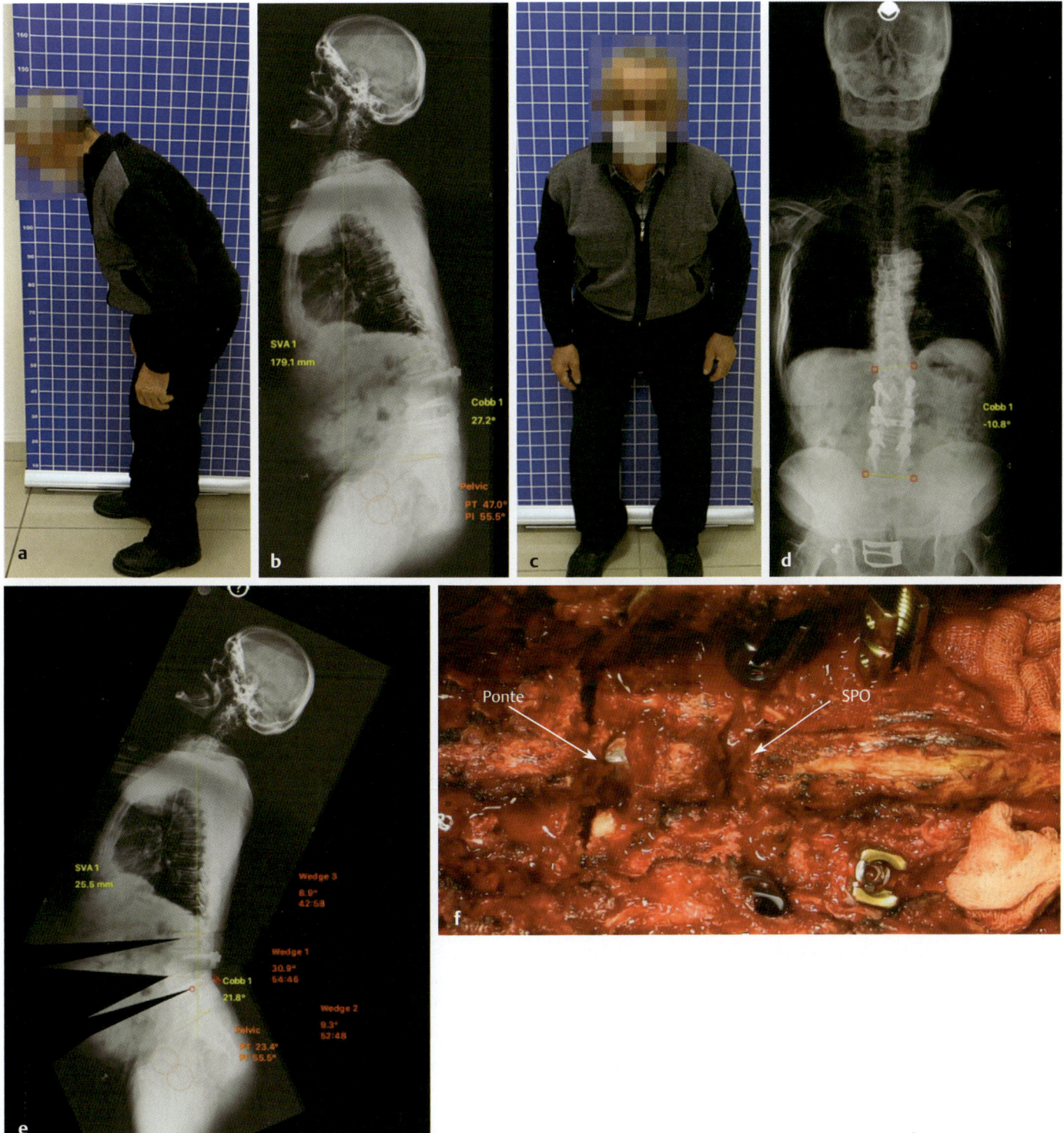

Fig. 12.2 A 67-year-old male patient applied to our outpatient clinic with complaints of low back pain, neurogenic claudication, difficulty in walking, and anteflexion posture. He had a history of lumbar spinal stenosis and a surgery involving L2–L4 stabilization 8 years ago. The patient had a kyphotic posture **(a, c)**. A preoperative whole-spine radiogram was taken to evaluate the kyphotic deformity **(b)**. Preoperative parameters were: sagittal vertical axis (SVA) = 17 cm, lumbar kyphosis angle = 27 degrees **(b)**. The preoperative coronal Cobb angle was 10.8 degrees **(d)**. Parametric measurements of the patient were evaluated in the digital environment with the help of assistive applications and amount of correction was planned **(e)**. The necessary osteotomy types and levels were decided to restore sagittal balance and provide lumbar lordosis. During revision surgery, the instruments placed during the previous surgery were removed. The kyphotic lateral fusion bone bar was released at all levels with a high-speed drill. T11–S1 posterior instrumentation, T12–L1 and L1–L2 Ponte osteotomy, and L2–L3 **Smith-Petersen osteotomy** (SPO) were performed **(f)**. (*Continued*)

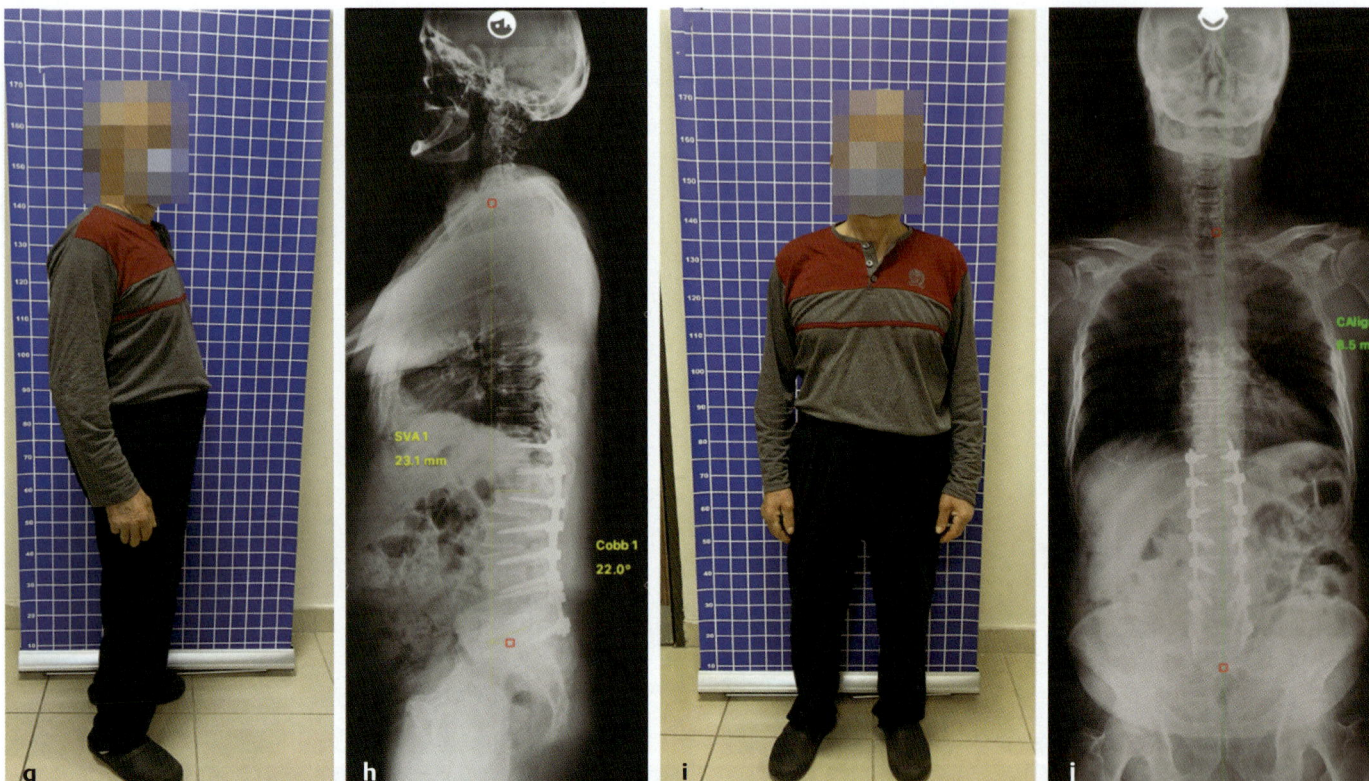

Fig. 12.2 (*Continued*) The authors observed the improvement of postoperative sagittal balance: SVA became 2 cm, lumbar kyphosis turned into lordosis, and the Cobb angle became 22 degrees **(h, j)**. The patient's postoperative posture improved, and his complaints resolved **(g, i)**.

inferior spine is removed. Hemorrhage problems may be overcome through bipolar cautery or compression with Spongostan. Too much compressive substance should not be used to prevent cord compression.

- *Neural compression*: Compression done to correct kyphosis would cause foraminal narrowing. So, root compression may develop in the foramen. This problem may be resolved with a large facetectomy.

- *Injury warning on the monitor* usually develops during a correction or insufficient decompression. This problem may be resolved with a large facetectomy.

- Removal of more anterior discs than necessary is usually seen in inexperienced surgery. The problem may be resolved by placing a graft in the anterior disc space.

Key Points

- PCO enables a 10-degree correction at every level.
- The anterior column is opened when the posterior column is closed.
- Care should be taken to avoid epidural venous hemorrhage.
- The posterior column may be decompressed by putting the table in deflexion without loading the system.

References

1. Smith-Petersen MN, Larson CB, Aufranc OE. Osteotomy of the spine for correction of flexion deformity in rheumatoid arthritis. J Bone Joint Surg 1945;27(1):1–11
2. Ponte A, Vero B, Siccardi GL, eds. Surgical Treatment of Scheuermann's Hyperkyphosis. Bologna: Aulo Gaggi; 1984
3. Shufflebarger HL, Clark CE. Thoracolumbar osteotomy for postsurgical sagittal imbalance. Spine 1992;17(8, Suppl): S287–S290
4. Cho KJ, Bridwell KH, Lenke LG, Berra A, Baldus C. Comparison of Smith-Petersen versus pedicle subtraction osteotomy for the correction of fixed sagittal imbalance. Spine 2005;30(18): 2030–2037, discussion 2038
5. Duan PG, Mehra RN, Wang M, Chou D. Posterior column osteotomy of the lumbar spine: 2-dimensional operative video. Oper Neurosurg (Hagerstown) 2020;19(4):E395
6. Holewijn RM, Schlösser TP, Bisschop A, et al. How does spinal release and Ponte osteotomy improve spinal flexibility? The law of diminishing returns. Spine Deform 2015;3(5):489–495
7. Wiemann J, Durrani S, Bosch P. The effect of posterior spinal releases on axial correction torque: a cadaver study. J Child Orthop 2011;5(2):109–113
8. Ponte A, Orlando G, Siccardi GL. The true Ponte osteotomy: by the one who developed it. Spine Deform 2018;6(1):2–11
9. Cheung ZB, Chen DH, White SJW, Kim JS, Cho SK. Anterior column realignment in adult spinal deformity: a case report and review of the literature. World Neurosurg 2019;123: e379–e386

13 Ponte Osteotomy

İsmail Bozkurt, Salim Şentürk, and Pedro Berjano

Introduction

Surgical management of spinal deformity has always been a complex problem. With the advancement in surgical approaches, the 20th century has seen tremendous surgery-related innovations.[1] However, each spinal deformity case is unique in its variables requiring equally unique approaches, surgical interventions, and instrumentation. The surgical approach aims to achieve the sagittal and coronal balance of the spine and pelvis, relieve pain, and prevent the deformity and symptoms from worsening. The instrumentation alone or with facet or ligament release is usually insufficient in correcting the deformity in these cases requiring spinal osteotomies.[2]

Although osteotomies were originally performed in anterior or anteroposterior approaches, with advanced surgical management and the spread of training for spinal surgeons, complex osteotomies are frequently performed in most clinics with a posterior-only approach. The advances in osteotomy techniques have caused some confusion as the techniques differed in slight details at times—the degree of posterior element resection, surgical procedure, type of pathology treated, etc.[3] For instance, the technique covered in this chapter has been interchangeably labeled as Smith-Petersen technique, although there are apparent differences between them. This chapter will focus on the osteotomy described by Ponte in 1984 to correct Scheuermann's kyphosis (SK),[4] and the authors will discuss additional use cases. Ponte proposed that hyperkyphosis consists of a short anterior column and a lengthened posterior column. At that time, the most accepted treatment for this condition was an anterior release and graft followed by posterior correction and fusion. In Ponte's view, preserving the anterior column and its load-sharing capacity while substantially shortening the posterior column would suffice for a stable correction, which remains the current practice for this condition.

Definition of the Technique

Ponte's osteotomy (PO), first described by Alberto Ponte in 1984 for the treatment of SK, is a resection osteotomy of the posterior column of the spine associated with shortening maneuvers on the posterior column. Although it was initially described to treat deformities in the thoracic spine, it can be applied to the treatment of sagittal, coronal, and combined deformities of the cervical[5] and lumbar spine. Some confusion exists regarding the distinction between PO and Smith-Petersen's osteotomy (SPO), the latter described for treating ankylosing spondylitis (AI). In both cases, the osteotomy is performed on the posterior column, and in both cases, the posterior column is shortened. The difference remains in the behavior of the anterior column: while in SPO, the anterior column is lengthened (typically in the fused and fragile bone of the vertebral bodies in AI), in PO, lengthening of the anterior column is avoided. Although some authors have reserved the term PO for posterior column osteotomies in the thoracic spine and SPO for those in the lumbar spine, it is our opinion that posterior shortening osteotomies without extension fracture of the anterior column should be identified as POs (independently of the spinal segment treated). In contrast, those coupled with extension fracture of the anterior column should be referred to as SPOs.[6]

Successful corrections with POs can be obtained under the condition that mobility is preserved or can be obtained at the disc at each level. Thus, anterior fusion or ankylosis should be ruled out with appropriate imaging (bolster extension X-rays or computed tomography [CT] scan).

During preoperative planning, the levels of the osteotomies are determined. In SK, three to six POs on consecutive levels centered on the apex of the kyphotic deformity are usually performed. In adult severe kyphosis cases, POs can be needed at virtually every level in the kyphotic area. In adult lumbar hypolordosis, POs are usually performed at every lumbar level. In collapsed, kyphotic, or air-filled discs, interbody cages are implanted to increase the correction. POs can help improve the flexibility of severe and rigid idiopathic scoliosis cases to obtain better correction. In these cases, the osteotomies are performed at four to six levels, centered in the apex of the stiff coronal curve.

Although osteotomies can be performed at any step of the surgical procedure, a sequence consisting of exposure, hemostasia, pedicle-screw implantation, preparation of rods, osteotomies, correction, decortication of fusion bed, and grafting is often the most efficient in terms of blood loss and hemodynamical stability of the patient.

A classical midline approach with subperiosteal exposures of the affected levels and one vertebra above and below is performed. The ligamentous structures of the levels above and below should be spared (**Fig. 13.1a**). PO is a full-thickness, side-to-side, segmental resection of the posterior column of the spine. The spinous process's inferior aspect and the interspinous and supraspinous ligament are removed using a standard rongeur. The removal of the base of the spinous processes allows for better visualization of the osseous borders. Ligamentum flavum is clearly visualized and thinned in the midline (where the posterior fat triangle protects the dura) using a Luer's rongeur. The midline raphe between the yellow ligaments is identified, and the yellow ligament is bilaterally removed in its totality using a small Kerrison rongeur while paying attention not to damage the dura. The descending facets are cut in line with the inferior border of the lamina with an osteotome, a high-speed burr, or a piezoelectric saw. After this, the ascending facets are resected from medial to lateral with a small Kerrison rongeur keeping its foot in contact with the ventral face of the facet to avoid damage to the epidural veins (which causes substantial bleeding) and the exiting root. The ascending facet removal is continued until no bony resistance is felt laterally. A nerve hook is used to ensure that the upper tip of the ascending facet has not been left "floating" in the foramen. Laminectomy is usually unnecessary as a 5 to 8 mm gap can be obtained by yellow ligament and facet resection. Preserving the lamina is advantageous as it allows

for a smaller opening after the closure of the osteotomy and a larger fusion bed (**Fig. 13.1b**) and preserves the laminae's mechanical resistance in case sublaminar wires or bands need to be employed. After completing the osteotomy, adequately sized (usually 0.5 × 4 cm) compressed cylinders of gelfoam are gently placed on the osteotomies to obtain hemostasis. In severe deformities, radical facetectomy and laminectomy extending cranially and caudally to the level of pedicles around the disc may be needed. At the end of the PO series, the spine will show a regular pattern of horizontal or slightly V-shaped osteotomies (**Figs. 13.2** and **13.3**).

Following the osteotomy session, posterior instrumentation should be ensured for proper correction and maintenance (**Fig. 13.1c**). The gaps created by the osteotomy should now allow for posterior flexion of the spine. However, this should be gradual, beginning at the apex and working toward the end of the deformity. In addition, semirigid rods may allow for better compression at each level,[5] and this should be distributed evenly throughout the deformity (**Fig. 13.1d**).

Indications

Although originally developed for the correction of thoracic hyperkyphosis, specifically SK (**Fig. 13.4**), the amount of release allowed by PO has proven to be useful in treating other spinal deformities in both the sagittal and coronal planes. It is indicated in severe (>70 degrees) and stiff curves in idiopathic scoliosis,[7,8] especially in mature

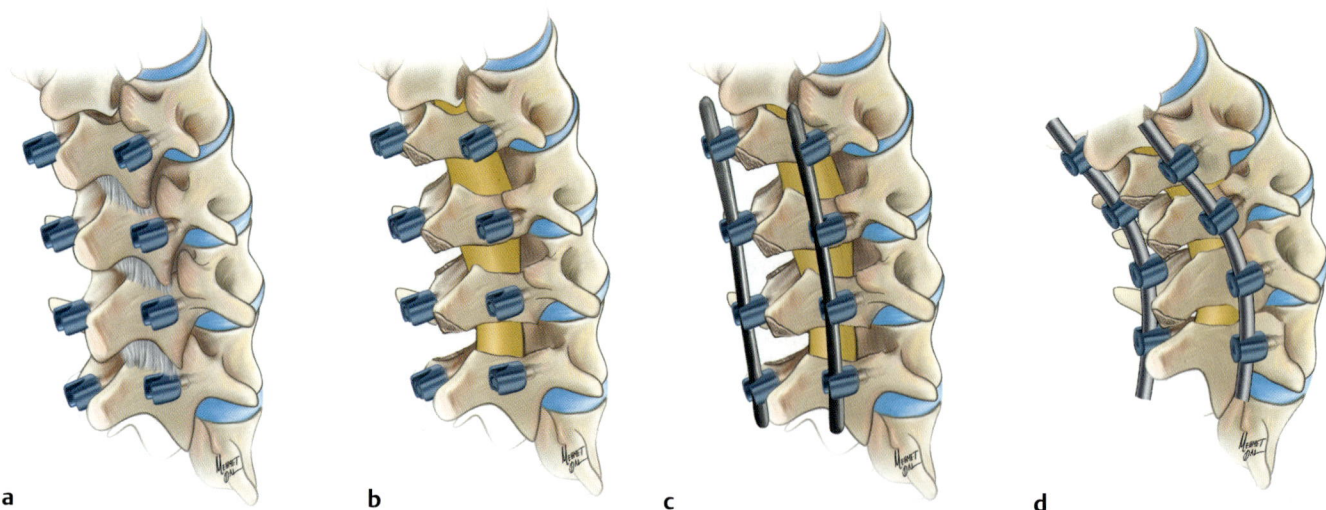

a   b   c   d

Fig. 13.1 Subperiosteal exposure should allow for a clear assessment of the vertebral anatomy, soft tissue-free fusion bed, and identification of the landmarks for implants and osteotomy **(a)**. Note the resection of facet joints, laminae, ligamentum flavum, and the base of spinous processes **(b)**. In situ posterior transpedicular instrumentation **(c)**. The amount of correction achieved by segmental correction of affected levels via a lordotic rod. Note the closure of the gaps, which allows for adequate lordosis **(d)**.

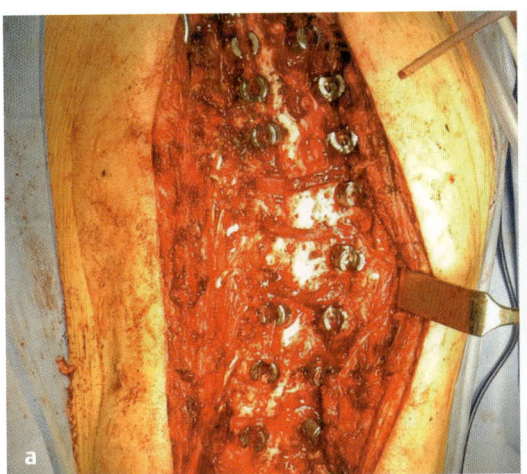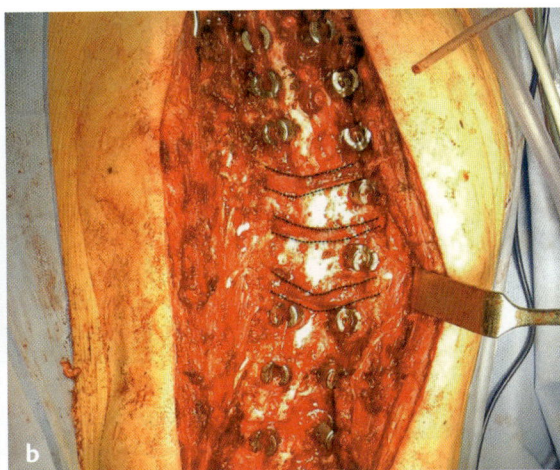

Fig. 13.2 Three Ponte's osteotomies (POs) at the apex of the scoliotic deformity have been done on a fusion mass to provide additional correction **(a)**. The osteotomies are depicted by the dotted lines **(b)**. (Note the horizontal and slightly V-shaped osteotomies.)

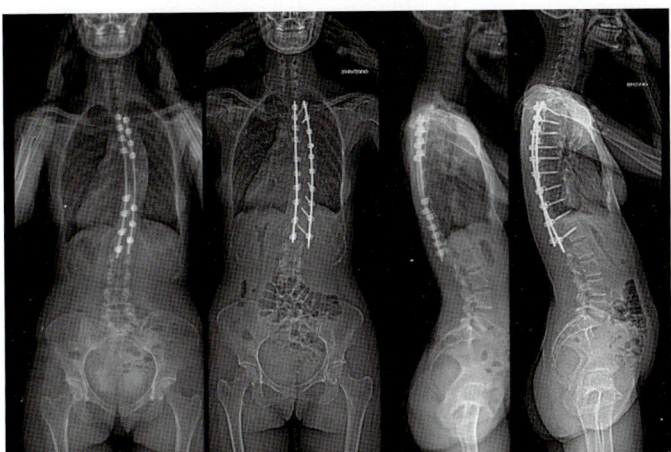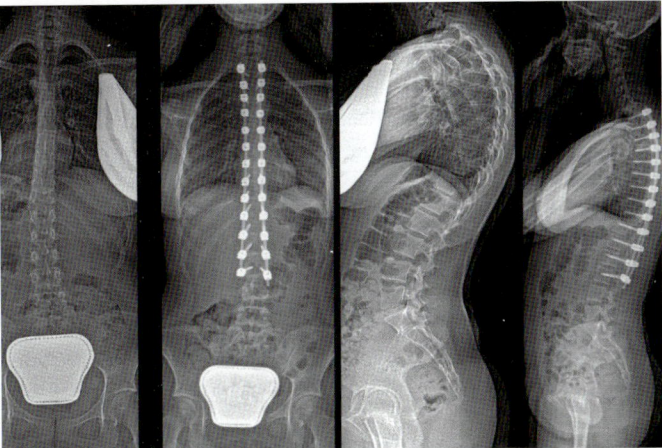

Fig. 13.3   The patient in **Fig. 13.2**. A 45-year-old woman with previous correction of thoracic scoliosis with a hook and rod construct presented with pain and increased deformity. The discs were not fused in the preoperative computed tomography (CT) scan. The implant was replaced with a pedicle-screw construct. Ponte's osteotomies were performed at the three apical levels. Two sublaminar bands were placed under the apical laminae for increased correction. Postoperatively, scoliosis has been reduced and kyphosis increased, improving the spinal alignment.

Fig. 13.4   A 21-year-old woman with Scheuermann's kyphosis presented with thoracic, low-back, and neck pain. Pedicle screws were implanted from T2 to the stable sagittal vertebra (L3). Six Ponte's osteotomies (POs) were done (T3–T9), and 5.5-mm cobalt-chrome (CoCr) rods pre-bent in moderate kyphosis were implanted from cranial to caudal, applying compression at each level to avoid a stretch of the spinal cord. At 2 years postoperatively, the patient has full activity as a medical student, and neck and back pain has resolved.

patients. Additional indications are syndromic scoliosis, especially when it is associated with hyperkyphosis (**Fig. 13.5**), restoration of lumbar lordosis in transforaminal lumbar interbody fusion (TLIF) procedures, degenerative disc disease or spondylolisthesis, or combined with hyperlordotic anterior lumbar interbody fusion (ALIF) at L5–S1. POs are increasingly considered in place of three-column osteotomies for correction of adult deformity with sagittal imbalance when the lumbar spine is mobile (**Fig. 13.6**), reducing morbidity compared to three-column osteotomies, which may be needed when the deformity is rigid.[2]

Complication Avoidance

It should be noted that PO, when compared with pedicle subtraction osteotomies, is less technically demanding, with shorter operative time and blood loss and less risk of neurological injury.[9] Intraoperatively, while performing laminectomy, facetectomy, or when removing the yellow ligament, caution must be taken of adhesions to the dura mater to avoid dural tears and neurological injury. This is especially true when spinal stenosis or yellow ligament calcifications are identified in the preoperative assessment.

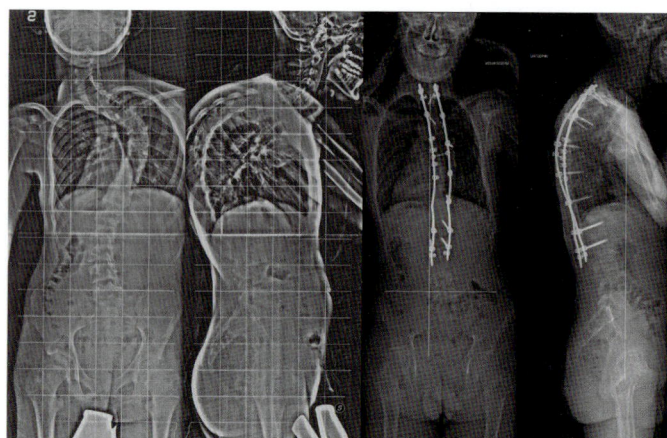

Fig. 13.5 This 15-year-old boy presented with severe and stiff kyphoscoliosis in Charcot-Marie-Tooth disease. The bone quality was poor. To reduce the risk of implant pull-out, the spine was instrumented with pedicle screws combined with sublaminar bands at the same vertebra at the cranial and caudal ends. A low-density pedicle screw construct was completed. Ponte's osteotomies were performed at seven levels, starting at T4, to reduce the stiffness. The correction was obtained with two 5.5 mm titanium rods connected with a cross-link at the apex of the scoliosis. Sublaminar bands were used at the apex of scoliosis to provide progressive correction.

In PO series of 78 patients treated with this technique, there were four cases of proximal junctional kyphosis. This could be avoided with intraoperative radiographic evaluation as the junctional kyphosis or excessive spine extension may create tension on the anterior longitudinal artery. This, in turn, can cause medullary ischemia leading to severe neurological complications. Ponte stressed the importance of intraoperative evaluation, and in cases of neurological impairment, complete clinical recovery was obtained by implant removal.[6] The risk of neurological deficit can also be substantially decreased with the employment of intraoperative neuromonitoring.

Tips and Tricks

- PO was initially described for the thoracic spine but can also be performed in the lumbar and cervical spine.
- The anterior column's stiffness may limit the spine's extension. Thus, the absence of fusion or ankylosis of the anterior column must be confirmed preoperatively.
- The amount of correction by the osteotomy level is modest, so POs are usually performed at multiple levels to provide the desired degree of correction.
- Additional techniques to maintain the length of the anterior column may be employed for enhanced

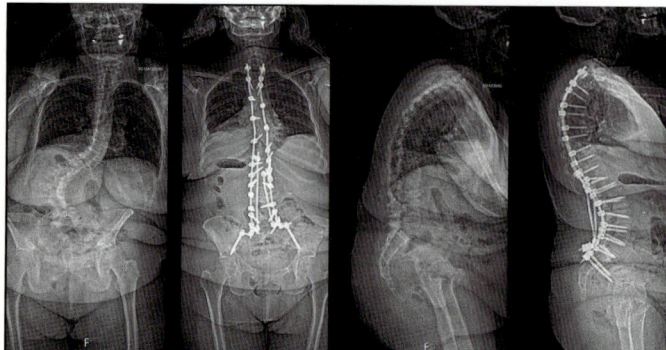

Fig. 13.6 A 56-year-old woman with severe lumbar scoliosis presented with coronal and sagittal imbalance. A T2 to pelvis construct with Ponte's osteotomies from T12 to L5 and arthrectomies at all levels provided sufficient release to obtain a satisfactory correction in both planes without using any three-column osteotomy. In addition, a delta-rod construct with two accessory rods was used to increase the mechanical resistance.

correction in the lumbar spine, usually with anterior interbody TLIF cages.

- Complete side-to-side excision of the bony components is needed for appropriate correction. Posterior bony remnants may block the posterior shortening and compromise the correction.
- A nerve hook or Penfield dissector should be used to assess that resections are completed in the entire width of the posterior spine.
- The gain in flexibility after the osteotomies can be verified by external compression on the apex of the deformity or with gentle use of a laminar spreader at each level.
- POs usually provide 7 to 10 degrees of correction per level.[10]

Key Points

- When PO is applied as a standalone procedure for kyphotic deformity, by preserving the anterior column by avoiding the opening of anterior disc spaces, the load-sharing capacity of the vertebral column is conserved, and the stability of correction is protected.[6]
- Lengthening of the anterior column must be avoided in the thoracic spine, as it can result in stretch ischemia of the spinal cord causing permanent neurological impairment. Level to level compression instead of cantilever correction must be ensured in these cases.
- Anterior column mobility is a requirement of POs. In cases with rigid anterior columns (i.e., AI), SPO or three-column osteotomies may be needed.

- For PO cases in the lumbar spine, when the disc has little mobility, disc release via diskectomy and increasing the length of the anterior column via interbody cage placement are recommended.

- Cases with pathologies related to the midthoracic region should be carefully evaluated before an anterior approach is made as a single anterior longitudinal artery supplies the anterior two-thirds of the spinal cord. Any iatrogenic disturbance creates a high risk for neurological deficits.

- PO was first described to correct cases of kyphosis. It is a valuable technique for lumbar hyperlordosis and severe or rigid thoracic or lumbar scoliosis.

References

1. Mohan AL, Das K. History of surgery for the correction of spinal deformity. Neurosurg Focus 2003;14(1):e1
2. Kose KC, Bozduman O, Yenigul AE, Igrek S. Spinal osteotomies: indications, limits and pitfalls. EFORT Open Rev 2017;2(3):73–82
3. Schwab F, Blondel B, Chay E, et al. The comprehensive anatomical spinal osteotomy classification. Neurosurgery 2014;74(1):112–120, discussion 120
4. Ponte A, Vero B, Siccardi GL. Surgical treatment of Scheuermann's kyphosis. In: Winter RB, ed. Progress in Spinal Pathology: Kyphosis. Bologna: Aulo Gaggi; 1984:75–80
5. Berjano P, Lamartina C. Ponte osteotomy. In: Heiko K, Robinson Y, eds. Cervical Spine Surgery: Standard and Advanced Techniques. Springer Nature Switzerland; 2019:549
6. Ponte A, Orlando G, Siccardi GL. The true Ponte osteotomy: by the one who developed it. Spine Deform 2018;6(1):2–11
7. Halanski MA, Cassidy JA. Do multilevel Ponte osteotomies in thoracic idiopathic scoliosis surgery improve curve correction and restore thoracic kyphosis? J Spinal Disord Tech 2013;26(5):252–255
8. Seki S, Yahara Y, Makino H, Kawaguchi Y, Kimura T. Selection of posterior spinal osteotomies for more effective periapical segmental vertebral derotation in adolescent idiopathic scoliosis—an in vivo comparative analysis between Ponte osteotomy and inferior facetectomy alone. J Orthop Sci 2018;23(3):488–494
9. Hyun SJ, Kim YJ, Rhim SC. Spinal pedicle subtraction osteotomy for fixed sagittal imbalance patients. World J Clin Cases 2013;1(8):242–248
10. Pérez-Grueso FS, Cecchinato R, Berjano P. Ponte osteotomies in thoracic deformities. Eur Spine J 2015;24(Suppl 1):S38–S41

14 Pedicle Subtraction Osteotomy

Kemal Paksoy and Onur Yaman

Introduction

Each level of pedicle subtraction osteotomy (PSO) allows nearly 30 degrees of correction.[1] PSO involves the use of a vertebral body wedge to remove posterior elements, shorten the spine posteriorly, and achieve sagittal plane correction as well as restore lumbar lordosis.[2] It was initially performed in cases of ankylosing spondylitis.[3] Nowadays, it is utilized to correct sagittal plane deformities in patients with degenerative conditions or who have previously undergone surgical procedures resulting in loss of lumbar lordosis.[4]

Indications

- Coronal and sagittal mismatch
- Need for lordosis correction of >25 degrees
- A rigid sagittal imbalance of >10 cm
- Rigid spine uncorrected on dynamic radiographs

Contraindications

- Patients with high medical comorbidities
- Patients with poor bone quality
- Patients requiring a sagittal correction of >40 degrees[5]

Multilevel Smith-Petersen osteotomies with fewer complications can be used as an alternative to PSO in patients with mobile disc structures. If a sagittal correction of >40 degrees is needed, the patients can benefit from an extended PSO that involves removal of two nonadjacent PSOs or resection of the vertebral column.[5]

Surgical Technique

- The patient is placed on the surgical table in the prone position.
- The abdomen should remain empty to prevent venous bleeding during surgery.

- The level at which surgery will be performed is determined by fluoroscopy.
- Following the patient's skin incision, the paravertebral muscles are stripped subperiosteally.
- The spinous processes, bilateral lamina, and facets of the level are exposed (**Fig. 14.1a**).
- Screws should be placed first to reduce bleeding during the procedure.

First, a total laminectomy is conducted to the level where the pedicle subtraction will be performed. The laminectomy site can be expanded to include the lower part of the upper lamina and the upper part of the lower lamina (**Fig. 14.1b**).

The pedicles on both sides of the level are exposed. After the roots emerging under the pedicle are decompressed bilaterally, the pedicles of both sides are removed by an osteotome or a high-speed motor.[6–8]

Bleeding originating from epidural veins, if any, is stopped with the help of bipolar coagulation, Surgicel, or Spongostan.

A triangular section is resected from the posterior side of the body with the help of an osteotome or a high-speed drill (**Fig. 14.1c**).

Closing the osteotomy site as rapidly as possible during this procedure will reduce the bleeding. The closing procedure is performed by deflection of the table or compression of the upper and lower screws[9,10] (**Fig. 14.1d, e**).

The posterior column is closed with the help of a compressor or by hyperextension of the surgical table (**Fig. 14.2**).

Neuromonitoring must be used during the closure of the posterior column. Changes in the neuromonitoring during the closing procedure should be checked frequently.[11]

During the closure procedure, care should be taken not to fold the dura mater. If folding occurs during the closure procedure, the laminectomy site should be expanded.[12]

Placing unilateral or bilateral rods will be helpful to prevent uncontrolled fracture during the closing procedure.[13]

In the post-PSO correction maneuver, the normal position of the spinal roots change; the position of the roots on the extracted pedicle shifts cranially, and the root becomes

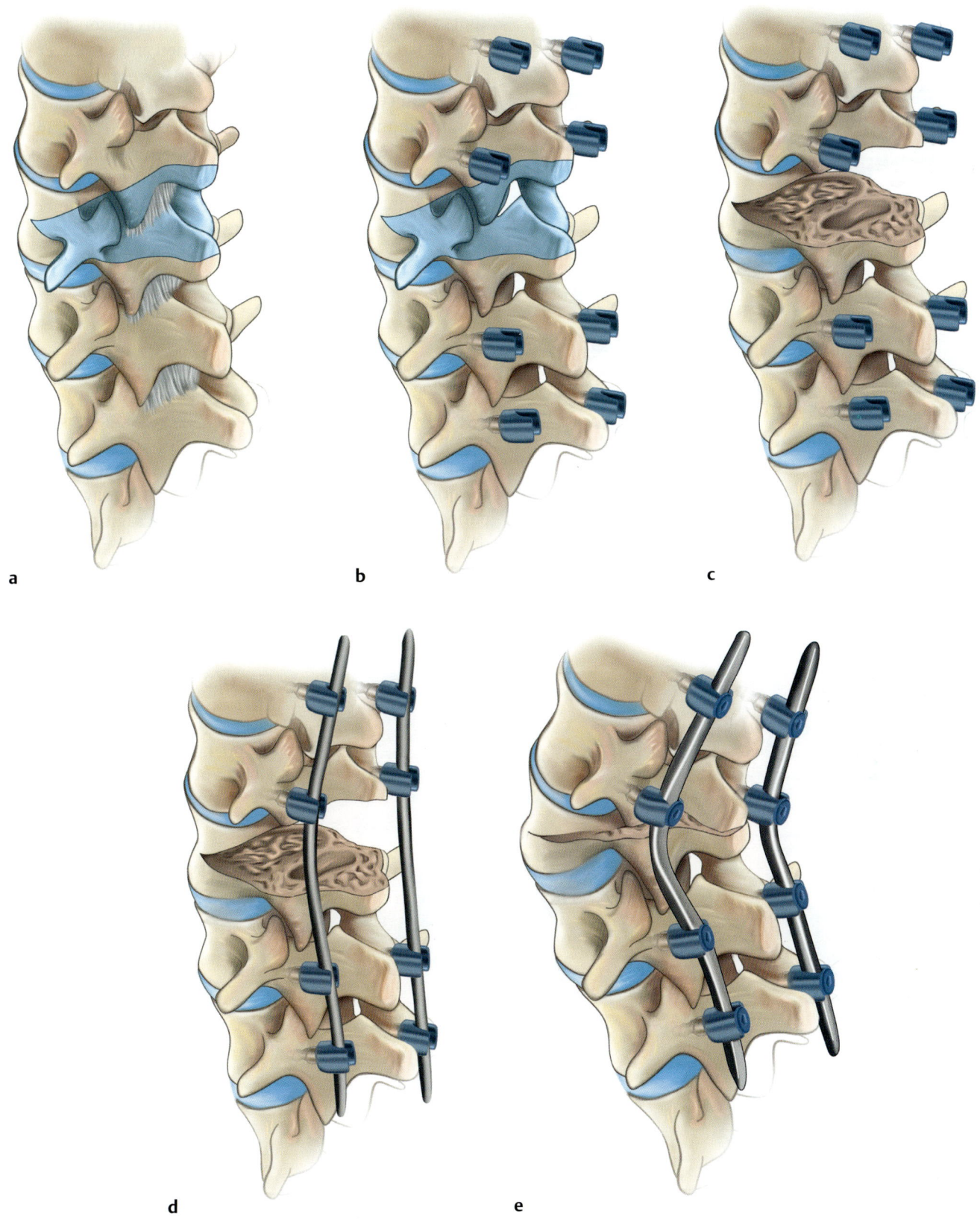

Fig. 14.1 **(a)** Spinous process, lamina, and facets are exposed. **(b)** Screws must be placed before pedicle subtraction is performed (area shaded in blue). **(c)** During pedicle subtraction osteotomy, a triangular bone fragment is resected from the posterior side of the body. **(d)** By adjusting the surgical table to hyperextension or with the help of the compression of the screws on the rod, the posterior column is closed **(e)**.

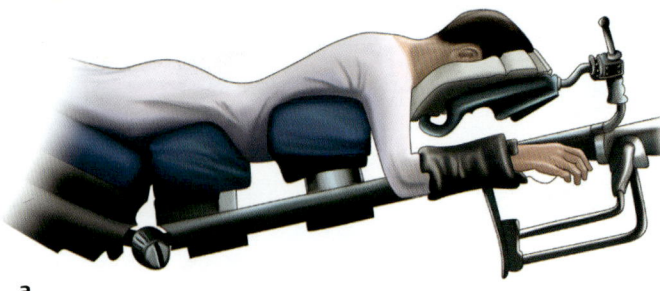

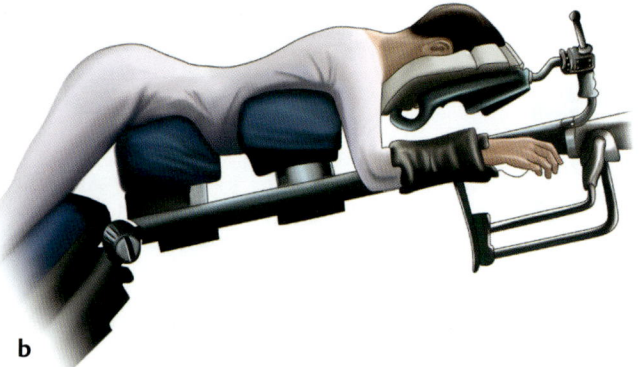

Fig. 14.2 The patient for whom pedicle subtraction osteotomy (PSO) is planned is in the flexion or neutral position **(a)**. The surgical table is adjusted to the deflection position to close the posterior column at the level of PSO **(b)**.

more vertical caudally. Likewise, the position of the lower roots shifts by ascending caudally. For this reason, the upper roots cause a sharp bend in the foramen and the lower roots on the pedicle of the lower adjacent vertebra. These sharp bends and stretches may impair the functions of the roots. Dural fold and root compression must be checked. In such a case, it is necessary to expand the laminectomy site. The lower part of the upper lamina and the upper part of the lower lamina are removed. Thus, two levels of laminectomy site width are obtained[4] (**Fig. 14.3**).

Tips and Tricks

In PSO surgery, attention should be paid to dural folds. Neurological injury involving the nerves around the osteotomy, dural defect, vascular injury, excessive bleeding, fusion, and instrumentation failure might occur as complications. Multilevel Smith-Petersen osteotomies with fewer complications can be used as an alternative to PSO in patients with mobile disc structures. If a sagittal correction of >40 degrees is needed, patients can benefit from an extended PSO that involves removal of two nonadjacent PSOs or resection of the vertebral column.[14]

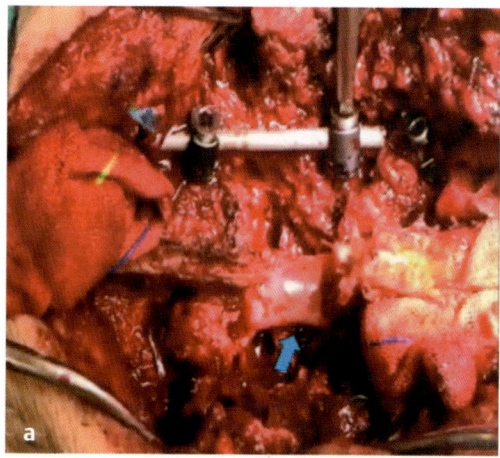
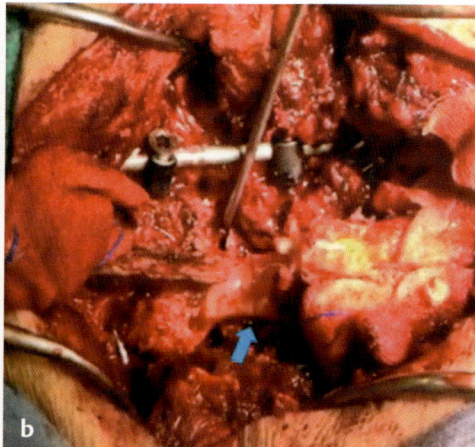

Fig. 14.3 The image of dura mater after pedicle subtraction osteotomy (PSO) in neutral position of operation table. There is no kinking of the dura (*blue arrow*) **(a)**. The image of the dura mater after PSO in hyperextension position of surgical table (blue arrow shows dural kinking) **(b)**.

Key Points

- PSO allows 30 degrees corrections for each level.

- Osteotomy shortens the posterior column.

- The osteotomy site should be closed as quickly as possible to reduce venous bleeding in the epidural space.

- While closing the posterior column, attention should be paid to the folding of the dura mater.

References

1. Bridwell KH, Lewis SJ, Lenke LG, Baldus C, Blanke K. Pedicle subtraction osteotomy for the treatment of fixed sagittal imbalance. J Bone Joint Surg Am 2003;85(3):454–463

2. Barrey C, Perrin G, Michel F, Vital JM, Obeid I. Pedicle subtraction osteotomy in the lumbar spine: indications, technical aspects, results and complications. Eur J Orthop Surg Traumatol 2014;24(1, Suppl 1):S21–S30

3. Thomasen E. Vertebral osteotomy for correction of kyphosis in ankylosing spondylitis. Clin Orthop Relat Res 1985;(194): 142–152

4. Le Huec JC, Aunoble S. Pedicle subtraction osteotomy for sagittal imbalance. Eur Spine J 2012;21(9):1896–1897

5. Alemdaroğlu KB, Atlihan D, Cimen O, Kilinç CY, Iltar S. Morphometric effects of acute shortening of the spine: the kinking and the sliding of the cord, response of the spinal nerves. Eur Spine J 2007;16(9):1451–1457

6. Gupta MC, Gupta S, Kelly MP, Bridwell KH. Pedicle subtraction osteotomy. JBJS Essential Surg Tech 2020;10(1): e0028.1–11

7. Hyun SJ, Kim YJ, Rhim SC. Spinal pedicle subtraction osteotomy for fixed sagittal imbalance patients. World J Clin Cases 2013;1(8):242–248

8. Menger RP, Davis DD, Bryant JH. Spinal Osteotomy. In: StatPearls [Internet]. Treasure Island, FL: StatPearls Publishing; January 2022

9. Lamartina C, Casero G. Bleeding control in pedicle subtraction osteotomy. Eur Spine J 2011;20(12):2284–2285

10. Daubs MD, Brodke DS, Annis P, Lawrence BD. Perioperative complications of pedicle subtraction osteotomy. Global Spine J 2016;6(7): 630–635

11. Lau D, Dalle Ore CL, Reid P, et al. Utility of neuromonitoring during lumbar pedicle subtraction osteotomy for adult spinal deformity. J Neurosurg Spine 2019;31(3):397–407

12. Hyun SJ, Rhim SC. Clinical outcomes and complications after pedicle subtraction osteotomy for fixed sagittal imbalance patients: a long-term follow-up data. J Korean Neurosurg Soc 2010;47(2):95–101

13. Watanabe K, Lenke LG, Daubs MD, et al. A central hook-rod construct for osteotomy closure: a technical note. Spine 2008;33(10):1149–1155

14. Choi HY, Hyun SJ, Kim KJ, Jahng TA, Kim HJ. Radiographic and clinical outcomes following pedicle subtraction osteotomy: minimum 2-year follow-up data. J Korean Neurosurg Soc 2020;63(1):99–107

15 Corner Osteotomy

Filippo Mandelli, Salvatore Petrone, and Pedro Berjano

Introduction

Spine deformity is a three-dimensional pathology, and planning corrective surgery should consider the coronal, sagittal, and axial planes. Normative values for spinopelvic parameters and sagittal alignment[1-4] should guide the preoperative surgical planning to reliably produce good results.[5-7] Sagittal misalignment has been correlated to disability, reduced quality of life, and poor outcomes after surgery.[8-10] Thus, restoring a normal sagittal alignment is mandatory to avoid high rates of poor outcomes and revision surgery.[11,12] Correction of severe misalignment with loss of lordosis is often performed through a pedicle subtraction osteotomy (PSO), especially in cases of rigid deformity (e.g., iatrogenic flat-back).[13,14] Insufficient correction in sagittal realignment procedures may happen even when a PSO is performed, leading to increased risks of failure and reoperation. PSO can correct around 25 to 30 degrees[15-17]; however, the main limiting factor of the ability to obtain a significant correction with PSO is the amount of posterior wall of the vertebra that can be resected. Although it is easy to remove the posterior wall between the upper end plate and 3 to 4 mm below the lower edge of the pedicle, extending the resection far below is difficult due to the presence of the exiting roots that run horizontally below the pedicle. Corner osteotomy is a modified PSO technique that allows more sagittal correction within the vertebra. The angular correction at the osteotomy is on average 20 degrees higher than PSO (with cases of as much as 56 degrees of correction at a single level).[18] The different shape of corner osteotomy determines a substantially more significant correction with the same resection in the height of the posterior wall. This is made possible by directing the osteotomy plane to a point posterior to the anterior cortex of the vertebral body and resecting the disc, leaving the closing hinge more dorsal to the anterior longitudinal ligament (**Figs. 15.1 and 15.2**). Furthermore, another potential advantage of corner osteotomy is that it provides direct bony contact between the end plate of the cranial vertebra and the osteotomy plane of the index vertebra, promoting interbody fusion. The corner osteotomy also has a similar safety profile to a classical PSO; thus, it should be considered a valid alternative, allowing easier achievement of the correction goals.

Definition of the Technique

Under general anesthesia, the patient is positioned prone on a spine table with a decompressed abdomen. The use of a table that allows for a reverse break is advisable to reduce the stress exerted on the implant during the closure of the osteotomy. Care must be taken to position the osteotomy level aligned with the hinge of the table. Neuromonitoring of motor and somatosensory-evoked potentials is routinely installed to monitor the spinal cord function. A standard midline posterior approach in the area to be instrumented is performed.

In this chapter, an L4 corner osteotomy will be described. After subperiosteal exposure, at least two levels above and two below should be instrumented with pedicle screws. Two rods are pre-bent to the final expected alignment, depending on the specific multi-rod construct chosen (deep-short satellite rod, delta rod, or other). Repeated contouring should be avoided to preserve the rods' mechanical properties. The spinous processes L3, L4, and L5 are resected, along with the inferior articular processes of L3 and L4 bilaterally. A high-speed burr is used to perform one horizontal trough just below the transverse processes of L3 and another above the transverse processes of L5. These are then completed with a Kerrison rongeur. Bleeding from the dorsal epidural plexus should be expected and controlled with hemostatic agents and bipolar coagulation. Complete resection of posterior bone elements between the two troughs is done. The L3 and L4 roots are well exposed in the foramina (**Fig. 15.3**). Bleeding from epidural veins is usual in this area and must be controlled with bipolar or hemostatic agents. Time is needed to obtain proper hemostasis. The authors usually proceed side to side. (Working on one side, coagulating vessels, applying hemostatic agents and compression, and proceeding to work on the opposite side, and in a similar manner alternating sides until the work is completed. This allows for enough action time to the hemostatic agents and reduces bleeding and surgical effort.) The exposure of the lateral wall of L4 begins with the osteotomy of the base of the L4 transverse process bilaterally with a Kerrison or an osteotome. Subperiosteal dissection is performed with a Cobb elevator, gently elevating the psoas muscle and the

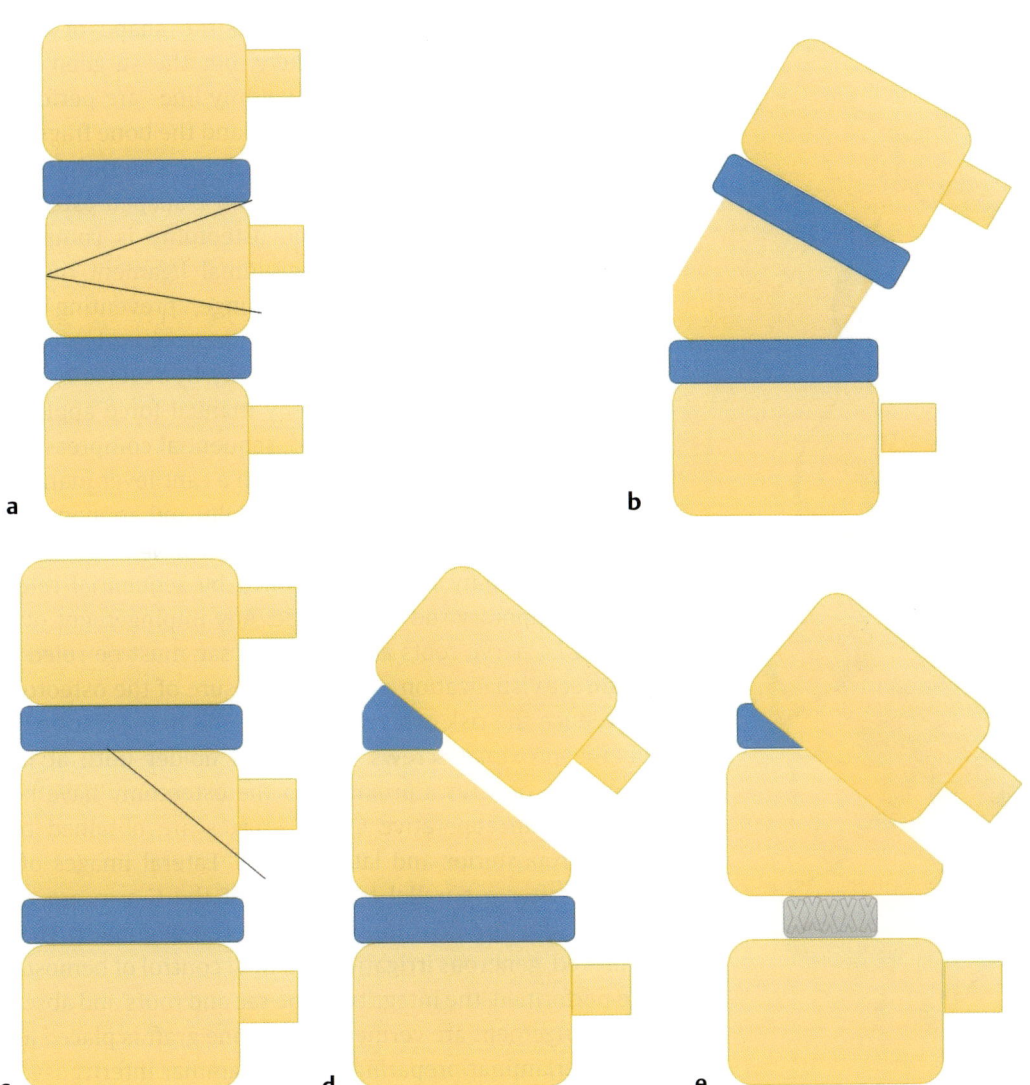

Fig. 15.1 Above: standard 30 degrees pedicle subtraction osteotomy (PSO): **(a)** osteotomy lines; **(b)** after the closure of osteotomy. Below: 40 degrees corner osteotomy: **(c)** osteotomy line; **(d)** after diskectomy and closure of osteotomy; **(e)** compression of osteotomy after implanting an interbody cage.

lumbar plexus. Care is taken not to injure the segmental vessels or the lumbar plexus. Inserting a large hemostatic sheet between the vertebral body and soft tissues lateral to it may help prevent excessive bleeding. The dural sac is retracted medially, exposing the L3–L4 disc, and annulectomy is performed from lateral to the most medial point that can be reached from each side. Then the annulotomy proceeds laterally. A large Penfield dissector is placed lateral to the disc and medial to the most lateral part of the exiting L3 root. A posterior annulotomy is performed extending the cut well lateral to facilitate the extraction of the lateral wall fragment after the osteotomy. After complete bilateral diskectomy, the caudal L3 end plate is prepared for fusion by removing the cartilage using shavers and curettes. After closing the osteotomy, this will allow contact between the end plate of L3 and the spongiosa of L4 and favor interbody fusion. For correct osteotomy shape, the plane of the inferior L3 end plate needs to be identified. We suggest inserting

a long straight instrument—a chisel or a rongeur—into the L3–L4 disc space as a reference and plan the angle of the osteotomy accordingly (**Fig. 15.4**). The osteotomy line starts below the inferior margin of the L4 pedicles. It is directed caudocranially to the intersection between the anterior one-third and posterior two-thirds of the L4 rostral end plate at an angle of approximately 20 to 40 degrees—depending on the planned correction—from the reference instrument. It can be performed with a 10- to 15-mm osteotome. Care must be taken to protect the L4 traversing nerve root with a large Penfield and the dural sac with a retractor. Then a vertical cut is made to the pedicle, and the first fragment is removed. The same two cuts are repeated more medially to complete the resection of the first half of the L4 vertebral body. Before addressing the contralateral side, profuse bleeding from the spongiosa should be prevented by placing hemostatic agents in the bone defect. A temporary rod is placed before proceeding to the opposite side to prevent an unplanned

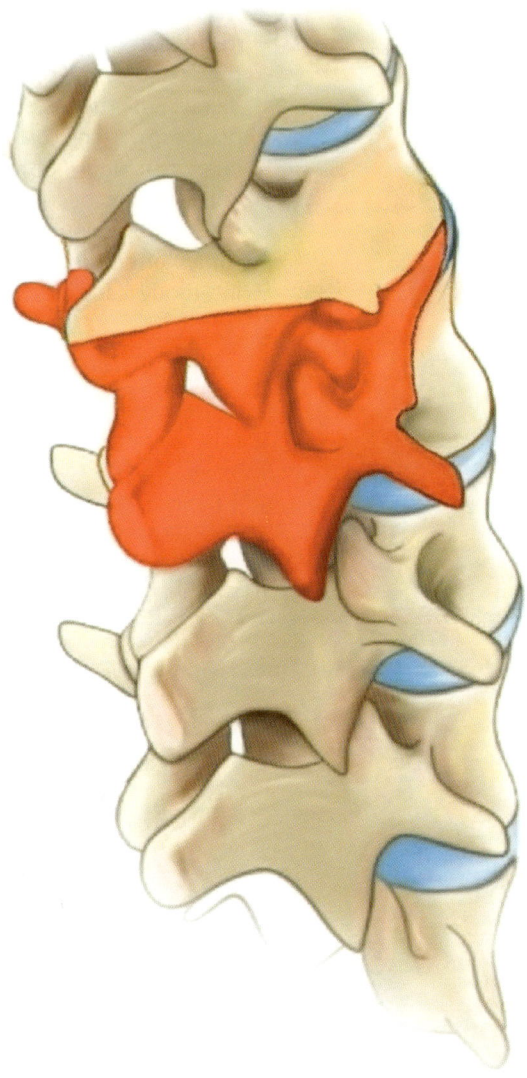

Fig. 15.2 Illustration of the corner osteotomy.

collapse of the osteotomy. Due to the shape of corner osteotomy, translation is unlikely, but the surgeon must, in any case, prevent it. The osteotomy lines are performed contralaterally in the same manner, and the bone fragments are removed. The remaining bridge of the posterior wall can be decancelled and impacted with an L-shaped osteotome below the dural sac. Once the osteotomy is completed, the anterior annulus and longitudinal ligament must be preserved since they act as a hinge, preventing spine dislocation. As mentioned regarding the positioning, closure of the osteotomy is performed mainly by reverse break of the table. This can be assisted by manual force applied to the spine from dorsal to ventral, sequential compression of the pedicle screws L3–L5, or through a cantilever maneuver by bilaterally securing the rods caudally and applying force to both rods. In cases with substantial instability, closure of the osteotomy can be controlled by sequential release of the temporary rod on one side. Any impingement of the L3 and L4 nerve roots and the dural sac must be ruled out by direct visualization during the closure of the osteotomy. To reduce the risk of screw pull-out, the rods must be held on the proximal screws with a rod holder until at least two pairs of screws proximal to the osteotomy have been engaged. Intraoperative C-arm images are obtained both in anteroposterior and lateral views. Lateral images of S1 and L1 after a parallel translation of the C-arm are used to measure the final lordosis. Once the alignment goal is achieved, generous irrigation and final control of hemostasis are performed, the integrity of the sac and roots and absence of impingement are verified, and a bone graft is placed after the interlaminar preparing the interlaminar intertransverse fusion bed. The authors prefer to systematically include an interbody fusion below the osteotomized vertebra (in this case at L4–L5) with an autologous graft and a cage. We prefer to perform a direct trans-psoas approach at the

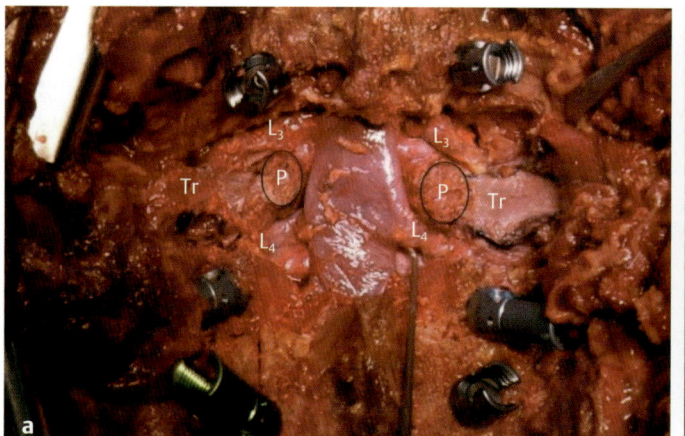
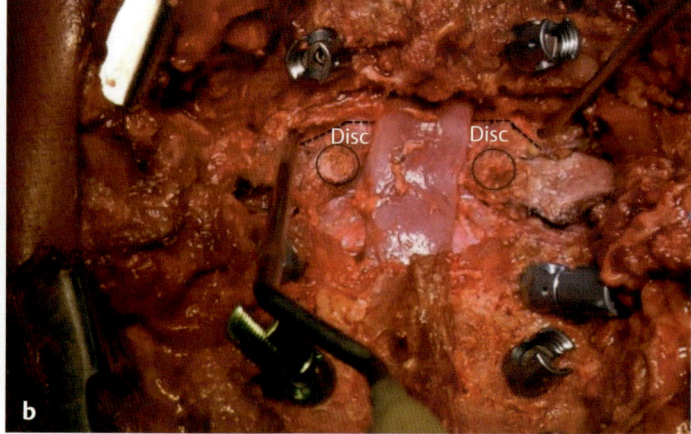

Fig. 15.3 The posterior elements were resected, and the nerve roots L3 and L4 are exposed **(a)**. The L3–L4 disc is visible after retraction of L3 nerve roots **(b)**. P, pedicle; Tr, transverse process.

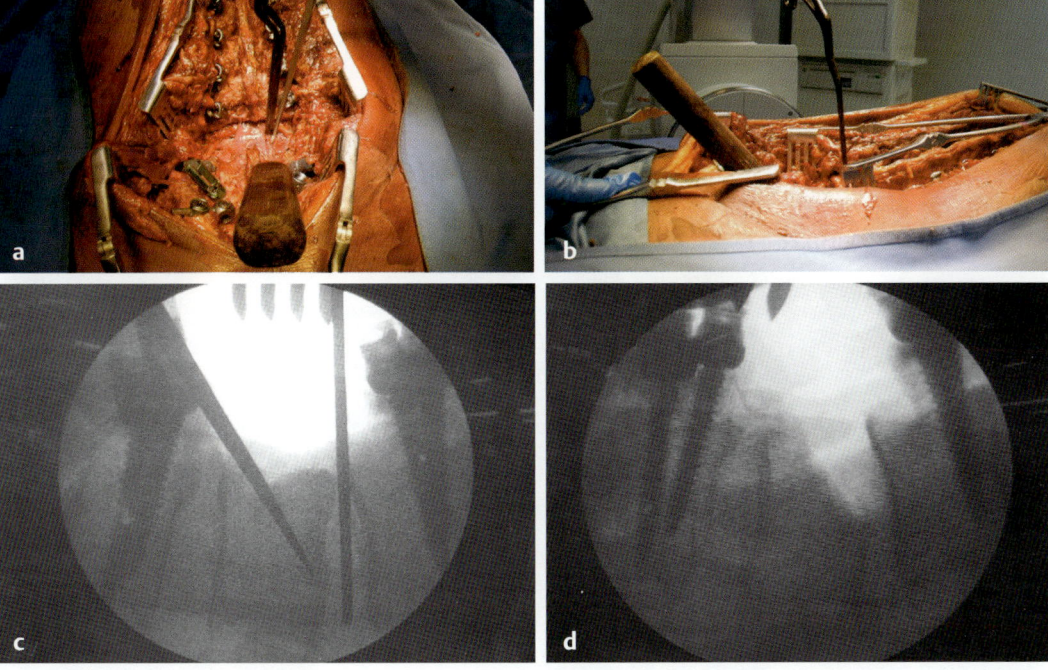

Fig. 15.4 A rongeur inserted as a reference into the disc space. An osteotome is used to perform the osteotomy starting under the pedicle of L4. Posterior view **(a)**, lateral view **(b)**, lateral C-arm view **(c)**, and lateral C-arm view after bone resection **(d)**.

end of the procedure in the same anesthesia, which can be done in prone decubitus position. This achieves interbody fusion with a large footprint cage and minimal blood loss. Additionally, implanting the cage after the closure of the posterior construct results in compression between the L3 lower end plate and the spongiosa of L4, increasing the chance of interbody fusion.

Indications

The primary indication for corner osteotomy is a rigid sagittal deformity, such as a post-traumatic kyphosis (**Fig. 15.5**), iatrogenic flat-back, ankylosing spondylitis, or rigid scoliosis (more frequent in the adult). In addition, deformity caused by tumors or infections may in some instances benefit from a corner osteotomy, but the underlying pathology must be properly addressed. In case of partially rigid deformity, efforts should be made to avoid a three-column osteotomy in favor of realignment procedures with anterior interbody cages, resection of the anterior longitudinal ligament, and posterior column osteotomies at multiple levels or multilevel posterior column osteotomy with or without posteriorly inserted interbody cages. However, a corner osteotomy is reasonable if the amount of correction at a given level cannot be achieved through an anterior column realignment.

Complication Avoidance

Complications of the corner osteotomy are similar to those encountered in classical PSO. Sufficient decompression of the spinal canal and the four nerve roots is essential to reduce the risk of neurologic injury, but excessive posterior bone resection preventing bone-to-bone laminar contact after the closure of the osteotomy increases instability resulting in the risk of nonunion. A stepwise closure of the osteotomy with repetitive nerve roots checking should prevent impingement of neural structures. Concomitant use of neuromonitoring is highly recommended. Excess dural scar should be removed as well to avoid dural buckling. Inadequate bone resection may block the closing of the osteotomy like in PSO; however, given the geometrical shape of the corner osteotomy, achieving enough sagittal correction is less of a concern. Meticulous hemostasis is necessary to avoid excessive bleeding, which in cases requiring an osteotomy is usually around 1,400 mL.[18] The use of a high-speed burr reduces bleeding from the bone. Epidural bleeding should be expected from the dorsal and ventral venous plexus and the area of the foramina; hemostatic agents and bipolar should be used to control it. After the resection of the posterior elements and before the osteotomy of the vertebral body, it is recommended to insert temporary rods across the index

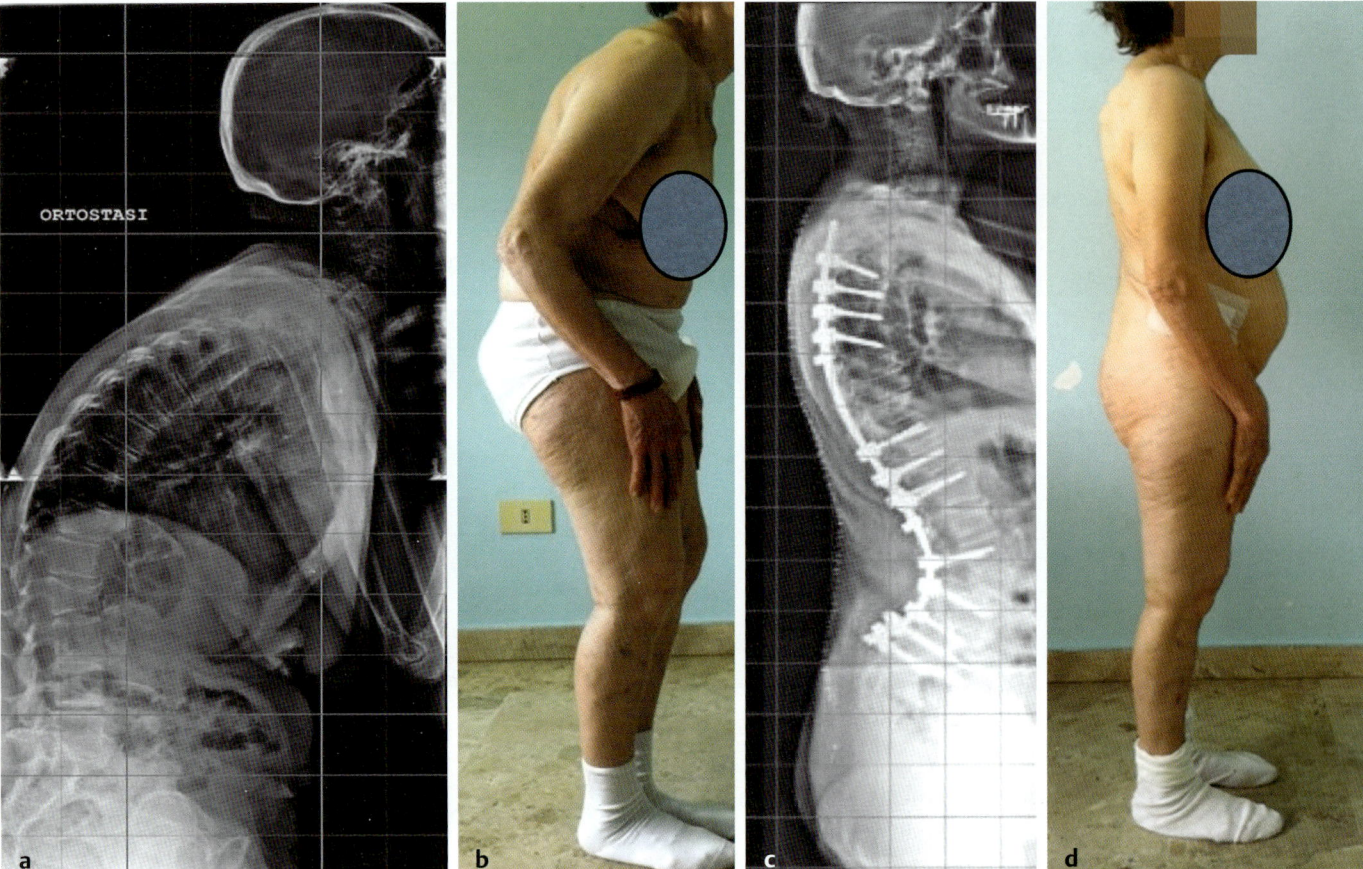

Fig. 15.5 A 75-year-old woman with severe back pain and claudication. Preoperative standing radiograms and image **(a, b)**. Postoperative results after L4 corner osteotomy (53 degrees) **(c, d)**.

vertebra to avoid inadvertent translation of the floating vertebra. Breaking the table in extension is the easiest way to close the osteotomy. However, additional maneuvers are often needed, such as pushing the spine anteriorly or compressing on the screws. In this last case, care must be taken not to overstress the implants causing pull-out of the screws. A cantilever technique using persuaders from caudal to cranial or two rods on each side connected by side-to-side connectors helps dissipate the forces on more screws and prevent pull-out. Cement augmentation of screws can improve pull-out resistance in osteoporotic patients, though preoperative medical optimization is mandatory in such patients.

Tips and Tricks

By closing the osteotomy, the end plate of L3 and the spongiosa of L4 below the osteotomy should come in contact.

To better visualize the plane of the caudal end plate of L3, we suggest inserting a long straight instrument like a

chisel or rongeur into the L3–L4 disc space as a reference and planning the angle of the osteotomy accordingly.

Closure of the osteotomy is performed mainly by reverse break of the table. This can be assisted by manual force applied to the spine from dorsal to ventral, sequential compression of the pedicle screws L3–L5, or a cantilever maneuver by bilaterally securing the rods caudally using pressure to both rods.

Key Points

- A Jackson table allowing reverse break of the table at the osteotomy level will assist in closure and reduce the stress on the implants.

- Extend the posterior annulotomy to the lateral annulus while protecting the exiting nerve root.

- Bilaterally expose the exiting and traversing nerve roots checking for any impingement throughout the closing maneuvers.

- Insert a straight instrument into the disc space above the osteotomy as a reference for the end plate's direction and align the osteotomy plane with the desired angle.
- Perform a 30 to 35 degrees osteotomy starting just below the lower limit of the pedicles and reaching the cranial end plate at the union of the posterior two-thirds and the anterior one-third.
- Protect the osteotomy with multi-rod constructs.
- Meticulously control bleeding from the bone and epidural veins.

References

1. Roussouly P, Nnadi C. Sagittal plane deformity: an overview of interpretation and management. Eur Spine J 2010;19(11): 1824–1836
2. Boulay C, Tardieu C, Hecquet J, et al. Sagittal alignment of spine and pelvis regulated by pelvic incidence: standard values and prediction of lordosis. Eur Spine J 2006;15(4):415–422
3. Jackson RP, McManus AC. Radiographic analysis of sagittal plane alignment and balance in standing volunteers and patients with low back pain matched for age, sex, and size. A prospective controlled clinical study. Spine 1994;19(14): 1611–1618
4. Mac-Thiong JM, Roussouly P, Berthonnaud E, Guigui P. Sagittal parameters of global spinal balance: normative values from a prospective cohort of seven hundred nine Caucasian asymptomatic adults. Spine 2010;35(22):E1193–E1198
5. Lafage R, Schwab F, Glassman S, et al; International Spine Study Group. Age-adjusted alignment goals have the potential to reduce PJK. Spine 2017;42(17):1275–1282
6. Yilgor C, Sogunmez N, Boissiere L, et al; European Spine Study Group (ESSG). Global alignment and proportion (GAP) score: development and validation of a new method of analyzing spinopelvic alignment to predict mechanical complications after adult spinal deformity surgery. J Bone Joint Surg Am 2017;99(19):1661–1672
7. Pizones J, Moreno-Manzanaro L, Sánchez Pérez-Grueso FJ, et al; ESSG European Spine Study Group. Restoring the ideal Roussouly sagittal profile in adult scoliosis surgery decreases the risk of mechanical complications. Eur Spine J 2020;29(1):54–62
8. Lafage V, Schwab F, Patel A, Hawkinson N, Farcy JP. Pelvic tilt and truncal inclination: two key radiographic parameters in the setting of adults with spinal deformity. Spine 2009; 34(17):E599–E606
9. Smith JS, Shaffrey CI, Berven S, et al; Spinal Deformity Study Group. Improvement of back pain with operative and nonoperative treatment in adults with scoliosis. Neurosurgery 2009;65(1):86–93, discussion 93–94
10. Kim MK, Lee SH, Kim ES, Eoh W, Chung SS, Lee CS. The impact of sagittal balance on clinical results after posterior interbody fusion for patients with degenerative spondylolisthesis: a pilot study. BMC Musculoskelet Disord 2011; 12:69
11. Berjano P, Bassani R, Casero G, Sinigaglia A, Cecchinato R, Lamartina C. Failures and revisions in surgery for sagittal imbalance: analysis of factors influencing failure. Eur Spine J 2013;22(Suppl 6):S853–S858
12. Malone A, Meldrum D, Gleeson J, Bolger C. Electromyographic characteristics of gait impairment in cervical spondylotic myelopathy. Eur Spine J 2013;22(11):2538–2544
13. Bridwell KH, Lewis SJ, Lenke LG, et al. Pedicle subtraction osteotomy for the treatment of fixed sagittal imbalance. J. Bone Joint Surg. Am 2003;85(3):454–63
14. Gupta MC, Gupta S, Kelly MP, Bridwell KH. Pedicle subtraction osteotomy. JBJS Essential Surg Tech 2020;10(1):e0028
15. Lafage V, Schwab F, Vira S, et al. Does vertebral level of pedicle subtraction osteotomy correlate with degree of spinopelvic parameter correction? J Neurosurg Spine 2011;14(2): 184–191
16. Berven SH, Deviren V, Smith JA, Emami A, Hu SS, Bradford DS. Management of fixed sagittal plane deformity: results of the transpedicular wedge resection osteotomy. Spine 2001;26(18):2036–2043
17. Bridwell KH, Lewis SJ, Edwards C, et al. Complications and outcomes of pedicle subtraction osteotomies for fixed sagittal imbalance. Spine 2003;28(18):2093–2101
18. Berjano P, Pejrona M, Damilano M, Cecchinato R, Aguirre MF, Lamartina C. Corner osteotomy: a modified pedicle subtraction osteotomy for increased sagittal correction in the lumbar spine. Eur Spine J 2015;24(Suppl 1):58–65

16 Vertebral Column Resection Osteotomy

Nuri Demirci, Çağlar Yılgör, and Ahmet Alanay

Introduction

In severe and rigid deformities, osteotomies can be used when the amount of correction achieved with instrumentation alone would be inadequate. Vertebral column resection (VCR) is a challenging osteotomy technique used to reconstruct such deformities. VCR provides the most correction compared to various osteotomy techniques,[1,2] thereby playing a pivotal role in fixed deformities in which sufficient correction may not be gained with less aggressive methods, such as angular osteotomies.

MacLennan first introduced VCR as a combined anterior–posterior procedure (AP-VCR) in 1922.[3] AP-VCR, as a circumferential anterior–posterior approach, has some disadvantages such as the long duration of operation and high volume of estimated blood loss, and the process may not be done under the same anesthetic procedure.[1] Therefore, in the early 2000s, Suk et al[2] described the posterior-only approach (P-VCR) to reduce operating time, blood loss, and the risk of related complications with circumferential VCR. Lenke popularized this approach in the later years.[4] The technique allows translational and rotational correction of the spinal column and controlled modification of both the anterior and posterior columns simultaneously, using a single approach. Shortened duration of operation leads to less intraoperative instability of the spine; thus, intraoperative neurological complication risks can be diminished.[2] P-VCR is currently the gold standard last-resort osteotomy for correcting severe structuralspinal deformities.[5]

The VCR procedure entails total excision of one or more vertebral segments, including the posterior components, the whole vertebral body, and the adjacent discs. The number of vertebral bodies to be removed is determined by the spinal deformity's rigidity and characteristics. It is used to treat a variety of conditions, including Type 1 congenital kyphosis, sagittal decompensation with Type 2 coronal malalignment, hemivertebra with its adjacent discs, sharp angular thoracic deformity, spondyloptosis, previously fused and severely misaligned deformity, and spinal tumor.[6]

In several studies that included pediatric and adult patients, VCR was found to be effective in correcting curves. Suk et al[7] reported corrections of 59% for the main curve and 51% for the minor curve. Lenke et al[4] noted scoliosis, global kyphosis, angular kyphosis, and congenital scoliosis curve improvements ranging from 51 to 60%. Hamzaoglu et al[8] reported a mean correction of 62% in the coronal and 72% in the sagittal planes. In a recent study, Jeszenszky et al[9] reported average correction of scoliosis to be 57%, and that of kyphosis to be 51% in a series of four patients with a mean age of 3.7 years.

VCR is a technically challenging treatment with a high incidence of neurological injury. It should only be performed by an experienced spine surgeon and spine team while neurological monitoring is in place.

Definition of the Technique

A VCR can be performed as an anterior–posterior circumferential surgery or as a posterior-only treatment, depending on the surgeon's experience with various methods.

In the surgical procedure, pedicle screws are placed except for the level(s) to be resected (**Fig. 16.1**). On one side, a temporary rod that mimics the shape of the deformity is used to connect the screws in order to prevent instability or damage to the neural structures (**Fig. 16.2**). Once the osteotomy is completed on this side, another temporary rod is placed on the contralateral side, and the first rod is removed. If the working side is switched several times, so should the temporary rods.

A wide lateral dissection is performed to remove the transverse process in the lumbar spine or the rib in the thoracic spine. Wide laminectomy is performed at the levels of planned resection as well as one level above and one level below to prevent postcorrection neural impingement. The exposed nerve roots are ligated at the thoracic level to prevent spinal cord compression. It is essential to prepare the lateral aspect of the vertebral body. On the working site (opposite to the stabilizing rod), subperiosteal dissection is performed to follow the lateral wall of the vertebral body till the anterior part is palpable. The soft tissues and great vessels anterior to the vertebral body are protected by retractors.

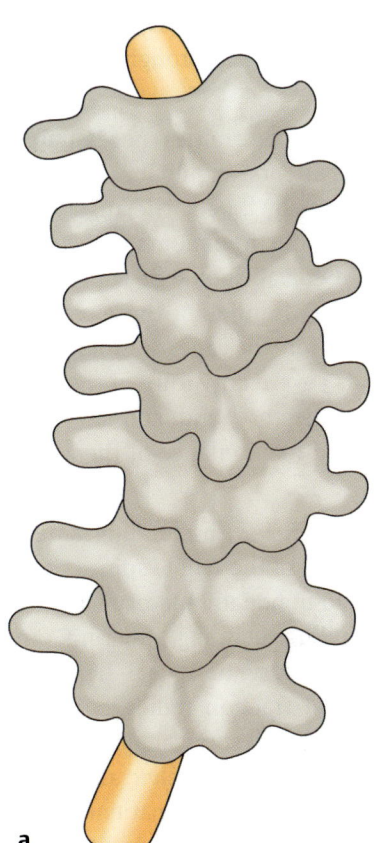

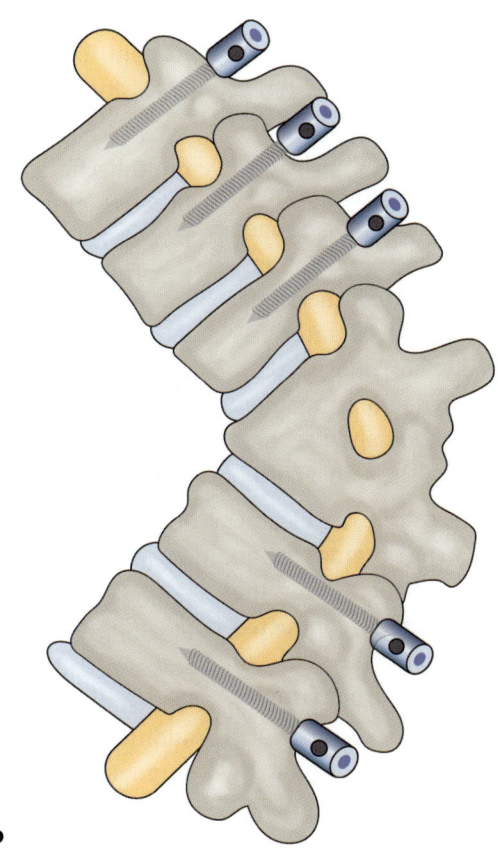

Fig. 16.1 A rigid deformity with some scoliosis (a) and a significant kyphosis (b) can be a candidate for vertebral column resection.

a   b

Typically, it is more convenient to initiate the osteotomy on the concave side. Otherwise, bleeding from the convex side may obscure the vision, making it challenging to resect the bony structures on the concave side (**Fig. 16.2**). Resecting the concave pedicle first may also help prevent impingement of the spinal cord at this side with increasing instability while working on the convex side. Then discs below and above the chosen resection level(s) are removed piecemeal, and the pedicle and vertebral body on the convex side are resected using rongeurs, curettes, osteotomies, and a high-speed drill. A thin bone shell at the anterior cortex and the anterior longitudinal ligament are kept to avoid translation, and the dura is protected by preserving the posterior bone wall. Generally, a reverse curette is utilized to remove the thin shell of the posterior bone on the working site adjacent to dura.

After the posterior wall has been resected, a second temporary rod is inserted with a minor amount of compression in both rods in order to shorten the vertebral column and to relieve the stresses on the cord. A precorrection, thorough assessment of the spinal canal is conducted to ensure that no bone or disc tissue remains that might compress the nerves during or after the correction maneuvers.

Correction of the deformity is achieved gradually by compression, in situ contouring, and the replacement of

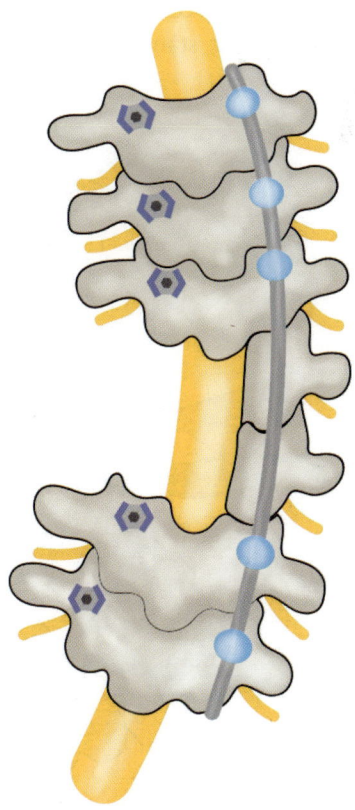

Fig. 16.2 Starting with removal of the concave side has some advanatges. The temporary rod is placed on the convex side.

deformed rods with rods precontoured to the physiological contours (**Fig. 16.3**). Monitoring the spinal cord is crucial during these maneuvers. Unlike other osteotomy types, VCR typically does not provide a bone-to-bone contact and necessitates structural allografts, autografts, or cages to reconstruct the vertebral column.[10] After resection, a mesh cage may be necessary to fill the gap and is often positioned anteriorly to prevent overshortening of the spinal column, which may cause dural buckling that endangers the spinal cord (**Fig. 16.4**). Additionally, a mesh cage placed anteriorly may enhance rotational stability. In kyphoscoliosis cases, lengthening the anterior column by using lamina spreaders or distractable cages aids in better correction and prevents dural buckling and excessive shortening of the spinal cord.

There is usually a laminectomy defect after the closure of anterior bony sites, and structural strip rib grafts or an H-shaped structural allograft can be implanted over the laminectomy site, and a final compression is conducted to secure stability.[8] Covering the osteotomy site with an H-shaped allograft may limit the development of hematomas and enhance fusion rates.

Preoperative Evaluation

A comprehensive history and examination of the patient's overall health and the locomotor system should be evaluated. Children's sitting, standing, and walking abilities

are examined.[11] Hip joint evaluation is also essential due to its contribution to the sagittal plane. A thorough neurologic assessment is required.

Severe and structural spine deformities necessitate a multidisciplinary approach. Patients should be evaluated in terms of general health status by a pediatrician. It is not rare to have a low body mass index in patients with severe deformities. In such cases, a dietician should be consulted.[12] A pulmonologist's evaluation is essential for these patients. Before surgery, it is crucial for the anesthesiologist to check the patient's airway, as severe curvature of the spine can sometimes affect the trajectory and course of the trachea, making intubation and maintenance of the airway challenging.[12]

Radiographic assessment begins with standing antero-posterior and lateral radiographs of the whole spine (sitting radiographs may be performed in nonambulatory patients). Flexibility radiographs including bending, fulcrum, and traction radiographs are mandatory to reveal flexibility. Under general anesthesia, axial traction radiographs give additional data about flexibility.[13,14] In surgical planning, the surgeon must account for the global spinopelvic alignment. The preoperative plan also considers the patient's chief complaint, neurological status, medical comorbidities, and the anticipated natural progression of the deformity. Due to the high prevalence of pseudarthrosis and complications, additional care should be taken with older patients in particular.[15,16]

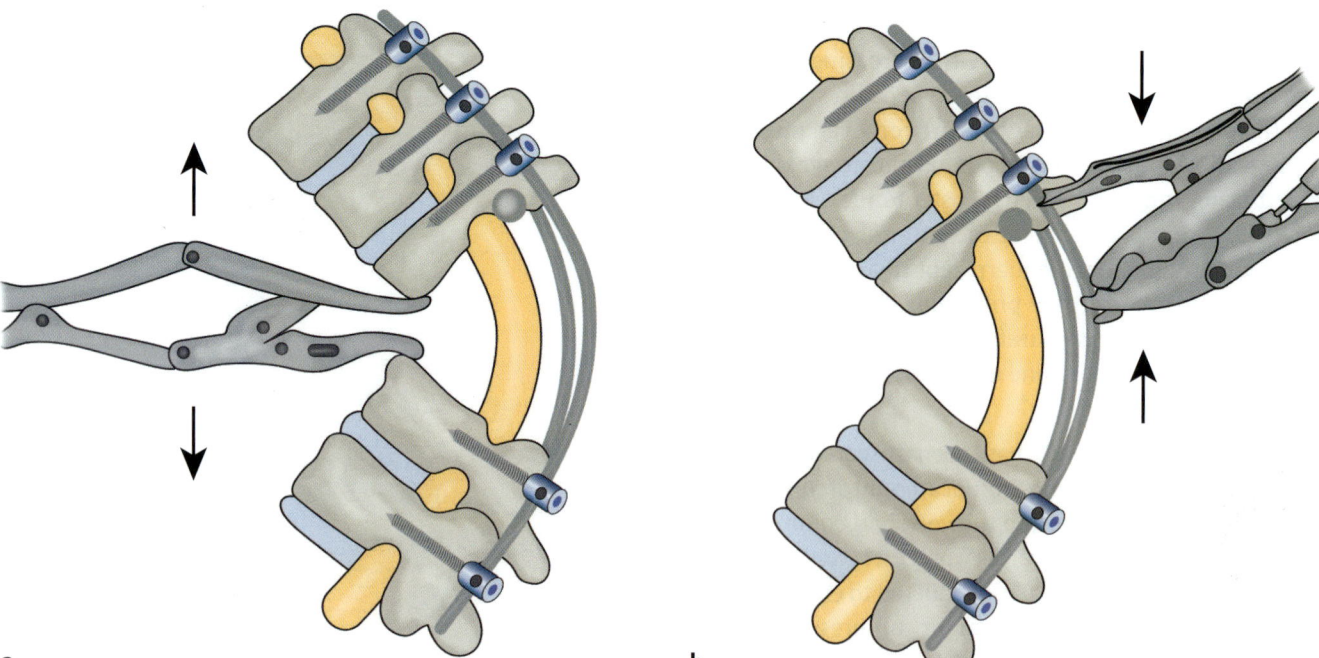

a   b

Fig. 16.3 Reduction can be achieved by a spreader at the anterior side (**a**) and a compressor at the posterior side (**b**) with shortening of the posterior column.

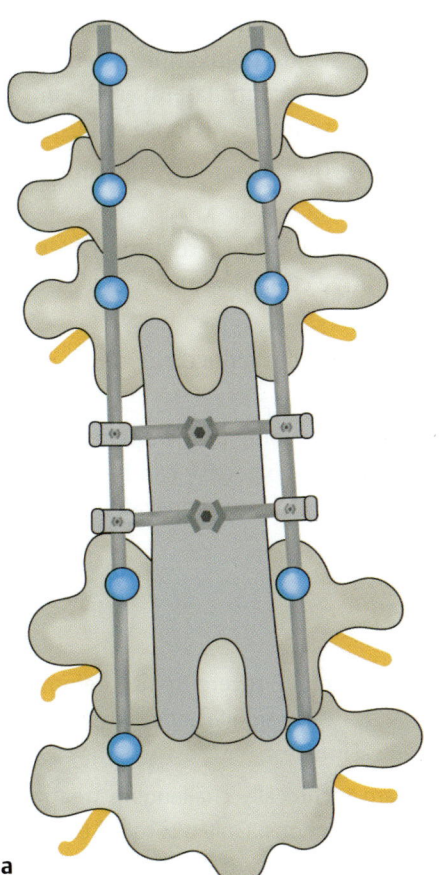 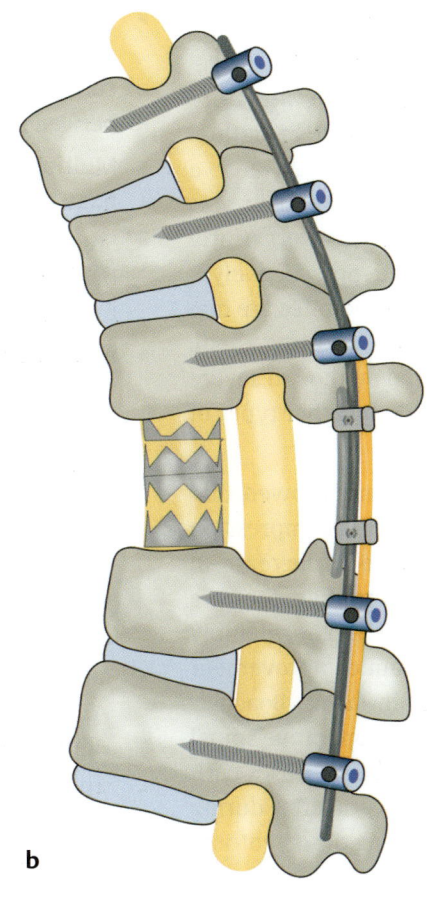

Fig. 16.4 The construction is completed by posterior grafts **(a)** and anterior cage **(b)** application.

a

b

Indications

VCR is generally reserved for deformities that cannot be corrected by less invasive osteotomies. The type of deformity is one of the most critical criteria in deciding the correction method and degree. The surgeon must be convinced that posterior column-based osteotomies are insufficient to correct the deformity and to achieve a well-aligned spine, and that the spine must be translated as well as shortened, which can only be provided by the excision of the vertebral body. Other clinical findings to drive indications can be neurological and/or functional deficit, cosmesis, pain (mainly in adults because of the degeneration), and progression of deformity (especially in pediatric patients because of the undone growth of the spine).

VCRs are indicated for severe (more than 90 degrees), rigid (less than 20% flexible), and angular deformities, according to the Kunming consensus.[17] Type 1 congenital kyphosis, a sagittal decompensation with a Type 2 coronal malalignment,[6] a hemivertebra,[18] a sharp angular thoracic deformity, spondyloptosis at L5,[19] and a resectable spinal tumor are commonly accepted indications. A fixed coronal plane deformity is another common reason to perform VCR.

Complication Avoidance

VCR complications can be divided into two, namely, intraoperative and postoperative complications. Lenke et al[20] reported the most prevalent complication to be loss of spinal cord monitoring signals or actual spinal cord or nerve root deficits. The same study also shows that the second most prevalent intraoperative complication was an estimated blood loss of more than 2 liters, and the most common postoperative complication was respiratory-related complications. Other common non-neurological complications were reported to be cardiovascular and implant failures.[17]

The overall and neurological complication rates associated with VCRs were reported to be relatively high in earlier studies. Suk et al[7] reported an overall rate of 34.3% and 17.1% for neurological complications. Lenke et al[4] reported an overall complication rate of 40% and a neurological complication rate of 11.4%. More recent studies indicate decreased risks of neurological complications. Hamzaoglu et al[8] reported a 1.96% rate of transient nerve palsies in 102 patients. Lenke et al[20] reported a rate of intraoperative spinal cord monitoring change of 27%; nevertheless, no patient was reported to have permanent complete paraplegia. Jeszenszky et al[9] reported no complications related to the spinal cord.

The rate of neurological complications in the literature is likely underreported due to their retrospective nature. Comparing the results of a prospective study and a retrospective one with identical inclusion criteria, it was concluded that rates of new neurological deficits were nearly twice as high when data were captured prospectively.[21] However, it is also likely that the low reported rates are due to very experienced centers and surgeons reporting them. All in all, VCR should only be the preferred method in severe and fixed cases that could not be managed by other types of osteotomies and halo-gravity traction.

A recent study involving pediatric patients showed that neuromonitoring alterations that occur after decompression and bone resection are often responsive to an increase in blood pressure.[22] However, in severe deformities, the rate of neuromonitoring changes during VCR is considerably higher and may be resistant to hemodynamic improvement since cord compression may be the main factor. Boachie-Adjei et al reported that 8 patients had intraoperative spinal cord monitoring alerts among 13 patients (61.5%) with highly severe deformities.[23] Unresponsive alerts during osteotomy closure are managed by reopening the osteotomy to adjust the cage and reduce the correction amount,[22] or decompression by additional bony and ligamenteous release if there is compression on the spinal cord. A surgeon should be calm, consider all possible scenarios causing neuromonitoring changes, and take all possible actions until the signals improve. Using checklists may help in standardization and ensure no step is missed.

Tips and Tricks

- Preoperative health optimization in terms of pulmonary and aerobic training, nutrition, and stretching is important.
- Gradual and partial correction using halo-gravity traction prior to the VCR approach can be helpful.[23]
- Preoperative three-dimensional CT scans and spine models printed in three dimensions are key in understanding the anatomy in order to perform a safer surgery. This will help in planning preoperatively and navigating intraoperatively.
- In the presence of prior fusion mass and/or weak screw purchase, construct-to-construct corrective maneuvers using dominos might be superior to individual screw manipulations and help avoid catastrophic screw–bone interface failure.

- It is important to have both temporary rods in place as soon as possible to avoid subluxation. Even during correction maneuvers, the contralateral rod can lay between the tulips of the screws with loose nuts.
- Multiple rods spanning the osteotomy site might aid fixation.
- Staged VCR surgery, particularly in revision cases, can help prevent perioperative complications and is strongly recommended.
- Antifibrinolytic agents can help reduce blood loss during VCR procedures.
- Planning skin closure before going to the operating room is essential. Plastic surgeon's expertise can be utilized in severe and multiple-times previously operated cases.

Key Points

- VCR is effective in correcting severe spinal deformities. A posterior-only VCR can significantly improve the radiographic and clinical images.
- AP-VCR and P-VCR are technically challenging treatments with risk of severe complications. Only a surgical team with extensive experience should perform VCR surgeries.
- Spinal cord neuromonitoring is required during the surgery to help prevent neurological injuries.
- VCR should be reserved for deformities that cannot be corrected by less invasive osteotomies. Alternatives including halo-gravity traction and multiple posterior column osteotomies can often obviate the need for VCR.

References

1. Bradford DS, Tribus CB. Vertebral column resection for the treatment of rigid coronal decompensation. Spine 1997;22(14):1590–1599
2. Suk SI, Kim JH, Kim WJ, Lee SM, Chung ER, Nah KH. Posterior vertebral column resection for severe spinal deformities. Spine 2002;27(21):2374–2382
3. MacLennan A. Scoliosis. BMJ 1922;2(3227):864–866
4. Lenke LG, O'Leary PT, Bridwell KH, Sides BA, Koester LA, Blanke KM. Posterior vertebral column resection for severe pediatric deformity: minimum two-year follow-up of thirty-five consecutive patients. Spine 2009;34(20):2213–2221
5. Saifi C, Laratta JL, Petridis P, Shillingford JN, Lehman RA, Lenke LG. Vertebral column resection for rigid spinal deformity. Global Spine J 2017;7(3):280–290
6. Bridwell KH. Decision making regarding Smith-Petersen vs. pedicle subtraction osteotomy vs. vertebral column resection for spinal deformity. Spine 2006;31(19, Suppl):S171–S178
7. Suk SI, Chung ER, Kim JH, Kim SS, Lee JS, Choi WK. Posterior vertebral column resection for severe rigid scoliosis. Spine 2005;30(14):1682–1687

8. Hamzaoglu A, Alanay A, Ozturk C, Sarier M, Karadereler S, Ganiyusufoglu K. Posterior vertebral column resection in severe spinal deformities: a total of 102 cases. Spine 2011;36(5): E340–E344

9. Jeszenszky D, Haschtmann D, Kleinstück FS, et al. Posterior vertebral column resection in early onset spinal deformities. Eur Spine J 2014;23(1):198–208

10. Gokcen B, Yilgor C, Alanay A. Osteotomies/spinal column resection in paediatric deformity. Eur J Orthop Surg Traumatol 2014;24(Suppl 1):S59–S68

11. Enercan M, Ozturk C, Kahraman S, Sarier M, Hamzaoglu A, Alanay A. Osteotomies/spinal column resections in adult deformity. Eur Spine J 2013;22(Suppl 2):S254–S264

12. Sucato DJ. Management of severe spinal deformity: scoliosis and kyphosis. Spine 2010;35(25):2186–2192

13. Davis BJ, Gadgil A, Trivedi J, Ahmed NB. Traction radiography performed under general anesthetic: a new technique for assessing idiopathic scoliosis curves. Spine 2004;29(21): 2466–2470

14. Liu RW, Teng AL, Armstrong DG, Poe-Kochert C, Son-Hing JP, Thompson GH. Comparison of supine bending, push-prone, and traction under general anesthesia radiographs in predicting curve flexibility and postoperative correction in adolescent idiopathic scoliosis. Spine 2010;35(4):416–422

15. Cho W, Lenke LG. Vertebral osteotomies—review of current concepts. Musculoskeletal Rev 2010;5:46–49

16. Dorward IG, Lenke LG. Osteotomies in the posterior-only treatment of complex adult spinal deformity: a comparative review. Neurosurg Focus 2010;28(3):E4

17. Xie JM, Chen ZQ, Shen JX, et al. Expert consensus for PVCR in severe, rigid and angular spinal deformity treatment: the Kunming consensus. J Orthop Surg (Hong Kong) 2017; 25(2):2309499017713939

18. Bradford DS, Boachie-Adjei O. One-stage anterior and posterior hemivertebral resection and arthrodesis for congenital scoliosis. J Bone Joint Surg Am 1990;72(4):536–540

19. Gaines RW. L5 vertebrectomy for the surgical treatment of spondyloptosis: thirty cases in 25 years. Spine 2005;30(6, Suppl):S66–S70

20. Lenke LG, Newton PO, Sucato DJ, et al. Complications after 147 consecutive vertebral column resections for severe pediatric spinal deformity: a multicenter analysis. Spine 2013;38(2): 119–132

21. Kelly MP, Lenke LG, Godzik J, et al. Retrospective analysis underestimates neurological deficits in complex spinal deformity surgery: a Scoli-RISK-1 Study. J Neurosurg Spine 2017;27(1):68–73

22. Jarvis JG, Strantzas S, Lipkus M, et al. Responding to neuromonitoring changes in 3-column posterior spinal osteotomies for rigid pediatric spinal deformities. Spine 2013; 38(8):E493–E503

23. Boachie-Adjei O, Sacramento-Dominguez C, Ayamga J, et al; FOCOS Spine Research Group. Characterization of complex vertebral transposition (gamma deformity)>180 degrees: clinical and radiographic outcomes of halo gravity traction and vertebral column resection (VCR). Spine Deform 2021;9(2):411–425

17 Y-Shaped Osteotomy

Nicat Bayram, Salim Şentürk, and Onur Yaman

Introduction

Fixed sagittal imbalance (FSI) is a syndrome in which the patient can only stand with shifts to the anterior areas at the posterior side of L5–S1 intervertebral disc space and the sagittal vertical axis of 2 cm or more and 6 cm or more, respectively. This syndrome can occur secondary to many etiologies. A typical group of patients is those with a history of inflammatory kyphosis processes such as ankylosing spondylitis (AS), infectious disease (e.g., tuberculosis), degenerative kyphosis, and thoracolumbar fractures which remained untreated with secondary kyphotic deformity.[1–5] The other group of patients is those with previous spinal surgery, such as posterior arthrodesis for lumbar scoliosis using distractive hypo-lordosis techniques, lumbar spinal fusions with "residual flatback deformity," and multilevel laminectomies.

Physicians recommend several osteotomy procedures, which are common ways to repair fixed plane sagittal imbalance of the vertebral column. One of these osteotomy techniques was developed by Smith-Petersen named open wedge osteotomies, which are suitable for young patients with mobile intervertebral discs (Zilke) and middle-age patients with ossification of the disc (Smith-Petersen). Another technique is pedicle subtraction osteotomies (PSOs), which is beneficial in patients with immobile discs who already have osteoporosis. Scuedes and others have described closing wedge osteotomy (CWO) as a single-level procedure, which is limited by a single vertebral body's anterior cortex and offers approximately 25 degrees correction of the thoracic vertebral column and 35 degrees correction of the lumbar vertebral column.[4] The previously mentioned two osteotomy techniques (Zilke and Smith-Petersen) lengthen the anterior vertebral column. Zilke osteotomies can achieve a more significant lengthening than Smith-Petersen osteotomies. However, neurovascular complications are a possibility to consider. CWOs are differentiated from Smith-Peterson osteotomies (SPOs) in terms of the effect on the anterior column. They do not lengthen the anterior vertebral column as in the other techniques. In a meta-analysis published by Liu et al,[6] in 2015, both SPO and PSO were found to be effective in correcting thoracolumbar kyphotic deformity in AS and have a similar risk of most complications. Vertebral column resection (VCR) is a more aggressive surgery primarily used in tumor resections and in patients with severe nonflexible deformities. Although it is an aggressive surgery type, the VCR technique can be used by the surgeon as just a posterior or anterior–posterior combined technique.[7–9]

There is another spinal osteotomy technique known as Y-shaped osteotomy. It is a mixed technique that includes VCR, SPO, PSO, and eggshell techniques. Y shape provides a more significant adjustment of both coronal and sagittal imbalance and makes possible adjustments for all three columns. It also can offer more substantial adjustment for a single-level vertebral osteotomy site in a safer way.[10–13]

This technique is an effective treatment option for AS, severe rigid congenital kyphoscoliosis, posttraumatic kyphosis, postsurgical kyphosis, and kyphotic deformity in Pott's patients.[10–13]

The osteotomy required for the patient should be planned before surgery. Otherwise, excessive or incomplete correction may be encountered, and major complications (such as rod breakage and pseudoarthrosis) may occur due to sagittal balance insufficiency. In addition, with technological advances, measurements of sagittal–coronal spinal parameters and osteotomy simulations (using Surgimap Spine, etc.) can be performed. This significantly contributes to preoperative surgical planning.[14]

Surgical Procedure

Instrument Preparation

Spine osteotome set, pedicle screw and rod set and general set.

Anesthesia

General anesthesia with endotracheal intubation.

Patient Position

The patient is placed in prone position, and the abdomen is left free to reduce intraoperative epidural bleeding. Any radiolucent table can be used for this surgery type. The operating table may be set as an inverted V shape according to the severity of the patients' kyphosis. For patients who have severe kyphosis, the waist bridge and the shoulders need to be elevated. A special cushion should be used for shoulder elevation. The head of the patient should be placed on the head frame that can be adjusted automatically, and the feet should be fixed on the end of the table. Pads should be used to fill the space under the ventral side; thus, after osteotomy the pads are to be removed or the table to be set flat to close the osteotomy site and straighten the trunk (if required).

Neuromonitoring

All surgeries should be performed with somatosensory-evoked potentials and transcranial motor-evoked potentials for neurophysiologic monitoring.

Surgery

A standard posterior midline incision is made at the predetermined level. The spine is exposed by dissection lateral to the costotransverse joint at the thoracic level and the lumbar transverse process. Pedicle screws are placed above and below the osteotomy site. Bleeding is controlled by electric cauterization and hemostatic gauze. The spinal canal opens laterally, and the posterior elements, including the spinous process, bilateral lamina, transverse process, and the adjacent facet joints at the vertebra, are osteotomized and removed as needed. And then Y-shaped osteotomy is performed (**Fig. 17.1a**). Related levels of nerve roots are identified on both sides, and medial retraction is done to expose the pedicles' inner cortex. Pilot holes are created into the pedicles of related level, which are then enlarged by the pedicle probe and drill. A careful decompression is performed to prevent nerve impingement while closing the osteotomy. A short temporary protection rod is secured on the heads of the screws above and below on one side to prevent premature osteotomy closure. Through the pedicle holes, the decancellous procedure is performed using a rongeur, curette, or osteotome on the posterior half of the target vertebra. The vertebral osteotomy is then performed using an osteotome, curette, and rongeurs on the opposite side of the temporary protection rod. The posterior cortical bone of the osteotomized vertebra is removed with the help of a Kerrison, and osteoclasis of the anterior cortex and lateral walls is then achieved using gentle manual extension when closing the posterior wedge space. The middle column is preserved as a hinge. The same procedure transposes the temporary rod on the opposite side. Hohmann retractors are placed around the body bilaterally to expose the lateral surface of the pedicles and corpus of vertebrae. This placement is a reference point for depth. Protecting the vascular structures and measuring the degree of osteotomy are necessary. Controlling the depth and width of the surgery is essential to prevent over/under-adjustments.

The position of the patient and operating table is adjusted for correction. Afterward, the middle vertebral column is closed by using the table's gradual extension and with the help of steady pressure on the pedicle screws superior and inferior of the osteotomy. The protection rod is removed, and the definitive rods are fixed to the screws. If more adjustment is necessary, it is achieved by bending the rods at the osteotomy site. Initially, the hinge is on the anterior column. Subsequently, the hinge is removed from the anterior column to the middle vertebral column at the last surgery (**Fig. 17.1b, c**). The V-shaped wedge is closed at this stage. Conversion from the "V-shaped" to "Y-shaped" ultimate position of the osteotomy is completed. To confirm the degree of adjustment and pedicle screws, lateral X-ray graphics are used. The bone graft of the excised vertebrae, matrix of the demineralized bone, and posterior elements are used for fusion. A drainage tube is left in the procedure area, and the scar is closed. Patient mobilization is provided using a custom-built thoracolumbosacral orthosis (TLSO) brace for about 8 to 12 weeks.

Complications

It is divided into two groups, intraoperative and postoperative.

Intraoperative Complications

Intraoperative complications include dural, vascular, and nerve root injuries, and lamina–pedicle fracture.

Postoperative Complications

As a result of instrumentation, pulmonary problems, pseudoarthrosis, infection, Bos fistula, ileus, and sacroiliac joint degeneration can be seen.

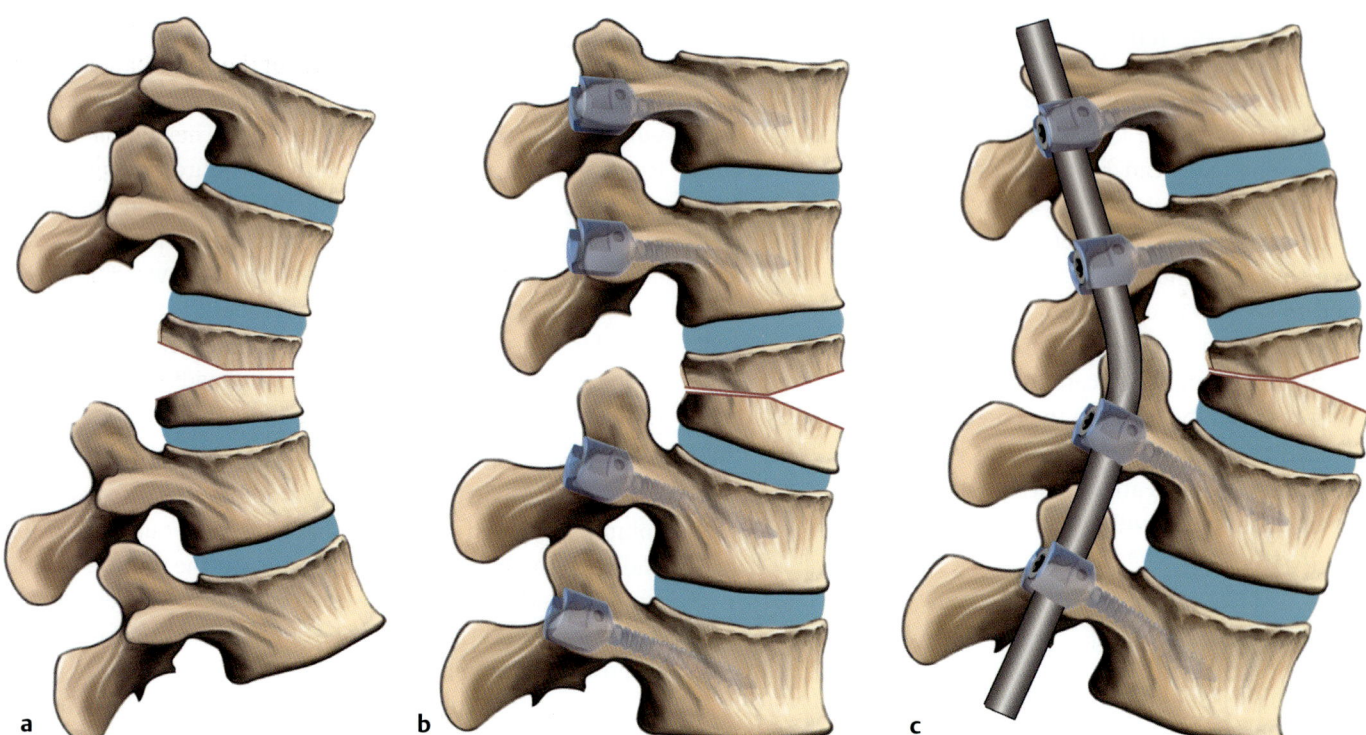

a   b   c

Fig. 17.1 Schematic illustration of Y-shaped osteotomy. **(a)** The anterior and middle columns of the vertebra are removed as little as possible, and the posterior column is completely removed. Thus, a Y-shaped osteotomy is performed. **(b, c)** With some pressure on upper and lower pedicle screws, the anterior column serves as the hinge at the beginning, and then the hinge moves to the middle column at the end of this procedure.

Key Points

- Biomechanically, restoring sagittal balance is to shift the center of gravity of the trunk on the hip axis. Common ways to operate thoracolumbar kyphosis are PSO, SPO, and VCR techniques. SPO with an open wedge osteotomy is an adequate method for patients with flexible kyphotic deformities. However, this method is not strongly suggested for rigid deformities such as AS. Transpedicular wedge osteotomy and PSO are the primary choice for AS patients. In a closing wedging osteotomy, the anterior column of the corpus vertebrae is used as a hinge. Shortening the posterior and middle columns without lengthening the anterior column is a negative aspect of the PSO technique. Although VCR is the most robust technique in correcting spinal deformity, it has disadvantages such as technical difficulty and a high rate of complications.[15–22]

- In "Y-shaped" osteotomies, the most remarkable point is the removing a relatively smaller amount from the posterior half than the other half of the osteotomy column. Moreover, the middle column is mostly preserved as the hinge in this osteotomy technique, which serves as the adjustment "leverage" to get better stability and greater fusion during the adjustment. Opening the anterior column leads to a larger correction angle. This greater angle reduces the posterior column shortening need and the neurological sequel and sagittal axis translation.[23] It is believed that the complications of opening the anterior column formed in Y-shaped osteotomies are acceptable since it creates a smaller anterior column opening than the wedge formed in other osteotomy types (i.e., SPO). In addition, decancellation of the vertebral column procedure from the inside to outside (similar to the eggshell technique) is applied in Y-shaped osteotomy, which in most cases does not require exposing the segmental vessels and reduces the risk of vascular complications.[24]

- Hu et al,[12] in their series of 36 patients with AS with kyphotic deformity, corrected patients' kyphosis with Y-shaped osteotomy and emphasized that Y-shaped osteotomy is a safe and effective technique in the AS patients who have a kyphotic deformity.

- In 2015, Mehdian et al[10] reported that Y-shaped osteotomy in a series of 10 patients with rigid kyphotic deformity provided a safe correction of up to 45 degrees in a single osteotomy region in patients with rigid kyphotic deformity and for corrections below the conus region.

- Zhang et al,[11] in their series of 36 patients with AS with kyphotic deformity, suggested that Y-shaped osteotomy is a new promising technique for adjusting rigid thoracolumbosacral orthosis (TLCO) in AS patients. The most significant advantage of this adjustment style is achieving convincing adjustment, which prevents sagittal translation by controlled anterior column opening and posterior column closing.

References

1. Kubiak EN, Moskovich R, Errico TJ, Di Cesare PE. Orthopaedic management of ankylosing spondylitis. J Am Acad Orthop Surg 2005;13(4):267–278

2. Glassman SD, Bridwell K, Dimar JR, Horton W, Berven S, Schwab F. The impact of positive sagittal balance in adult spinal deformity. Spine 2005;30(18):2024–2029

3. Bridwell KH, Lewis SJ, Lenke LG, Baldus C, Blanke K. Pedicle subtraction osteotomy for the treatment of fixed sagittal imbalance. J Bone Joint Surg Am 2003;85(3):454–463

4. Bridwell KH. Decision making regarding Smith-Petersen vs. pedicle subtraction osteotomy vs. vertebral column resection for spinal deformity. Spine 2006;31(19, Suppl):S171–S178

5. Lagrone MO, Bradford DS, Moe JH, Lonstein JE, Winter RB, Ogilvie JW. Treatment of symptomatic flatback after spinal fusion. J Bone Joint Surg Am 1988;70(4):569–580

6. Liu H, Yang C, Zheng Z, et al. Comparison of Smith-Petersen osteotomy and pedicle subtraction osteotomy for the correction of thoracolumbar kyphotic deformity in ankylosing spondylitis: a systematic review and meta-analysis. Spine 2015;40(8):570–579

7. Roy-Camille R, Mazel C. Vertebrectomy through an enlarged posterior approach for tumors and malunions. D.R. Bridwell KH. 1st ed. Philadelphia: Lippincott; 1991:1243–1256

8. Suk SI, Kim JH, Kim WJ, Lee SM, Chung ER, Nah KH. Posterior vertebral column resection for severe spinal deformities. Spine 2002;27(21):2374–2382

9. Bradford DS, Tribus CB. Vertebral column resection for the treatment of rigid coronal decompensation. Spine 1997;22(14):1590–1599

10. Mehdian H, Arun R, Aresti NA. V-Y vertebral body osteotomy for the treatment of fixed sagittal plane spinal deformity. Spine J 2015;15(4):771–776

11. Zhang X, Zhang Z, Wang J, et al. Vertebral column decancellation: a new spinal osteotomy technique for correcting rigid thoracolumbar kyphosis in patients with ankylosing spondylitis. Bone Joint J 2016;98-B(5):672–678

12. Hu W, Yu J, Liu H, Zhang X, Wang Y. Y shape osteotomy in ankylosing spondylitis, a prospective case series with minimum 2 year follow-up. PLoS One 2016;11(12):e0167792

13. Xin Z, Zheng G, Huang P, Zhang X, Wang Y. Clinical results and surgery tactics of spinal osteotomy for ankylosing spondylitis kyphosis: experience of 428 patients. J Orthop Surg Res 2019;14(1):330

14. Akbar M, Terran J, Ames CP, Lafage V, Schwab F. Use of Surgimap Spine in sagittal plane analysis, osteotomy planning, and correction calculation. Neurosurg Clin N Am 2013;24(2):163–172

15. Song K, Zheng G, Zhang Y, Zhang X, Mao K, Wang Y. A new method for calculating the exact angle required for spinal osteotomy. Spine 2013;38(10):E616–E620

16. Smith-Petersen MN, Larson CB, Aufranc OE. Osteotomy of the spine for correction of flexion deformity in rheumatoid arthritis. Clin Orthop Relat Res 1969;66(66):6–9

17. Thomasen E. Vertebral osteotomy for correction of kyphosis in ankylosing spondylitis. Clin Orthop Relat Res 1985;(194):142–152

18. Xi YM, Pan M, Wang ZJ, et al. Correction of post-traumatic thoracolumbar kyphosis using pedicle subtraction osteotomy. Eur J Orthop Surg Traumatol 2013;23(Suppl 1):S59–S66

19. Zheng GQ, Song K, Zhang YG, et al. Two-level spinal osteotomy for severe thoracolumbar kyphosis in ankylosing spondylitis. Experience with 48 patients. Spine 2014;39(13):1055–1058

20. Qian BP, Wang XH, Qiu Y, et al. The influence of closing-opening wedge osteotomy on sagittal balance in thoracolumbar kyphosis secondary to ankylosing spondylitis: a comparison with closing wedge osteotomy. Spine 2012;37(16):1415–1423

21. Bridwell KH, Lewis SJ, Edwards C, et al. Complications and outcomes of pedicle subtraction osteotomies for fixed sagittal imbalance. Spine 2003;28(18):2093–2101

22. Suk KS, Kim KT, Lee SH, Kim JM. Significance of chin-brow vertical angle in correction of kyphotic deformity of ankylosing spondylitis patients. Spine 2003;28(17):2001–2005

23. Murrey DB, Brigham CD, Kiebzak GM, Finger F, Chewning SJ. Transpedicular decompression and pedicle subtraction osteotomy (eggshell procedure): a retrospective review of 59 patients. Spine 2002;27(21):2338–2345

24. Arun R, Dabke HV, Mehdian H. Comparison of three types of lumbar osteotomy for ankylosing spondylitis: a case series and evolution of a safe technique for instrumented reduction. Eur Spine J 2011;20(12):2252–2260

18 Sacral Derotation Osteotomy

Bronek Boszczyk

Introduction

Deformities of the sacrum are uncommon entities. The most common reason for performing lumbosacral operations in deformity surgery is for the correction of spondylolisthesis. Rarely, however, sacral hyperkyphosis can also lead to an increased pelvic incidence with overall sagittal plane disbalance, which develops in childhood. This needs to be recognized in addition to any existing spondylolisthesis. Typically, by the age of 10, the pelvic incidence is fixed within the pelvis.[1]

Indications

In the event of sacral hyperkyphosis and excessive pelvic incidence, corrective options are limited to osteotomies. Here, the conventional techniques are either a subtraction osteotomy around the S1 pedicles of the sacral vertebral body or a derotation osteotomy through the lateral masses. The author has experienced one case with sacral derotation osteotomy[2] due to these entities being uncommon. Describing this technique in detail may benefit others in case they encounter a similar entity.

Definition of the Technique

The principle of sacral derotation osteotomy lies in vertical osteotomies through the lateral mass of the sacrum bilaterally from S1 right through to the sciatic notch. At this moment, the central portion of the sacrum is detached from the pelvis bilaterally. The neural foramen remains medial to the osteotomy, reducing the risk of neural involvement or injury. To avoid translation of the sacrum and to facilitate controlled rotation around a transverse axis, a transverse screw, bolt, or large K-wire needs to be placed ideally through the S1 vertebral body. The reduction is then achieved through instrumentation of the pelvis and lower lumbar spine, whereby the lower lumbar spine is reduced to the pelvis around the transverse rotational axis placed through the S1 vertebral body. In principle, the degree of the rotation can be chosen freely, and large degrees of derotation can be achieved to balance pelvic incidence.

Operative Steps

This procedure is best done on a radiolucent table. It is essentially done in prone position with draping to allow access to the lateral part of the pelvis for placement of the trans-sacral screw or K-wire. The author prefers an inverted U-shaped incision for lumbar–pelvic pathologies. At this moment, a U-shaped flap is lifted, which is centered across L3 with the lateral margins of the incision crossing the iliac crest of either side. This flap is lifted caudally so that the iliac crest, thoracolumbar fascia, and posterior wall of the sacrum are exposed. The next step is to incise the thoracolumbar fascia close to the midline in the standard technique. This allows exposure of the multifidus muscle across the entire sacrum. The multifidus muscle is carefully dissected out of its bed from the distal portions of the sacrum to the lumbosacral junction where the lateral muscle tract is formed. Lifting the multifidus muscle preserves structural integrity and provides excellent exposure to the entire posterior aspect of the sacrum (**Fig. 18.1**). The multifidus muscle at the lumbosacral junction also naturally runs into the typical "Wiltse" muscles splitting plane. Continuing the split allows the exposure of the pedicle entry sites

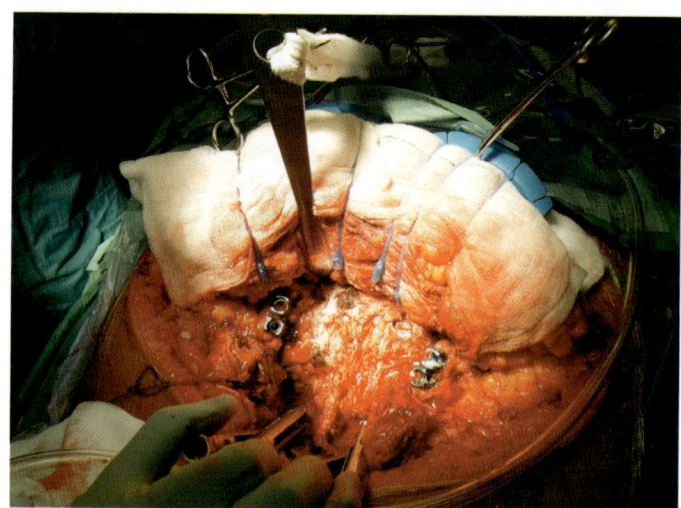

Fig. 18.1 Posterior exposure of sacrum: Via an inverted "U"-shaped incision, a flap has been mobilized inferiorly (covered with swabs). The sacrum is fully exposed after the multifidus muscle has been elevated cranially. Screws have been placed in the iliac bone bilaterally.

at the intersection between the transverse and articular processes. This is no different from conventional muscle splitting techniques. The next step consists of placing the pedicle screws in the lumbar spine, typically L3/L4 or L4/L5. By splitting the muscle, a high degree of conversion can be achieved. Screws are also placed in the pelvis in the conventional technique. Here, it is helpful to place two pelvic screws bilaterally. It is now possible to place a screw, bolt, or K-wire across the posterior ring of the pelvis through S1. For this step, the image intensification is adjusted in the lateral position. The vertebral body of S1 is visualized with the posterior cortex of S1, and the contours of the anterior vertebral body and anterior border of the sacral lateral mass are seen. Details of the anatomical landmarks have been published previously.[3] In brief, the following are the safe borders for the placement of the K-wire: The S1 root passes across the inferior posterior corner of the S1 vertebral body and needs to be avoided. The L5 root crosses the superior anterior corner of the S1 vertebral body as it passes along the projected line of the lateral mass of the sacrum. Central placement within S1 is safe, however. Passage of the K-wire is completed under anteroposterior (AP) and lateral image intensification. Starting in a lateral position allows for ideal centralization in S1; alternating views are used to verify the positioning. The K-wire needs to be passed all the way across the contralateral sacroiliac joint. Once the K-wire has been placed satisfactorily, the osteotomy of the sacrum can be performed (**Fig. 18.2**). This can be performed either with a high-speed burr down to the anterior cortex of the sacrum with the cortex being resected with Kerrison rongeurs or alternatively utilizing an ultrasonic bone scalpel. Care needs

to be taken to avoid contact of the tools directly with the trans-sacral K-wire or another device. If the sacrum is too deep for a regular bone scalpel blade, the posterior portion of the sacrum can be opened with a high-speed burr to create a trough for the ultrasonic bone scalpel. **Fig. 18.3** demonstrates the screw placement of the pelvis and the reduction tube placement in the lumbar spine. The pelvis is now instrumented with two trans-sacral bars whereby the screws from the pelvis are connected bilaterally. Placing two bars allows for a solid fixation and closes the posterior ring of the pelvis. The longitudinal rods are mounted to these trans-sacral bars at the angle estimated to be desirable for the derotation correction. Once this has been achieved, the lumbar spine screws are reduced to the rod through reduction tubes (**Fig. 18.4**). By reducing the lumbar screws to the rods, the spine can be derotated around the trans-sacral rotational axis. This is monitored under image intensification (fluoroscopy) and the reduction can be adjusted to allow correction to the optimal pelvic incidence. If necessary, a bone graft can be placed from the lumbar spine to the sacrum. There is no need for bone grafting across the sacrum osteotomy as the osteotomy sites have excellent fusion properties. Deep drains are inserted under the flap, and closure is performed in the usual technique. It is helpful to place deep sutures under the flap to avoid the formation of a postoperative seroma. Typically, the drains are left in situ for 3 to 4 days. With a solid fixation, patients can bear weight immediately after surgery. Running and jumping should be avoided. If there is concern regarding the bone quality, then crutches for 6 to 8 weeks to offset the load to the sacrum and pelvis should be considered.

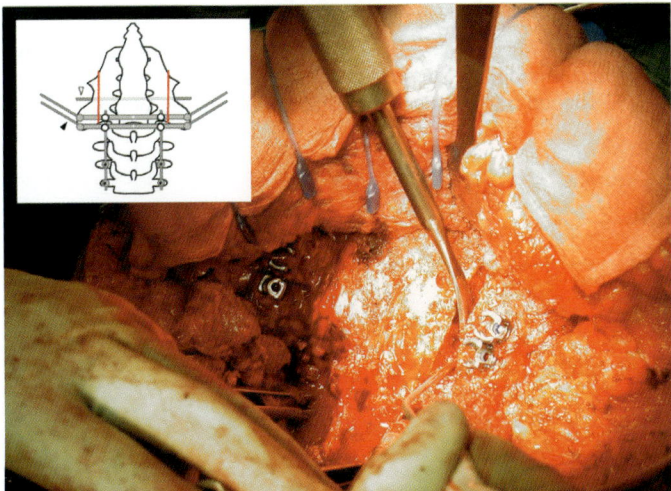

Fig. 18.2 Bilateral osteotomy of the sacrum: The osteotomy has been completed bilaterally. The tip of the Cobb instrument is in the osteotomy. The inset shows the osteotomy lines across the sacrum in the picture's orientation.

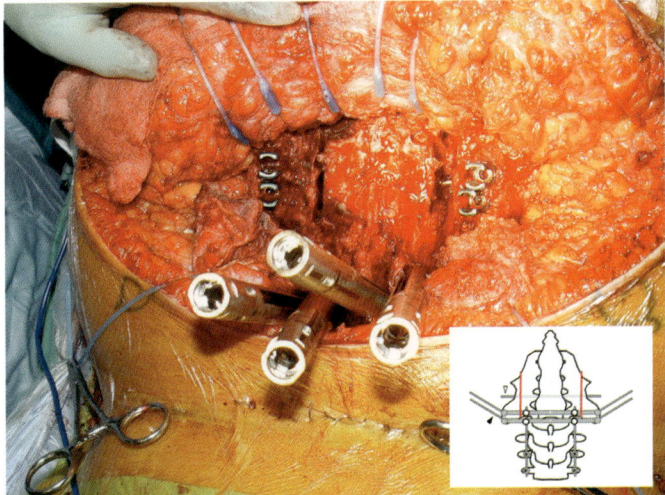

Fig. 18.3 Overview of the instrumentation before reduction: Two pelvic screws are placed bilaterally. Downtubes are mounted to the instrumented lumbar vertebrae.

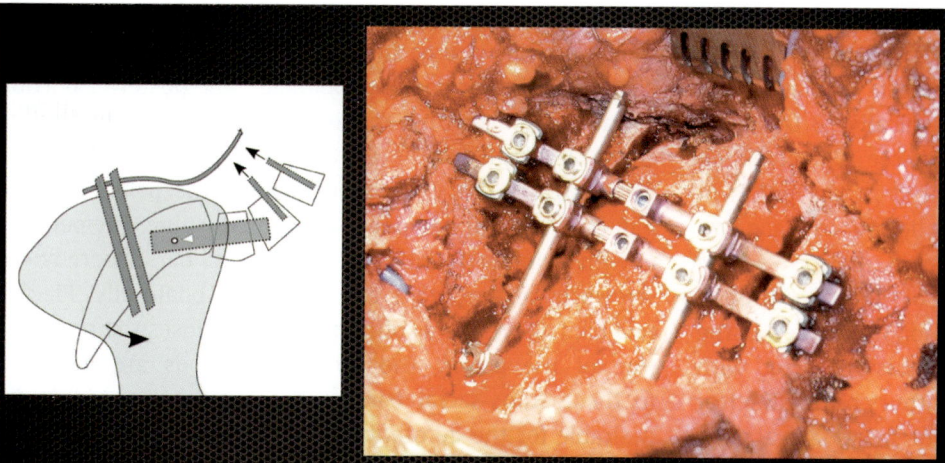

Fig. 18.4 Derotation of the sacrum: The sacrum is derotated by reducing the lumbar spine to the rods. Double rods across the sacrum prevent loss of correction.

Typical complications beyond those familiar to spinal surgery include the formation of a seroma under the flap. This can be aspirated using ultrasonic guidance.

Although the author has only performed the actual derotation in one selected case (**Fig. 18.5**), the exposure and sacrum osteotomy technique has been used in several cases for various spinal and sacrum pathologies, including tumors and fractures.

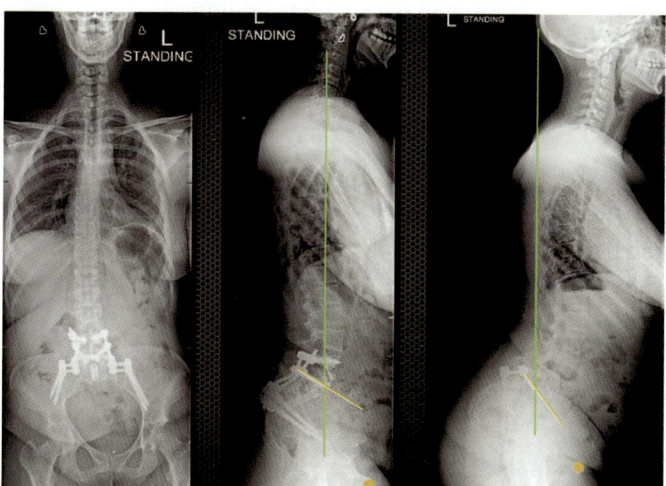

Fig. 18.5 Example of sacral rotation in a patient with previous lumbar fusion: The orange marking on the symphysis in relation to the instrumented lumbar spine. Pelvic incidence has been reduced close to normal with the restoration of sagittal balance.

References

1. Marty C, Boisaubert B, Descamps H, et al. The sagittal anatomy of the sacrum among young adults, infants, and spondylolisthesis patients. Eur Spine J 2002;11(2):119–125
2. Czyz M, Forster S, Holton J, Shariati B, Clarkson DJ, Boszczyk BM. New method for correction of lumbo-sacral kyphosis deformity in patient with high pelvic incidence. Eur Spine J 2017;26(8):2204–2210
3. König MA, Seidel U, Heini P, et al. Minimal-invasive percutaneous reduction and transsacral screw fixation for U-shaped fractures. J Spinal Disord Tech 2013;26(1):48–54

Part IV

Sagittal Plane Correction Techniques

J. Manuel Sarmiento, Frank Schwab, and Virginie Lafage

Introduction

The human spine is comprised of the cervical, thoracic, lumbar, and sacral regions each of which has inherent curvatures. The "normal" lumbar curve is lordotic, the thoracic and sacral curves are kyphotic, while the cervical alignment can be neutral, lordotic, or mildly kyphotic. The progression from a primal "C-shape" spinopelvic configuration to the "S-shape" composed of the aforementioned inherent curves, along with progressive widening and retroversion of the pelvic ring, has permitted humans to evolve into a bipedal species and successfully adopt a neutral upright posture. Spinal alignment is therefore unique to *Hominidae* species.

There is a wide range of cervical lordosis in asymptomatic individuals, so a meaningful discussion of this parameter should be in relation to the thoracic spine. Thoracic kyphosis can be defined as the angle between the upper endplate of T4 vertebra and the lower endplate of the T12 vertebra. The average T4–T12 thoracic kyphosis in an asymptomatic adult subject typically varies from 34 to 44 degrees. However, the normal kyphotic range of the thoracic spine can span from 20 to 70 degrees. The normal range of lumbar lordosis (LL) can range from 40 to 80 degrees and sometimes even higher.[1-4] The sagittal alignment of the thoracolumbar junction is relatively neutral. LL is instrumental for modern humans to maintain an upright, properly aligned posture, and the amount of segmental lordosis increases with each level in the lumbar spine.[5] Approximately two-thirds of the normal LL is generated by the L4–S1 levels. It is important to emphasize that these reference parameters are age-specific (and dependent upon pelvic morphology) and not meaningful in isolation. Rather, they should be measured and analyzed in relation to each other to appropriately assess the global sagittal alignment of the spine.

The three principal spinal curves (cervical, thoracic, and lumbar) harmoniously balance one another to maintain the head centered over the shoulders, and the shoulders centered just over the sacrum and pelvis with minimal energy expenditure. This ideal neutral posture configuration was described by Dubousset in his "cone of economy" (**Fig. 19.1**), referring to the standing alignment range where the body remains balanced with minimal muscle action.[6] Upright human posture requires the center of gravity to fall over a narrow range between the feet while maintaining a horizontal gaze.[7]

Definition of Spinopelvic Parameters

Evaluation of Spinopelvic Alignment on Radiographs

The evaluation of the spinopelvic alignment begins with full-length standing coronal and sagittal radiographs. Patients should maintain a neutral, upright position with the hips and knees in a comfortable posture. The elbows should be flexed with fingertips placed on the clavicles. This is the optimal patient stance for obtaining a lateral 36″ radiograph because it provides the best overall visualization of important spinal landmarks without inducing changes in sagittal curvatures (**Fig. 19.2**).[8] The spine should be visible above the level of C2,

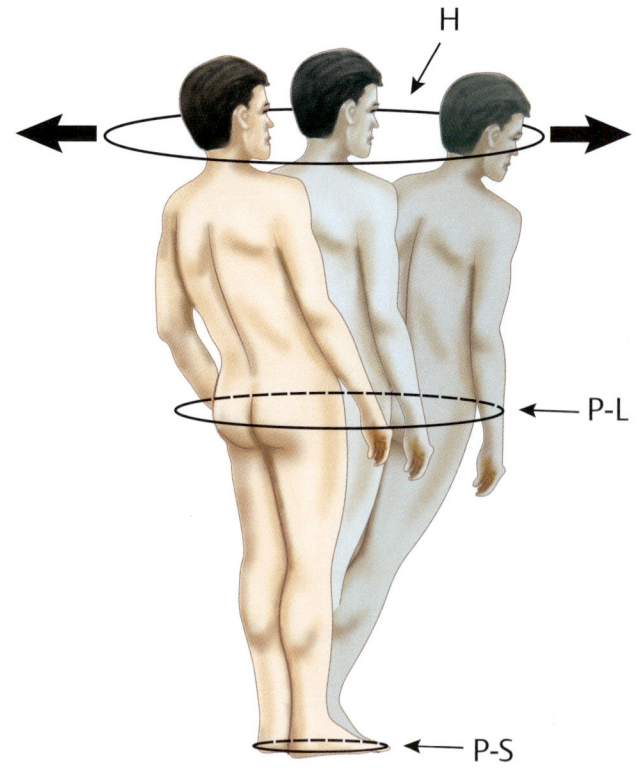

Fig. 19.1 Dubousset's "cone of economy." H, head; P-L, pelvic level; P-S, polygon of sustentation.[6]

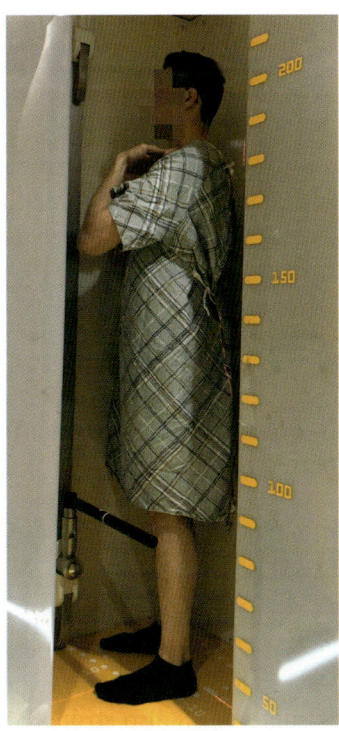

Fig. 19.2 The clavicle position for obtaining lateral 36" or EOS radiographs is shown. The elbows are flexed, the wrists are flexed, and the fingers are placed into the supraclavicular fossae. There is no external support needed with this position.

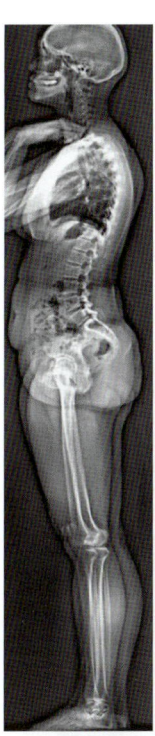

Fig. 19.3 The ideal sagittal spinopelvic alignment is shown here, where the patient maintains a horizontal gaze with a vertical trunk and little-to-no compensation.

and the femoral heads should be visualized in the same film. The ideal sagittal spinopelvic alignment is one where the patient is able to maintain a horizontal gaze with a vertical trunk and no engagement of compensatory mechanism (**Fig. 19.3**).

Sagittal Spinopelvic Parameters

The Pelvis: Foundation of the Spine

One can think of the pelvis as the foundation of the spine. The pelvis has been termed "the pedestal of the spine" by Le Huec, and it provides an important link between the spine and lower extremities.[9] Since the spine starts at the pelvis, it can be thought of as the regulator of the sagittal plane. Ginette Duval-Beaupere's work[10] on the influence of pelvic morphology on spinal alignment highlighted three critical parameters to evaluate the pelvis: pelvic incidence (PI), pelvic tilt (PT), and sacral slope (SS). These three parameters are related according to the following formula: PI = PT + SS (**Fig. 19.4**).

Pelvic Incidence: The Starting Point of the Spine

The PI is a fixed anatomical parameter defined as the angle between a perpendicular line at the midpoint of the sacral

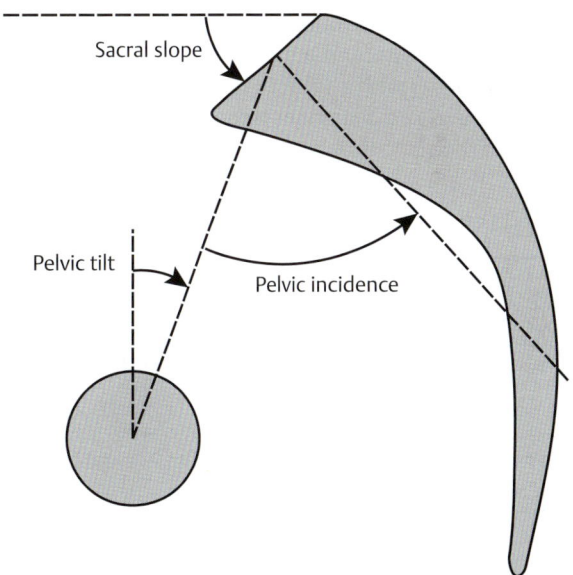

Fig. 19.4 The relation between the three pelvic parameters (PI = PT + SS), with PI = pelvic incidence, PT = pelvic tilt, and SS = sacral slope.

plate and a line connecting this point to the center of the femoral head.[11] PI essentially measures the orientation of the sacrum within the pelvis. PI is considered a morphological, fixed parameter that is unaffected by the spatial orientation of the pelvis (**Fig. 19.5**). The reported average value in asymptomatic adults is 52 degrees (range 35–85 degrees).

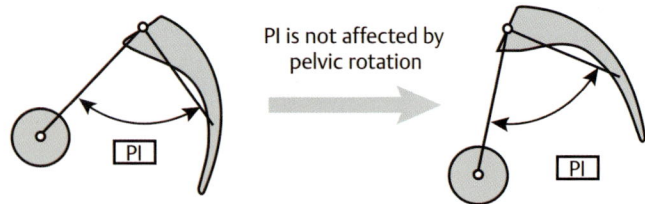

Fig. 19.5 Impact of rotation on pelvic incidence (PI) and example of PI measurements.

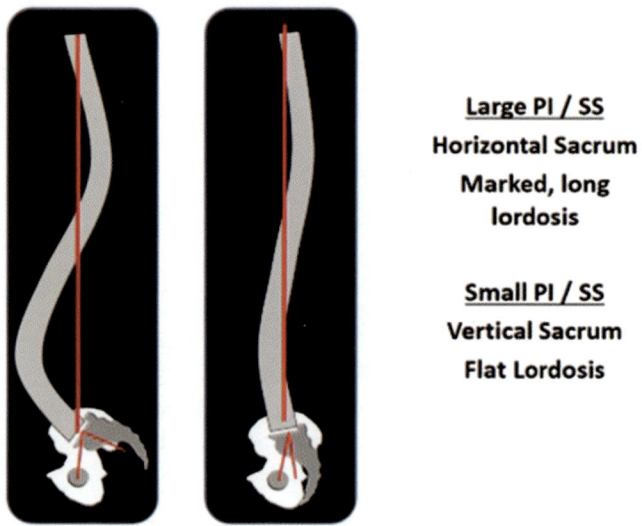

Large PI / SS

Horizontal Sacrum

Marked, long lordosis

Small PI / SS

Vertical Sacrum

Flat Lordosis

Fig. 19.6 Patients with a large pelvic incidence (PI) tend to have a more horizontal position of the sacrum within the pelvis, a large lumbar lordosis, and a more elevated curvatures of the spine (left). Patients with a small PI tend to have a more vertical sacrum, a relatively small lumbar lordosis, and less pronounced curvatures of the spine (right).

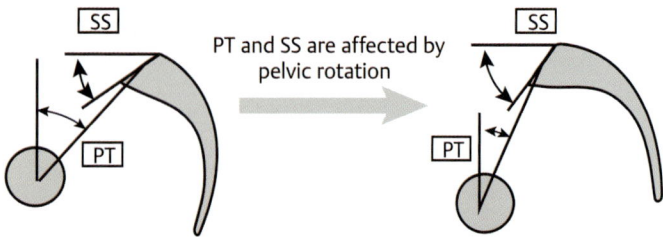

PT and SS are affected by pelvic rotation

Fig. 19.7 Impact of rotation on pelvic tilt (PT) and sacral slope (SS) and example of measurements.

Though there is wide variation in the PI range, there does not seem to be any actual pathological PI value.[12] However, extreme PI values have been associated with Scheuermann's kyphosis (low PI) and spondylolisthesis (high PI).[13-15] In general, patients with a small PI tend to have vertical sacrum, relatively small LL, and less spinal curvature. Conversely, patients with a large PI tend to have horizontal sacrum, large LL, and more spinal curvature (**Fig. 19.6**).

Pelvic Tilt and Sacral Slope

The pelvis freely rotates around the femoral heads, and its anterior angular orientation (anteversion) and posterior angular orientation (retroversion) can be assessed by the PT and SS. PT and SS are both dynamic parameters that change with patient positioning, specifically by rotation of the pelvis around the hip axis (**Fig. 19.7**).

The SS corresponds to the sagittal inclination of the sacral endplate; it is defined as the angle between the sacral endplate of the S1 vertebra and a line in the horizontal plane. In asymptomatic subjects, SS also strongly correlates with PI (**Fig. 19.8**), with an average value reported to be 41 ± 8 degrees.[12] Since the sacral endplate serves as the basis for the entire spine, SS measures the slope of lordosis at S1 and therefore influences the position and alignment of the lumbar spine.

The PT is defined as the angle between a vertical line at the center of the femoral head axis, and a line that connects to the midpoint of the sacral plate. When the femoral heads are not precisely aligned and superimposed over each other, a line is drawn between the centers of both femoral heads and the midpoint of this line is used to measure the PT (**Fig. 19.9**). The average PT in asymptomatic adult subjects is 13 ± 6 degrees. PT is used to quantify the degree of compensatory pelvic retroversion recruited by a patient to maintain/restore a global sagittal alignment (**Fig. 19.10**). Positive values of PT indicate a posterior rotation of the pelvis (retroversion) and negative values indicate an anterior rotation (anteversion).

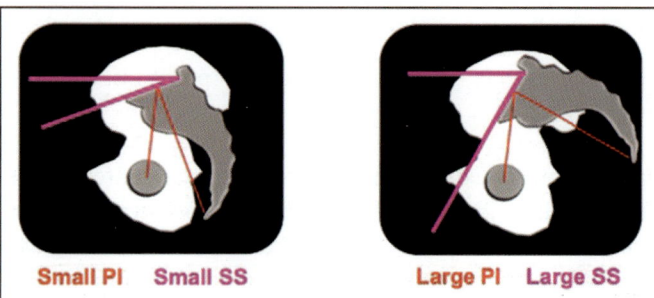

Small PI   Small SS   **Large PI   Large SS**

Fig. 19.8 Sacral slope (SS) correlates with pelvic incidence (PI).

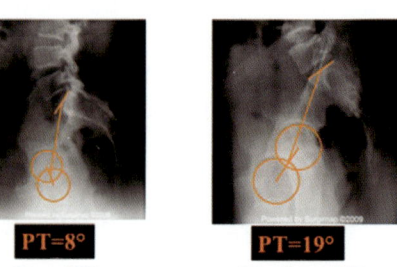
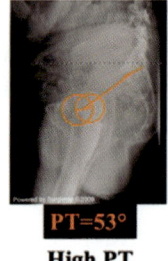

PT=8°   PT=19°   PT=53°

Low PT   **Medium PT**   **High PT**

Fig. 19.9 Variation of pelvic tilt (PT) and example of measurements when femoral heads are not aligned.

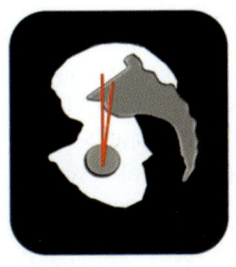

Low PT
Low or no pelvic retroversion

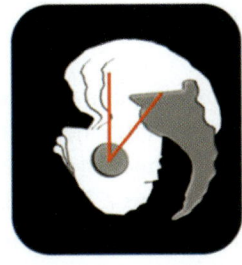

High PT
High pelvic retroversion

Fig. 19.10 The pelvis can rotate around the femoral heads (measure of pelvic tilt [PT]) and serve as one of the most effective mechanisms of sagittal plane regulation.

Lumbar Lordosis

The lumbar curvature is quantified by the LL angle using the Cobb method proposed by John Robert Cobb in 1948.[16] LL is measured by the Cobb angle between the upper endplate of the L1 vertebra and upper endplate of the S1 vertebra. The mean reported values for LL in asymptomatic adult subjects ranges from 40 to 63 degrees with a standard deviation of 10 degrees, but extreme values may extend from 30 degrees to over 80 degrees range. As discussed later, the appropriate amount of LL needed for any given patient should be estimated based on the patient's PI and age. A simple and acceptable rule of thumb when determining how much LL is needed during surgical planning is to match LL with the patient's PI. This rule will hold true as long as the patient's thoracic kyphosis or PI is within the normal ranges.

The "pelvic incidence minus lumbar lordosis" parameter quantifies the mismatch between the pelvis' inherent morphology and the patient's lumbar curve. PI-LL is defined as the difference between the PI and the LL (**Fig. 19.11**). A target PI-LL below the 10 degrees threshold achieves a satisfactory spinopelvic alignment.[17] This relationship allows the surgeon to estimate the required amount of LL needed to match a patient's fixed PI and properly align them in the sagittal plane. The simple PI-LL < 10 degrees relationship requires modification for patients with abnormal PI ranges and high thoracic kyphosis.[7] Patients with low PI require an LL that is larger than their PI (LL = PI + 10 degrees) and patients with large PI require an LL that is smaller than their PI (LL = PI − 10 degrees) (**Fig. 19.12**). Patients with high thoracic kyphosis require an LL larger than the theoretically calculated one in order to accommodate their hyper-thoracic kyphosis. These findings were incorporated into a more developed formula to account for patients with these characteristics, where LL = (PI + TK)/2 + 10.

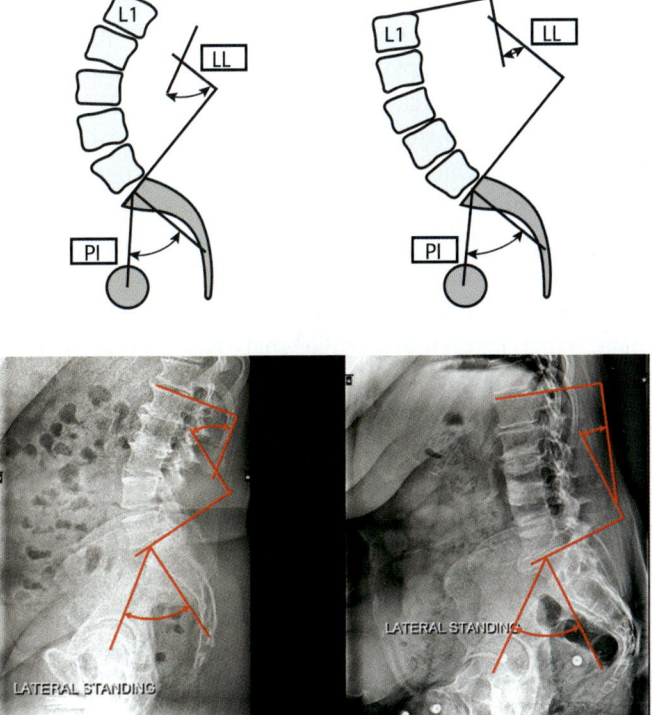

Fig. 19.11 Pelvic incidence minus lumbar lordosis (PI-LL).

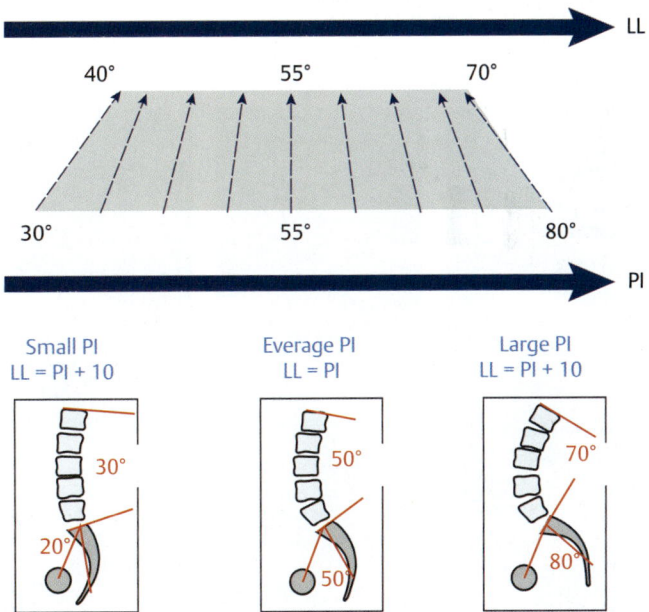

Fig. 19.12 Lumbar lordosis (LL) required across different ranges of pelvic incidence (PI).

There is a variation of lumbar segmental lordosis in asymptomatic adults that is related to the PI. Pesenti et al studied anatomic landmarks in asymptomatic adult volunteers to define normative values of segmental lordosis at each level according to PI.[18] They found that an increase of PI correlated with a proximal migration of the apex of LL.

The lordosis within the proximal portion of the lumbar spine (defined as the angle between the superior endplate of L1 and the superior endplate of L4) increased with increasing PI (**Fig. 19.13**). In fact, in patients with high PI, proximal lordosis was responsible for almost half of the total lordosis. Distal lordosis, which was defined as the angle between the superior endplates of L4 and S1, was nearly constant and independent of the PI (**Fig. 19.14**). By understanding that PI strongly influences the proximal portion of LL, surgeons may plan lumbar fusions accordingly to restore proper lumbar shape using segmental angular goals based on a patient's pelvic morphology.

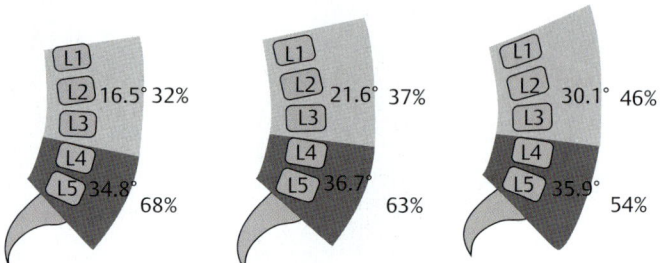

Low pelvic incidence   Average pelvic incidence   HIgh pelvic incidence

Fig. 19.13 The proximal lordosis increases with pelvic incidence (PI). The distal lordosis remains relatively constant in spite of changes in PI.

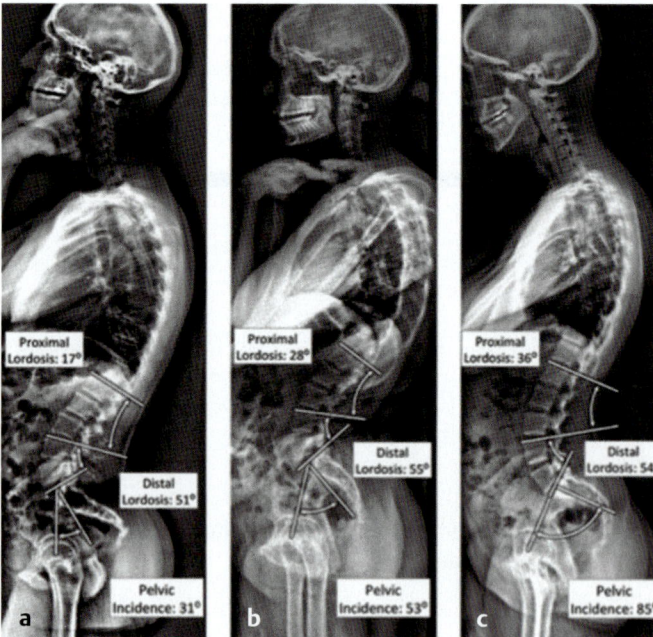

Fig. 19.14 Clinical examples of increasing proximal lordosis correlating with increasing pelvic incidence (PI). In patients with low **(a)** and average **(b)** PI, the main part of the lordosis occurs within the distal vertebra, whereas in patients with high PI **(c)**, 36% of the total lordosis is located within the proximal vertebra. Note that the distal lordosis was nearly constant in these three patients, irrespective of the PI value. (Adapted with permission from Pesenti et al.[18])

Sagittal Vertical Axis (SVA)

The most common parameter used to assess a patient's global spinopelvic alignment is the sagittal vertical axis (SVA). The SVA is defined as the distance of a horizontal plumb line dropped from C7 vertebral body to the posterosuperior corner of the sacral plate (**S1**). It is used to determine if a patient is in neutral, positive, or negative sagittal alignment. It has been proposed that the spine is positively malaligned when the C7 plumb line falls in front of the posterosuperior corner of S1 in excess of 5.0 cm.[19] Importantly, the SVA measurement is influenced by patient's position and patient's PT (**Fig. 19.15**). This means that a truly malaligned spine may be masked by a compensatory pelvic retroversion (i.e., an increase in PT).

Cervical Spine

Cervical lordosis is defined as the angle between the inferior endplate of C2 and the inferior endplate of C7.[20] There is a wide range in cervical lordosis in asymptomatic adult subjects, up to 30% of the normal population have a kyphotic

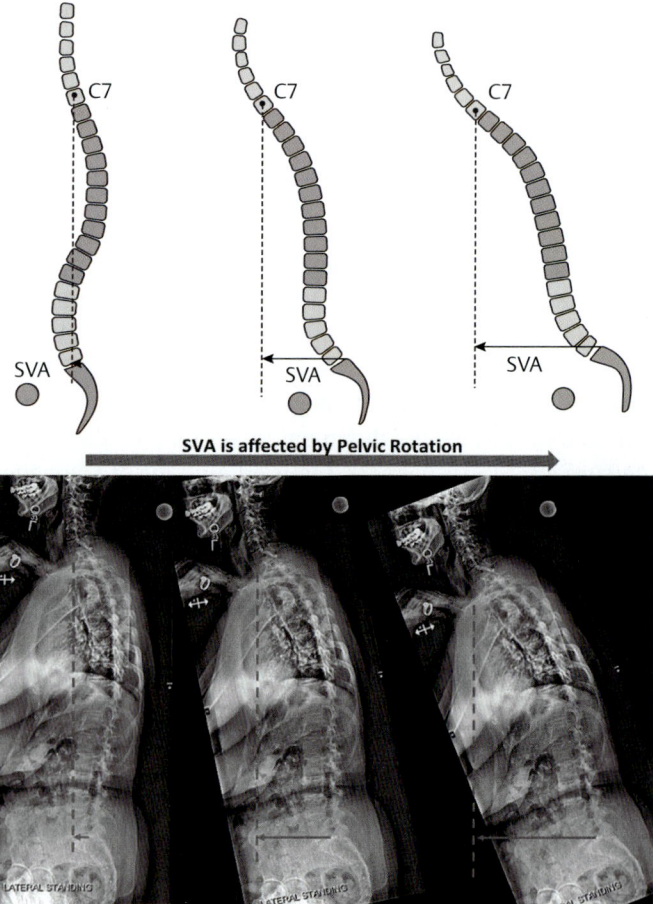

Fig. 19.15 Sagittal vertical axis measurement and impact of rotation.

cervical curve.[21] Therefore, measuring cervical lordosis as a standalone parameter is of questionable utility. The cervical sagittal vertical axis (cSVA) quantifies the regional alignment of the cervical spine. It is defined as the distance between a plumb line dropped from the center of C2 and the posterior superior aspect of C7. The threshold C2–C7 SVA value beyond which the neck disability index is adversely affected is 4.0 cm. However, the true interpretation of this value is complex because cSVA is highly affected by the orientation of the thoracic, lumbar, and pelvic regions (**Fig. 19.16**). Therefore, cervical spinal deformity is difficult to define, especially when there is a concurrent thoracolumbar deformity. The relationship between the T1 slope and cervical lordosis is used to define primary cervical spinal deformity and identify patients who also have a concurrent thoracolumbar deformity. T1 slope is the angle formed between a line in the horizontal plane and the T1 upper endplate.[22]

Cervical lordosis should generally be proportional to the T1 slope (**Fig. 19.17**). Thus, just as PI is used to determine the optimal LL, the ideal cervical lordosis is determined by the T1 slope.[23] A large T1 slope correlates with a lordotic cervical curve, while a small T1 slope correlates with a kyphotic cervical curve. The "T1 slope minus cervical lordosis" parameter is used to quantify the mismatch between the orientation of T1 and the cervical lordosis (**Fig. 19.18**). The T1-CL should be less than 17 degrees. A great mismatch between T1-CL means the greater the difference between T1 and CL values, the greater the degree of cervical malalignment and disability.[24]

Mechanisms of Compensation

The musculoskeletal system recruits conscious and unconscious spinopelvic compensatory mechanisms in response to segmental, regional, or global alignment changes. These alignment changes may come from pathologic etiologies or simply from the normal aging process. As we age, degenerative changes in our spine result in disc degeneration, increased thoracic kyphosis, and loss of LL; all of these factors contribute to progressively positive sagittal alignment.[25] In response to these changes, during stance, we recruit compensatory mechanisms to maintain the gravity line over a small area between the feet and maintain a horizontal gaze. The most common compensatory mechanisms are hyperextending the lumbar curvature, flattening of the thoracic kyphosis, pelvic retroversion, knee flexion, and pelvic shift (**Fig. 19.19**). It is paramount to differentiate the driver of the spinal deformity from compensatory mechanisms during surgical planning so that the true cause of the deformity is targeted and corrected.

Loss of LL is the most common cause of sagittal malalignment. A regional compensation for loss of normal

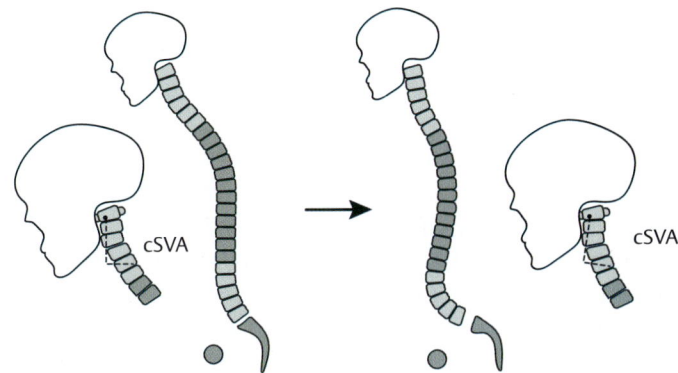

Fig. 19.16   Cervical sagittal vertical axis (cSVA) and impact on thoracolumbar deformity and correction.

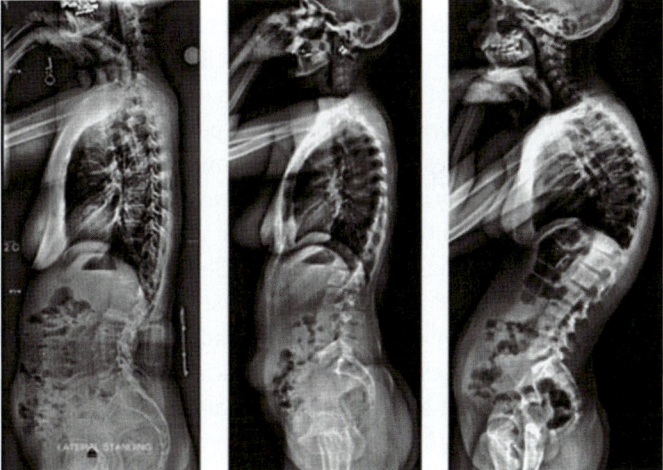

Fig. 19.17   Cervical lordosis increases with T1 slope.

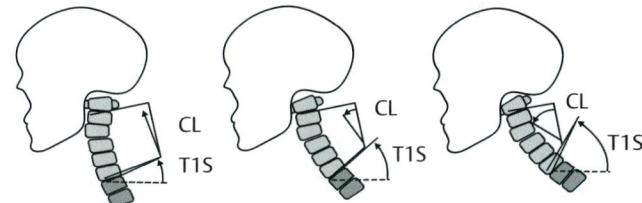

Fig. 19.18   T1 slope minus cervical lordosis (TS-CL): increase in CL with increase of T1 slope to maintain and horizontal gaze TS-CL.

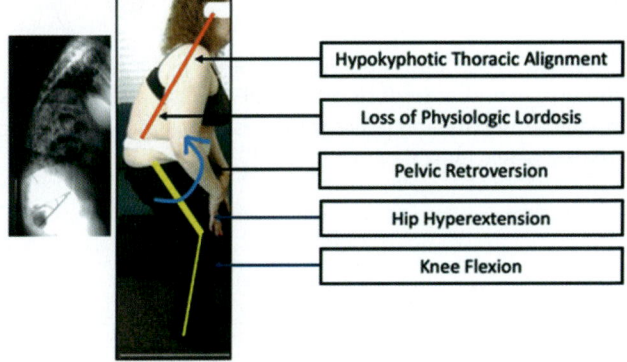

Fig. 19.19   Compensatory mechanisms in response to spinal sagittal malalignment.

LL involves the adjacent functional spinal units in the lumbar spine. These adjacent segments compensate by hyperextension to limit the consequence of the loss of lordosis. Young patients with a flexible spine and strong musculature may flatten their thoracic kyphosis to limit the anterior shift of the trunk. Pelvic retroversion (backward rotation) is arguably one of the most effective compensatory mechanisms against sagittal malalignment, largely because of the high mobility of the hip joint.[26] In an attempt to bring the spine back into neutral sagittal alignment, the body recruits the aide of the pelvis by retroversion (quantified by an increase in PT) in order to increase the LL (**Fig. 19.20**). However, the degree of pelvic retroversion is ultimately exhausted as the spinopelvic mismatch (PI-LL) increases.[7]

Another common compensation mechanism for spinal sagittal malalignment is knee flexion, but it generally appears after exhaustion of earlier compensatory mechanisms such as lumbar hyperextension and pelvic retroversion. Knee flexion requires constant activation of thigh muscles, which inadvertently affects gait pattern, increases energy expenditure, and ultimately decreases walking autotomy (**Fig. 19.21**). The magnitude of knee flexion is measured by the knee flexion angle, which is the angle between a line from the center of the femoral heads to the center of two femoral condyles and the mechanical axis of the tibia. The posterior pelvic shift is a compensatory mechanism to maintain the gravity line position in the sweet-spot position over a small area between the feet in the setting of a positive malalignment (**Fig. 19.21**).[1] Pelvic shift is defined as the distance between the S1 posterior superior corner plumb line and the anterior cortex of the distal tibia. The pelvic shift is the combination of PT and knee flexion.

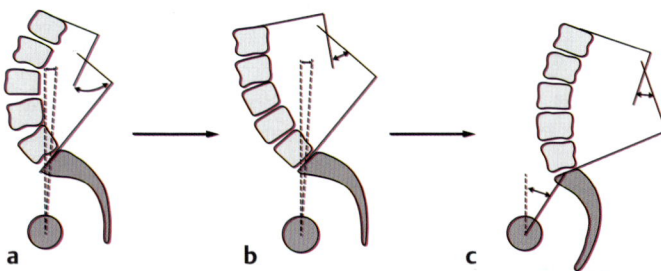

Fig. 19.20 Asymptomatic lumbar and pelvic tilt position with normal lumbar lordosis and no PI-LL mismatch **(a)**, loss of lumbar lordosis **(b)**, and pelvic retroversion exemplified through increased pelvic tilt **(c)**.

Age-Specific Sagittal Alignment Thresholds

It is important to understand spinal alignment not just in the context of mechanical posture and balance, but also according to each patient's age. For example, elderly patients tend to have slightly increased SVA and pelvic retroversion. Therefore, the goal of surgical correction for adult spinal deformity should be to find the optimum range of alignment that correlates to the least amount of disability for each patient. Lafage et al defined age-specific alignment targets for sagittal spinopelvic realignment in the setting of adult spinal deformity.[27] The authors utilized regression models to generate radiographic parameters (PT, PI-LL, SVA, and T1 pelvic angle [TPA]) based on age-specific health-related qualify of life outcomes (ODI, SF-36) (**Table 19.1**). They showed that optimal spinopelvic alignment values that correlated to patient-reported outcomes increased with age (**Fig. 19.22**). Therefore, preoperative planning should incorporate the patients' age-adjusted alignment when setting targets for surgical realignment. Younger patients generally require a more aggressive spinal reconstructions than older patients to reach age-specific ideal alignment.

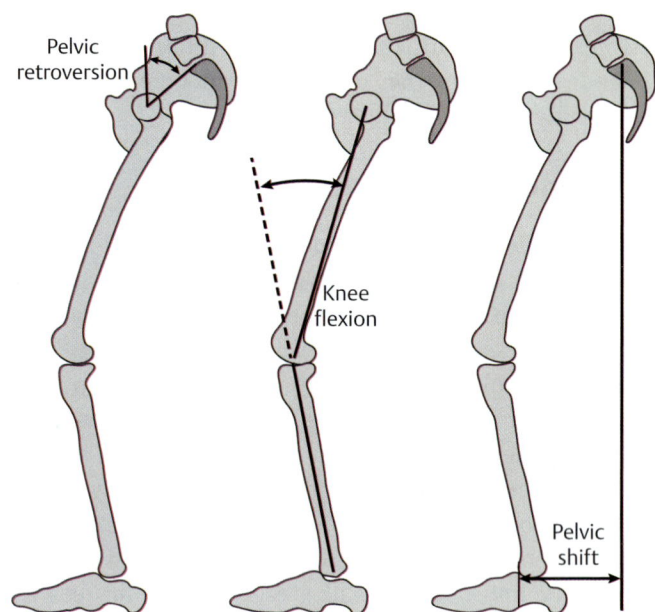

Fig. 19.21 Pelvic and lower extremity compensation mechanisms.

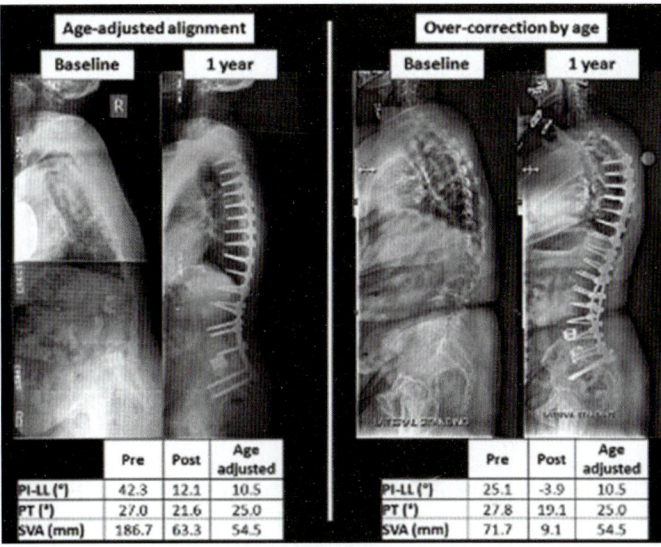

	Pre	Post	Age adjusted
PI-LL (°)	42.3	12.1	10.5
PT (°)	27.0	21.6	25.0
SVA (mm)	186.7	63.3	54.5

	Pre	Post	Age adjusted
PI-LL (°)	25.1	-3.9	10.5
PT (°)	27.8	19.1	25.0
SVA (mm)	71.7	9.1	54.5

Fig. 19.22 Case examples (baseline and 1-year postoperatively) of two patients with nearly identical ages (65 and 66 years old), type of surgery (pelvic fixation, interbody fusion, length of fusion construct), and age-adjusted alignment ideals. The patient on the left was surgically realigned to a sagittal alignment that was similar to age-adjusted ideals. The patient on the right was overcorrected past the age-adjusted thresholds. Figure adapted from Lafage et al.[27]

Tips and Tricks

- Always be mindful to restore the proper amount and distribution of LL when correcting sagittal plane deformities. Patients with a high PI and low LL are at risk for adjacent segment disease. Patients with such PI-LL mismatch exhibit a 10 times higher risk for undergoing revision surgery than controls if sagittal malalignment is maintained after lumbar fusion surgery.[28]

- Maintaining the relationship between PI and LL in the setting of a fusion eliminates the need for compensatory modification below the fusion and is less likely to result in long-term complications.

- Always look for clinical signs of compensatory mechanisms that may mask a sagittal plane deformity. Adolescent patients may tolerate spinal deformities well until their compensatory mechanisms are eventually exhausted. Therefore, the clinical impact of their longstanding deformity may become apparent only in adulthood. Adults may eventually also lose their compensatory mechanism reserves over time as their muscular endurance and strength diminishes.

Table 19.1 Radiographic spinopelvic alignment values increased with age. For example, the PT ranged from 11 degrees in patients younger than 35 years old to 29 degrees in patients over 74 years old.

Age group	% in database	Mean age in database	ODI US norms*	PT	PI-LL	LL-TK	SVA	TPA
Radiographic thresholds based on age-specific ODI US norms								
<35	17.7	26.2	9.49	11.1	-11.3	29.2	-29.1	4.4
35–44	8.8	40.7	11.77	15.5	-6.2	21.9	-4.0	10.0
45–54	19.9	51.2	15.43	18.9	-1.7	16.4	16.5	14.5
55–64	28.0	60.5	20.87	22.1	3.3	11.1	37.0	18.8
65–74	19.5	69.7	24.62	25.2	7.5	6.1	55.6	22.8
≥74	6.2	79.6	32.54	28.8	13.7	0.2	79.9	27.8
Note: *Value extrapolated using the PCS US norm.								
Radiographic thresholds based on age-specific SF-36 PCS US norms								
<35	17.7	26.2	53.72	10.8	-9.7	29.8	-31.9	4.0
35–44	8.8	40.7	52.15	15.2	-3.0	22.3	-7.0	9.6
45–54	19.9	51.2	49.64	18.6	2.6	16.5	13.6	14.1
55–64	28.0	60.5	45.9	21.9	8.3	11.1	34.6	18.5
65–74	19.5	69.7	43.33	24.9	13.4	5.9	53.4	22.5
≥74	6.2	79.6	37.89	28.7	20.2	-0.2	78.6	27.7

Abbreviations: LL-TK, lumbar lordosis minus thoracic kyphosis; ODI US norms, oswestry disability index United States normative data; SF-36 PCS US norms, short form (SF)-36 physical component score United States normative data; PI-LL, pelvic incidence minus lumbar lordosis; PT, pelvic tilt; SVA, sagittal vertical axis; TPA, T1 pelvic angle.
Note: Figure adapted from Lafage et al.[27]

This results in markedly increased muscular effort to maintain the cone of economy and daily function that will generate fatigue and disability.

- Long-term success in the spinal deformity surgery depends primarily on achieving the appropriate range of correction in the sagittal plane. Studies have reported high correlations between SVA and health-related quality of life in adult spinal deformity patients.[29] Therefore, significant attention should be directed at re-establishing a balanced global sagittal spinopelvic alignment, especially in patients with large or multiple coronal curves that may distract the surgeon from evaluating sagittal malalignment.

Key Points

- The pelvis is the regulator of sagittal spinopelvic harmony.

- PI is a fixed pelvic parameter that does not change with position and is determined by how each person's sacrum is oriented within the pelvis.

- In most cases, the degree of LL needed is contingent on the PI based on the PI-LL < 10 degrees rule.

- The pattern of compensatory mechanisms recruited to restore sagittal spinal alignment must be differentiated from the actual driver of the spinal deformity.

- Restoration of global sagittal alignment, not coronal alignment, has been associated with improving health-related quality of life outcomes.

- Preoperative planning should incorporate the patients' age-adjusted alignment when setting targets for surgical realignment. Younger patients generally require a more aggressive alignment than older patients to reach age-specific ideal alignment.

References

1. Schwab F, Lafage V, Boyce R, Skalli W, Farcy JP. Gravity line analysis in adult volunteers: age-related correlation with spinal parameters, pelvic parameters, and foot position. Spine 2006;31(25):E959–E967

2. Iyer S, Lenke LG, Nemani VM, et al. Variations in sagittal alignment parameters based on age: a prospective study of asymptomatic volunteers using full-body radiographs. Spine 2016;41(23):1826–1836

3. Roussouly P, Gollogly S, Berthonnaud E, Dimnet J. Classification of the normal variation in the sagittal alignment of the human lumbar spine and pelvis in the standing position. Spine 2005;30(3):346–353

4. Roussouly P, Nnadi C. Sagittal plane deformity: an overview of interpretation and management. Eur Spine J 2010;19(11): 1824–1836

5. Been E, Barash A, Marom A, Kramer PA. Vertebral bodies or discs: which contributes more to human-like lumbar lordosis? Clin Orthop Relat Res 2010;468(7):1822–1829

6. Dubousset J. Three-Dimensional Analysis of the Scoliotic Deformity. The Pediatric Spine: Principles and Practice. New York, NY: Raven Press; 1994

7. Lafage V, Diebo B, Schwab F. Sagittal Spino-Pelvic Alignment: From Theory to Clinical Application. Madrid, Spain: Editorial Medica Panamerica; 2014

8. Horton WC, Brown CW, Bridwell KH, Glassman SD, Suk SI, Cha CW. Is there an optimal patient stance for obtaining a lateral 36" radiograph? A critical comparison of three techniques. Spine 2005;30(4):427–433

9. Le Huec JC, Saddiki R, Franke J, Rigal J, Aunoble S. Equilibrium of the human body and the gravity line: the basics. Eur Spine J 2011;20(Suppl 5):558–563

10. Boulay C, Tardieu C, Hecquet J, Benaim C, Mouilleseaux B, Marty C, Prat-Pradal D, Legaye J, Duval-Beaupère G, Pélissier J. Sagittal alignment of spine and pelvis regulated by pelvic incidence: standard values and prediction of lordosis. Eur Spine J. 2006;15(4):415–22

11. Legaye J, Duval-Beaupère G, Hecquet J, Marty C. Pelvic incidence: a fundamental pelvic parameter for three-dimensional regulation of spinal sagittal curves. Eur Spine J 1998;7(2):99–103

12. Vialle R, Levassor N, Rillardon L, Templier A, Skalli W, Guigui P. Radiographic analysis of the sagittal alignment and balance of the spine in asymptomatic subjects. J Bone Joint Surg Am 2005;87(2):260–267

13. Jiang L, Qiu Y, Xu L, et al. Sagittal spinopelvic alignment in adolescents associated with Scheuermann's kyphosis: a comparison with normal population. Eur Spine J 2014; 23(7):1420–1426

14. Tyrakowski M, Mardjetko S, Siemionow K. Radiographic spinopelvic parameters in skeletally mature patients with Scheuermann disease. Spine 2014;39(18):E1080–E1085

15. Oh YM, Choi HY, Eun JP. The comparison of sagittal spinopelvic parameters between young adult patients with L5 spondylolysis and age-matched control group. J Korean Neurosurg Soc 2013;54(3):207–210

16. Cobb JR. Outline for the study of scoliosis. American Academy of Orthopaedic Surgeons Instructional Course Lecture. Vol. 5; 1948:261–275

17. Schwab F, Patel A, Ungar B, Farcy JP, Lafage V. Adult spinal deformity-postoperative standing imbalance: how much can you tolerate? An overview of key parameters in assessing alignment and planning corrective surgery. Spine 2010; 35(25):2224–2231

18. Pesenti S, Lafage R, Stein D, et al. The amount of proximal lumbar lordosis is related to pelvic incidence. Clin Orthop Relat Res 2018;476(8):1603–1611

19. Jackson RP, McManus AC. Radiographic analysis of sagittal plane alignment and balance in standing volunteers and patients with low back pain matched for age, sex, and size. A prospective controlled clinical study. Spine 1994;19(14): 1611–1618

20. Ames CP, Blondel B, Scheer JK, et al. Cervical radiographical alignment: comprehensive assessment techniques and potential importance in cervical myelopathy. Spine 2013;38(22, Suppl 1):S149–S160

21. Grob D, Frauenfelder H, Mannion AF. The association between cervical spine curvature and neck pain. Eur Spine J 2007; 16(5):669–678

22. Lee SH, Son ES, Seo EM, Suk KS, Kim KT. Factors determining cervical spine sagittal balance in asymptomatic adults: correlation with spinopelvic balance and thoracic inlet alignment. Spine J 2015;15(4):705–712

23. Staub BN, Lafage R, Kim HJ, et al; International Spine Study Group. Cervical mismatch: the normative value of T1 slope minus cervical lordosis and its ability to predict ideal cervical lordosis. J Neurosurg Spine 2018;30(1):31–37

24. Hyun SJ, Kim KJ, Jahng TA, Kim HJ. Relationship between T1 slope and cervical alignment following multilevel posterior cervical fusion surgery: impact of T1 slope minus cervical lordosis. Spine 2016;41(7):E396–E402

25. Gelb DE, Lenke LG, Bridwell KH, Blanke K, McEnery KW. An analysis of sagittal spinal alignment in 100 asymptomatic middle and older aged volunteers. Spine 1995;20(12):1351–1358

26. Jackson RP, Peterson MD, McManus AC, Hales C. Compensatory spinopelvic balance over the hip axis and better reliability in measuring lordosis to the pelvic radius on standing lateral radiographs of adult volunteers and patients. Spine 1998;23(16):1750–1767

27. Lafage R, Schwab F, Challier V, et al; International Spine Study Group. Defining spino-pelvic alignment thresholds: should operative goals in adult spinal deformity surgery account for age? Spine 2016;41(1):62–68

28. Rothenfluh DA, Mueller DA, Rothenfluh E, Min K. Pelvic incidence-lumbar lordosis mismatch predisposes to adjacent segment disease after lumbar spinal fusion. Eur Spine J 2015;24(6):1251–1258

29. Schwab FJ, Blondel B, Bess S, et al; International Spine Study Group (ISSG). Radiographical spinopelvic parameters and disability in the setting of adult spinal deformity: a prospective multicenter analysis. Spine 2013;38(13):E803–E812

20 Correction Techniques for Scheurmann's Kyphosis

Sleiman Haddad, Susana Nuñez-Pereira, and Ferran Pellisé

Introduction

Scheurmann's kyphosis (SK) is considered as a rigid thoracic or thoracolumbar—primarily sagittal—spinal deformity.[1] It is defined by the presence of more than three consecutive wedged vertebrae (>5 degrees kyphosis at each level) with characteristic endplate changes.

SK is divided into two types: Type 1 (apex above T10) and type 2 (apex below T10).

Epidemiology

Prevalence of SK is about 0.4 to 8% in general population. Typical age of onset is 10 to 12 years of age. Male:female ratio is between 2:1 and 7:1.[1–3]

Clinical Presentation

Most patients are asymptomatic. Main concern is body image, self-image. Some patients present with thoracic, thoracolumbar, or lumbar pain, especially later on.

Radiological and Clinical Assessment

Whole spine front and lateral X-rays including femoral heads are needed for proper biplanar assessment and surgical planning. They will show the vertebral wedging and Schmorl's nodes. Supine lateral radiograph with patient lying in hyperextension over a bolster can help differentiate from postural/flexible kyphosis. Routine magnetic resonance imaging (MRI) is controversial and is done if a thoracic herniation or cyst is suspected (abnormal findings on neurological physical examination).

Surgical Technique

Posterior Surgical Correction with Multiple Posterior Column Osteotomies[4–10]

Indications

- Regular deformity spread over more than three levels.
- Posterior-only instrumentation with thoracic pedicle screws and segmental posterior column osteotomies reduce operative time, blood loss, and complication rates compared with anterior–posterior fusion.
- Correction obtained with posterior-only approach is not compromised especially in skeletally immature patients with regular deformities.
- Posterior-only approaches are able to "open"/increase anterior disc height with proper posterior osteotomies.[11]

Patient's Positioning

A standard radiolucent spinal surgical table is preferable. The upper pads should be placed caudal to the shoulder and the lower pads at the iliac crest to passively help correct the thoracic kyphosis. If needed as per ideal sagittal profiles, placing the hips in hyperextension helps to maintain lumbar lordosis (LL). The knees are flexed to relax the hamstrings (**Fig. 20.1**).

Surgical Approach

Posterior midline incision centered over selected levels is done. Meticulous dissection through anatomical planes and full exposure of the posterior arch and thoracic transverse processes are followed.

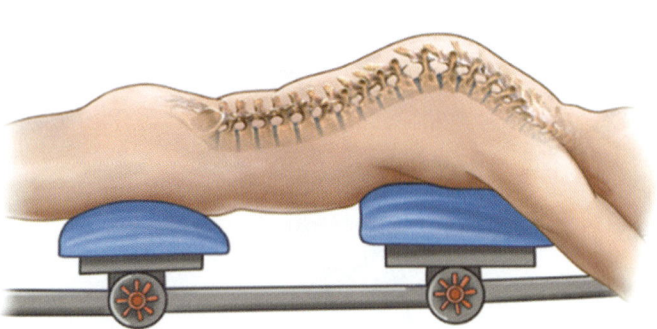

Fig. 20.1 Patient positioning: On a standard radiolucent spinal surgical table with the upper pads caudal to the shoulder and the lower pads at the iliac crest to passively help correct the thoracic kyphosis.

Screw Placement

Following the standard technique thoracic pedicle screws are placed. Starting with a partial/subtotal superior facet osteotomy can help to identify better the entry point and make the posterior column osteotomy easier to achieve. Strong anchorage at cranial and caudal foundations should be obtained with at least six bilateral pedicle screws over three vertebrae. Alternatively, hooks can be used at the upper instrumented vertebra protecting ligaments to prevent junctional failure with a "softer landing." Periapical bilateral pedicle screws are recommended for proper deformity correction and opening of the anterior spinal column. Hybrid instrumentation using sublaminar wires and hooks is associated with less curve correction and is coming to disuse (**Fig. 20.2**).

Periapical Ponte Type Posterior Column Osteotomy (PCO)

You should start by widely removing the interspinous processes and ligaments to expose the ligamentum flavum at each level. Then you can remove totally the inferior facet of the superior vertebra and then remove the ligamentum flavum entering the epidural space at the midline and progressing laterally on both sides until you reach the superior facet joint of the inferior vertebra. Afterwards, complete the bilateral Ponte, Schwab type 2, posterior column osteotomy (PCO) is performed by removing the superior facet of the inferior vertebra, exiting through the foramen bilaterally to fully mobilize each level. You can check if the osteotomy is satisfactory by compressing locally or exerting downward force and checking for segmental mobility (**Fig. 20.3**).

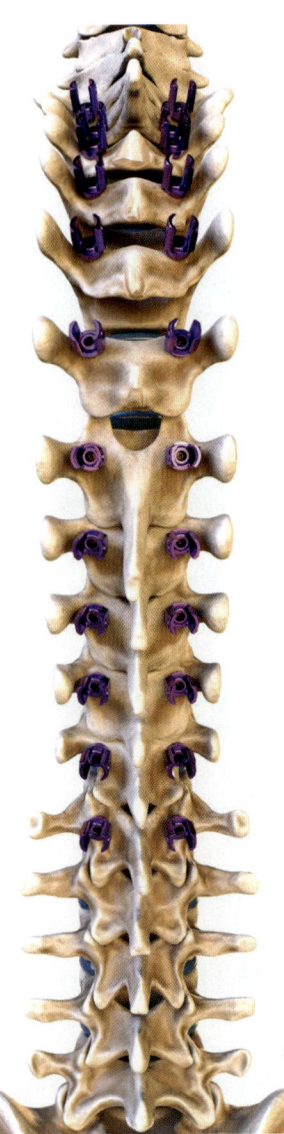

Fig. 20.2 Pedicle screws insertion: Strong anchorage at cranial and caudal foundations should be obtained with at least six bilateral pedicle screws over three vertebrae. Periapical bilateral pedicle screws are recommended for proper deformity correction and opening of the anterior spinal column.

Reduction Technique

A rod should be contoured to the desired sagittal alignment. The rod is inserted into the proximal or distal foundation and cantilevered progressively into the remaining screws using reduction screws, towers, or persuaders. After placing the rod, perform compression maneuver especially over the apex.

Closure of PCOs is done by shortening of posterior column. Wide Pontes or Smith-Peterson osteotomies (SPOs) allow

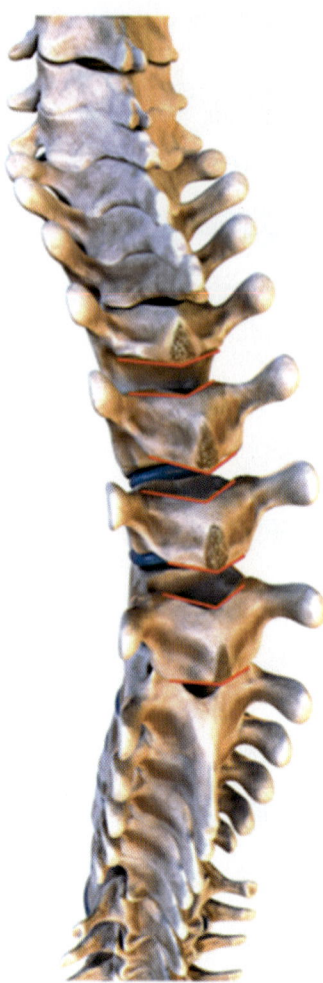

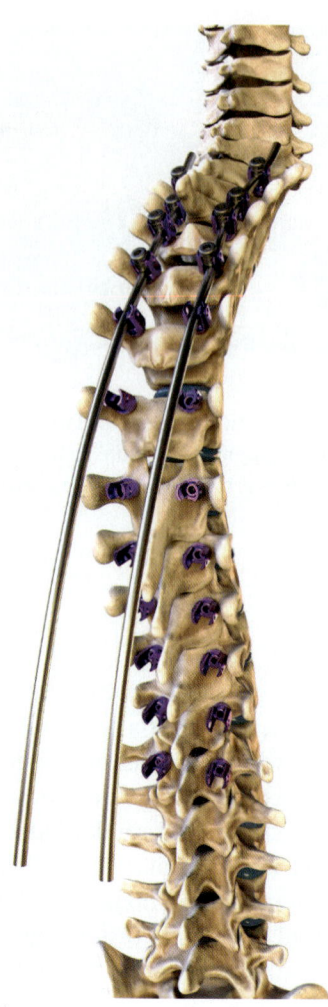

Fig. 20.3 Posterior column osteotomies: Complete the bilateral Ponte, Schwab type 2, posterior column osteotomies are shown with removal of the superior facet of the inferior vertebra, exiting through the foramen bilaterally to fully mobilize each level.

Fig. 20.4 Reduction maneuvers: The rod is inserted into the proximal or distal foundation and cantilevered progressively into the remaining screws using reduction screws, towers, or persuaders. After placing the rod, perform compression maneuver especially over the apex.

for larger corrections. You must check for intraoperative neuromonitoring (IONM) signals (**Fig. 20.4**).

Closure and Wound Care

After both the rods have been placed and reduction performed satisfactorily, the posterior arch is decorticated and local autograft and allograft are placed to favor fusion (**Fig. 20.5**).

Leave deep and superficial surgical drains. Then perform meticulous double closure of muscular plane and progressive closure of adjacent planes. Avoid using staples at apex. The authors recommend interrupted simple sutures using nylon or subcuticular continuous suture using a barbed suture. The authors recommend the use of vancomycin powder

in the superficial layer and a negative pressure dressing to decrease surgical site infections.

Anterior Release[12]

It is seldom needed. It can be done through a minimally invasive thoracoscopy technique with an open retropleural thoracic approach or through a limited apical costotransversectomy.[13] However, it increases morbidity by invading the thoracic chest and is associated with higher blood loss and more postoperative pain and complications.[4–7] It should better be reserved for patients having evidence of calcification of the anterior longitudinal ligaments or adult patients with major deformities (>100 degrees).

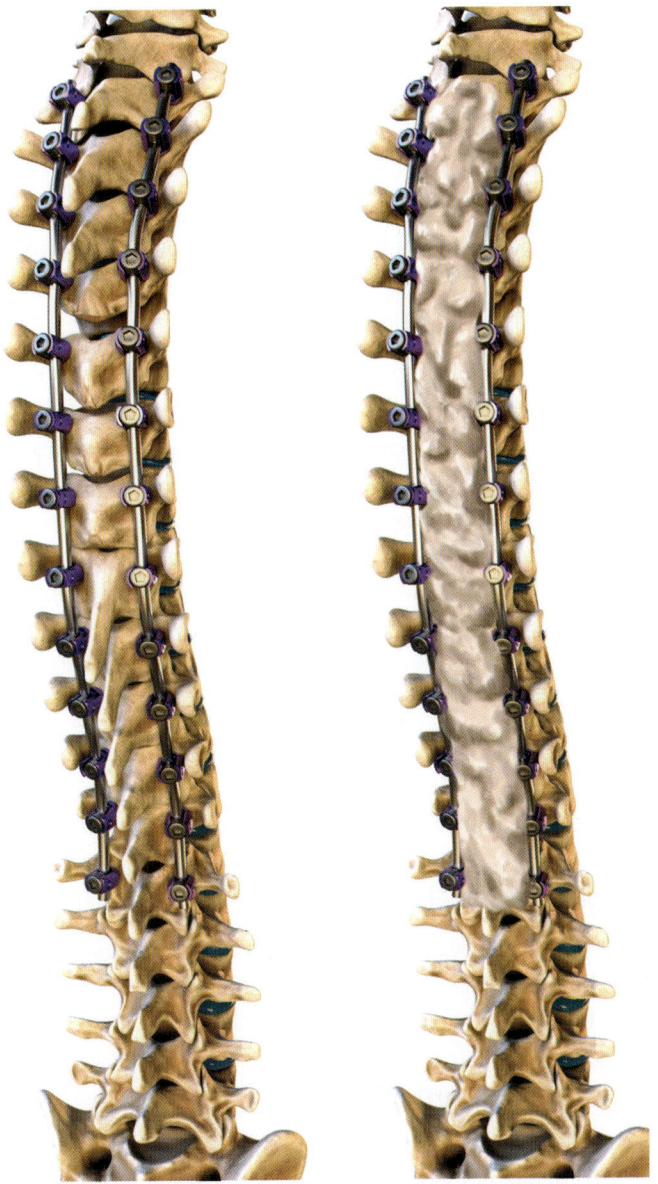

Fig. 20.5 Final aspect after closure of the posterior column osteotomies and placement of graft.

Posterior Vertebral Column Resection (PVCR) or Posterior Subtraction Osteotomy (PSO)

PVCR is preferred over PSO due to the degree of correction obtained. Both the techniques entail a higher risk of neurological injury reaching 10% and major blood loss. While PCO provides a regular harmonious kyphosis correction, 3CO concentrate the correction at the apex and can alter the physiologic distribution of thoracic kyphosis. They should therefore be reserved for patients having angular and rigid deformities (more than 40 degrees over one to two segments).

Indications

Patient selection should be based on the following criteria:

- The main drivers for deformity correction are patient's concern over body image and pain both linked to the magnitude of the deformity itself.
- Other indications of surgery include deformity progression.
- Rarely does SK cause any neurological deficit (thoracic disc herniation, epidural cysts, or a severe kyphosis [>100 degrees]).
- Surgery is usually thought in deformities greater than 75 degrees, or less in the presence of pain.
- However, radiological figures should be considered in relationship to the pelvic incidence (PI) and not as absolute figures (i.e., thoracic kyphosis of 70 degrees can be at the upper limit of normality for a patient with a PI of 80 degrees and is a severe deformity for someone with a PI of 30 degrees).

Surgical planning must have the following items:

- Alignment goals: The physiologically accepted thoracic kyphosis varies greatly with the PI. To avoid mechanical failures, it is advisable to correct SK less than 50% and maintain thoracic kyphosis adjusted to its physiological magnitude according to PI.[14–17] We must avoid reducing LL excessively in patients with high PI.[16]

Fusion levels must be prepared according to the following criteria:

- Upper instrumented vertebra (UIV): Final cranial vertebra of the kyphosis as measured by the Cobb angle, typically T2.
- Lowest instrumented vertebra (LIV): Extend the fusion to the stable sagittal vertebra (SSV), defined as the most cranial vertebra whose body is intersected by the vertical line traced from the posterosuperior corner of S1.[18–20]

Alternatively, LIV could be identified as the vertebra just caudal to the first lordotic disc. It has been shown that in 50% of the cases this is inferior to the SSV; it increases fusion length but decreases distal junctional failures (DJK).[21–23]

- Osteotomy sites: Periapical at the apex and at the three adjacent cranial and caudal levels or where the deformity is centered.
- Indication for anterior release: Calcification of the anterior longitudinal ligaments or adult patients with major deformities.
- Indications of PVCR: Angular and rigid deformities of more than 40 degrees over one to two segments.

Complication Avoidance

Complications are known to have a long-lasting effect on patient's quality of life and should be prevented. Total incidence of complications is 14.5% as per the Scoliosis Research Society (SRS) morbidity report.[24]

The most common complication was wound infection (3.8%), followed by implant-related complications (2.5%), acute neurological deficit (1.9%), and death (0.6%).

The overall incidence of surgical complications was more common in adults (21.7%) compared with patients in their teens (11.8%).

Junctional problems proximal junctional kyphosis/distal junctional kyphosis (PJK/DJK) are underestimated in the SRS report (mainly addressing acute complications) and are the major cause for revision surgery (10–30%).[15,16,20,23] They are more common if excessive correction is performed (>50% of curve), if the LIV is above SSV, or if the LL is flattened in patients with high PI.

Preoperative Screening and Optimization

Proper consent of the patient and family by assessing the patient's expectations (pain, cosmetics, function) and providing a realistic and evidence-based feedback is necessary.

Optimizing the patient physically and medically should be sought whenever possible.

Check for locally or distally active acne lesions and perform a dermatological consult or prophylactically treat with guided antibiotic prior to surgery.

Surgical Planning

Proper surgical planning defining fusion levels and amount of correction needed as well as picking up the right strategy to achieve it is fundamental to avoiding predictable complications.

Perform whole-spine X-ray and hyperextension lateral films over bolsters with or without MRI and computed tomography (CT) scans to assess flexibility, identify the UIV and LIV, assess pedicles, and need for "aggressive releases."

Intraoperative Measures

Intraoperative Neuromonitoring[25]

The relative risk of spinal cord injury with posterior osteotomies is relatively less in SK than in adolescent idiopathic scoliosis (AIS) due to the anterior location of the spinal cord with kyphosis.

IONM is performed using motor-evoked potentials (MEP), somatosensory-evoked potentials (SSEP), and electromyography (EMG).

It is useful to detect early signal change in relation to improper screw placement while performing vertebral osteotomies or when applying corrective forces on the lever arm for the final reduction and correction.

The incidence of complete loss of mixed evoked potentials during surgery can be up to 21%.

If sustained and irreversible changes appear, surgical correction should be released, and instrumentation should be checked and removed if in doubt. The intervention should be concluded if changes persist, and no cause is identified. An MRI should be obtained in the immediate postoperative period and surgery rescheduled accordingly.

Tranexamic Acid[26]

Routine use of tranexamic acid can reduce intraoperative blood loss and blood transfusions as well as reduce postoperative complications.

Cell Salvage Techniques

Performing surgery under conditions of hypotension and the use of blood salvage proved useful in reducing intraoperative blood loss and reducing the need for blood transfusion.

Radiological Control

The use of a radiolucent surgical table is advisable to allow for intraoperative control of screw placement (whenever needed) and surgical correction.

The introduction of navigation can improve safety and allow for better estimation of obtained surgical correction than uniplanar fluoroscopy.

Postoperative Care

Wound Care and Drains

Using negative pressure wound dressing reduces external contamination of the wound and enhances wound healing.

Perform change of surgical dressings when needed under sterile conditions.

Remove surgical drains as soon as possible. The authors recommend removing them as soon as the debit in each drain is inferior to 30 to 50 cc.

Postoperative Workup

Perform a full blood test at the 2nd operative day to check for anemia after volume redistribution. Perform a standing X-ray as soon as the patient is able to bear weight.

Postoperative Control

Schedule for the patient to have a radiological control at 6 weeks to check for surgical correction, reciprocal changes, and early signs of implant failures.

The use of a postoperative brace is controversial and should be reserved for patients at risk for early mechanical complication such as those with poor screw purchase or inadequate surgical correction.

Case Example

An 18-year-old male with thoracic kyphosis (TK) of 97 degrees, PI 55 degrees, and SSV at L3. Note the severe anterior thoracoabdominal crease. He underwent all posterior surgical correction with instrumentation from T2 to L3 (SSV) obtaining a 37% correction (55 degrees) reducing LL to 48 degrees. We avoided a hypercorrection due to the relatively high PI in this patient and obtained good clinical outcome and no junctional failures at 5 years (X-ray) (**Fig. 20.6**).

Tips and Tricks

- The supraspinous ligament and facet joints at the most cranial level(s) should be preserved to prevent proximal junctional kyphosis.

- It is important to properly resect the inferior facet of superior vertebrae and anterior capsule of facet joint to fully mobilize each segment and maximize segmental correction.
- Wide SPOs allow for more posterior column shortening and therefore better correction.
- Use hemostatic agents such as porcine sterile gelatin sponge (Spongostan ™), oxidized regenerated cellulose (Surgicel™), or human thrombin (Floseal™) especially at the osteotomy site to decrease blood loss.
- Use thick cobalt–chrome rods and bend them using in-situ benders to obtain the most homogeneous contour possible, decreasing rod stress points.
- Confirm proper rod contouring using a sterile protractor or sextant to avoid overcorrection and risk of junctional kyphosis.
- Preferably use reduction screws—or alternatively towers or persuaders—for better deformity correction through cantilever maneuver.
- During cantilever maneuver, spread the corrective force over the maximum number of distal screws and precede sequentially as to decrease pullout.

Key Points

- SK is defined as a rigid thoracic or thoracolumbar sagittal deformity with three consecutive wedged vertebrae with characteristic endplate changes.
- Surgical correction is indicated for deformity correction and improvement of pain and function.

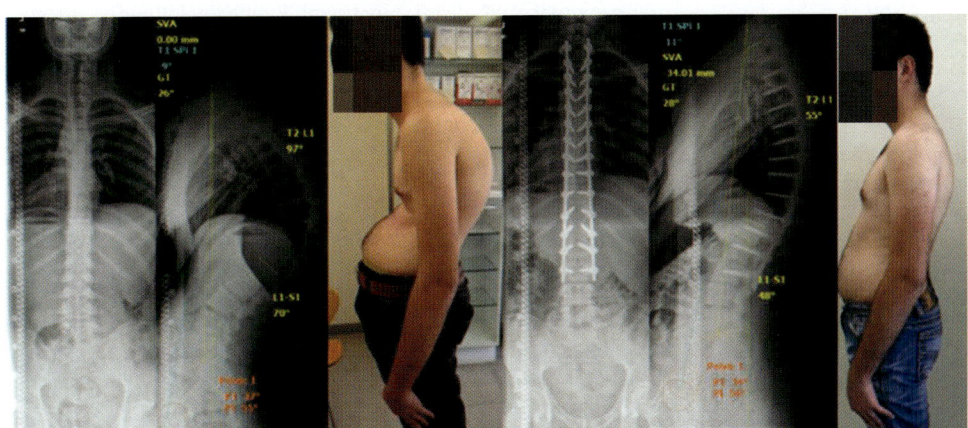

Fig. 20.6 An 18-year-old male with thoracic kyphosis (TK) of 97 degrees, pelvic incidence (PI) 55 degrees, and stable sagittal vertebra (SSV) at L3. Note the severe anterior thoracoabdominal crease. He underwent all posterior surgical correction with instrumentation from T2 to L3 (SSV) obtaining a 37% correction (55 degrees) reducing LL to 48 degrees. We avoided hyper-correction due to the relatively high PI in this patient and obtained good clinical outcome and no junctional failures at 5 years (X-ray).

- Multiple posterior column shortening osteotomies with pedicle screws can achieve excellent deformity correction with acceptable risk profile.

- Anterior release and PVCR are associated with increased surgical risks and are reserved for specific cases (anterior longitudinal ligament [ALL] calcification and angular deformities respectively).

- Adequate surgical planning including proper UIV and LIV choice as well as undercorrection to less than 50% and adjusting for PI does reduce rates of mechanical failures.

- Specific strategies should be put in place to decrease neurological complications, blood loss, and surgical site infections.

References

1. Tribus CB. Scheuermann's kyphosis in adolescents and adults: diagnosis and management. J Am Acad Orthop Surg 1998;6(1):36–43

2. SØRENSEN, K. Harry. Scheuermann's juvenile kyphosis: clinical appearances, radiography, aetiology, and prognosis. Munksgaard, 1964

3. Murray PM, Weinstein SL, Spratt KF. The natural history and long-term follow-up of Scheuermann kyphosis. J Bone Joint Surg Am. 1993;75(2):236–48

4. Etemadifar M, Ebrahimzadeh A, Hadi A, Feizi M. Comparison of Scheuermann's kyphosis correction by combined anterior-posterior fusion versus posterior-only procedure. Eur Spine J 2016;25(8):2580–2586

5. Riouallon G, Morin C, Charles YP, et al; French Scoliosis Study Group. Posterior-only versus combined anterior/posterior fusion in Scheuermann disease: a large retrospective study. Eur Spine J 2018;27(9):2322–2330

6. Lee CH, Won YI, San Ko Y, et al. Posterior-only versus combined anterior-posterior fusion in Scheuermann disease: a systematic review and meta-analysis. J Neurosurg Spine 2020;34(4):608–616

7. Lee SS, Lenke LG, Kuklo TR, et al. Comparison of Scheuermann kyphosis correction by posterior-only thoracic pedicle screw fixation versus combined anterior/posterior fusion. Spine 2006;31(20):2316–2321

8. Otsuka NY, Hall JE, Mah JY. Posterior fusion for Scheuermann's kyphosis. Clin Orthop Relat Res 1990;(251):134–139

9. Geck MJ, Macagno A, Ponte A, Shufflebarger HL. The Ponte procedure: posterior only treatment of Scheuermann's kyphosis using segmental posterior shortening and pedicle screw instrumentation. J Spinal Disord Tech 2007;20(8):586–593

10. Lonner BS, Newton P, Betz R, et al. Operative management of Scheuermann's kyphosis in 78 patients: radiographic outcomes, complications, and technique. Spine 2007;32(24):2644–2652

11. Tsutsui S, Pawelek JB, Bastrom TP, Shah SA, Newton PO. Do discs "open" anteriorly with posterior-only correction of Scheuermann's kyphosis? Spine 2011;36(16):E1086–E1092

12. Yun C, Shen CL. Anterior release for Scheuermann's disease: a systematic literature review and meta-analysis. Eur Spine J 2017;26(3):921–927

13. Herrera-Soto JA, Parikh SN, Al-Sayyad MJ, Crawford AH. Experience with combined video-assisted thoracoscopic surgery (VATS) anterior spinal release and posterior spinal fusion in Scheuermann's kyphosis. Spine 2005;30(19):2176–2181

14. Lowe TG, Kasten MD. An analysis of sagittal curves and balance after Cotrel-Dubousset instrumentation for kyphosis secondary to Scheuermann's disease. A review of 32 patients. Spine 1994;19(15):1680–1685

15. Ghasemi A, Stubig T, A Nasto L, Ahmed M, Mehdian H. Distal junctional kyphosis in patients with Scheuermann's disease: a retrospective radiographic analysis. Eur Spine J 2017;26(3):913–920

16. Nasto LA, Perez-Romera AB, Shalabi ST, Quraishi NA, Mehdian H. Correlation between preoperative spinopelvic alignment and risk of proximal junctional kyphosis after posterior-only surgical correction of Scheuermann kyphosis. Spine J 2016;16(4, Suppl):S26–S33

17. Debnath UK, Quraishi NA, McCarthy MJH, et al. Long-term outcome after surgical treatment of Scheuermann's kyphosis (SK). Spine Deform 2022;10(2):387–397

18. Cho KJ, Lenke LG, Bridwell KH, Kamiya M, Sides B. Selection of the optimal distal fusion level in posterior instrumentation and fusion for thoracic hyperkyphosis: the sagittal stable vertebra concept. Spine 2009;34(8):765–770

19. Xu Y, Hu Z, Zhang L, et al. Selection of the optimal distal fusion level for Scheuermann kyphosis with different curve patterns: when can we stop above the sagittal stable vertebra? Eur Spine J 2022;31(7):1710–1718

20. Lundine K, Turner P, Johnson M. Thoracic hyperkyphosis: assessment of the distal fusion level. Global Spine J 2012;2(2):65–70

21. Dikici F, Akgul T, Sariyilmaz K, et al. Selection of distal fusion level in terms of distal junctional kyphosis in Scheuermann kyphosis. A comparison of 3 methods. Acta Orthop Traumatol Turc 2018;52(1):7–11

22. Yanik HS, Ketenci IE, Coskun T, Ulusoy A, Erdem S. Selection of distal fusion level in posterior instrumentation and fusion of Scheuermann kyphosis: is fusion to sagittal stable vertebra necessary? Eur Spine J 2016;25(2):583–589

23. Denis F, Sun EC, Winter RB. Incidence and risk factors for proximal and distal junctional kyphosis following surgical treatment for Scheuermann kyphosis: minimum five-year follow-up. Spine 2009;34(20):E729–E734

24. Coe JD, Smith JS, Berven S, et al. Complications of spinal fusion for scheuermann kyphosis: a report of the Scoliosis Research Society morbidity and mortality committee. Spine 2010;35(1):99–103

25. Cheh G, Lenke LG, Padberg AM, et al. Loss of spinal cord monitoring signals in children during thoracic kyphosis correction with spinal osteotomy: why does it occur and what should you do? Spine 2008;33(10):1093–1099

26. Alajmi T, Saeed H, Alfaryan K, Alakeel A, Alfaryan T. Efficacy of tranexamic acid in reducing blood loss and blood transfusion in idiopathic scoliosis: a systematic review and meta-analysis. J Spine Surg 2017;3(4):531–540

21 Correction Techniques for Lumbar Kyphosis

Nikolay Peev, Joseph S. Butler, Shahswar Arif, Zarina Brady, and Sandra O'Malley

Introduction

Spinal deformity is one of the pathologies described quite early in history. Due to the lack of safe surgical options, initially, these problems were treated conservatively with different traction methods or bracing with dubious effect. With the advancement of modern surgical techniques, spinal surgeons have now a large armamentarium of safe surgical options for the correction of spinal deformities.[1,2] Surgical correction procedures for spinal deformities are still technically challenging and highly demanding for surgeons and patients.[3–6]

Interbody fusion approaches, such as posterior lumbar interbody fusion (PLIF), transforaminal lumbar interbody fusion (TLIF), extreme lateral interbody fusion (XLIF), oblique lumbar interbody fusion (OLIF) L2–L5, anterior lumbar interbody fusion (ALIF), and OLIF L5–S1, have shown to be efficacious in correcting deformity.[7,8]

Posterior Lumbar Interbody Fusion

PLIF has undergone significant evolution since its first description by Briggs and Milligan in 1944.[9] PLIF outcomes have improved significantly with the development of more choices of autologous bone grafting, fusion techniques and implants, including the wide range of cages in use today, and the use of pedicle screws.[10–13] In adult spinal deformity correction surgery, multilevel PLIF has shown to be efficacious; however, compromise of neural function and high blood loss are major drawbacks.[14]

It is a less popular option nowadays due to a high risk of associated complications such as neural compromise as well as interbody graft failures and inferior fusion rates, excessive blood loss, and prolonged surgical timing.[15,16]

Definition of the Technique

In PLIF surgery, the patient is in prone position on the operating table promoting the lordotic position of the lumbar spine. A longitudinal midline incision (length can vary according to the number of segments being operated) is performed, followed by the division of fascia and muscle.

With the use of retractors, the operator exposes the vertebral laminae. A complete laminectomy and foraminotomy is usually performed to create access point for the interbody spacer used.[17] To get access to intervertebral discs, the visible dura is retracted medially together with the traversing nerve roots. The disc is then excised, and the adjacent vertebral body end plates are prepared. Insertion of interbody cage packed with bone graft is performed under direct vision and imaging control, aiming to enable fusion across the level. To complete the surgery a posterolateral fixation with pedicle screw and rods is performed.[17,18]

Indications

The main indication for a PLIF is spinal fusion and correction of spinal deformity. Other indications include surgical management of recurrent lumbar disc herniation, failed spinal fusion surgery, and diskogenic intractable lower back pain.[19]

Complications and Avoidance

PLIF carries a significant risk of retraction damage to the nerve roots and has high incidence of radiculopathy—up to 10% of the cases will have transient postoperative radiculopathy and in up to 50% of them it will remain permanent.[20–22] Furthermore, it is challenging to correct coronal imbalance and restore lordosis due to the cage design. Blood loss due to prolonged surgical times is another drawback.[23] A key to reduce the complication rate will be a good exposure of the neural structures and proper mobilization to avoid stretching during the manipulation and cage insertion. The cage size also should be carefully planned according to the available anatomical spaces. Cage insertion under direct visualization and good illumination, ideally with operating microscope or surgical loupes, is a prerequisite for successful and complication-free surgery.

Tips and Tricks

As PLIF is one of the more conventional lumbar approaches, most spinal surgeons are well trained to perform it. PLIF enables a good visualization of the nerve roots and good decompression options.[24] In addition, PLIF allows 360-degree fusion and at the same time optimal neural decompression via a single posterior surgery access and bilateral approach.[14] Good visualization of the structures and wide approach allow cage insertion under direct visualization and good illumination which are key to reduce complications rate. Careful and meticulous end plate preparation will increase the chance for achieving a good interbody fusion.

Key Points

- The PLIF surgery allows good circumferential fusion via bilateral posterior approach. The technical aspects of PLIF surgery contribute to a relatively high rate of nerve root injury—10% transient and 5% permanent nerve root injury and radiculopathy. Previous lumbar surgery at the level increases the risk of nerve root injury due to the scar tissue formation preventing nerve mobilization and it is a relative contraindication.[16]

- Careful and wide decompression of the neural structures, use of magnification and illumination, cage insertion under direct vision and X-ray control, and meticulous preparation of the end plates are prerequisites for successful and complication-free surgery.

Transforaminal Lumbar Interbody Fusion

To tackle some of the intrinsic drawbacks associated with PLIF, Harms and Rolinger introduced placing the interbody bone graft and subsequently interbody cage through a transforaminal approach; so the technique is named TLIF, standing for transforaminal lumbar interbody fusion.[25] It decreases the necessity of bilateral dissection and retraction of paraspinal muscles to access the transverse processes and potentially lead to lower estimated blood loss and postoperative pain. Alternatively, there is an option for the surgery to be performed via paraspinal Wiltse approach, which will preclude the necessity of wide dissection of the muscles, further lowering blood loss and muscle trauma. TLIF also allows entrance to the spinal canal more laterally, preventing the need for midline dura exposure, thus reducing the risk of inadvertent tear of the dura and associated issues.[26] The lateral entry of the canal also gives an alternative clean (free of scar) route in the setting of previous surgery. With a TLIF approach, to achieve entry to the intervertebral disc, only unilateral hemilaminectomy and facetectomy are needed at the fusion level.[18]

Definition of the Technique

In TLIF, similar to the PLIF approach, the patient is placed in prone position on the operating table promoting the lordotic position of the lumbar spine. TLIF involves approaching the spine via the conventional (posterior) midline incision or alternatively with a paramedian incision over the Wiltse plane. Decompression is then started with a hemilaminectomy, leading to the removal of the whole facet. On resection of posterior bony elements and ligaments, the dura and neural anatomy are well visualized with the exposure of the lateral dura, the traversing nerve root medially, and the exiting nerve root laterally and above, forming a space known as Kambin's triangle, named after the author who first described it—Parviz Kambin, an American spinal surgeon originating from Iran. The Kambin's triangle, after being exposed, is a space wide enough to access the disc and to perform diskectomy, end plate preparation, and insertion of interbody bone graft or interbody cage for the necessary interbody fusion. A suitable size interbody cage is usually possible to be inserted in the prepared disc space with minimum or no retraction of the adjacent neural structures, and this lowers the chance of nerve root from overstretching and the resulting neuropathy. The cage insertion is ideally performed under X-ray control and direct visualization and illumination with an operating microscope or surgical loupes. Following decompression and cage insertion, the level is fixed with posterolateral fixation using pedicle screws.[27]

Indications

Indications for TLIF are similar to PLIF surgery—spinal fusion and correction of spinal deformity. Other indications include surgical management of recurrent lumbar disc herniation, failed spinal fusion surgery, and diskogenic intractable back pain. Unlike the PLIF however, where the technique specificity (retraction) limits its application only to the lower lumbar levels, due to the limited or no retraction with the TLIF route, the transforaminal interbody fusion can be applied to thoracic levels as well.

Complication Avoidance

Due to the unique access route that the TLIF technique is using, compared with the PLIF, the complication rates are significantly reduced, especially in terms of nerve roots injury which is reported to be up to 1 to 2% in different series, representing a significant reduction in comparison to the 5 to 10% with PLIF. A key factor to further reduce the likelihood of neural compromise is proper exposure of the Kambin's triangle, which leaves enough space for insertion of an optimum size cage without significant or no retraction of the traversing/exiting nerve roots. The dura is exposed only marginally in its lateral margin which gives an advantage, especially in cases with previous decompression surgery at the index level and with similar scar tissue formation. Accessing the canal laterally gives the surgeon the advantage of a new pristine surgical trajectory without interference from the scar tissue, which will be normally in the way in midline approaches.

When used with Wiltse approach, the TLIF technique decreases the necessity of dissecting laterally and retracting paraspinal muscles to access the transverse processes and potentially lead to lower estimated blood loss and postoperative pain. The lateral access of the canal also prevents the need for midline dural exposure and mobilization, thus reducing the risk of inadvertent tear of the dura and associated issues.[26,28]

Partial inferior articulating process removal, leaving an overhang over the exiting nerve root, provides protection of the nerve when the cage and other instruments are driven in and out of the disc space (**Figs. 21.1** and **21.2**).

Some of the limitations of the TLIF approach, particularly associated with young and inexperienced spinal surgeons, are partial removal of intervertebral disc, poor vertebral end plate preparation and low fusion rates, potential occult damage to the exiting nerve root when the access is not properly centered, and inadequate central decompression when needed. However, such complications and shortfalls get infrequent with experience.

As TLIF is a single-sided approach, it does not decompress the opposite nerve root directly, but indirectly due to the distraction with the cage insertion. However, if needed, a simple contralateral facetectomy or over the top contralateral decompression from the same unilateral approach can be considered, which requires more experience from the performing surgeon.[18]

Key Points

- TLIF surgery provides a significant advantage compared to the PLIF approach.[29]
- By moving the access trajectory laterally to the PLIF route, the surgeon enters the spinal canal more laterally which gives several advantages: no need for retraction of the neural structures and the dura, which significantly reduces the risk for dural tears and neural compromise, especially in revision cases and cases with previous one or more surgeries at the index level. With the available minimally invasive options and use of the Wiltse plane, there is no necessity of muscle retraction which improves the postoperative pain, blood loss, and functional recovery significantly.[15] The newly available expandable cage technology significantly increases the potential for deformity correction with minimal risk for the neural elements and still maintaining the benefits of the posterolateral surgical approach in comparison with the significant morbidity of the anterior approaches.

Extreme Lateral Interbody Fusion

XLIF is a relatively new technique introduced to achieve minimally invasive circumferential spinal fusion. Although XLIF was introduced by Pimenta in 2001, it gained popularity nearly a decade later.[30–34] XLIF allows access to the lumbar spine via a lateral transpsoas approach.[35]

Retrospective studies comparing XLIF with TLIF have shown comparable results with regards to rates of complications, estimated blood loss, length of hospital stay, and 6-month mortality rate.[36]

Studies have reported XLIF to be more efficacious in improving/maintaining lumbar lordosis and sagittal and coronal alignment.[30,33,37,38] XLIF was also reported to be superior with regards to postoperative pain (visual analog scale [VAS] score).[32,37–42] Pimenta et al[32] reported the average reduction in VAS score to be 5.17, and Oswestry disability index (ODI) score almost halved. Results have shown XLIF surgery to be very efficacious in correcting (single plane) deformity in patients.[39]

XLIF surgery has proven its potential to reduce approach-related trauma to the musculature, blood loss, and length of stay at the hospital and as such represents a good minimally invasive option in the armamentarium of the spinal surgeon.

Definition of the Technique

XLIF involves approaching the spine through a lateral angle; thus the patient is in a lateral position. It is a true lateral retroperitoneal access to the spine with the possibility to access the whole lumbar spine without L5–S1 and up to the upper thoracic spine (up to T5). The access trajectory toward the lumbar spine involves going through the psoas muscle. The skin incision is planned with the help of X-ray in lateral position. The incision must be projected over the desired level, or in between the two desired levels in surgery aiming for more than one level. The length of the incision is normally 3 to 4 cm. Care must be taken to make sure that no anterior extension is done as this would risk damage to peritoneal structures and vascular anatomy.[43]

Neurological monitoring is recommended during the surgery to protect the lumbar plexus.[32,44,45] To ensure optimal decompression of nerve roots as well as to prevent lumbar plexus stretching, a free running electromyography (EMG) is used to monitor the neurological function throughout the surgery.

The nature of the technique involves a muscle-splitting approach with the use of progressive dilators to generate the working route via the psoas muscle using neuromonitoring of the lumbar plexus.[46] The bilateral annulus fibrosus release

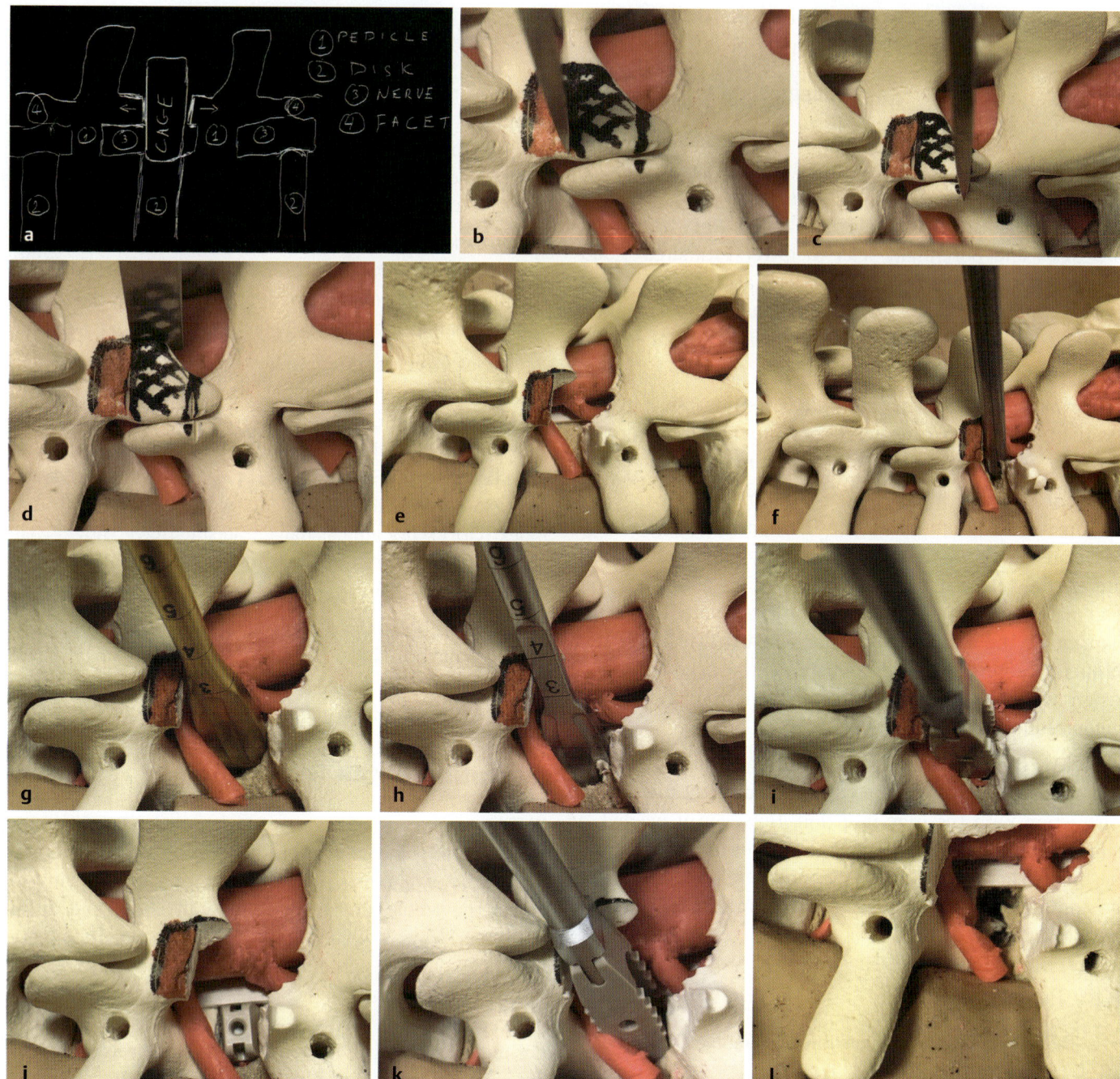

Fig. 21.1 Transforaminal lumbar interbody fusion (TLIF) technique for nerve root injury avoidance. The relational anatomy of the pedicle, disc, nerve root, and facet during cage insertion (**a**). Superior articular process partially resected by an osteotome (**b–e**). The bony overhang is protecting the exiting nerve root (**f**). After diskectomy and curettage of the disc, the disc space is prepared and a cage is inserted by distraction (**g–j**). Beware not to damage the exiting nerve root by the cage (**k, l**).

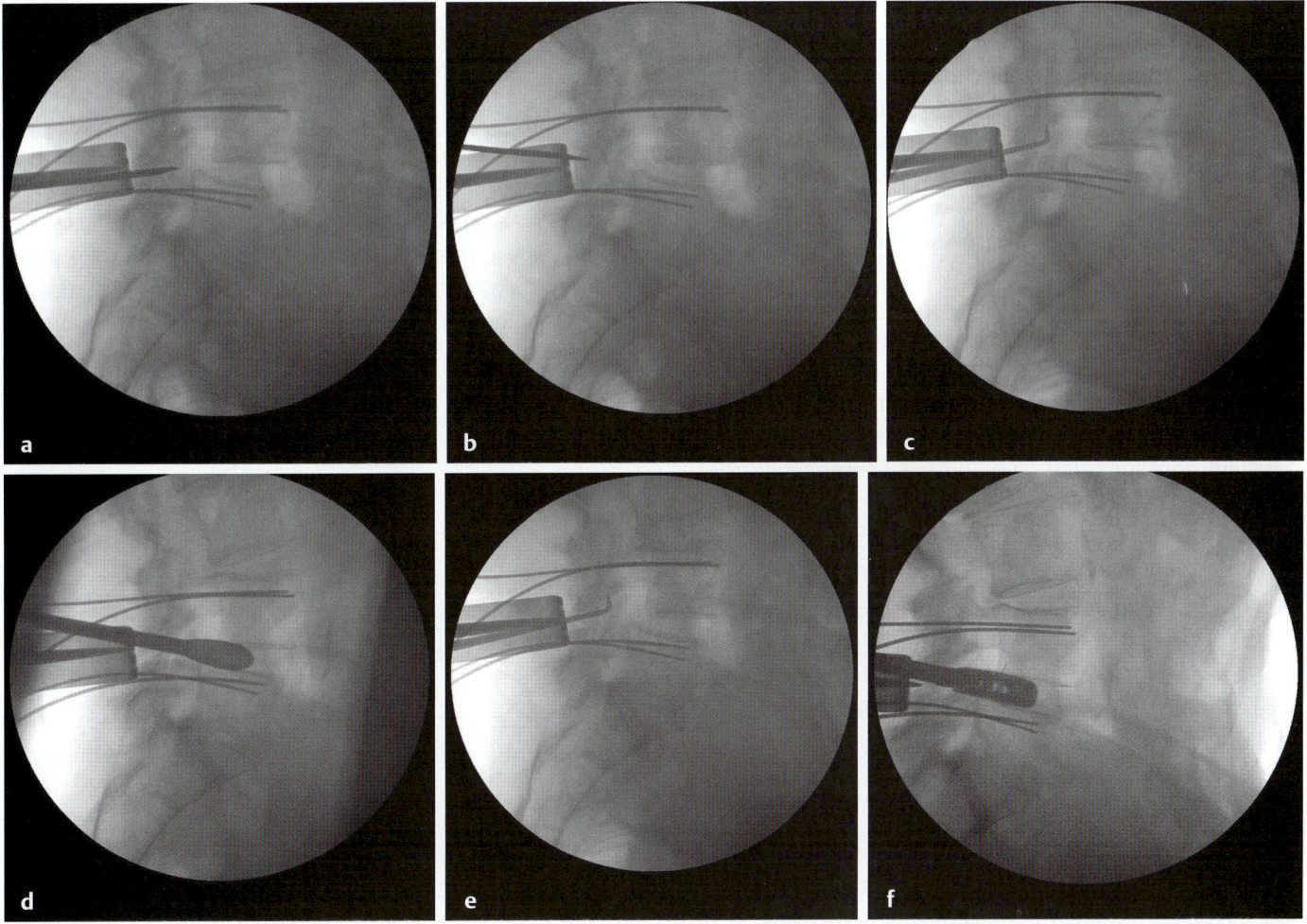

Fig. 21.2 X-ray image of the inferior articulating process—cut in line with the superior margin of the lower pedicle **(a)**. X-ray image of the superior articulating process—partial superior articulating process osteotomy performed in order to leave a bony overhang to protect the nerve root **(b)**. X-ray image demonstrating partial removal of the superior articulating process—the probe is demonstrating the bony overhang **(c)**. X-ray image of instrument driven into the disc space—the left bony overhang after the partial superior articulating process osteotomy is protecting the exiting nerve root (blue star) **(d)**. X-ray image demonstrating partial removal of the superior articulating process—the probe is demonstrating the bony overhang **(e)**. X-ray image of interbody cage driven into the disc space—the left bony overhang after the partial superior articulating process osteotomy is protecting the exiting nerve root (blue star) **(f)**.

in combination with lateral insertion of wide cages aids in restoration of coronal alignment. This technique has gained popularity for deformity correction in older cohorts, as it has the potential to restore end plate asymmetry almost bloodlessly and with minor injury to the tissues.[47]

Indications

Indications of the technique include symptomatic, unstable, degenerative disc pathologies, adjacent segment disease, degenerative spondylolisthesis, revision disc herniation surgery, and degenerative scoliosis.[43]

XLIF may not be suitable for patients with high-grade spondylolisthesis, as well as patients with bilateral scarring

behind the abdominal cavity owing to prior surgical intervention or infection.[48]

Complication Avoidance

The most common postoperative complications in XLIF cohort include transient anterior thigh pain, hypoesthesia, dysesthesia, and weakness.[49]

In comparison to the conventional anterior interbody fusion techniques, XLIF has significant advantages: XLIF reduces the risk of sexual dysfunction in terms of retrograde ejaculation; there is no need of retracting the peritoneum and for great vessels mobilization with the associated risks.[50–53] When compared with ALIF, XLIF allows much safer access to the retroperitoneal space and disc space in cases with a history of open abdominal surgery, when the anterior approach (ALIF) would be difficult or impossible. Compared with TLIF and PLIF, XLIF allows a more thorough diskectomy, osteotomy, and insertion of larger interbody devices. XLIF avoids dissection of paraspinal musculature and provides an alternative route for cage insertion and diskectomy in cases with significant epidural scar formation following multiple previous surgeries.[31,37,40,54]

Tips and Tricks

Prior to surgical intervention, it is pertinent to set feasible expectations with the patient, as XLIF often leads to transient anterior thigh pain and weakness, hypoesthesia, and dysesthesia (due to trauma or stretching of the femorocutaneous nerve) but a majority of patients improve within 6 weeks postoperatively.

Nerve root damage and deficit is a major issue, especially at L4–L5 level. The use of EMG during any maneuvers that have the potential to cause injury to the roots and avoiding excessive retraction are crucial to avoid nerve root damage. Shallow retractor docking and direct visualization are important surgical techniques to avoid neural elements damage.[48]

Positioning of the patient on the operating table is crucial for the X-ray orientation and for successful and safe surgery. The patient is positioned strictly lateral with the left side up and the right side dependent. The true lateral positioning of the patient should be ascertained and verified with anteroposterior (AP) and lateral X-rays taken intraoperatively. Repositioning the operating table under guidance for each disc to allow optimal access can limit the risk of canal penetration, misplacement of the cage, and any vascular or visceral trauma.[48]

Key Points

- XLIF is thought to be a good alternative to conventional anterior approaches to the lumbar spine. XLIFs usually do not require a general surgeon for access, as well as the need for any retraction of peritoneum or necessity of mobilization of the great vessels. Thus, it can be performed by a majority of spinal surgeons or neurosurgeons.[30,33,41,48]

- XLIF is not suitable for L5–S1 level pathology and in the case the L5–S1 level needs to be addressed, an alternative approach should be used—anterior to psoas lateral approach or classic anterior approach.

Oblique Lateral Interbody Fusion (Anterior to Psoas Lumbar Interbody Fusion)

The OLIF approach was introduced by Michael Mayer more than 40 years ago.[55] It utilizes minimally invasive access to the disc space through a space behind the peritoneum and between the great retroperitoneal vessels and psoas muscle using an oblique path to the spine, unlike the XLIF approach where the approach is strictly lateral and through the psoas. The approach could be viewed as a modification of the XLIF approach by moving the access trajectory from direct lateral transpsoas to oblique and anterior to psoas. The aim of OLIF is to attain neural decompression and correction of lumbar lordosis by placing a larger cage into the disc space.[56]

Definition of the Technique

For the anterior to psoas approach (also known by the commercial name OLIF [oblique lumbar interbody fusion]), the patient is positioned laterally, on either side based on the operator's choice, unlike the XLIF approach where the dependent side is usually the right side and the left side is up.[57,58] The true lateral position is also very important for the proper orientation and for complication avoidance. The proper positioning should be ascertained and verified with AP and lateral X-rays.[59] As the space anterior to the psoas muscle is utilized for access, neuromonitoring is usually not required.

Studies have shown that OLIF does yield sufficient lumbar lordosis correction in the management of major lumbar kyphosis. The technique could be combined with posterior osteotomy techniques if required for sufficient correction of sagittal imbalance for cases with major kyphotic deformity.[56]

A systematic review conducted by Zhu et al revealed that OLIF yielded major improvement in back and leg VAS and ODI scores.[56,60]

Indications

Indications of the technique include all degenerative pathologies, similar to the XLIF approach. OLIF is suitable for correcting sagittal and coronal deformity, in particular lumbar degenerative scoliosis with antero- or latero-listhesis and foraminal stenosis. Contraindications include cases with severe central canal stenosis and high-grade spondylolisthesis.[56] Also similar to the XLIF technique, the anterior to psoas approach is not recommended in cases of previous abdominal surgery with retroperitoneal extension or previous history of abdominal infective or malignant process. Unlike the XLIF approach, the anterior to psoas route could be used for L5–S1 pathology as well with a modification of the approach allowing access in between the iliac vessels.

Complication Avoidance

OLIF's average complication rate is reported to be around 3 to 5%, with the most often reported complications being transient numbness or pain in the thigh (often linked to pulling and stimulating the psoas muscle during the surgery, or postoperative hematoma), cage movement, and proximal junctional kyphosis (could be due to osteoporosis and fusion to pelvis).[61] As a vast majority of the complications linked with OLIF were transient, it is considered a safe approach.

Proper implementation of the surgical technique and recognition of the surgical anatomy are the main key points for complication avoidance. True lateral positioning of the patient and proper fixation to prevent intraoperative movement of the patient are important for acquisition of reliable X-ray of the anatomy and to prevent malposition of the hardware toward the spinal canal causing neurological compromise or malposition toward the abdominal cavity causing major vessel or abdominal organ injury. Recognition of the respective surgical anatomy would prevent abdominal organ injury or major bleeding.

Tips and Tricks

OLIF facilitates minimally invasive surgery with quick postoperative mobility, enables correction of major deformities, and yields high rates of fusion with significant clearance of disc space.[62–64] OLIF has a very low risk of lumbar plexus and psoas injury as the dissection is performed anterior to the psoas. Thorough preoperative planning and meticulous surgical technique are prerequisite for successful and safe surgery. Patient positioning in true lateral position with radiological confirmation on true AP and lateral X-rays is important for complication avoidance. In the setting of proper implementation of the surgical technique, it is not necessary to use neuromonitoring to prevent neurological injury of the patient. The patient can be positioned on the left lateral or right lateral position, depending on the surgeon's preference and pathology addressed. Usually, the spine is accessed from the concave side.

Key Points

OLIF is thought to be a good alternative to conventional anterior approaches to the lumbar spine. It usually does not require a general surgeon for access, as well as the need for any retraction of peritoneum or necessity of mobilization of the great vessels; thus, it can be performed by a majority of spinal surgeons or neurosurgeons.[56,58] OLIF is suitable for L5–S1 level pathology in case the L5–S1 level needs to be addressed, with the patient being in the same lateral position.

Anterior Lumbar Interbody Fusion (ALIF) Using Anterolateral Approach

Anterior fusion has been found to be effective in lower back pain due to degenerative disc disease and adult spinal deformity as it facilitates excellent segmental correction with increased disc height loss and improved lordosis.[65]

Surgeons have traditionally accessed the L3–S1 intervertebral disc spaces through a direct anterior approach. However, this is associated with complications, including vascular injury, retrograde ejaculation, postoperative colonic obstruction, lymphocele, and sympathetic chain injury,[66,67] with access to the intervertebral disc spaces cranial to L5–S1 requiring mobilization of the great vessels.

Definition of the Technique

This technique is a reproducible single-incision, muscle-splitting, anterolateral pre-psoas surgical approach to the lumbar spine from L1 to S1. An anterolateral pre-psoas retroperitoneal approach has been used for many years for ALIFs from L1 to L5.[68] This provides a slightly oblique trajectory to the intervertebral disc spaces of L1 to L5, with a separate Pfannenstiel approach required for access to the L5–S1 intervertebral disc space.

Indications

ALIF is indicated for single or multilevel segments vertebral deformity (**Fig. 21.3**) between L1 and S1,[68] for asymmetric diskopathy, isthmic spondylolisthesis, or degenerative spondylolisthesis and scoliosis dislocation.[69] It is also indicated for sequelae of posterior decompression, and isolated modic 1 or 2 degenerative diskopathy with or without interbody collapse and sagittal imbalance.[70]

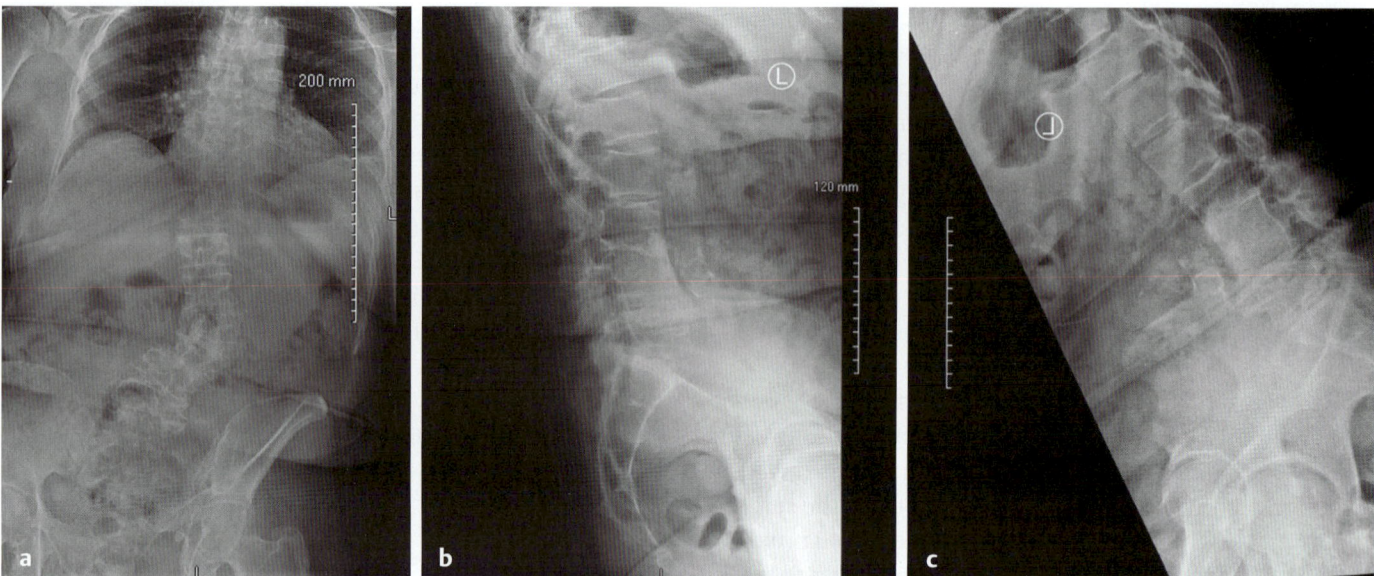

Fig. 21.3 **(a–c)** Preoperative anteroposterior (AP) and lateral flexion extension radiographic imaging for degenerative multilevel lumbar spondylosis and scoliosis.

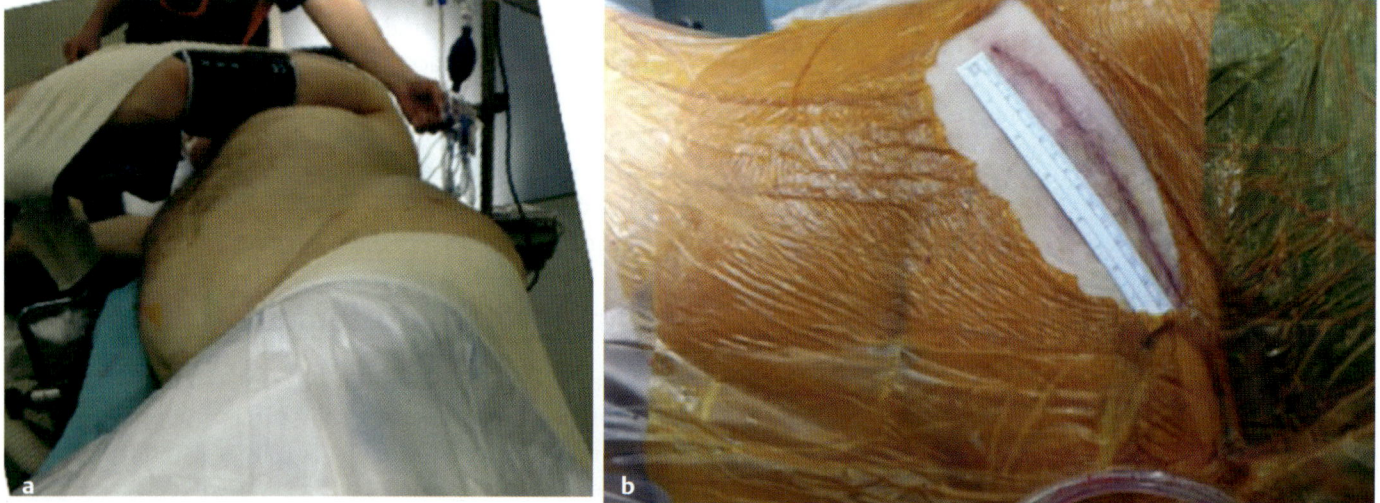

Fig. 21.4 **(a)** Semilateral position. **(b)** Anterolateral incision. (Reproduced with permission from Molloy et al.[68])

Position

The patient is placed in a semilateral decubitus position, on a beanbag positioner, and tilted 30 degrees posteriorly (**Fig. 21.4**). The table is broken to increase the space between the T12 rib and the iliac crest, enhancing access and facilitating instrumentation. A left-sided approach is preferred as it is safer from a vascular perspective to deal with more robust great arteries than more vulnerable great veins. The patient is held in position with table straps and taped over the greater trochanter and shoulder. The upper arm is placed in a gutter, and all pressure areas are protected.

Surgical Approach

An oblique (posterior superior to anterior inferior) anterolateral incision is made, 4 cm anterior to the anterior iliac spine, centered over the levels of interest. The length is determined by the number of levels to be instrumented. The external oblique muscle is split, and the tendinous portion of the anterior rectus sheath is cut in the line of the external oblique muscle fibers. Both internal oblique and transversus abdominis muscles are split in a similar fashion. The ilioinguinal and iliohypogastric nerves are preserved as they emerge through the muscle.

The retroperitoneum is approached by sweeping the posterior peritoneum away from the psoas muscle and iliac vessels. The spermatic cord and the round ligament along with their contents are preserved. The lumbar spine, from L1 to L5, may be approached through one or two separate access windows in the muscles, depending on the number of levels to be instrumented; one window is used to facilitate access for L1–L3 and a separate window for L3–L5.

The great vessels are retracted anteromedially to expose the intervertebral disc spaces. When approaching the L4–L5 disc, the iliolumbar vein is often encountered and can be preserved. If improved access to L4–L5 is required or injury to the iliolumbar vein is a concern, then it can be ligated. A dissection plane is developed between the sympathetic chain and anterior border of the psoas muscle, which is retracted posteriorly.[71] This exposes the anterior longitudinal ligament (ALL), which should be preserved from L1 to L5. Diskectomy is performed posterior to the ALL, and the interbody cage is inserted in a slightly oblique fashion.

The anterolateral retroperitoneal approach described provides a number of clear advantages. It is a single-incision, muscle-splitting approach, avoiding the need for patient repositioning and a separate incision to access the L5–S1 disc space. It has a short operative time and is associated with minimal intraoperative blood loss, with no ligation of major vessels or iliolumbar vessels.[72] It allows for a more limited mobilization of the great vessels compared with the direct anterior approach, enabling access to the intervertebral

discs from L1 to S1 and maintaining the integrity of the ALL between L1 and L5 (**Fig. 21.5**).

The anterior approach provides superior visualization of the disc space and offers an advantage over PLIF and TLIF in a number of ways.[73–75] It allows excellent access for the preparation of the end plates for fusion. It also has the ability to restore foraminal height, local disc angle, and lumbar lordosis (**Fig. 21.6**).[76] It has been suggested that ALIF may be less likely to lead to adjacent segment degeneration than PLIF.[77] ALIF, either alone or with a posterior instrumented spinal fusion, has gained popularity as a means of addressing degenerative disc disease, spondylolisthesis, and complex lumbar deformity.

Complication Avoidance

The use of spinal navigation as part of 360-degree fusion[72] has been shown to be a safe and effective strategy for multilevel ALIF as part of a two-stage, 360-degree lumbosacral fusion. The first stage of ALIF can be carried out as described above; the second stage involves open midline approach and computer navigated pedicle screw insertion technique using O-arm imaging and navigation system.

Although ALIF can provide significant deformity correction, there is a complication associated with this approach particularly when there is a need to mobilize the great vessels. An approach surgeon (vascular) should be utilized to minimize high-risk complications such as major vascular, ureter, and/or bowel/bladder injury.

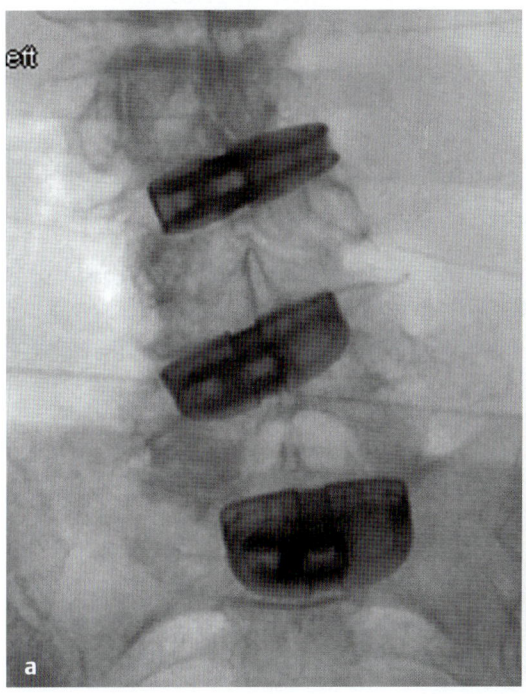
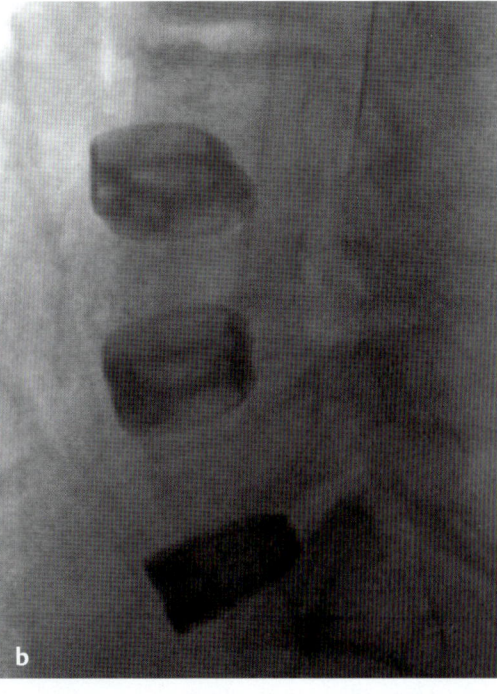

Fig. 21.5 (a, b) Intraoperative anteroposterior (AP) and lateral imaging during stage 1, multilevel, L3–S1, anterior body lumbar interfusion.

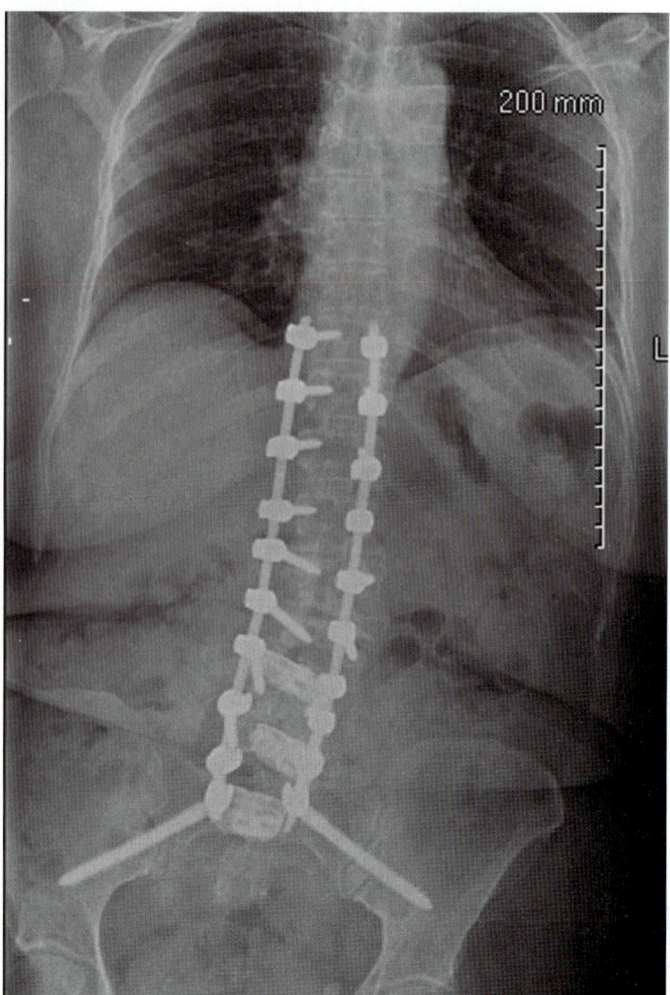

Fig. 21.6 Postoperative imaging 8 weeks after two-stage lumbar spine reconstruction. The patient underwent stage 1 multilevel L3–S1 anterior body lumbar interfusion and stage 2 T10–pelvis decompression, deformity correction, and instrumented fusion. Goals of the surgery were to restore spinal balance, obtain solid fusion, and relieve pain.

Tips and Tricks

Positioning

Deflate the beanbag after the table is broken. The body should be moved toward the anterior side of the table and tilted slightly backwards so that imaging will not be hampered by the edges of the table. Place pillows under the upper leg to avoid adducting the leg (helping relative position of the psoas).

Surgical Approach

Perform the retroperitoneal incision from the anterior side. After the oblique skin incision, the external oblique (EO) aponeurosis incision should be in line with the skin incision. The internal oblique (IO) incision is a perpendicular window, best chosen after visualizing the neurovascular segments and going between them. One IO incision will cover L2–L5, but a separate IO incision is required for L5–S1.

Pull the peritoneum anteriorly, but push the loose fat posteriorly. Leave the genitofemoral nerve on the psoas; the ureter comes anteriorly with ease. Approach the psoas–spine interval with a pledget and bipolar. Identify the ascending lumbar vein; tie medially first which makes it small, then clip, then double clip laterally, and then cut the suture. Use the Cobb dissector on the psoas gently.

Diskectomy

The direction of the disc in the concavity will be vertically down. So, the diskectomy, trial, and cage will be the same. Start the disc dissection with a monopolar vertical opening incision from within the disc. This identifies the end plates and is safe from the side of the monopolar hitting off the vein below. Operate from the caudal side of the assistant, from the back. Narrow paddles are great for levering open the disc. But be sure that they are not inserted through the posterior longitudinal ligament (PLL) into the canal.

Imaging

Leave the blade in when screening the level with the spinal needle in the disc space. If there is a buckle on the needle then it tells where the needle is entering the disc, thus showing how anterior the entry point is, as the mistake is to go too anteriorly. The synframe can be in the way; thus, consider placing one half of the frame and attaching the connectors to this. Only lateral views are required. Use Floseal on the side of the cage to reduce friction against the vein.

L5–S1

There is always a posterior lip on the S1 upper end plate. Use this to stop migration into the canal, particularly if doing an ALIF plus posterior reduction.

Ensure that the trial engages both end plates posteriorly to know that the trial is opening the foramina but beware of over-distracting a disc with previous scarred nerve.

Key Points

ALIF offers a direct midline view of the disc space with extensive lateral exposure of the vertebral bodies.

- This reduces deformity with superior disc space clearance, rapid end plate preparation, and potential for better fusion than posterior interbodies (TLIF/PLIF).

- ALIF allows anterior access to the disc space and facilitates maximal implant size and surface area to provide aggressive correction of local foraminal height and restoration of segmental lordosis with more lordotic cage options.

- There is avoidance of significant morbidity of traditional open posterior surgery (muscle split, postoperative pain, slow to mobilize resulting in a longer length of stay).

Oblique Lumbar Interbody Fusion (OLIF) L5–S1

OLIF as described previously can be used for access to L2–L5.[57] In certain cases, a pre-psoas oblique retroperitoneal approach which is described here can be used to access L5–S1.

Definition of the Technique

In 1997, Mayer first described an oblique approach to the lumbar spine, L2–L5.[78] Since then, to access L5–S1 an anterior transabdominal approach was recommended to avoid interference and serious complication with the aortic bifurcation at the L5–S1 level. However, it was not used until Silvestre et al reported a minimally invasive technique in 2012 using an oblique retroperitoneal approach to L5–S1.[57]

Indications

OLIF is indicated for surgical correction in the lumbar spine in the presence of mild to moderate central canal stenosis, loss of coronal and sagittal balance, lumbar spondylolisthesis, and previous spinal surgery at that level.[79–81] It is a single-incision, muscle-splitting technique that can offer access to multiple levels. Similar to ALIF and in contrast to PLIF, it reduces the risk of dural tears and avoids the need to retract nerve roots.

Complication Avoidance

Care should be taken to avoid the sensory branches of the lumbar plexus descending between the internal oblique and transverse muscles. Care must be taken not to mistake it for the quadratus lumborum as there would be risk of injuring the lumbar nerve roots. The anterior edge of the psoas is followed leading directly to the transverse process of the spine. The ureter should be located and retracted forward along with the peritoneum.

Tips and Tricks

The patient can be positioned in the semi-lateral decubitus position to facilitate exposure of the entire anterior L5–S1 disc space. Usually, the hip is flexed to relax the psoas; however, for access to L5–S1 the hip should be extended.

A separate window is used to access the L5–S1 intervertebral disc space. This window is through the incision made in the lateral aspect of the anterior rectus sheath (**Fig. 21.7**).

The external and internal oblique and transverse muscle fibers are dissociated along their long axis. Once the transverse muscle has been crossed, the retroperitoneal fatty tissue is visible and should be pushed back toward the midline with the peritoneal sac by tampons then valves until the psoas becomes visible, which is an essential landmark, sometimes lying more anteriorly than one might expect.

The rectus muscle and the posterior peritoneum are reflected medially, exposing the great vessels and the anterior aspect of the L5–S1 disc below the bifurcation.

The spine is visible on the medial aspect of the psoas. The genitofemoral nerve will be seen in the angle between the spine and psoas. The left common iliac artery and vein should be located; the common iliac artery can be palpated anterior to the psoas and should be used as a landmark to identify the iliac vein. The iliac vein lies behind the artery, usually in contact with the spine. For L4–L5 and L5–S1, it is indispensable to ligate or clip the ascending lumbar vein.[82] Once the anterolateral side of the spine has been exposed, exposure should be maintained using Steinmann nails in the vertebral bodies. Apart from the incision being on the anterolateral side of the annulus, the diskectomy technique is the same for both the anterior and oblique approach. A cage is inserted in the standard ALIF manner.

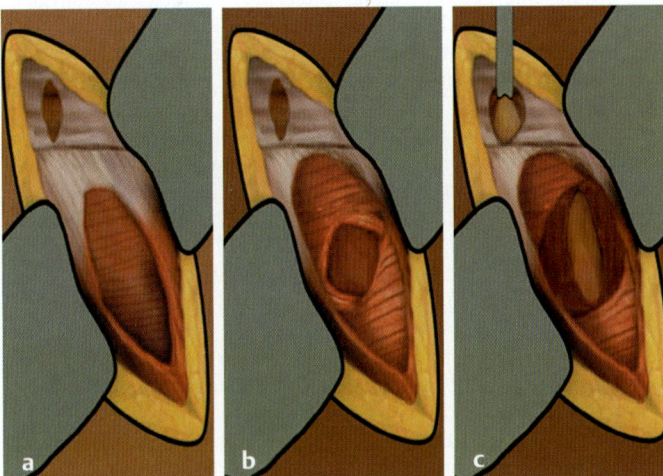

Fig. 21.7 **(a)** Access windows for L3–L5 and L5–S1. Superficial dissection splitting fibers of external oblique muscle. **(b)** Split fibers of internal oblique and **(c)** split fibers of transversus abdominus. (Reproduced with permission from Molloy et al.[68])

Key Points

- OLIF is indicated for lumbar pathology at L2–L5 and further caudal to L5–S1. Access via OLIF for L5–S1 can be used in certain cases if anatomy allows, that is, low bifurcation of vessels and a low iliac crest.

- L5–S1 OLIF is a relatively new technique. Outcomes are thought to be comparable to other approaches to this level; for example, OLIF avoids the complications associated with a transabdominal approach. Preoperative planning should determine the appropriateness of this technique at the L5–S1 disc space.

References

1. Meccariello L, Muzii VF, Falzarano G, et al. Dynamic corset versus three-point brace in the treatment of osteoporotic compression fractures of the thoracic and lumbar spine: a prospective, comparative study. Aging Clin Exp Res 2017;29(3):443–449

2. Ailon T, Shaffrey CI, Lenke LG, Harrop JS, Smith JS. Progressive spinal kyphosis in the aging population. Neurosurgery 2015;77(Suppl 4):S164–S172

3. Smith-Petersen MN, Larson CB, Aufranc OE. Osteotomy of the spine for correction of flexion deformity in rheumatoid arthritis. Clin Orthop Relat Res 1969;66(66):6–9

4. Smith-Petersen MN, Larson CB, Aufranc OE. Osteotomy of the spine for correction of the flexi on deformity in rheumatoid arthritis. J Bone Joint Surg 1945;27:1–11

5. Thomasen E. Vertebral osteotomy for correction of kyphosis in ankylosing spondylitis. Clin Orthop Relat Res 1985;(194):142–152

6. Hehne HJ, Zielke K, Böhm H. Polysegmental lumbar osteotomies and transpedicled fixation for correction of long-curved kyphotic deformities in ankylosing spondylitis. Report on 177 cases. Clin Orthop Relat Res 1990;(258):49–55

7. Gelalis ID, Kang JD. Thoracic and lumbar fusions for degenerative disorders: rationale for selecting the appropriate fusion techniques. Orthop Clin North Am 1998;29(4):829–842

8. Gupta MC. Degenerative scoliosis. Options for surgical management. Orthop Clin North Am 2003;34(2):269–279

9. Briggs H, Milligan P. Chip fusion of the low back following exploration of the spinal canal. J Bone Joint Surg Am 1944;26:125–130

10. Cloward RB. The treatment of ruptured lumbar intervertebral discs by vertebral body fusion. I. Indications, operative technique, after care. J Neurosurg 1953;10(2):154–168

11. Ray CD. Threaded titanium cages for lumbar interbody fusions. Spine 1997;22(6):667–679, discussion 679–680

12. Branch CL, Branch CL Jr. Posterior lumbar interbody fusion with the keystone graft: technique and results. Surg Neurol 1987;27(5):449–454

13. Simmons JW. Posterior lumbar interbody fusion with posterior elements as chip grafts. Clin Orthop Relat Res 1985;(193):85–89

14. Iwamae M, Matsumura A, Namikawa T, et al. Surgical outcomes of multilevel posterior lumbar interbody fusion versus lateral lumbar interbody fusion for the correction of adult spinal deformity: a comparative clinical study. Asian Spine J 2020;14(4):421–429

15. Dorward IG, Lenke LG, Bridwell KH, et al. Transforaminal versus anterior lumbar interbody fusion in long deformity constructs: a matched cohort analysis. Spine 2013;38(12):E755–E762

16. Kim DH, Vaccaro A, Henn J, Dickman C. Surgical Anatomy & Techniques to the Spine. Saunders; 2006

17. Spoonamore MJ. Posterior Lumbar Interbody Fusion (PLIF) & Transforaminal Lumbar Interbody Fusion (TLIF). University of Southern California. Accessed at: https://www.uscspine.com/treatement-options/back-treatment/lumbar-interbody-fusion/

18. Hey HW, Hee HT. Lumbar degenerative spinal deformity: surgical options of PLIF, TLIF and MI-TLIF. Indian J Orthop 2010;44(2):159–162

19. Sekhon L, Sears W. Posterior Lumbar Interbody Fusion (PLIF): Advantages and Indications. Accessed at: https://www.spineuniverse.com/treatments/surgery/minimally-invasive/posterior-lumbar-interbody-fusion-plif-advantages-indications

20. Fan SW, Hu ZJ, Fang XQ, Zhao FD, Huang Y, Yu HJ. Comparison of paraspinal muscle injury in one-level lumbar posterior interbody fusion: modified minimally invasive and traditional open approaches. Orthop Surg 2010;2(3):194–200

21. Humphreys SC, Hodges SD, Patwardhan AG, Eck JC, Murphy RB, Covington LA. Comparison of posterior and transforaminal approaches to lumbar interbody fusion. Spine 2001;26(5):567–571

22. Zhang Q, Yuan Z, Zhou M, Liu H, Xu Y, Ren Y. A comparison of posterior lumbar interbody fusion and transforaminal lumbar interbody fusion: a literature review and meta-analysis. BMC Musculoskelet Disord 2014;15:367

23. Mobbs RJ, Phan K, Malham G, Seex K, Rao PJ. Lumbar interbody fusion: techniques, indications and comparison of interbody fusion options including PLIF, TLIF, MI-TLIF, OLIF/ATP, LLIF and ALIF. J Spine Surg 2015;1(1):2–18

24. Lestini WF, Fulghum JS, Whitehurst LA. Lumbar spinal fusion: advantages of posterior lumbar interbody fusion. Surg Technol Int 1994;3:577–590

25. Avila MJ, Baaj AA, Navarro-Ramirez R, et al. Transforaminal lumbar interbody fusion (TLIF). In: Manjila SV, Mroz TE, Steinmetz MP, et al, eds. Lumbar Interbody Fusions. Elsevier; 2019:59–62

26. Harms J, Rolinger H. [A one-stager procedure in operative treatment of spondylolistheses: dorsal traction-reposition and anterior fusion (author's transl)]. Z Orthop Ihre Grenzgeb 1982;120(3):343–347

27. Gum JL, Reddy D, Glassman S. Transforaminal lumbar interbody fusion (TLIF). JBJS Essential Surg Tech 2016;6(2):e22

28. Yadla S, Maltenfort MG, Ratliff JK, Harrop JS. Adult scoliosis surgery outcomes: a systematic review. Neurosurg Focus 2010;28(3):E3

29. Hackenberg L, Halm H, Bullmann V, Vieth V, Schneider M, Liljenqvist U. Transforaminal lumbar interbody fusion: a safe technique with satisfactory three to five year results. Eur Spine J 2005;14(6):551–558

30. Pimenta L. Lateral endoscopic transpsoas retroperitoneal approach for lumbar spine surgery. Presented at the Eighth Brazilian Spine Society Meeting; 2001; Belo Horizante, Brazil

31. Pimenta L, Díaz RC, Guerrero LG. Charité lumbar artificial disc retrieval: use of a lateral minimally invasive technique. Technical note. J Neurosurg Spine 2006;5(6):556–561

32. Pimenta L, Lhamby J, Gharzedine I, et al. XLIF approach for the treatment of adult scoliosis: 2-year follow-up. Spine J 2007;7:52S–53S

33. Pimenta L, Oliveira L, Coutinho E, et al. Minimally invasive surgery for degenerative scoliosis. Spine J 2009;9:131S

34. Ozgur BM, Aryan HE, Pimenta L, Taylor WR. Extreme lateral interbody fusion (XLIF): a novel surgical technique for anterior lumbar interbody fusion. Spine J 2006;6(4):435–443

35. McAfee PC, Shucosky E, Chotikul L. Anterior MIS rod instrumentation with XLIF deformity, techniques and results. Presented at the Society of Lateral Access Surgeons Annual Meeting; June 2011; San Diego, CA

36. Rodgers WB, Gerber EJ, Rodgers JA. Lumbar fusion in octogenarians: the promise of minimally invasive surgery. Spine 2010;35(26, Suppl):S355–S360

37. Isaacs RE, Hyde J, Goodrich JA, Rodgers WB, Phillips FM. A prospective, nonrandomized, multicenter evaluation of extreme lateral interbody fusion for the treatment of adult degenerative scoliosis: perioperative outcomes and complications. Spine 2010;35(26, Suppl):S322–S330

38. Diaz R, Phillips F, Pimenta L. XLIF for lumbar degenerative scoliosis: outcomes of minimally invasive surgical treatment out to 3 years postoperatively. Spine J 2006;6(5):75S

39. McAfee PC, Garfin SR, Rodgers WB, Allen RT, Phillips F, Kim C. An attempt at clinically defining and assessing minimally invasive surgery compared with traditional "open" spinal surgery. SAS J 2011;5(4):125–130

40. Akbarnia B, Varma V, Bess S. Extreme lateral interbody fusion (XLIF) safely improves segmental and global deformity in large adult lumbar scoliosis: Preliminary results on 13 patients. Presented at the 15th Annual Meeting of International Meeting of Advanced Spine Technologies; July 2008; Hong Kong

41. Kepler C, Sharma A, Huang RC, et al. Correction of sagittal and coronal plane degenerative lumbar deformity using the extreme lateral interbody fusion (XLIF) technique. Spine J 2009;9:59S

42. Schwab F, Dubey A, Gamez L, et al. Adult scoliosis: prevalence, SF-36, and nutritional parameters in an elderly volunteer population. Spine 2005;30(9):1082–1085

43. McAfee PC, Shucosky E, Chotikul L, Salari B, Chen L, Jerrems D. Multilevel extreme lateral interbody fusion (XLIF) and osteotomies for 3-dimensional severe deformity: 25 consecutive cases. Int J Spine Surg 2013;7:e8–e19

44. Dakwar E, Cardona RF, Smith DA, Uribe JS. Early outcomes and safety of the minimally invasive, lateral retroperitoneal transpsoas approach for adult degenerative scoliosis. Neurosurg Focus 2010;28(3):E8

45. Tormenti MJ, Maserati MB, Bonfield CM, Okonkwo DO, Kanter AS. Complications and radiographic correction in adult scoliosis following combined transpsoas extreme lateral interbody fusion and posterior pedicle screw instrumentation. Neurosurg Focus 2010;28(3):E7

46. Berjano P, Lamartina C. Minimally invasive lateral transpsoas approach with advanced neurophysiologic monitoring for lumbar interbody fusion. Eur Spine J 2011;20(9):1584–1586

47. Berjano P, Lamartina C. Far lateral approaches (XLIF) in adult scoliosis. Eur Spine J 2013;22(Suppl 2):242–253

48. London Spine Care. XLIF - Extreme Lateral Interbody Fusion. Accessed at: https://www.londonspinecare.co.uk/xlif-extreme-lateral-interbody-fusion-trauma-orthopaedic-surgeon-london.html

49. Akbarnia BA, Mundis G, Bagheri R, et al. Lateral approach for interbody fusion (LIF) is a safe and effective technique to reconstruct the anterior spinal column in complex adult spinal deformity: a minimum 2-year follow-up study. In: Proceedings of the 4th annual SOLAS (Society of Lateral Access Surgery) research meeting, March 31–April 2, 2011, San Diego, California

50. Benglis DM, Vanni S, Levi AD. An anatomical study of the lumbosacral plexus as related to the minimally invasive transpsoas approach to the lumbar spine. J Neurosurg Spine 2009;10(2):139–144

51. Hyde JA. Clinical application: degenerated/collapsed disc. In: Goodrich JA, Volcan IJ, eds. eXtreme Lateral Interbody Fusion (XLIF). St Louis, MO: QMP Publishing; 2008:127–142

52. Leary SP, Regan JJ, Lanman TH, Wagner WH. Revision and explantation strategies involving the CHARITE lumbar artificial disc replacement. Spine 2007;32(9):1001–1011

53. Smith W, Malone K. Complications in extreme lateral interbody fusion: one surgeon's experience with 566 patients and 1550 levels. Spine J 2009;9:178S–179S

54. Rodgers WB, Tohmeh A, Hyde J, et al. A prospective, multi-center, non-randomized evaluation of XLIF in the treatment of adult scoliosis: Mid-term radiographic outcomes. Spine J 2009;9(10):156S–157S

55. Mobbs RJ, Phan K, Malham G, Seex K, Rao PJ. Lumbar interbody fusion: techniques, indications and comparison of interbody fusion options including PLIF, TLIF, MI-TLIF, OLIF/ATP, LLIF and ALIF. J Spine Surg 2015;1(1):2–18

56. Zhu L, Wang JW, Zhang L, Feng XM. Outcomes of oblique lateral interbody fusion for adult spinal deformity: a systematic review and meta-analysis. Global Spine J 2022;12(1):142–154

57. Silvestre C, Mac-Thiong JM, Hilmi R, Roussouly P. Complications and morbidities of mini-open anterior retroperitoneal lumbar interbody fusion: oblique lumbar interbody fusion in 179 patients. Asian Spine J 2012;6(2):89–97

58. Ohtori S, Orita S, Yamauchi K, et al. Mini-open anterior retroperitoneal lumbar interbody fusion: oblique lateral interbody fusion for lumbar spinal degeneration disease. Yonsei Med J 2015;56(4):1051–1059

59. Ohtori S, Mannoji C, Orita S, et al. Mini-open anterior retroperitoneal lumbar interbody fusion: oblique lateral interbody fusion for degenerated lumbar spinal kyphoscoliosis. Asian Spine J 2015;9(4):565–572

60. Kim KT, Jo DJ, Lee SH, Seo EM. Oblique retroperitoneal approach for lumbar interbody fusion from L1 to S1 in adult spinal deformity. Neurosurg Rev 2018;41(1):355–363

61. Zeng ZY, Xu ZW, He DW, et al. Complications and prevention strategies of oblique lateral interbody fusion technique. Orthop Surg 2018;10(2):98–106

62. Zhang Y, Tao L, Hai Y, et al. One-stage posterior multiple-level asymmetrical Ponte osteotomies versus single-level posterior vertebral column resection for severe and rigid adult idiopathic scoliosis: a minimum 2-year follow-up comparative study. Spine 2019;44(20):E1196–E1205

63. Shi B, Zhao Q, Xu L, et al. SRS-Schwab Grade 4 osteotomy for congenital thoracolumbar kyphosis: a minimum of 2 years follow-up study. Spine J 2018;18(11):2059–2064

64. Glassman SD, Bridwell K, Dimar JR, Horton W, Berven S, Schwab F. The impact of positive sagittal balance in adult spinal deformity. Spine 2005;30(18):2024–2029

65. Riouallon G, Lachaniette CHF, Poignard A, Allain J. Outcomes of anterior lumbar interbody fusion in low-grade isthmic spondylolisthesis in adults: a continuous series of 65 cases with an average follow-up of 6.6 years. Orthop Traumatol Surg Res 2013;99(2):155–161

66. Baker JK, Reardon PR, Reardon MJ, Heggeness MH. Vascular injury in anterior lumbar surgery. Spine 1993;18(15):2227–2230

67. Lindley EM, McBeth ZL, Henry SE, et al. Retrograde ejaculation after anterior lumbar spine surgery. Spine 2012;37(20):1785–1789

68. Molloy S, Butler JS, Benton A, Malhotra K, Selvadurai S, Agu O. A new extensile anterolateral retroperitoneal approach for lumbar interbody fusion from L1 to S1: a prospective series with clinical outcomes. Spine J 2016;16(6):786–791

69. Flouzat-Lachaniette CH, Ratte L, Poignard A, et al. Minimally invasive anterior lumbar interbody fusion for adult degenerative scoliosis with 1 or 2 dislocated levels. J Neurosurg Spine 2015;23(6):739–746

70. König MA, Ebrahimi FV, Nitulescu A, Behrbalk E, Boszczyk BM. Early results of stand-alone anterior lumbar interbody fusion in iatrogenic spondylolisthesis in patients. Eur Spine J 2013;22(12):2876–2883

71. Davis TT, Hynes RA, Fung DA, et al. Retroperitoneal oblique corridor to the L2-S1 intervertebral discs in the lateral position: an anatomic study. J Neurosurg Spine 2014;21(5):785–793

72. Butler JS, Lui DF, Malhotra K, et al. 360-degree complex primary reconstruction using porous tantalum cages for adult degenerative spinal deformity. Global Spine J 2019;9(6):613–618

73. Jiang SD, Chen JW, Jiang LS. Which procedure is better for lumbar interbody fusion: anterior lumbar interbody fusion or transforaminal lumbar interbody fusion? Arch Orthop Trauma Surg 2012;132(9):1259–1266

74. Tang S. Does TLIF aggravate adjacent segmental degeneration more adversely than ALIF? A finite element study. Turk Neurosurg 2012;22(3):324–328

75. Videbaek TS, Egund N, Christensen FB, Grethe Jurik A, Bünger CE. Adjacent segment degeneration after lumbar spinal fusion: the impact of anterior column support: a randomized clinical trial with an eight- to thirteen-year magnetic resonance imaging follow-up. Spine 2010;35(22):1955–1964

76. Rahn KA, Shugart RM, Wylie MW, Reddy KK, Morgan JA. The effect of lordosis, disc height change, subsidence, and transitional segment on stand-alone anterior lumbar interbody fusion using a nontapered threaded device. Am J Orthop 2010;39(12):E124–E129

77. Min J-H, Jang J-S, Lee S-H. Comparison of anterior- and posterior-approach instrumented lumbar interbody fusion for spondylolisthesis. J Neurosurg Spine 2007;7(1):21–26

78. Mayer HM. A new microsurgical technique for minimally invasive anterior lumbar interbody fusion. Spine 1997;22(6):691–699, discussion 700

79. Herkowitz HN. Degenerative lumbar spondylolisthesis: evolution of surgical management. Spine J 2009;9(7):605–606

80. Phan K, Mobbs RJ. Oblique lumbar interbody fusion for revision of non-union following prior posterior surgery: a case report. Orthop Surg 2015;7(4):364–367

81. Li R, Li X, Zhou H, Jiang W. Development and application of oblique lumbar interbody fusion. Orthop Surg 2020;12(2):355–365

82. Allain J, Dufour T. Anterior lumbar fusion techniques: ALIF, OLIF, DLIF, LLIF, IXLIF. Orthop Traumatol Surg Res 2020;106(1S):S149–S157

22 Sacropelvic Fixation Techniques

Mehmet Zileli, Habib Canberk Karakoç, and Onur Yaman

Introduction

Allen and Ferguson first described lumbopelvic fixation in 1982.[1] The authors used a bent rod to enter the iliac wing and connect to the lumbar and upper levels by wires. They called this technique as "Galveston rod technique." The rods are bent to give an "L" shape; then they are inserted into the ilium through the posterior superior iliac spine. However, they are associated with a high pseudoarthrosis rate (36%).[2] Significant limitations were implant prominence, loosening of the rods, which causes pain, and a "windshield wiper" effect that may be seen radiographically.[3] Gokaslan et al modified the technique in 1997 by using pedicle screws in the lumbar spine.[4] Because of the disadvantages, such as high pseudoarthrosis rates, these techniques were replaced by more advanced techniques. Achieving a solid fusion of the lumbosacral region of the spine is challenging for spine surgeons.

The sacrum of adult patients is cancellous in structure and has short S1 pedicles; for this reason, the sacrum is a weak structure for fixation. Biomechanically, the lumbosacral pivot point is at the dorsal L5–S1 annulus fibrosus level. This point is between the mobile lumbar spine and the relatively less mobile pelvis and carries shearing motions. McCord et al pointed out that the pivot point represents the axis about which the lumbosacral region flexes and extends.[5] Nonunion at the lumbosacral junction is a common complication of long instrumentations. By using S1 promontory screws, the nonunion incidence ranges between 5 and 44%.[6–8] If the fixation points are extended to L3 and above, the nonunion risk increases.[9] To decrease the risk of nonunion, anterior interbody support or iliac fixation is recommended.[10,11] However, without anchors extending anterior to the pivot point of the spine, such as pelvic fixation, adding anterior support does not decrease the pressure on S1 screws.[9] Anchors extending anterior to the pivot point of the spine decreases flexion and shear loads distally, reducing slippage.[12] Indications for instrumentation down to the pelvic ring are long segment fusions extending to the sacrum, revision of previous fusions, deformities requiring three-column osteotomies in the lumbar spine, high-grade spondylolisthesis, sacrectomies, and severe osteoporosis.[13] O'Brien et al described a classification system for sacropelvic fixation.[14] They divided the sacropelvic area into three zones.

Zone 1 is the S1 vertebral body and the upper sacral ala; zone 2 is the lower sacral ala and body of S2 and coccyx; zone 3 is the bilateral ilia.[14] The strength of the construct increases as fixation involves all three zones.[15] There are many methods used for spinopelvic fixation. However, the most popular spinopelvic fixation techniques are iliac screw fixation and S2 alar iliac screw fixation.

The iliac screws' strength is three times greater than Galveston rod technique.[16]

Indications

The main indications of sacropelvic fixation are below:

- Adult spinal deformity patients with osteoporosis require a long construct spinopelvic fixation.[17] Patients with deformity and high-grade spondylolisthesis are the most common indications. Neuromuscular scoliosis patients having pelvic imbalance are also candidates.

- Sacral tumor removal
    - ➢ Total sacrectomy (bilateral sacroiliac [SI] joint removal)[18]
    - ➢ Partial sacrectomy (>50% of bilateral SI joint removal or resection of one SI joint)[19]
    - ➢ Lack of quality sacral bone due to the destruction of tumor[20]

- Sacral U-shaped fracture type 3 of Roy Camille[21]
- Pyogenic infection of the lumbosacral area
- Revision surgery for L5–S1 nonunion (S1 screw loosening and pseudoarthrosis) and cases with L5–S1 fusion with severe osteoporosis

Definition of the Technique

Iliac Screw Placement

The entry point of the iliac wing screw can be selected on any part of the iliac wing. However, an entry point selected distal to the S1 screw will help during rod placement.

There are three options for iliac screwing: (a) traditional entry point, (b) anatomical entry point, and (c) sacral entry point (**Fig. 22.1**).

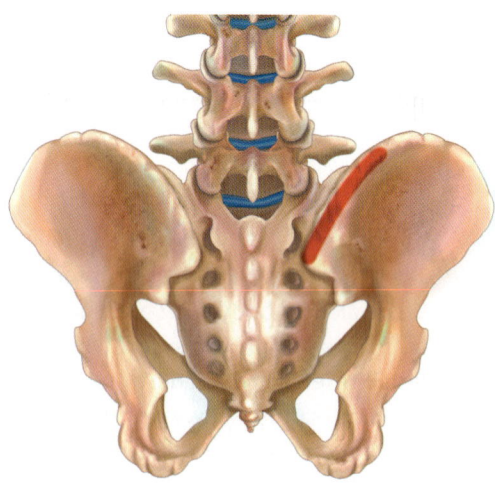

Fig. 22.1 Any part of the iliac crest can be selected as an entry point (red line). However, three options are most used: traditional entry point (a), anatomical entry point (b), and sacral entry point (c).

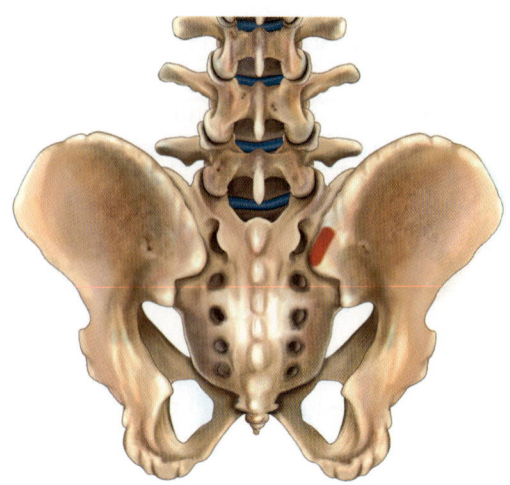

Fig. 22.2 The traditional entry point. You can remove a small piece of bone to decrease the profile of the screw head and prevent a threat to the skin. Besides, choosing an entry point caudal to the S1 screw is useful for rod placement.

Traditional Entry Point

- The entry point for the iliac screw is the superior edge of the posterior superior iliac crest. Its trajectory must target the anterior superior iliac spine or the superior acetabular notch. We must remove the superior prominence to let the screw head to stay in a deeper position within the ilium. Removal of the prominence permits bone graft harvesting (**Figs. 22.2–22.5**).

An offset connector or a slotted connector can be used to connect laterally located iliac screws to more medially located lumbosacral screws. This method has a higher fusion rate than the Galveston technique and is biomechanically superior.[22] Pain caused by the protrusion of the screw into the skin, further dissection of the tissues, and the need for various connector systems are the main drawbacks.[13] Additionally, instrument failure and loosening of the screw have been reported to be 17.3 and 11.8%, respectively.[23]

Anatomical Entry Point

This is below the traditional entry point (**Fig. 22.1**).

Technique for Traditional Entry Point and Anatomical Entry Point

Position

The patient is placed on the radiolucent table in a prone position. A C-arm is placed; the position of the C-arm should be easily adjustable (**Fig. 22.5a**).

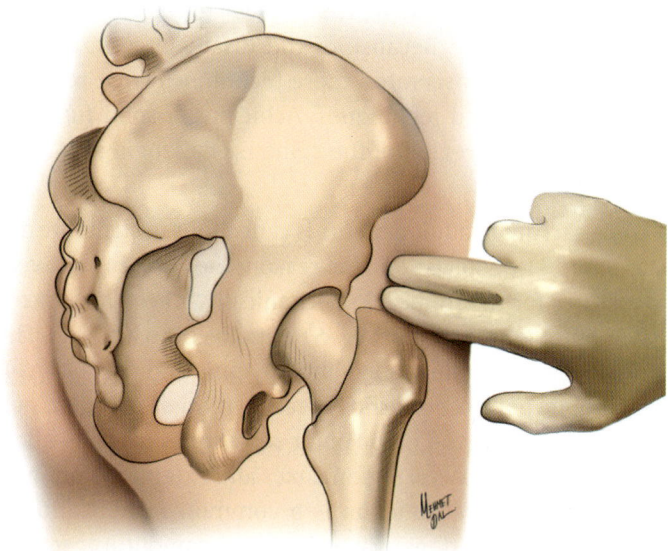

Fig. 22.3 Determining the iliac wing screw according to palpation of the trochanter major.

Surgical Technique

A midline skin incision down to S2 level is necessary. Following the skin incision, paravertebral muscles are dissected subperiostally. Borders of iliac wings need to be determined. Iliac screws can be placed easily from the opposite side.

The entry point for the "traditional" technique is 1 cm above the inferior process of the posterior superior iliac spine (PSIS).

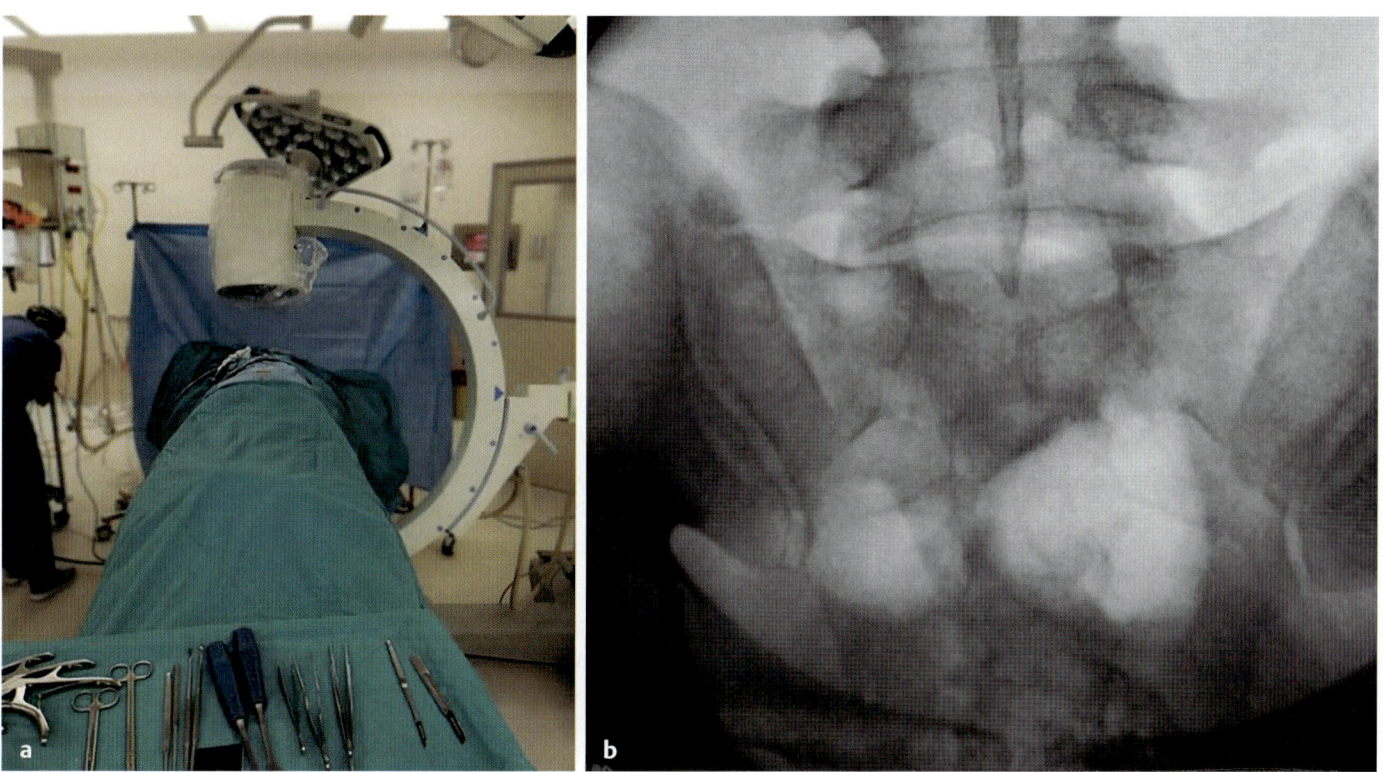

Fig. 22.4   (a, b) Sacral inlet C-arm views may be helpful during iliac screw placement.

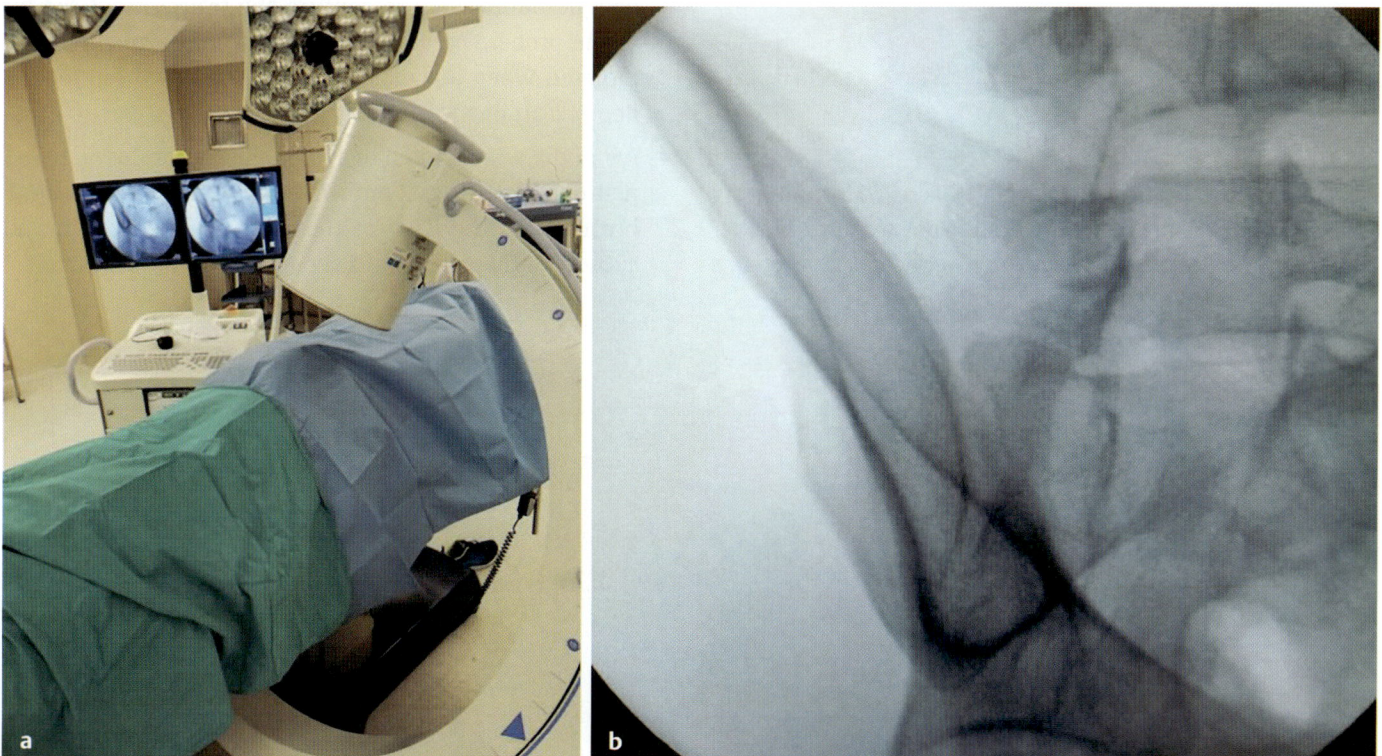

Fig. 22.5   (a, b) Position of C-arm for obturator oblique view. The screw must be in the teardrop part.

Direction

Anterior inferior iliac spine (AIIS) should be the target. The trajectory of iliac wing screws can be determined according to trochanter major palpation (**Fig. 22.3**).

- Screw trajectory should be far away from the sciatic notch. This is because the bone just over the sciatica notch (1–2 cm above) is cortical and is much stronger than the spongy bone.
- The angulation of the probe should be 30 to 45 degrees in the coronal plane and 25 to 45 degrees in the axial plane. A pedicle probe with a bent tip should proceed into the cancellous bone. The line between PSIS and AIIS is the thickest part of the ilium.
- For a powerful grip, you must pass the sciatic notch level.
- Sacral inlet and obturator oblique C-arm views may be helpful during iliac screw placement (**Figs. 22.4** and **22.5**).
- Pedicle finder must be in the bone and checked with a controller for proper screw placement (**Fig. 22.6**).
- Iliac screw (6–8 mm diameter, 70–100 mm length) can be placed according to the trajectory (**Fig. 22.7a**). The iliac screw can be attached to the rod with the help of a connector (**Fig. 22.7b**). The screw head should not be felt from the skin.

Sacral Entry Point

S1 Alar Screw Placement

The main indication for the S1 alar iliac is S1 promontory screw failure. This technique does not require further dissection of the S2 pedicle, which reduces the surgery's duration and bleeding. Considering that the entry point of the screws is located more medially compared to traditional sacral screw fixation, this technique does not need connectors. It mainly preserves the tissues surrounding the sacral ala. However, it has not been proven that this type of screw is more advantageous than S1 promontory screws biomechanically.[24]

Surgical Technique

The entry point should be aligned with the L5 screws. A 2-mm burr or an awl is used to create a hole at the entry point. To prevent an anterior sacral breach, the pedicle probe is directed caudally. The caudal angulation of the probe should be 35 to 45 degrees, whereas horizontal angulation should be 20 degrees in the coronal plane.

- First, pedicle probe is inserted 3 to 5 cm until it reaches the cortical bone at the SI joint. Then the SI joint is pierced through by the pedicle finder; subsequently, the curved probe is rotated 180 degrees facing ventrally.
- Using a long iliac probe and avoiding the surrounding soft tissues are favored. A 20 degrees horizontal angulation should be kept when inserting the probe.
- Teardrop-like image of the ischial body is obtained with oblique fluoroscopy to confirm the trajectory of the tip of the probe. The center of the teardrop sign should be targeted when advancing the probe until the intended depth is attained (generally ≥75 mm).
- Avoid the sciatic notch to avoid injuring the vascular and neuronal structures. Confirm the absence of cortical wall breach with the K-wire; then tap the screw path and subsequently place the screw in the traditional fashion.[24]

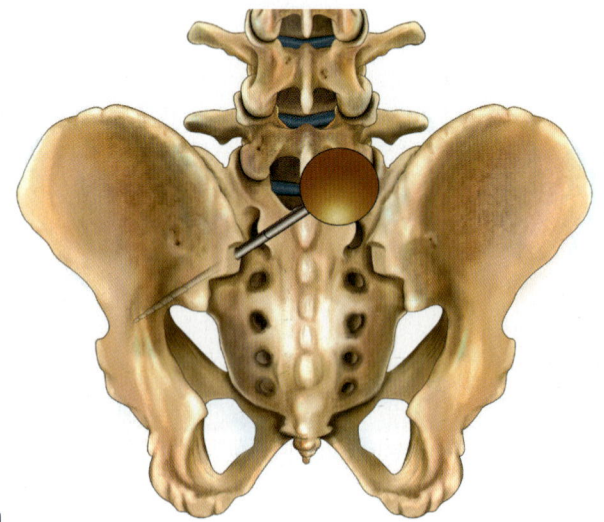
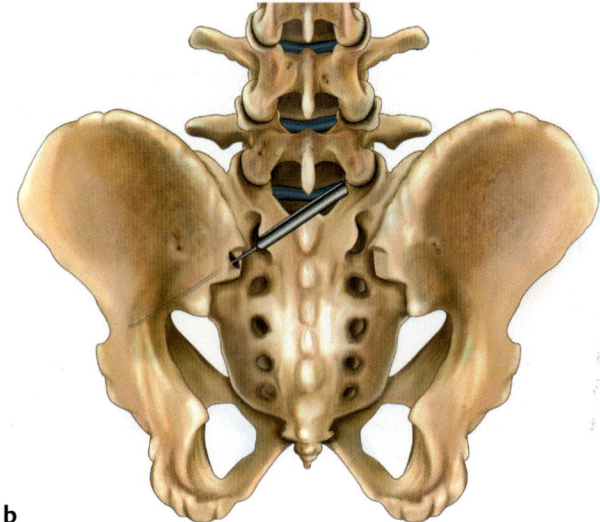

a   b

Fig. 22.6 A pedicle finder is introduced into the bone **(a)** and checked with a controller for proper screw placement **(b)**. The pedicle finder must be over the sciatica notch, and the direction has to be to trochanter major.

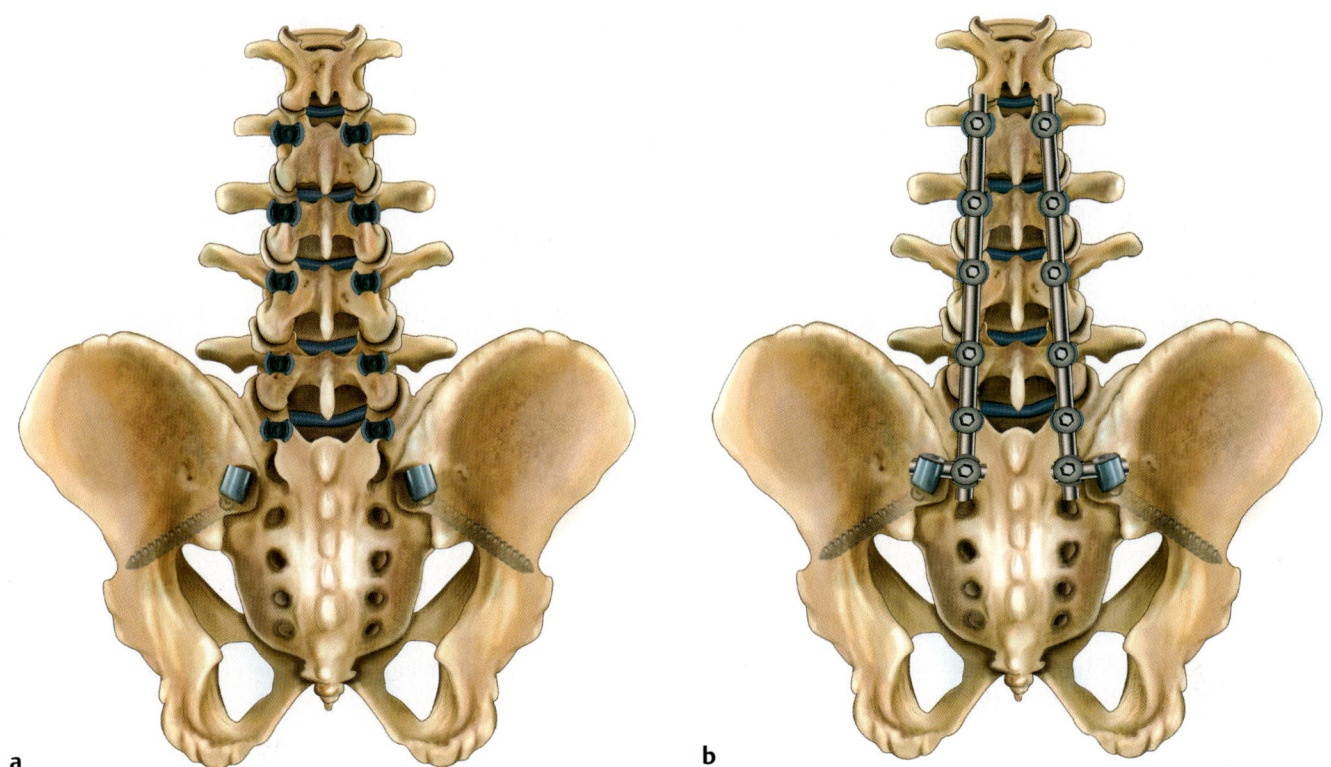

Fig. 22.7 Bilateral iliac screws are placed according to anatomical landmarks **(a)**, and construction is completed using offset connectors to both rods **(b)**.

S2 Alar Screw Placement

Khaled M. Kebaish demonstrated using S2 alar iliac (S2AI) screws in adult patients, while Paul D. Sponseller described the procedure in the pediatric group.[13] The S2AI screw is inserted 1.5 mm deeper than the iliac screw so that the screw is felt less through the skin.[10] Positive aspects of S2AI screws are less need for offset connectors due to the alignment with the S1 pedicle, higher pullout strength and requiring minor soft tissue dissection, and lower wound infection rates as compared to iliac screws (22.8%). Extensive dissection of the lumbosacral fascia surrounding PSIS may be the cause of higher wound infection rates.[18] In a cadaveric study, O'Brien et al reported that the rate of SI joint cartilage violation by the S2AI screw is 60%.[7] However, SI joint pain rates are not as high among the patients who received S2AI screws.[6] SI joint fixation by the screw which crosses the SI joint may be the underlying cause.[25] Early clinical outcome studies demonstrated that S2AI screws cause fewer complications, have superior fusion rates, and provide further correction of pelvic obliquity as compared to iliac screws.[26]

Surgical Technique

- Entry point should be the lateral part of the midpoint of S1 and S2 foramina (**Fig. 22.8**). It is approximately 2 mm medial to the sacral lateral protuberance and inferolateral to the S1 foramen. This makes head of the screw compatible with the S1 screw for rod placement.

- S2 alar screw trajectory can be easily determined according to the trochanter major. Attention should be paid to the sciatica notch.

- Pedicle finder should be used according to the anatomical structure of the bone (**Fig. 22.9a**).

- With the help of the controller, the trajectory of the pedicle finder is checked (**Fig. 22.9b**).

- S2 alar screw should be placed after checking the bone walls (**Fig. 22.10a**). The S2 alar screw head can be easily placed into the rod, and an offset connector is not necessary (**Fig. 22.10b**).

If parallel double screws are necessary, the second screws can be inserted in the iliac bone 1 to 3 cm above the last screw and proceed similarly. Angulated dual screws are another option. In this case, the second screw is in a superolateral direction. Both the screws may be shorter (40–50 mm) (Armitta technique).

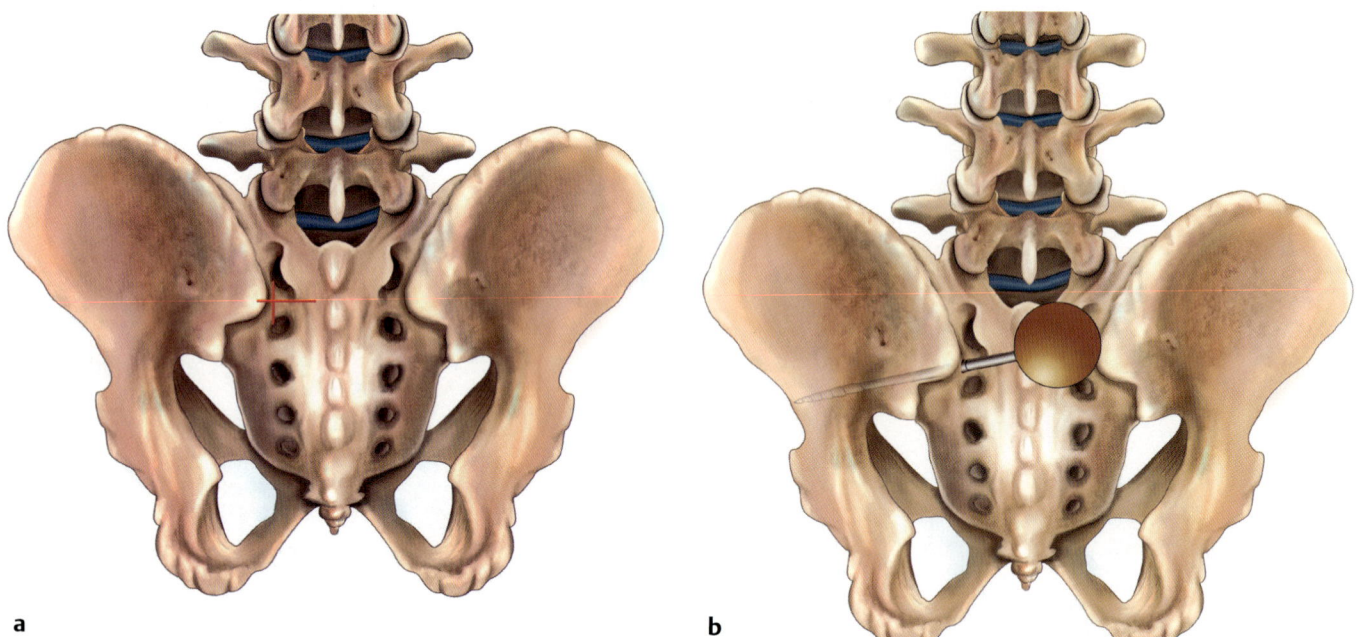

Fig. 22.8 The entry point for the S2 alar screw is the intersection of the S1 and S2 foraminal line **(a)**. Therefore, the pedicle finder should be above the sciatica notch **(b)**.

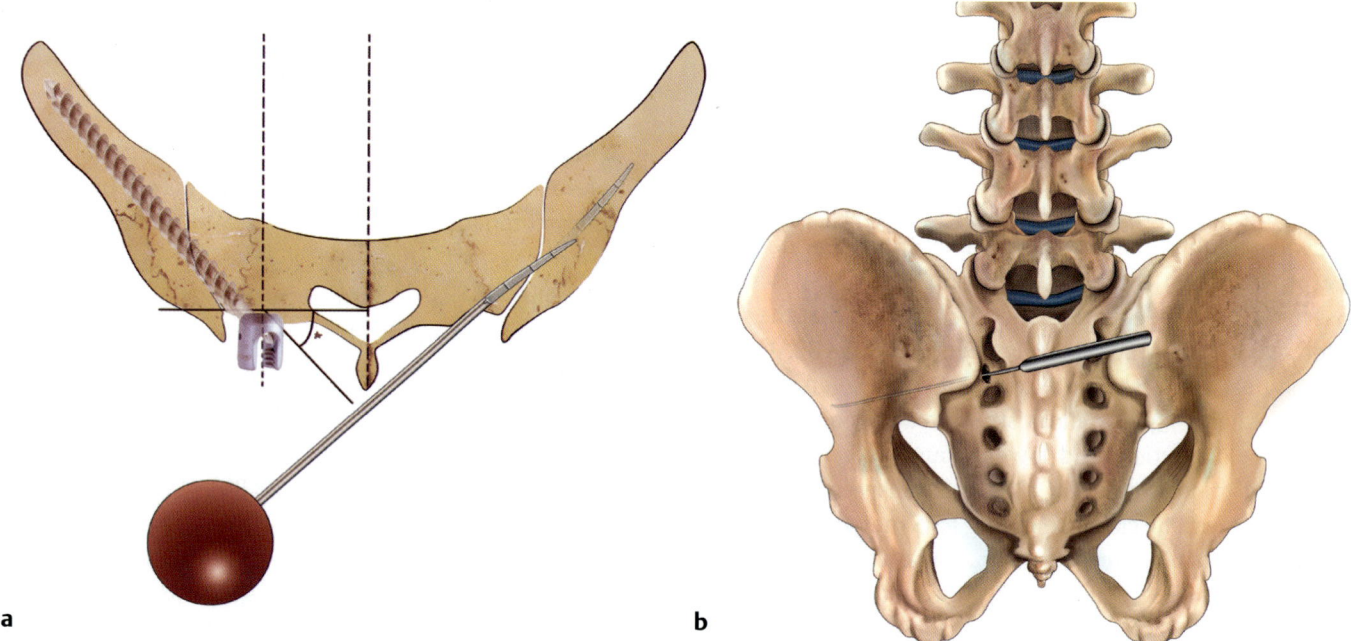

Fig. 22.9 Axial view of the S2 alar screw placement depicting the pedicle finder passing through the sacroiliac joint **(a)**. A K-wire or controller checks the trajectory of the pedicle finder **(b)**.

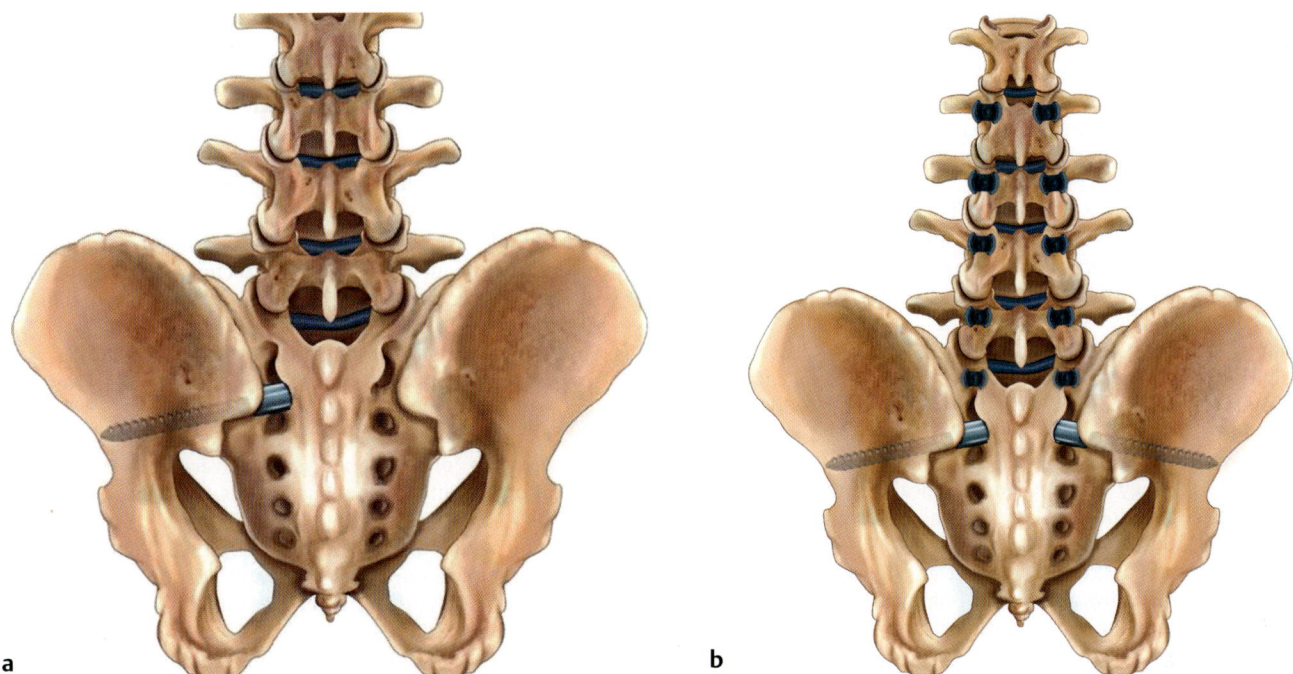

Fig. 22.10 S2 alar screw is placed following the check of bone walls **(a)**. Connection of S2 alar screw with the rod can be made directly without using an offset connector **(b)**.

Tips and Tricks

- Screw direction must be considered according to the sciatica notch. For a proper order of the screw, the anterior inferior iliac spine must be felt. If not, the screw should be directed toward the upper part of the femur head.
- Proceed using a probe. Then use a tap with a conic tip screw.
- Proceed stepwise by controlling the walls using a K-wire/ probe. Pelvic bone resistance must be controlled during all screw placements.
- C-arm fluoroscopy is necessary. Sacral inlet and obturator oblique views are the ideal positions for pelvic imaging.
- Preoperative computed tomography (CT) scan must be used to determine screw length.
- Offset connectors are used for classical and anatomical entry points. S1AI screws are connected directly to the rod.

Conclusion

Although various fixation techniques have been described, lumbosacral joint stabilization is still challenging for surgeons due to this joint's biomechanical features and the region's complex anatomy. Despite not knowing the long-term effect of S2AI screws on the SI joint, biomechanical studies have shown that including the pelvis to the long segment lumbar fusion is beneficial in patients who need fusion from thoracolumbar region to the sacrum, patients who undergo osteotomies involving three columns, and patients who have osteoporosis.

References

1. Allen BL Jr, Ferguson RL. The Galveston technique for L rod instrumentation of the scoliotic spine. Spine 1982;7(3): 276–284
2. Emami A, Deviren V, Berven S, Smith JA, Hu SS, Bradford DS. Outcome and complications of long fusions to the sacrum in adult spine deformity: Luque-Galveston, combined iliac and sacral screws, and sacral fixation. Spine 2002;27(7):776–786
3. Broom MJ, Banta JV, Renshaw TS. Spinal fusion augmented by Luque-rod segmental instrumentation for neuromuscular scoliosis. J Bone Joint Surg Am 1989;71(1):32–44
4. Gokaslan ZL, Romsdahl MM, Kroll SS, et al. Total sacrectomy and Galveston L-rod reconstruction for malignant neoplasms. Technical note. J Neurosurg 1997;87(5):781–787
5. McCord DH, Cunningham BW, Shono Y, Myers JJ, McAfee PC. Biomechanical analysis of lumbosacral fixation. Spine 1992;17(8, Suppl):S235–S243
6. Park YS, Hyun SJ, Park JH, Kim KJ, Jahng TA, Kim HJ. Radiographic and clinical results of freehand S2 alar-iliac screw placement for spinopelvic fixation: an analysis of 45 consecutive screws. Clin Spine Surg 2017;30(7):E877–E882

7. O'Brien JR, Yu WD, Bhatnagar R, Sponseller P, Kebaish KM. An anatomic study of the S2 iliac technique for lumbopelvic screw placement. Spine 2009;34(12):E439–E442

8. Finger T, Bayerl S, Onken J, Czabanka M, Woitzik J, Vajkoczy P. Sacropelvic fixation versus fusion to the sacrum for spondylodesis in multilevel degenerative spine disease. Eur Spine J 2014;23(5):1013–1020

9. Sutterlin CE III, Field A, Ferrara LA, Freeman AL, Phan K. Range of motion, sacral screw and rod strain in long posterior spinal constructs: a biomechanical comparison between S2 alar iliac screws with traditional fixation strategies. J Spine Surg 2016;2(4):266–276

10. Chang TL, Sponseller PD, Kebaish KM, Fishman EK. Low profile pelvic fixation: anatomic parameters for sacral alar-iliac fixation versus traditional iliac fixation. Spine 2009;34(5): 436–440

11. Harimaya K, Mishiro T, Lenke LG, Bridwell KH, Koester LA, Sides BA. Etiology and revision surgical strategies in failed lumbosacral fixation of adult spinal deformity constructs. Spine 2011;36(20):1701–1710

12. Hart RA, Domes CM, Goodwin B, et al. High-grade spondylolisthesis treated using a modified Bohlman technique: results among multiple surgeons. J Neurosurg Spine 2014;20(5): 523–530

13. Kebaish KM. Sacropelvic fixation: techniques and complications. Spine 2010;35(25):2245–2251

14. O'Brien MF, Kuklo TR, Lenke LG. Sacropelvic instrumentation: anatomic and biomechanical zones of fixation. Semin Spine Surg 2004;16(2):76–90

15. El Dafrawy MH, Kebaish KM. Spinopelvic fixation techniques. In: Vaccaro AR, Baron EM, eds. Operative Techniques: Spine Surgery. Elsevier; 2012:240–255

16. Schwend RM, Sluyters R, Najdzionek J. The pylon concept of pelvic anchorage for spinal instrumentation in the human cadaver. Spine 2003;28(6):542–547

17. Ebata S, Ohba T, Oba H, Haro H. Bilateral dual iliac screws in spinal deformity correction surgery. J Orthop Surg Res 2018;13(1):260

18. Mindea SA, Chinthakunta S, Moldavsky M, Gudipally M, Khalil S. Biomechanical comparison of spinopelvic reconstruction techniques in the setting of total sacrectomy. Spine 2012;37(26):E1622–E1627

19. Yu BS, Zhuang XM, Li ZM, et al. Biomechanical effects of the extent of sacrectomy on the stability of lumbo-iliac reconstruction using iliac screw techniques: What level of sacrectomy requires the bilateral dual iliac screw technique? Clin Biomech (Bristol, Avon) 2010;25(9):867–872

20. Fujibayashi S, Neo M, Nakamura T. Palliative dual iliac screw fixation for lumbosacral metastasis. Technical note. J Neurosurg Spine 2007;7(1):99–102

21. König MA, Jehan S, Boszczyk AA, Boszczyk BM. Surgical management of U-shaped sacral fractures: a systematic review of current treatment strategies. Eur Spine J 2012;21(5): 829–836

22. Moshirfar A, Rand FF, Sponseller PD, et al. Pelvic fixation in spine surgery. Historical overview, indications, biomechanical relevance, and current techniques. J Bone Joint Surg Am 2005;87(Suppl 2):89–106

23. Kim JW, Oh CW, Oh JK, et al. The incidence of and factors affecting iliosacral screw loosening in pelvic ring injury. Arch Orthop Trauma Surg 2016;136(7):921–927

24. Wang Z, Boubez G, Shedid D, Yuh SJ, Sebaaly A. Is S1 alar iliac screw a feasible option for lumbosacral fixation?: A technical note. Asian Spine J 2018;12(4):749–753

25. Mattei TA, Fassett DR. Low-profile pelvic fixation with sacral alar-iliac screws. Acta Neurochir (Wien) 2013;155(2):293–297

26. Sponseller PD, Zimmerman RM, Ko PS, et al. Low profile pelvic fixation with the sacral alar iliac technique in the pediatric population improves results at two-year minimum follow-up. Spine 2010;35(20):1887–1892

23 Surgery for Kyphosis in Patients with Sharp Angle Deformity and Neurological Deficit

Marcos Masini, Joao Amorim, and Mehmet Zileli

Introduction

The physiological angle in thoracic spine kyphosis (between T2 and T12) varies between 30 and 50 degrees. Kyphosis is a sagittal spine deformity that may cause significant disability, pain, and neurological deficits.[1] Kyphosis can be classified based on its etiology, presence of neurological deficit, or angulation.

Using etiology as a parameter one can classify kyphosis as congenital, postural, Scheuermann's disease, paralytic, ankylosing spondylitis, trauma, infection, tumor, degenerative, and postlaminectomy. Authors have used other parameters too. They can be classified as kyphosis without neurological deficits, kyphosis with neurological deficits, sharp-angled kyphosis, and smooth-angled kyphosis.

Kyphosis Classification

During the clinical evaluation of the patient, one should focus mainly on pain, impairment in quality of life, respiratory failure, kyphosis angle, and neurological deficit. These findings are essential for determining conservative or surgical treatment.

The indications for surgical treatment vary a lot depending on the etiologies of kyphosis, but the main and general ones are related to the presence of neurological deficit, pain unresponsive to conservative therapy, respiratory failure, and kyphosis with an angle greater than 75 degrees[1] (**Fig. 23.1**).

The etiology that presents the best results with conservative approach to kyphosis is Scheuermann's disease. The conservative treatment of this pathology is based on the use of brace wear and physical therapy. The brace must be worn for at least 20 hours a day for 18 months and can be reduced to 12 to 14 hours a day after kyphosis correction.[2] The focal neurological deficit is closely related to excessively acute angles in kyphosis. Defining the exact angle necessary for the development of neurological deficits is difficult. Still, in experimental models, it has been described that an angle of 50 degrees is likely to initiate spinal cord compression. An angle of 90 degrees produces severe spinal cord compression.[3] Therefore, for patients with focal neurological deficits and sharp-angle kyphosis, the surgical approach is mandatory to prevent disease progression and a worse outcome in the future.

In patients with surgical indications, the choice of surgical approach is a multifactorial one, mainly considering

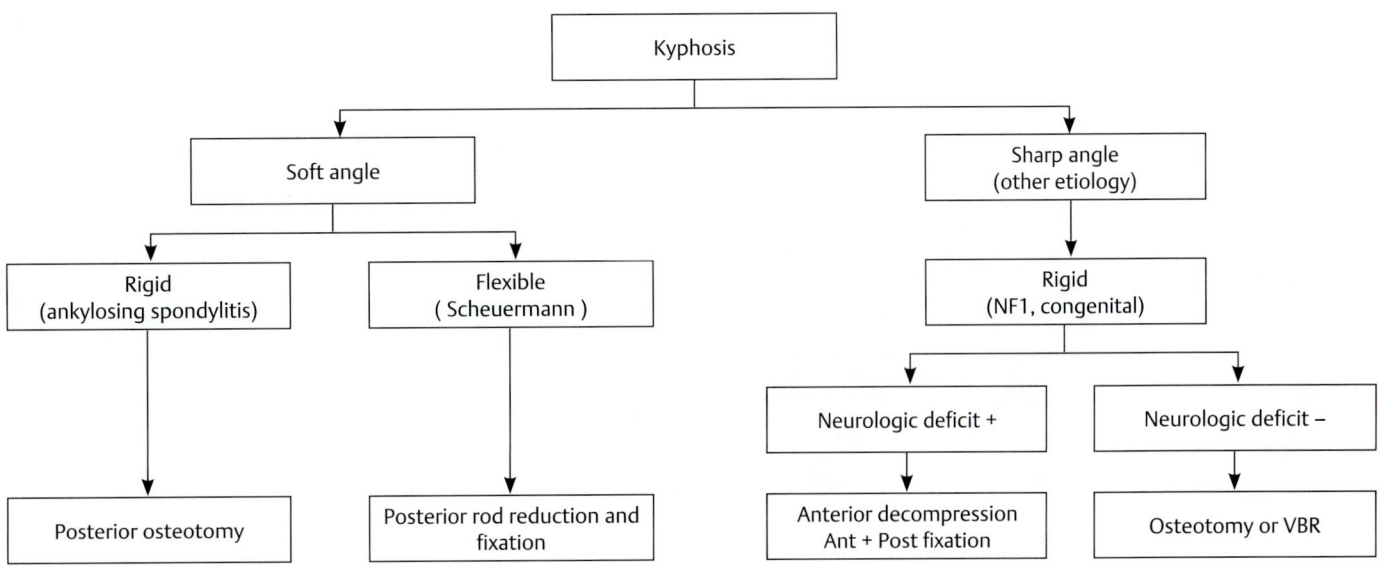

Fig. 23.1 Algorithm which may be used for the treatment of kyphosis.

the presence of neurological deficit, kyphosis angulation, and other pathologies or limitations of the patient. For example, the preferred route is usually the posterior one for patients with open-angle or acute-angle kyphosis and without the presence of neurological deficit. On the other hand, for patients with neurological deficits and acute-angle kyphosis, the preferred approach is the anterior approach.[1]

Congenital kyphosis can be due to a lack of segmentation or an anomalous segmentation (**Fig. 23.2**). Traction applied before surgery may be effective only in flexible kyphosis (**Fig. 23.3**).

Surgery

The surgical treatment methodology is closely related to the biomechanical and morpho-pathological characteristics of the deformity and the presence of compression of nervous structures. Therefore, the flexibility of kyphosis is a significant concern. There are many technical options to solve this problem.[4] For the patient with a neurological deficit and a sharp angle, the direct approach is decompression via an anterior approach and anterior and/or posterior fixation of the spine.[1]

Surgical Technique

The principle of the surgery must be to decompress the apex of the kyphotic deformity. At the same session, deformity correction may also be tried. You may use traction or distraction systems. During this procedure, it is essential to have neurophysiological monitoring. Kyphosis due to trauma, Pott's disease, and some congenital diseases are the most frequent reasons for kyphosis with neurological deficits. Pain may be the only symptom of congenital diseases. Respiratory problems are late complications of severe kyphosis. Traction reduction maneuvers cannot be a choice for an external reduction in cases of congenital kyphosis due to the risk of deficit aggravation (**Fig. 23.3**).

If there is a neurologic deficit, a thoracotomy is performed from the convex side of the deformity. After decompressive osteotomy, anterior strut grafting has also been advocated to reduce the angle and support the anterior column after releasing the compression and discs two levels above and below the deformity. Although the combined anterior–posterior osteotomy may be chosen, the risk of increased instability may worsen the neurological deficit. Bone chips may be put in between the strut grafts (**Fig. 23.4**). An anterior cage can be placed during posterior reduction and fixation if the surgery aims for a radical corpectomy or a vertebral body resection (**Fig. 23.5**).

In the past, surgeons placed rib grafts between the vertebral bodies to provide an in-situ ventral fusion without correcting deformities (**Fig. 23.6**).

As in Scheuermann's disease, flexible kyphosis can be corrected using a rod reduction and fixation technique. First, pedicle screws are placed on the cranial and caudal segments; after tightening both the rods on the upper vertebra, the rods are pushed ventrally and placed on the lower screws, thus achieving some kyphosis correction (**Fig. 23.7**).

There are also different osteotomy techniques used for kyphosis reduction. It may be by multiple posterior osteotomies (**Fig. 23.8**) or one-level pedicle subtraction osteotomy (**Fig. 23.9**). One of the maneuvers used for kyphosis reduction is the deflexion of the operating table (**Fig. 23.10**). In addition, a C7 pedicle subtraction osteotomy can be used to reduce cervicothoracic kyphosis (**Fig. 23.11**).

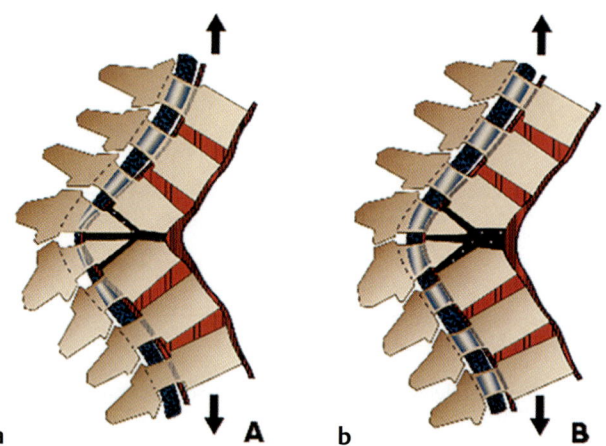

Fig. 23.3 Effects of traction on kyphosis. **(a)** In the case of a rigid kyphosis, the apical area will not change with traction, but the adjacent spine will be lengthened. The spine and, thus, the spinal cord will lengthen with increased tension in the spinal cord and aggravate neurologic loss. **(b)** When the kyphosis is flexible, traction will improve the apical area and reduce the pressure of the bone anteriorly on the spinal cord.

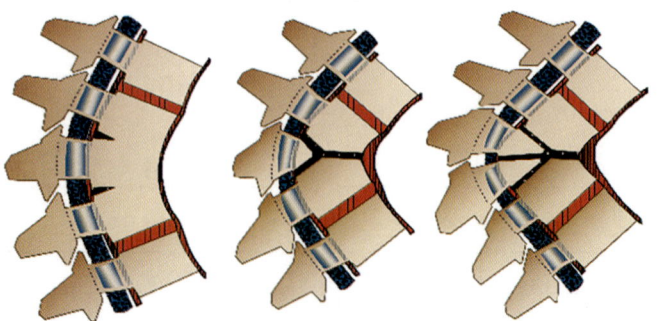

Fig. 23.2 Congenital kyphosis can result from a lack of segmentation or an anomalous segmentation.

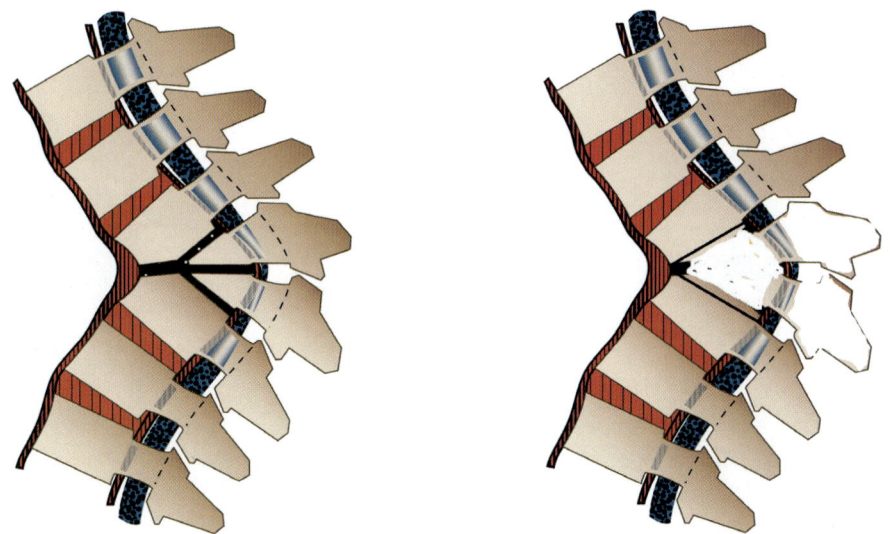

Fig. 23.4 Removing the apex of the kyphosis by corpectomy aims to decompress the spinal cord and provide a flexible deformity to correct easily.

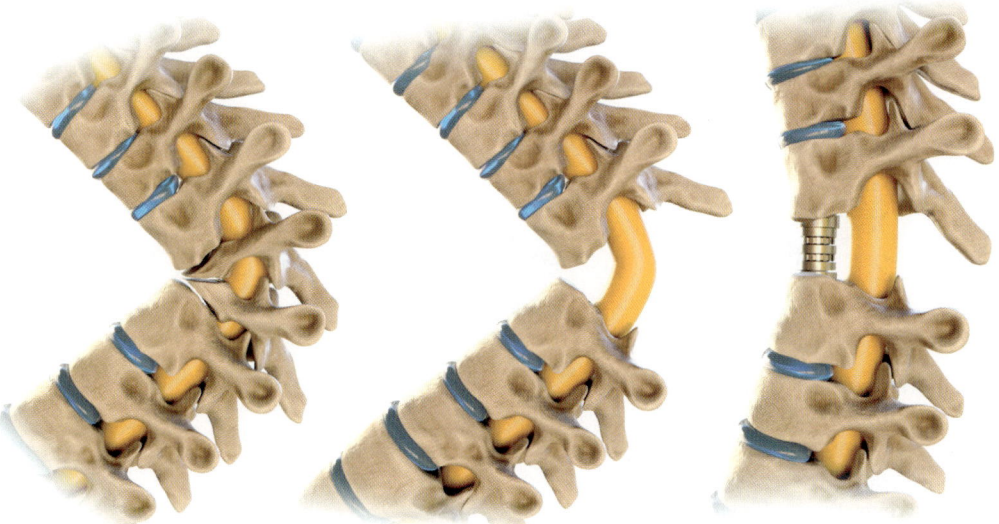

Fig. 23.5 After vertebral body resection, an anterior cage can be placed during posterior reduction and fixation.

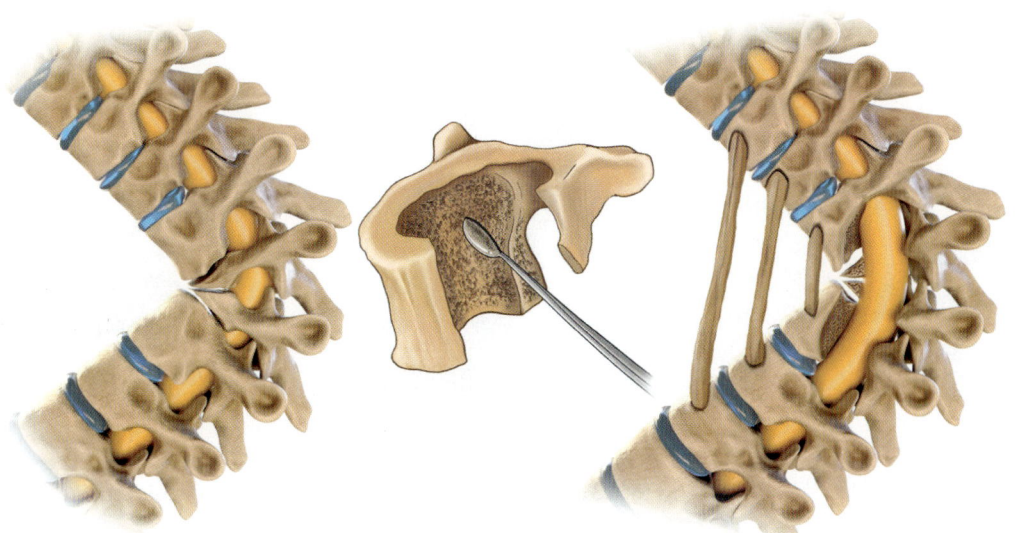

Fig. 23.6 Another option is to provide in-situ fusion without correction after decompression. In the past, surgeons have used rib grafts for ventral fusion.

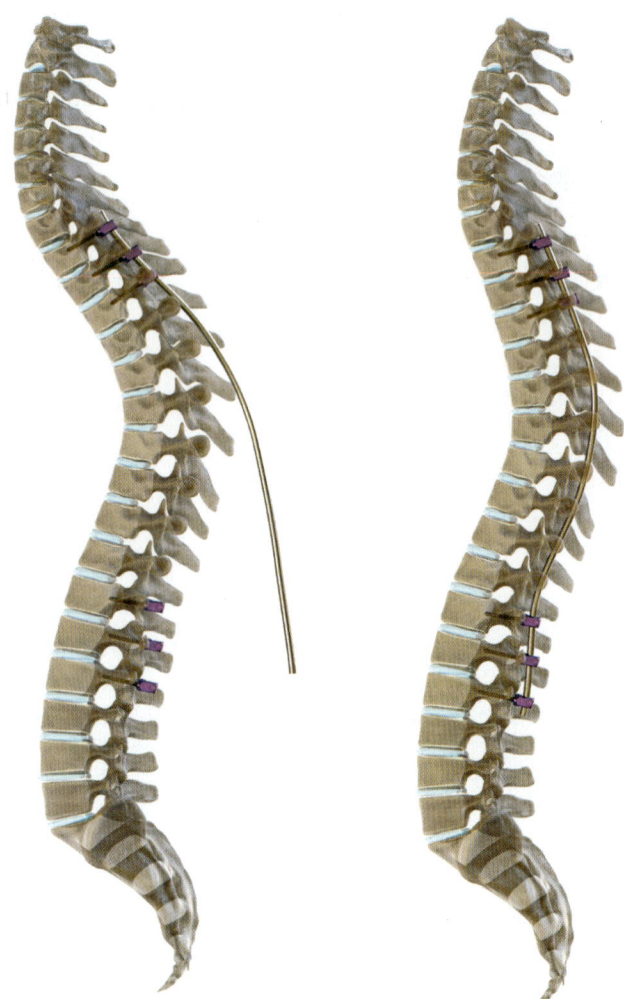

Fig. 23.7 Flexible kyphosis can be corrected using a rod reduction and fixation technique. Screws and/or hooks anchor the cranial and caudal kyphotic segments; after placing and tightening both the rods on the upper vertebra, the rods are pushed ventrally and placed on the lower screws, thus achieving some kyphosis correction.

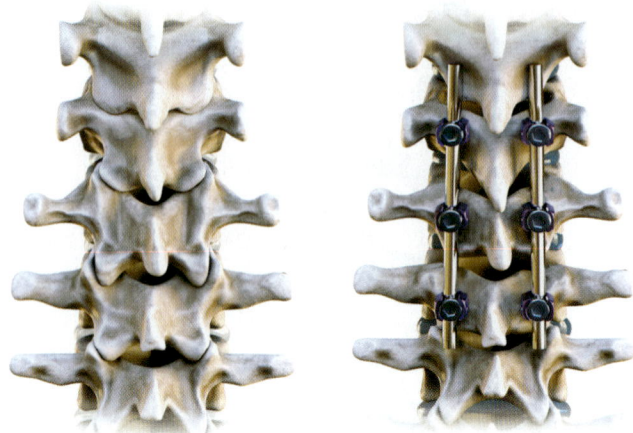

Fig. 23.8 Reduction achieved by multiple posterior osteotomies.

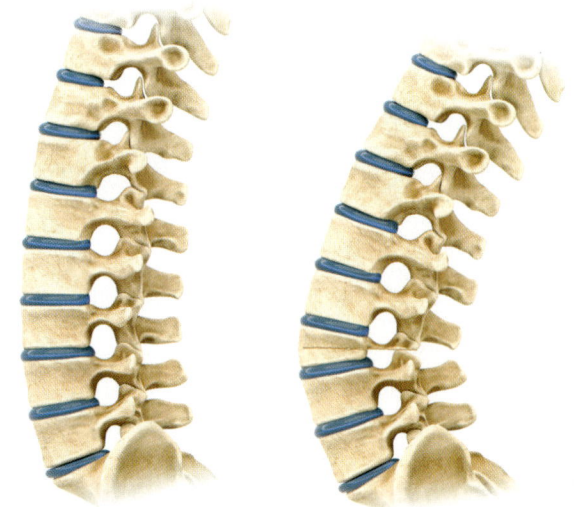

Fig. 23.9 Reduction by one-level pedicle subtraction osteotomy.

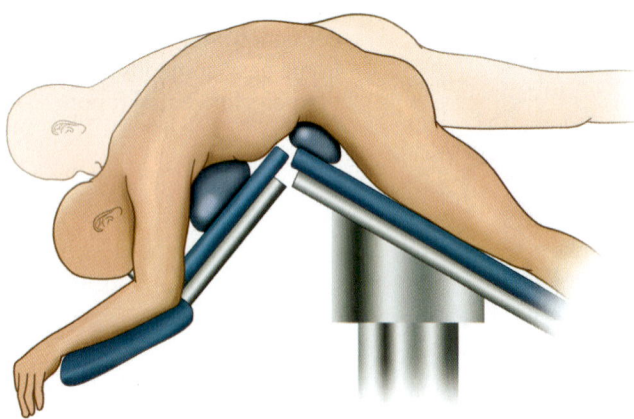

Fig. 23.10 Deflexion of the operating table helps to close the osteotomy site and reduce kyphosis.

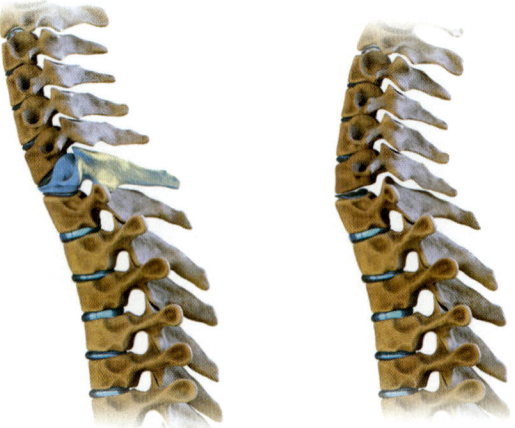

Fig. 23.11 Reduction of cervicothoracic kyphosis by C7 pedicle subtraction osteotomy.

Complications and Outcome

- Neurologic compromise could result from spinal cord compression due to inadequate decompression or subluxation.

- Aorta rupture and death: This complication was reported in earlier series with posterior osteotomies with the section of the anterior longitudinal ligament that loads stretching forces to the aorta.

- Respiratory problems: This is possible especially in patients with preoperative restriction of lung capacity. Preoperative respiratory physiotherapy can be preventive.

- Infection is a common complication in long-lasting and instrumented spine surgeries.

- Loss of correction may happen for many reasons such as inappropriate surgical planning, pseudarthrosis, osteopenia, and smoking.

Personal Series

Between 1980 and 2010, 10 patients with thoracic acute angle kyphosis with neurological deficits were surgically treated. The mean age was 15 (between 9 and 21 years); the male/female ratio was 5/5. The etiology of all kyphosis was congenital (10). None of the patients had a previous laminectomy. The mean kyphosis angle was 77 degrees (50–133 degrees), and the mean associated scoliosis was 42 degrees (9–100 degrees). The level involved was T4 to T8, with a fulcrum in T7. Associated pathologies were syringomyelia, cerebral palsy, and epilepsy. Surgery performed was thoracotomy in nine cases and costotransversectomy in one case. The patients had anterior decompression of the spinal cord and posterior fusion. We had postoperative complications—one case of pneumonia and one case with colon Volvo (torsion). The Frankel scale was used for neurological evaluation. No patient was classified in A; two were classified in B, five in C, and three in D. Postoperative evaluation at 1 month showed significant improvement, with one patient in B, two patients in C, and seven patients in D. After 1 year, one patient remained in B, one in C, one in D, and seven in E. It is an extraordinary recovery outcome.

Case Report

A 10-year-old male child had a walking impairment for the last 4 years. His condition was progressively worsening, and he needed help for walking. He had bilateral clonus and Babinski sign. He had a computed tomography (CT) myelogram followed by anterior decompression and fusion. At the last follow-up he was walking independently and classified in Frankel D (**Fig. 23.12**).

Key Points

- Nonoperative treatment for kyphosis can be tried in some flexible cases.

- Surgery should better be tailored according to flexibility and rigidity of the deformity, smooth or sharp angle kyphosis, presence of neurological deficits, the quality of bone, and the age and morbidities of the patient.

- Smooth angled kyphosis, especially in cases with ankylosing spondylitis, may be managed by posterior osteotomies.

- Anterior decompression and posterior fixation surgery is better in sharp angled kyphosis with neurological deficits, especially in cases with 70 degrees or more kyphosis angle.

- In case a vertebral body resection is done, a ventral support using a cage would provide a better construct.

- In-situ decompression without kyphosis reduction may also be an option for some rigid kyphosis.

Conclusions

Surgical management of kyphosis needs consideration of various aspects of the deformity, such as neurological status, spinal cord compression, angle of the kyphosis, quality of bone, and monitoring of diseases. In case of significant cord compression and neurological compromise, a ventral decompression should be prioritized. Although the physical outcome of surgical treatment is beneficial, risks and complications exist which must be considered.

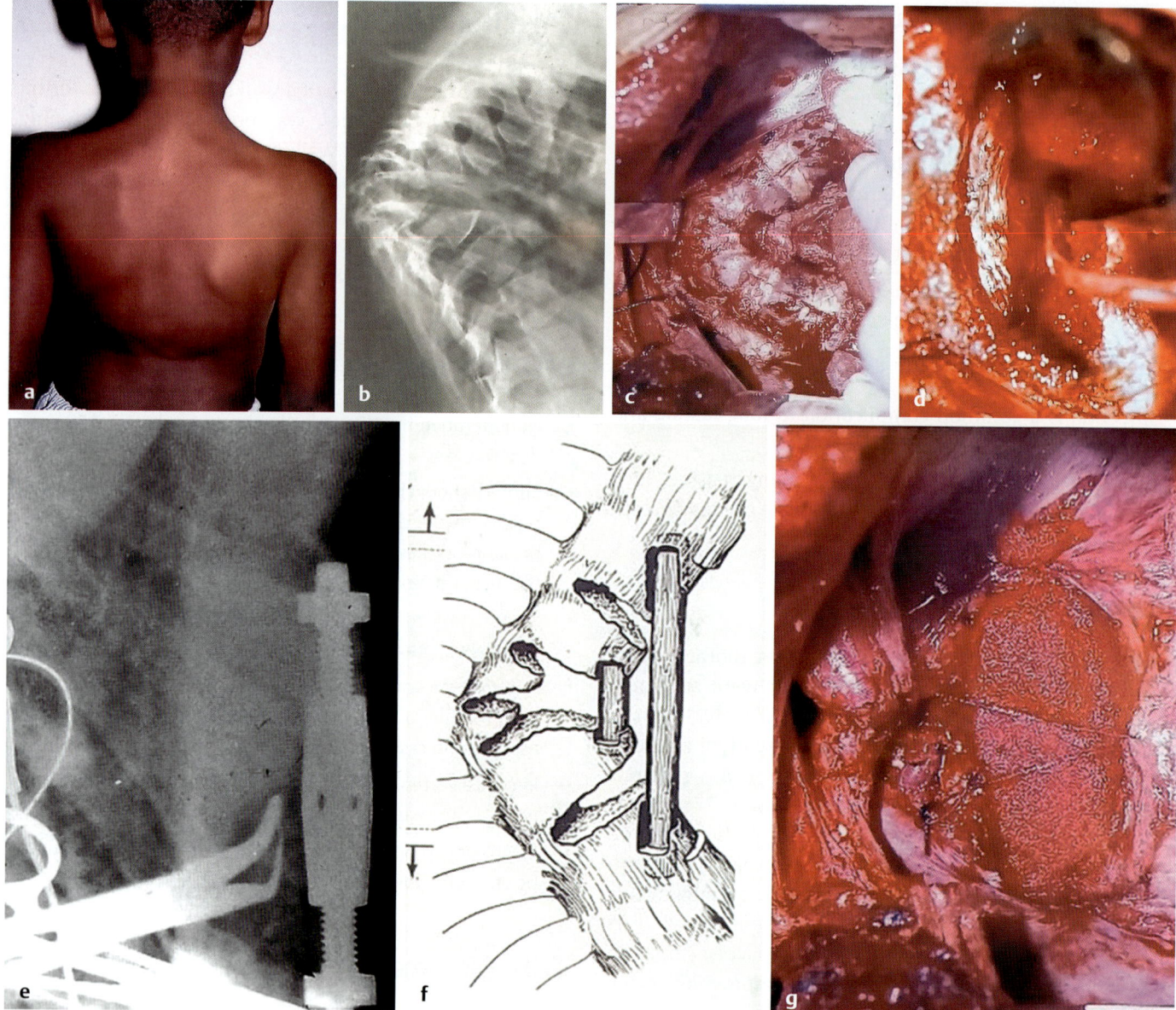

Fig. 23.12 A 10-year-old male with progressive spastic paraparesis for the last 4 years **(a, b)**. An anterior decompression and fusion were performed **(c–g)**.

References

1. Zileli M. Surgery for kyphosis. Adv Tech Stand Neurosurg 2014;41:71–103
2. Yaman O, Dalbayrak S. Kyphosis and review of the literature. Turk Neurosurg 2014;24(4):455–465
3. Masini M, Maranhão V. Experimental determination of the effect of progressive sharp-angle spinal deformity on the spinal cord. Eur Spine J 1997;6(2):89–92
4. Defino HLA, Rodriguez-Fuentes AE, Piola FP. Tratamento cirúrgico da cifose patológica. Acta Ortopédica Brasileira 2002, 10/1:10–16

Part V

Coronal Plane Correction Techniques

Jean Charles Le Huec, Abhishek Mannem, Emanuele Quarto, Wendy Thompson, Lisa Boue, and Stéphane Bourret

Introduction and Terminology

The three-dimensional deformity in the axial, coronal, and sagittal plane is termed as scoliosis.[1] The health-related quality of life is decreased due to the disability and pain associated with scoliosis.[2] Attainment of a balanced spine in both sagittal and coronal planes[3,4] is the primary objective of treating patients with scoliosis surgically (**Fig. 24.1**). Although patient-related outcomes have been greatly affected by sagittal alignment, the satisfaction rates of patients could also be affected negatively by the imbalance in the coronal plane.[5] Guidance regarding coronal techniques and coronal correction is lacking in literature. "Coronal malalignment or alignment" and "coronal imbalance or balance" are the other terms used for referring to coronal deformity. Obeid et al posited that measurements made on static sitting X-rays or standing X-rays are termed as alignment, whereas a patient's function, pain, and position influences the dynamic concept of balance.[6] Coronal balance is improved in patients with adolescent idiopathic scoliosis (AIS) (secondary to an idealistic choice of fusion levels) among whom the phenomenon of correcting the compensatory curve is spontaneous and common.[7] Postural compensation from back pain related to decreased paraspinal muscle density, facet joint degeneration, and spinal stenosis

causes coronal malalignment (CM) in adult spinal deformity (ASD).[8] Depending on the series, the range of estimated preoperative prevalence of CM in ASD is between 15 and 35%. Ploumis et al posited that CM defined as coronal vertical axis (CVA) was more than 4 cm, wherein preoperative CM was at 20.4%.[9] Bao et al reported preoperative CM as 34.8% in their study on 284 patients with ASD.[10] Xu et al identified a preoperative CM of 29.2% in a study of 130 patients with ASD, wherein CVA of more than 3 cm threshold was utilized.[11] A CVA threshold of 3 cm with a preoperative CM rate of 31.3% was reported by Zhang et al. However, it could be challenging to restore postoperative coronal balance in patients with ASD involving long deformity corrections.[12] The capability of attaining postoperative coronal balance is affected by preoperative factors, such as larger coronal curve magnitude, osteoporosis, and high body mass index (BMI). Similar to the preoperative CM rate at 6 weeks, a postoperative CM was reported by Ploumis et al[9] in 11 of their 54 cases (20.4%); however, no preoperative CM was found among 4 patients.[9] Postoperative CM of 30.4% from 34.8% preoperatively was reported by Bao et al.[10] With a mean follow-up of 41.3 months Xu et al found postoperative CM among 20% of patients with ASD.[11] Postoperative coronal balance might be affected by technical tricks, such as ability to level distal lumbar segments relative to the pelvis, offset connectors, and magnitude of correction. The objectives of the current chapter are to understand the definition of coronal imbalance in deformity surgery, analyses of clinical and radiological CM, surgical planning, find the predictors of postoperative CM, and know the salvage options.

Definition and Analysis of Coronal Balance

Coronal imbalance is diagnosed by physical examination and a comprehensive history. Patients usually complain of abnormal posture with a truncal tilt to one side alongside back pain and leg pain. Physical examinations reveal abnormal shoulder levels, hump in the back, loin folds, pelvic obliquity, and limb length discrepancy (**Fig. 24.2**). Spinal EOS standing anteroposterior radiographs are obtained for all these patients. CM can be global, involving patient's

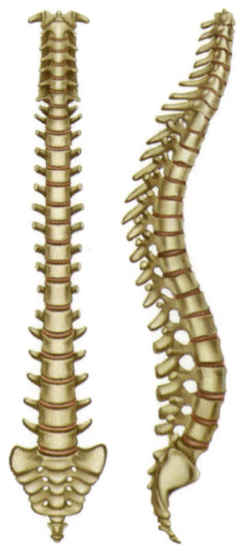

Fig. 24.1 Illustration of optimal coronal and sagittal balance.

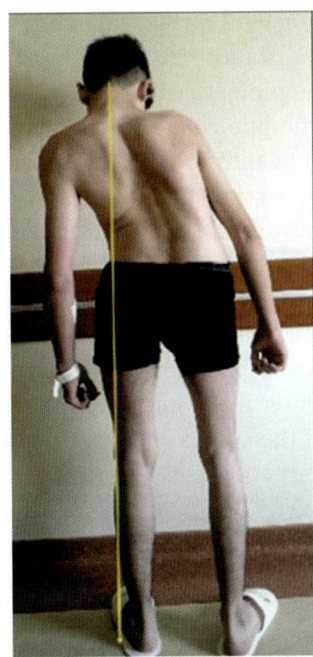

Fig. 24.2 Image of a patient with scoliosis showing severe left shift, shoulder imbalance, and leg discrepancy.

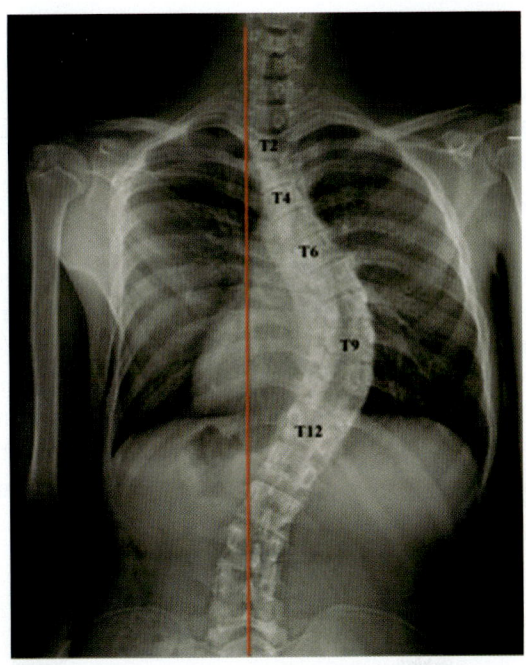

Fig. 24.3 Radiogram of a patient with scoliosis and main thoracic curve.

overall posture determined on EOS long film radiographs, or regional, where curves are restricted to the lumbosacral (LS), thoracolumbar/lumbar (TL/L), thoracic (T), proximal thoracic (PT), or cervicothoracic (CT) areas. Few researchers in the past have delineated CM in terms of present or absent binary variable. Further, a continuous variable is developed to assess the quantum of CM, which is found by measuring the distance between the C7 plumbline (C7PL) or C2 plumbline (C2PL) and the central sacral vertical line (CSVL) (**Fig. 24.3**).[13] The other terminology used in this chapter for these measurements is CVA or coronal balance distance (CBD). The C7PL or C2PL is a vertical line that is dropped downwards from the middle of the C7 or C2 vertebral body. The CSVL is vertically drawn upwards through the sacrum's center (**Fig. 24.4**). Ames et al[14] proposed that a C7PL is positive to the right of CSVL and a C7PL is negative to the left of CSVL (**Fig. 24.5**). This type of measurement helps calculate the postoperative changes. Most research in the past has defined CM by using a threshold value of 3 cm. Bao et al suggested a CBD-based classification system and determined three types of coronal imbalance,[10] namely, Type A (CBD < 3 cm), Type B (CBD > 3 cm) (C7PL shifted to the curve's concave side), and Type C (CBD > 3 cm) (C7PL shifted to the curve's convex side). The SRS-Schwab coronal categorization has classified patients as Type D patients (double major curve with each curve > 30 degrees), Type L patients (TL/L curve [apex ≤ T10] > 30 degrees), Type T patients (thoracic major curve > 30 degrees), or Type N patients (no coronal curve > 30 degrees).[15] Obeid et al suggested three major patterns of

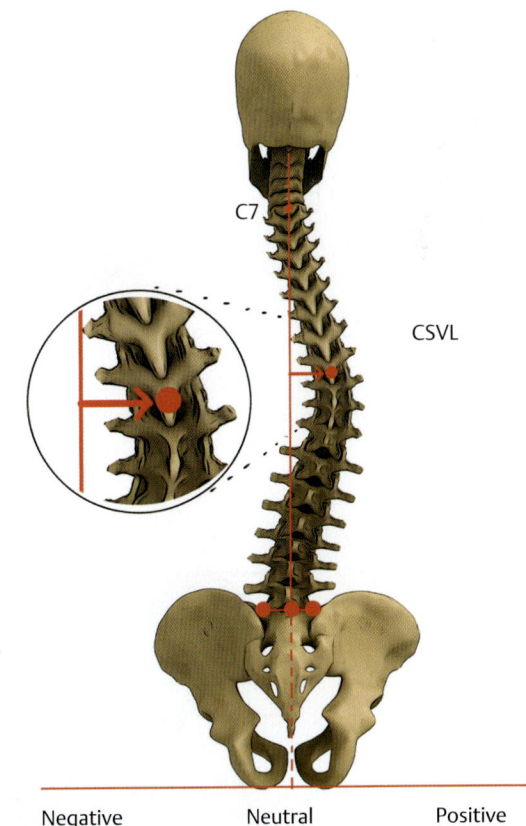

Fig. 24.4 Illustration of the central sacral vertical line (CSVL). A vertical line from C7 to symphysis pubis is drawn. The part of the vertebra shifting away from the CSVL is considered as positive balance. The part shifting toward the CSVL is considered a negative balance.

Negative   Neutral   Positive

CM, namely, Type 0 (CVA ≤ 3 cm), Type 1 (CM with CVA > 3 cm and coronal T1 plumbline falling on the concavity of the main coronal curve), and Type 2 (CM with CVA > 3 cm and coronal T1 plumbline falling at the side on the convexity of the main coronal curve).[6]

The researchers suggested that the reduction in CM was coupled with correction of the main curve in the case of concave CM. Conversely, increase in CM in convex CM is caused by the main curve's correction. Further, they developed treatment-oriented classification by classifying each type into four subtypes. The major drawback of this classification is the lack of reproducibility, and no multicentric validation has been obtained for this treatment-oriented classification. Zhang et al suggested a new angular index called coronal T1 pelvic tilt (CTPT) for overcoming the defects of distance parameters and for analyzing global coronal alignment (GCM).[16] CTPT is defined as the angle between the line connecting the midpoint of the S1 endplate to the T1 centroid and the vertical line (**Fig. 24.6**). CTPT was strongly correlated with GCM, also termed C7 migration, by Zhang et al. This had a similar correlation with the major Cobb angle, fractional curve, L5 coronal tilt, and L4 coronal tilt. CTPT has been proven as a practical index to evaluate GCM and is superior to CVA, as it is not subject to variability of body habitus and calibration is not required. These classifications allow surgeons to identify patterns of natural course of the curves and propose helpful treatment algorithms for correcting CM.

Surgical Planning

Like any ASD surgery, age, medical comorbidities, and patient goals should be given the utmost importance. Magnetic resonance imaging (MRI) of the whole spine is performed in all these patients to look for cord morphology and stenosis. Computed tomography (CT) of the whole spine is performed to assess for levels of corrections for posterior column osteotomies (PCOs) and for anterior fusions and understand the bony morphology of the deformity. Presence of pelvic obliquity, presence of leg length discrepancy, presence of fractional curve, and direction of CM (as curves toward convexity have increased risk for postoperative CM) are the parameters that need to be considered on EOS standing radiographs.[17] The presence of pelvic obliquity and leg length discrepancy may sometimes result in a false interpretation of coronal balance. Supine and bending radiographs are used to assess the CM and coronal curve flexibility.

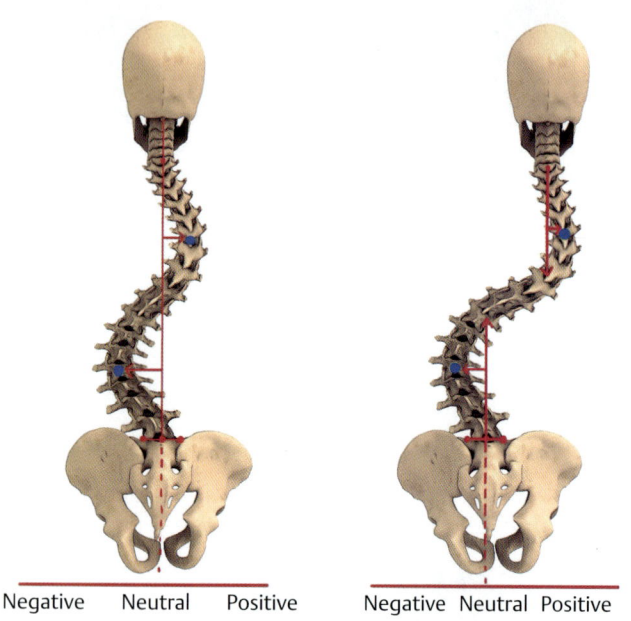

Negative   Neutral   Positive   Negative   Neutral   Positive

Fig. 24.5 Illustration of the central sacral vertical line (CSVL) showing examples of positive and negative coronal balance.

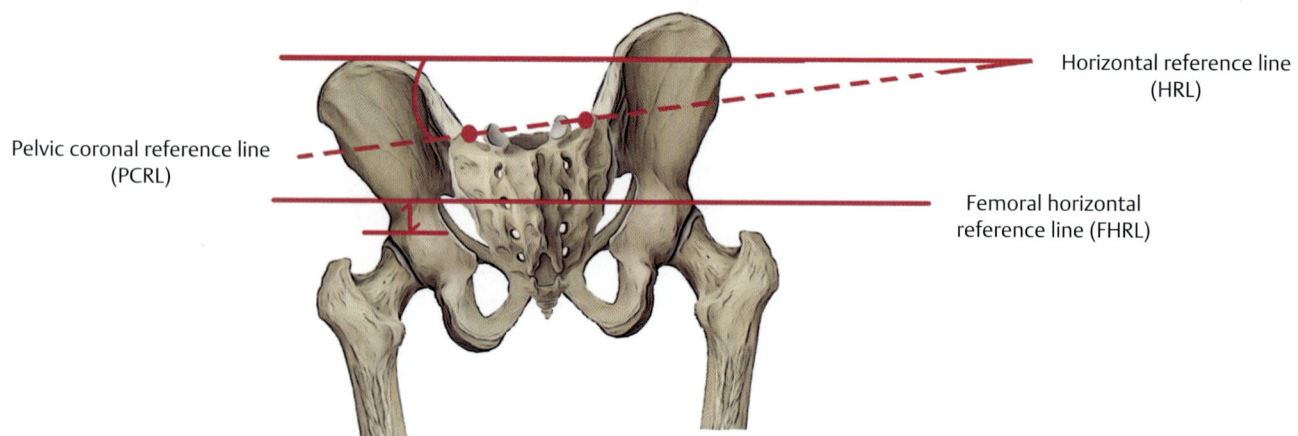

Horizontal reference line (HRL)

Pelvic coronal reference line (PCRL)

Femoral horizontal reference line (FHRL)

Fig. 24.6 Illustration of the pelvis demonstrating pelvic tilt.

Predictors of Postoperative Coronal Malalignment

Several studies have been published in the past outlining the risk factors and predictors for developing postoperative CM. Zhang et al, from their study of 67 patients with ASD, reported that the postoperative coronal plane balance would be affected by the modified Cobb angle from pre-Cobb to post-Cobb and the preoperative coronal plane balance after ASD patients were operated.[12] It was also found that patients with Type C Bao curves had more postoperative CM. Tanaka et al, in their series of 121 patients, reported that CM was significantly correlated with L5 coronal tilt angle postoperatively.[18] This further led to the concept of "oblique take-off" (a straight spine on an oblique foundation—resulting from an L5 coronal tilt angle). Oblique take-off is considered as one of the leading causes of postoperative CM. In their study on coronal imbalance following three-column osteotomy (in thoracolumbar congenital kyphoscoliosis), Xu et al found that immediate postoperative LIV tilt of ≥12.3 degrees and preoperative LIV tilt of ≥23.5 degrees were found to have CM at the latest follow-up.[11] Bao classification suggests the association of higher rates of CM with a preoperative Type C curve, when compared to Types A and B. During the straightening of the major coronal curve, it is likely that the shoulders would be moved away from the CSVL and toward the convexity, especially without the correction of fractional curve, because of the deviation of the preoperative curve toward the convexity. CM could be perpetuated by the postoperative and persistent L4 and L5 tilt, which is enabled due to the easy correctability and flexibility of the main TL/L curves when compared to fractional lumbosacral curves. A positive correlation is found between the magnitude of coronal CM and factors, namely, L4 and L5 tilt angles, and pelvic obliquity, postoperatively. Jimbo et al reported that pre-existing degenerative lumbar scoliosis progressed due to the predictor of L4 tilt.[19] Schwab et al demonstrated a significant correlation between pain in patients with adult scoliosis and L3 and L4 obliquities.[20] Lewis et al, from their series of 47 patients, proposed that after ASD surgery with fusions extending to the pelvis, better self-reported image scores and better coronal balance were caused by the horizontal leveling of L4 and L5.[8] They also observed a positive correlation between coronal imbalance magnitude and residual L4 and L5 tilt magnitudes. Ploumis et al reported that changes in coronal balance were predicted by two significant factors, namely, combination of anterior approach surgery (with a history of previous surgery) and presence of osteoporosis.[9] A few underpowered studies reported that leg length discrepancy and pelvic obliquity are additional risk components for the growth of CM.

Impact on Outcomes

Rod fractures have been found to be the most common mechanical complications associated with CM. In a series of 121 patients with more than 2-year follow-up, 25 CM patients were found to have rod fractures and 96 patients were found with coronal alignment. Tanaka et al reported that the incidence of rod fractures was 17% in the non-CM group and 36% in the CM group.[18] Scheer et al conducted a predictive modeling study of 336 ASD patients and found that pseudoarthrosis was predicted by the third most important variable of maximum coronal Cobb angle; nevertheless, pseudoarthrosis was not significantly predicted by the global coronal balance.[21] It was evidenced through the 2012 SRS Schwab classification study that outcomes, excluding coronal balance parameters in the suggested alignment goals, were not significantly influenced by CM.[15] Likewise, four radiographic measurements and age (none included coronal alignment measures—relative spinopelvic alignment, lordosis distribution, relative lumbar lordosis, relative pelvic version) were used as the base by the Global Alignment and Proportion Score for describing three spinopelvic states, namely, severely disproportioned, moderately disproportioned, and proportioned.[22] Furthermore, reoperation rates and mechanical complications were not predicted by coronal alignment, as found in other studies. Glassman et al reported that patient-reported outcomes (PROs) improved significantly in ASD patients with CVA being more than 4 cm preoperatively.[23] In Bao's study,[10] patients with Type C curves have lower satisfaction rates postoperatively compared to Types A and B. Plais et al, from their study on 576 ASD patients, identified that patients with Type B curves have substantially worse SRS-22, SF-36, and Oswestry Disability Index (ODI) at baseline.[24] In a multicenter analysis of 483 patients, Acaroglu et al showed an independent association between worse postoperative SRS-22 scores and poor coronal alignment.[25] Bao et al reported that their 21 patients with postoperative CM had lower visual analog scale (VAS) and mean SF-36 scores when compared to postoperatively aligned patients.[26]

Tips and Trick

Correction of the fractional curve in the lumbar/lumbosacral region is the critical step in achieving a stable base. The goal is to achieve horizontal L4 and L5 endplates. This could be achieved by performing symmetric or asymmetric distal transforaminal lumbar interbody fusions (TLIFs). In addition to anterior column support, the lumbosacral fractional curve's coronal correction is provided by the fusion. Asymmetric TLIF could be used to level out a segment with coronal angulation. The coronal curves could be straightened by an interbody device on the concave side. Either oblique lumbar interbody fusion (OLIF) or lateral lumbar interbody fusion (LLIF) is preferred by some researchers. In patients with a concomitant sagittal imbalance to be addressed, the authors prefer to perform asymmetrical pedicle subtraction osteotomy (PSO). This can help correct the CVA by 5 to 7 cm from one level asymmetrical PSO. Usually, a four to six rods construct is preferred to stabilize the PSO level. A VCR could be performed on the coronal curve apex in the thoracolumbar or thoracic spine in cases where more bone removal is required for countering coronal imbalance with superimposed kyphosis. Rods are cantilevered cranially and locked caudally if the pelvis is involved in the fusion. Rods are cantilevered caudally and locked cranially if the pelvis is not involved in the fusion. The sagittal correction has to be performed first with cantilever forces. The rods must be placed on fractional curve convexity first, and compression forces address the coronal curve for creating coronal alignment and horizontalization of L4 and L5 levels. Following this, the rod is inserted on the concave side and distraction is performed further for optimizing the lumbar lordosis and for straightening the L3, L4, and L5 endplates. Contralateral concave distraction maneuverers are followed after the treatment of the main curve with compression forces and convex cantilever. The kickstand rod technique is an excellent alternative if significant pelvic obliquity or CM is observed after both the rods are inserted and tightened.

References

1. Aebi M. The adult scoliosis. Eur Spine J 2005;14(10):925–948
2. Diebo BG, Shah NV, Boachie-Adjei O, et al. Adult spinal deformity. Lancet 2019;394(10193):160–172
3. Yagi M, Rahm M, Gaines R, et al; Complex Spine Study Group. Characterization and surgical outcomes of proximal junctional failure in surgically treated patients with adult spinal deformity. Spine 2014;39(10):E607–E614
4. Schwab F, Patel A, Ungar B, Farcy J-P, Lafage V. Adult spinal deformity-postoperative standing imbalance: how much can you tolerate? An overview of key parameters in assessing alignment and planning corrective surgery. Spine 2010;35(25):2224–2231
5. Schwab FJ, Blondel B, Bess S, et al; International Spine Study Group (ISSG). Radiographical spinopelvic parameters and disability in the setting of adult spinal deformity: a prospective multicenter analysis. Spine 2013;38(13):E803–E812
6. Obeid I, Berjano P, Lamartina C, Chopin D, Boissière L, Bourghli A. Classification of coronal imbalance in adult scoliosis and spine deformity: a treatment-oriented guideline. Eur Spine J 2019;28(1):94–113
7. Ma Q, Wang L, Zhao L, et al. Coronal balance vs. sagittal profile in adolescent idiopathic scoliosis, are they correlated? Front Pediatr 2020;7:523
8. Lewis SJ, Keshen SG, Kato S, Dear TE, Gazendam AM. Risk factors for postoperative coronal balance in adult spinal deformity surgery. Global Spine J 2018;8(7):690–697
9. Ploumis A, Simpson AK, Cha TD, Herzog JP, Wood KB. Coronal spinal balance in adult spine deformity patients with long spinal fusions: a minimum 2- to 5-year follow-up study. J Spinal Disord Tech 2015;28(9):341–347
10. Bao H, Yan P, Qiu Y, Liu Z, Zhu F. Coronal imbalance in degenerative lumbar scoliosis: prevalence and influence on surgical decision-making for spinal osteotomy. Bone Joint J 2016;98-B(9):1227–1233
11. Xu L, Chen X, Qiao J, et al. Coronal imbalance after three-column osteotomy in thoracolumbar congenital kyphoscoliosis: incidence and risk factors. Spine 2019;44(2):E99–E106
12. Zhang Z, Song K, Wu B, Chi P, Wang Z, Wang Z. Coronal imbalance in adult spinal deformity following posterior spinal fusion with instrument: a related parameters analysis. Spine 2019;44(8):550–557
13. Mac-Thiong J-M, Transfeldt EE, Mehbod AA, et al. Can C7 plumbline and gravity line predict health related quality of life in adult scoliosis? Spine 2009;34(15):E519–E527
14. Ames CP, Smith JS, Scheer JK, et al. Impact of spinopelvic alignment on decision making in deformity surgery in adults: a review. J Neurosurg Spine 2012;16(6):547–564
15. Schwab F, Ungar B, Blondel B, et al. Scoliosis Research Society-Schwab adult spinal deformity classification: a validation study. Spine 2012;37(12):1077–1082
16. Zhang J, Wang Z, Chi P, Chi C. Coronal T1 pelvic tilt, a novel predictive index for global coronal alignment in adult spinal deformity. Spine 2020;45(19):1335–1340
17. Garg B, Mehta N, Bansal T, Malhotra R. EOS® imaging: concept and current applications in spinal disorders. J Clin Orthop Trauma 2020;8
18. Tanaka N, Ebata S, Oda K, Oba H, Haro H, Ohba T. Predictors and clinical importance of postoperative coronal malalignment after surgery to correct adult spinal deformity. Clin Spine Surg 2020;33(7):E337–E341
19. Jimbo S, Kobayashi T, Aono K, Atsuta Y, Matsuno T. Epidemiology of degenerative lumbar scoliosis: a community-based cohort study. Spine 2012;37(20):1763–1770
20. Schwab FJ, Smith VA, Biserni M, Gamez L, Farcy J-PC, Pagala M. Adult scoliosis: a quantitative radiographic and clinical analysis. Spine 2002;27(4):387–392
21. Scheer JK, Oh T, Smith JS, et al; International Spine Study Group. Development of a validated computer-based preoperative predictive model for pseudarthrosis with 91% accuracy in 336 adult spinal deformity patients. Neurosurg Focus 2018;45(5):E11
22. Yilgor C, Sogunmez N, Boissiere L, et al; European Spine Study Group (ESSG). Global alignment and proportion (GAP) score: development and validation of a new method of analyzing spinopelvic alignment to predict mechanical complications after adult spinal deformity surgery. J Bone Joint Surg Am 2017;99(19):1661–1672
23. Glassman SD, Berven S, Bridwell K, Horton W, Dimar JR. Correlation of radiographic parameters and clinical symptoms in adult scoliosis. Spine 2005;30(6):682–688
24. Plais N, Bao H, Lafage R, et al; International Spine Study Group. The clinical impact of global coronal malalignment is underestimated in adult patients with thoracolumbar scoliosis. Spine Deform 2020;8(1):105–113
25. Acaroglu E, Guler UO, Olgun ZD, et al; European Spine Study Group. Multiple regression analysis of factors affecting health-related quality of life in adult spinal deformity. Spine Deform 2015;3(4):360–366
26. Bao H, Liu Z, Zhang Y, et al. Sequential correction technique to avoid postoperative global coronal decompensation in rigid adult spinal deformity: a technical note and preliminary results. Eur Spine J 2019;28(9):2179–2186

25 Correction of Shoulder Balance for Adolescent Idiopathic Scoliosis

Emre Acaroğlu and Engin Çetin

Introduction

Shoulder balance is one of the biggest concerns of adolescent idiopathic scoliosis (AIS) patients. It is an important parameter that patients consider when evaluating their appearance and the cosmetic results of the surgery. It is remarkable in terms of patient and parent perception and satisfaction.[1,2] However, postoperative shoulder imbalance (PSI) is common, and its incidence has been reported to be as high as 25%.[3]

Numerous measurement methods have been described for the radiological evaluation of shoulder imbalance. The main ones are clavicle angle (CA), radiographic shoulder height (RSH), and T1 tilt angle (T1A). CA is the angle that is subtended between a line connecting the highest point of each clavicle and a horizontal reference line (**Fig. 25.1**). RSH is the linear distance in millimeters between the acromioclavicular joint and the soft tissue shadow directly above it. They are measured for both cephalad and caudal shoulders (**Fig. 25.2**). Finally, T1A is the angle that is subtended between a line drawn along the cephalad end plate of T1 or along the zenith of both first ribs (if the T1 end plate is not well visualized) and a horizontal reference line (**Fig. 25.3**). CA, T1A, and RSH differences measured with the left shoulder up are positive, while the values measured with the right shoulder up are negative.[4,5]

Kuklo et al described a clinical grading system for shoulder imbalance based on RSH. When the side-to-side shoulder height difference was <1 cm, it was defined as balanced, 1 to 2 cm was defined as minimal imbalance, 2 to 3 cm was defined as moderate imbalance, and >3 cm was defined as significant imbalance.[6] In the subsequent years, Ono et al reclassified shoulder imbalance into medial and lateral shoulder imbalance. They suggested that medial imbalance is reflected in trapezial prominence related to spinal deformity created by upward tilted proximal ribs and T1 tilt. In contrast, the lateral imbalance is reflected by CA and correlates weakly with radiographic measures. Correction of trapezial prominence may be more predictable than clavicle angulation after scoliosis surgery.[7] Kwan et al emphasized the importance of neck tilt and introduced a neck tilt grading system based on correctable neck tilt and trapezius height differences. They suggested that neck tilt has a poor correlation with shoulder imbalance. Neck tilt is correlated with cervical axis and T1 tilt, whereas shoulder imbalance is correlated better with CA, RSH, coracoid height difference, and clavicle rib intersection distance.[8] In the following years, neck tilt was investigated with shoulder imbalance in several studies. Lee et al reported that AIS patients with significant neck tilt and lateral shoulder imbalance were unhappy with their appearances. Neck tilt was associated more with larger T1A and cervical axis angles, whereas lateral shoulder imbalance was associated more with CA and RSH.[9]

It is not clear which components of the deformity are more critical when leveling the shoulders. Proximal spinal alignment and its relationship with shoulder balance and the effect of spinal deformity correction on shoulder alignment are among the most emphasized issues.[10] In the surgical treatment of AIS, selecting the upper instrumented vertebra (UIV) is an important strategy to obtain shoulder balance. Rose and Lenke recommended instrumentation to T2 for left shoulder elevation, T3 or T4 for level shoulders, and T4 or T5

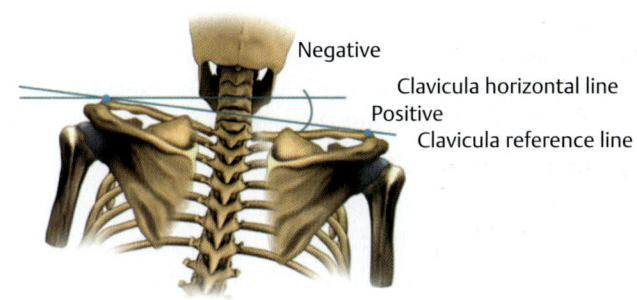

Fig. 25.1 Illustration of a positive clavicular angle.

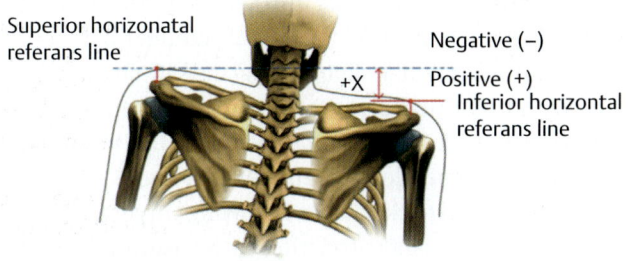

Fig. 25.2 Illustration of a positive radiographic shoulder height (RSH) difference.

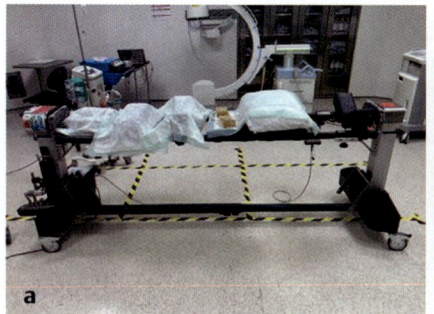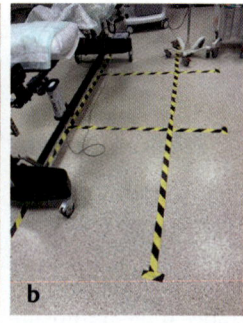

Fig. 25.3 Picture of the markings on the operating room (OR) floor as seen from the lateral side **(a)** and foot side **(b)** of the Jackson table.

concluded that lower postoperative main thoracic curve, a greater percentage of correction of the main thoracic curve, and higher postoperative sacral slope were independent risk factors of PSI in AIS patients. Shoulder balance and symmetry were not affected by the level of UIV selected.[19] Finally Yuan et al suggested that harmonizing the correction ratio of the proximal thoracic curve, main thoracic curve and lumbar curve should be recommended for intraoperative correction and postoperative compensation of PSI.[20]

Definition of the Technique

The authors' approach to correction and/or preservation of the shoulder balance in surgically treated AIS consists of recognizing the causes of shoulder imbalance following surgery, and active evaluation and application to achieve balanced shoulders.

First, as also suggested by the brief literature review above, the authors do not think that shoulder balance has a single cause located at the upper thoracic (UT) curve level. Therefore, whether the UT needs to be instrumented to achieve balance is irrelevant. Instead, the authors tend to think that the overall coronal balance and the shoulder balance are affected by the rigidity of the curves (be they instrumented or not) and whether a harmonious correction has been achieved by surgery. This means that, especially for selective fusions (thoracic or lumbar), the effort is usually to correct the instrumented curve, as much as possible, that causes the shoulder (and coronal) imbalance in most cases.

This said, the authors' technique depends on active evaluation of the coronal balance as well as the shoulders (as decided upon by T1 tilt and/or the levels of the first ribs) and on consequent increases or decreases in the correction rates of the instrumented curves. For this technique, it is essential to use an operating table under which the C-arm of the fluoroscopy machine may be placed and allows sliding of the C-arm throughout the entire trunk, from sacrum to T1. To this end, the authors marked the floor of their operating room (OR) so that the Jackson table and the C-arm fluoroscopy can be placed in a standard way so that they are parallel to each other (**Fig. 25.3**). They used regular operating tables on which the patient is placed at the upper or lower half of the radiolucent part of the table in the past, but the best results can only be achieved by using the totally radiolucent Jackson type of tables.

During surgery, once the placement of the screws and the initial correction of the curve(s) are achieved, the C-arm is introduced underneath the patient at a level appropriate to visualize the sacrum and the iliac crests (**Fig. 25.4**). At this

for right shoulder elevation for Lenke type 1 (main thoracic) deformities. The recommendations for Lenke type 2 (double thoracic) or type 4 (triple major) deformities were that the UIV should be T2 for left shoulder elevation, T2 or T3 for level shoulders, and T3 for right shoulder elevation.[11] Ilharreborde et al concluded that instrumentation of the entire proximal thoracic curve is unnecessary in every case of double thoracic curvature. They selected the UIV based on preoperative analysis of the rigidity of the proximal curvature, T1 tilt, and shoulder balance and on the anticipated effect of correcting the main curve on both T1 and the shoulders.[12] Trobisch and colleagues suggested instrumentation to T2 for left shoulder elevation, T3 for level shoulders, T4 for right shoulder elevation in Lenke type 1 deformities, and T2 for Lenke type 2 and 4 deformities.[13] Suk et al recommended that the proximal curve be included in the fusion when it is over 30 degrees, shoulders are leveled, or the left shoulder is elevated.[14]

On the other hand, Bjerke et al evaluated the current recommendations for UIV selection. They reported that they could not identify a set of UIV selection criteria that accurately predicted postsurgical shoulder balance.[15] Terheyden et al suggested that high preoperative left shoulder level, extensive correction of the distal thoracic curve, a structural proximal thoracic curve, and low preoperative Cobb angle in the lumbar curve are risk factors for left-sided shoulder elevation after surgery.[16] These factors outweighed the selection of UIV as significant predictors of PSI. Yang and colleagues also concluded that for Lenke type 2 patients, fusion to T2 is not a solution for lateral shoulder balance. It can only improve medial shoulder balance. A positive T1A is an indication for fusion to T2.[17] Chan et al proposed that selection of UIV is not an essential factor. Still, UIV tilt angle is an essential independent parameter that could affect the medial shoulder and neck balance following surgery, and UIV tilt angle has a significant correlation with postoperative T1A and cervical axis measurement.[18] Moorthy and colleagues

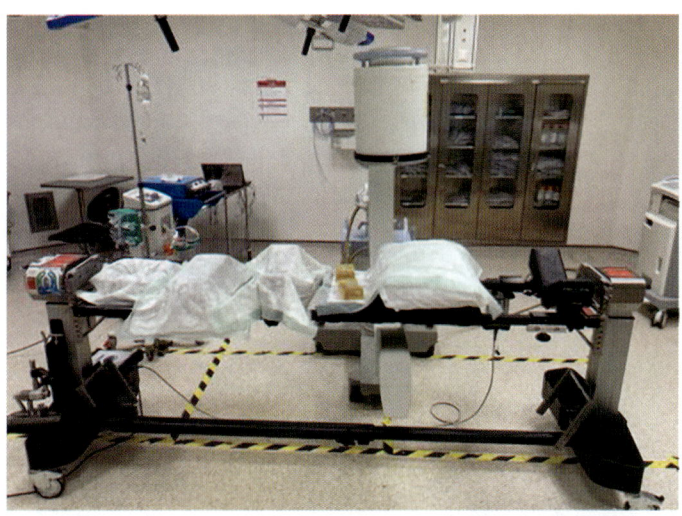

Fig. 25.4 Placement of the C-arm underneath the table to visualize the sacrum and iliac crests.

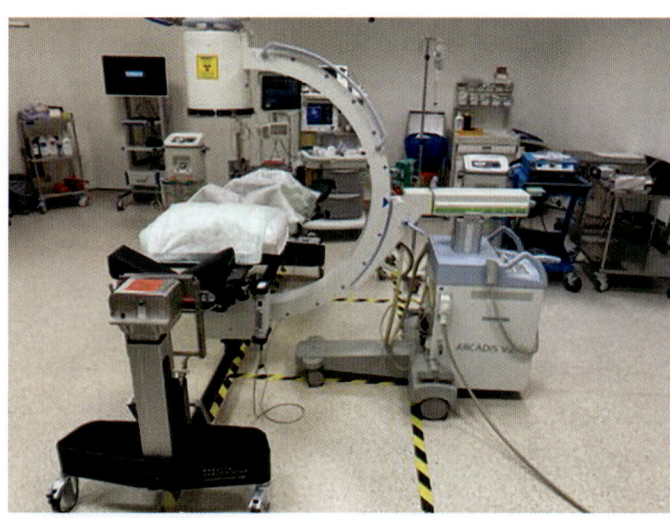

Fig. 25.5 Parallel placement of the table (and the patient) and the C-arm machine is ensured by the floor markings.

point, it is essential to have the C-arm strictly perpendicular to the table, and the floor markings can achieve this in the OR (**Fig. 25.5**). After placement, a single fluoroscopy shot of the sacrum is obtained and rotated 90 degrees (clockwise or counterclockwise depending on the side at which the C-arm is introduced) so that the sacrum and/or the iliac crests are seen in a coronal view, and the upper end plate of the sacrum (or in case there is a structural abnormality in the sacrum, the iliac crests or even the acetabulums) is perfectly horizontal (**Fig. 25.6**). The central sacral vertical line (CSVL) would be located at the midline of the screen. A second sacral fluoroscopy shot is taken at this point to ensure that this view is saved by the fluoroscopy machine (in the digital radiography mode). The C-arm is then slid cranially, parallel to the table, remaining strictly perpendicular to it at the level of T1 (**Fig. 25.7**), and a third fluoroscopy shot is taken (**Fig. 25.8**). On this view, the surgeon can evaluate the coronal location of T1 in relation to the CSVL (now that it has to be located at exactly the middle of the screen) as well as the T1 tilt or the levels of the first ribs. Ideally, T1 should be located on the midline of the screen, and it, as well as the first ribs, should appear horizontal. If this goal has been achieved, no further corrections or manipulations of the curves are attempted, and the curves are fused at this position. If, on the other hand, there are problems with either the location or angulation of T1 (ribs), the instrumentation is revisited, and correction of the relevant curves is increased or decreased through compressive and/or distractive forces until an ideal or, in case it is not possible, an acceptable positioning is obtained (please see the Tips and Tricks section below for more details) (**Fig. 25.9**).

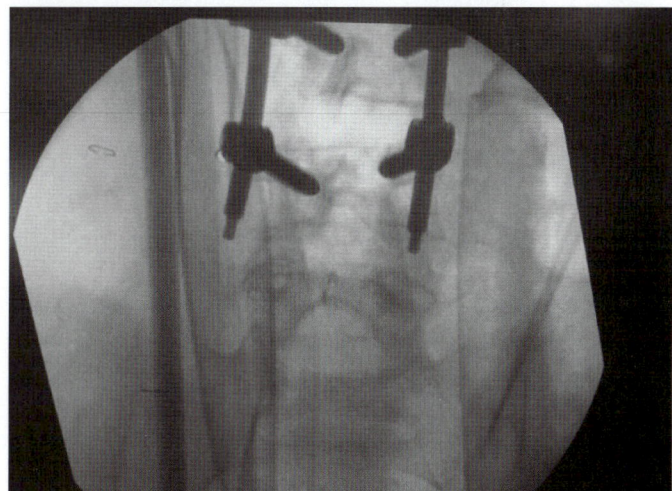

Fig. 25.6 The first C-arm shot taken at the level of the sacrum and posterior superior iliac spines. Please note that the image is rotated clockwise by 90 degrees, and the midpoint of the S1 upper end plate corresponds to the midline of the fluoroscopy screen.

Indications

This technique is indicated and used by the authors in all deformity cases where the coronal balance of the trunk or the shoulders will be intentionally or unintentionally changed. At this point, it may be beneficial to emphasize that this technique predominantly applies to definitive surgeries (i.e., with fusion) of coronal plane deformity, after which the coronal shape and/or the balance of the spinal

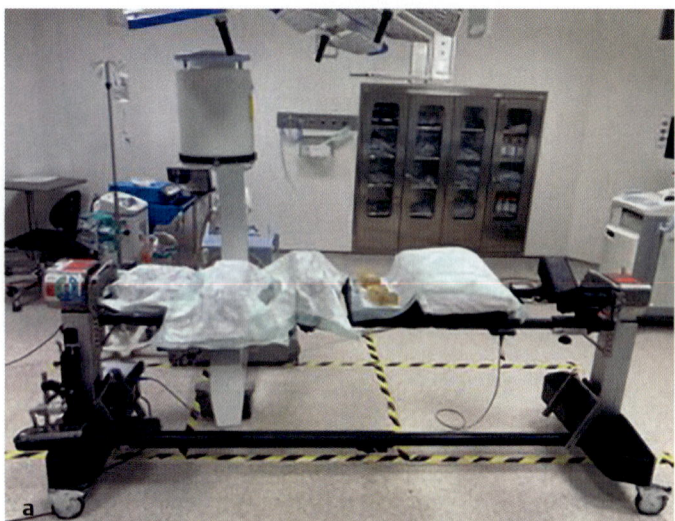
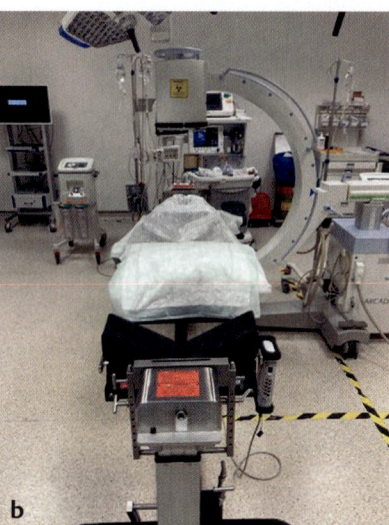

Fig. 25.7 Position of the side after being slided to the level of T1, seen from the lateral side **(a)** and the foot side **(b)**.

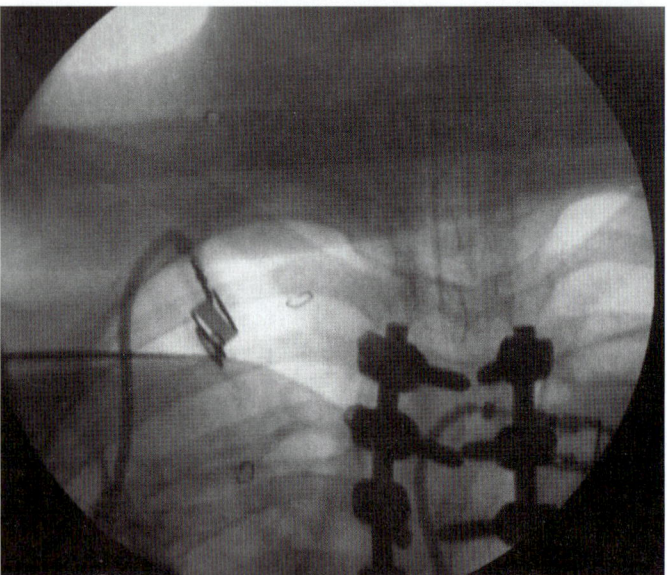

Fig. 25.8 The C-arm shot taken with the C-arm positioned as in **Fig. 25.7**. Note that although T1 appears completely horizontal, its midpoint is shifted to the right by 3 to 4 cm.

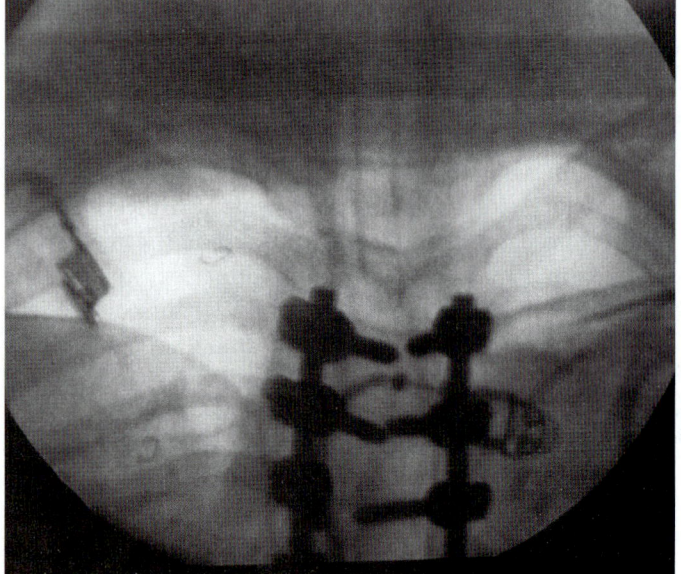

Fig. 25.9 The last C-arm shot taken with the C-arm positioned as in **Fig. 25.7**, following adjustments to correct the coronal shift of T1. For this patient, these adjustments consisted of distraction at the lower end of the instrumentation at the right side (to push T1 to the left) and distraction at the upper end of the instrumentation on the left side (to elevate the left side of T1, thereby preventing tilt). However, please note that this final position compromises T1 shift and tilt, the best correction of T1 shift, while ensuring that it stayed horizontal which was accepted as the optimum solution.

column is not expected to change, regardless of the etiology, be it idiopathic, congenital, neuromuscular, or any other. Therefore, it is not indicated in nonfusion surgeries which may be performed for early-onset pediatric deformity, from unilateral growth arrests to lengthening devices to the so-called vertebral body tethering.

Complication Avoidance

Complications are rare but they do exist. The main complication is failure to achieve acceptable balance and may be related to several factors:

- In cases where the placement and motion of the C-arm under the table is not ideal, achieving good balance becomes arbitrary or impossible. The most common cause of this problem is the initial incorrect positioning of the C-arm underneath the table (not perpendicular to the table) and/or inability to slide the C-arm perfectly parallel to the table. These may be related to human errors and shortcomings related to the OR, table, or C-arm machine.

- In cases with a deformity of the reference point (i.e., sacrum, iliac crests, or acetabulums) or a significant discrepancy of the lengths of the lower limbs that is not recognized preoperatively or during surgery, achievement of ideal standing (or, in cases of neuromuscular deformity, sitting) becomes impossible. One must realize that this technique aligns the spine and the shoulders on an "a priori" reference frame, and if this reference frame is wrong, the outcome will also be wrong.

- Although the radiographs taken on the surgical table have been shown to resemble the result accurately,[21] and the authors' experience suggests that this accuracy is applicable to the C-arm views described; there may be exceptions to this rule. One exception that the authors have identified is the rare patient in whom balance (or overall postural) control is compromised due to disorders of the central nervous system, like autistic children, Friedreich ataxia, and early forms of Parkinson's disease. In these patients, especially if the fusion will remain selective or semi-selective, any balance adjustments performed on the operating table may not necessarily be reflected in the clinical result.

Second, it may be argued that the use of C-arm fluoroscopy as such may increase the rate of infection and/or introduce unnecessary radiation exposure to the patient or the OR personnel.

Tips and Tricks

First, to achieve coronal trunk and shoulder balance, we need to recognize that the extent of fusion has to be commensurate with the expected or desired correction rate(s) of the curve(s) we intend to perform in the surgery. This is because most imbalance problems arise because of the overcorrection of one or two curves that cannot be accommodated or compensated for by the neighboring fractional/uninstrumented curves. In this regard, as an example, if the maximum achievable correction of a given main thoracic curve is aimed, it would be advisable to extend the fusion into the UT and, even at times, the lumbar curves so that these curves may be manipulated at the time of final surgical correction. This principle not only applies mainly to the UT curves, which almost always tend to be reasonably rigid due to their connections to the ribcage and sternum, but also may occasionally apply to some rigid lumbar curves. For this reason, the authors frequently instrument the UT curve up to a level past its apex (usually up to T3) in most cases of thoracic deformity correction. Alternatively, suppose the surgeon is reluctant to extend the instrumentation to the neighboring curves (mainly the lumbar curve), in that case, correction of the thoracic curve should be limited to a rate that the uninstrumented curves may compensate.

Second, how can we manipulate the coronal and shoulder balance during surgery? **Table 25.1** describes the possible outcomes of the initial series of fluoroscopy shots as described above and the necessary measures that need to be taken in each scenario.

Table 25.1 Potential problems in balance identified using C-arm during surgery and their proposed solutions

Scenario	T1/rib tilt	T1 displacement	Maneuver	Result
1	Horizontal	None (0–2 cm)	None	Ideal result
2	Horizontal	+ (>2 cm)	Distraction at the lower end of the instrumentation at the side of displacement	May achieve ideal result if the lumbar curve is very flexible, otherwise accept to end up with some trunk shift rather than shoulder imbalance
3	Tilted to one side	None (0–2 cm)	Distraction at the upper end of the instrumentation at the side T1 is tilted toward along with distraction at the lower end of the instrumentation at the opposite side	In this case, we want to eliminate T1 tilt as much as possible at the expense of accepting some T1 translation if it is not avoidable
4	Tilted to one side	+ (>2 cm) (to the same side)	Mild distraction at the lower and upper ends at the side of the displacement and tilt	Ideal result achievable in most cases; please note that distraction at both the upper and lower ends will result in a decrease in correction for at least one of the instrumented curves (i.e., it will be distracted at its convex side)
5	Tilted to one side	+ (>2 cm) (to the opposite side)	Mild distraction at the upper end of instrumentation aiming at the correction of the shoulder balance (i.e., on the side of the T1 tilt) and mild distraction at the lower end of the opposite side (i.e., on the side of T1 translation)	The ideal result is not achievable in most cases; it is advisable to prioritize correcting the shoulder balance (T1 tilt) and accepting compromise in trunk shift (T1 translation)

Key Points

- Achieving shoulder balance in deformity surgery is very important as shoulder imbalance is the most readily observable outcome of surgery. Therefore, it cannot be concealed.

- Shoulder imbalance may present as a problem of its own. Still, it is very frequently associated with other factors such as the coronal curve(s) rate of correction, whether the fractional curves have been included in the instrumentation, and overall coronal balance.

- In most cases, shoulder balance has more weight than coronal balance. If both cannot be corrected to within acceptable limits, shoulder balance (T1 or first rib tilt) should be prioritized.

References

1. Smith PL, Donaldson S, Hedden D, et al. Parents' and patients' perceptions of postoperative appearance in adolescent idiopathic scoliosis. Spine 2006;31(20):2367–2374

2. Chan CYW, Gani SMA, Lim MY, Chiu CK, Kwan MK. APSS-ASJ Best Clinical Research Award: is there a difference between patients' and parents' perception of physical appearance in adolescent idiopathic scoliosis? Asian Spine J 2019;13(2):216–224

3. Zhang S, Zhang L, Feng X, Yang H. Incidence and risk factors for postoperative shoulder imbalance in scoliosis: a systematic review and meta-analysis. Eur Spine J 2018;27(2):358–369

4. Kuklo TR, Lenke LG, Graham EJ, et al. Correlation of radiographic, clinical, and patient assessment of shoulder balance following fusion versus nonfusion of the proximal thoracic curve in adolescent idiopathic scoliosis. Spine 2002; 27(18):2013–2020

5. O'Brien MF, Kuklo TR, Blanke KM, et al. Radiographic Measurement Manual. Spinal Deformity Study Group (SDSG). Medtronic Sofamor Danek; 2004

6. Kuklo TR, Lenke LG, Won DS, et al. Spontaneous proximal thoracic curve correction after isolated fusion of the main thoracic curve in adolescent idiopathic scoliosis. Spine 2001; 26(18):1966–1975

7. Ono T, Bastrom TP, Newton PO. Defining 2 components of shoulder imbalance: clavicle tilt and trapezial prominence. Spine 2012;37(24): E1511–E1516

8. Kwan MK, Wong KA, Lee CK, Chan CYW. Is neck tilt and shoulder imbalance the same phenomenon? A prospective analysis of 89 adolescent idiopathic scoliosis patients (Lenke type 1 and 2). Eur Spine J 2016;25(2):401–408

9. Lee SY, Ch'ng PY, Wong TS, et al. Patients' perception and satisfaction on neck and shoulder imbalance in adolescent idiopathic scoliosis. Global Spine J 2021;21925682211007795. doi:10.1177/21925682211007795. Online ahead of print

10. Menon KV, Tahasildar N, Pillay HM, Anbuselvam M, Jayachandran RK. Patterns of shoulder imbalance in adolescent idiopathic scoliosis: a retrospective observational study. J Spinal Disord Tech 2014;27(7):401–408

11. Rose PS, Lenke LG. Classification of operative adolescent idiopathic scoliosis: treatment guidelines. Orthop Clin North Am 2007;38(4): 521–529, vi

12. Ilharreborde B, Even J, Lefevre Y, et al. How to determine the upper level of instrumentation in Lenke types 1 and 2 adolescent idiopathic scoliosis: a prospective study of 132 patients. J Pediatr Orthop 2008;28(7):733–739

13. Trobisch PD, Ducoffe AR, Lonner BS, Errico TJ. Choosing fusion levels in adolescent idiopathic scoliosis. J Am Acad Orthop Surg 2013;21(9): 519–528

14. Suk S-I. Pedicle screw instrumentation for adolescent idiopathic scoliosis: the insertion technique, the fusion levels and direct vertebral rotation. Clin Orthop Surg 2011;3(2):89–100

15. Bjerke BT, Cheung ZB, Shifflett GD, Iyer S, Derman PB, Cunningham ME. Do current recommendations for upper instrumented vertebra predict shoulder imbalance? An attempted validation of level selection for adolescent idiopathic scoliosis. HSS J 2015;11(3):216–222

16. Terheyden JH, Wetterkamp M, Gosheger G, et al. Predictors of shoulder level after spinal fusion in adolescent idiopathic scoliosis. Eur Spine J 2018;27(2):370–380

17. Yang H, Im GH, Hu B, et al. Shoulder balance in Lenke type 2 adolescent idiopathic scoliosis: should we fuse to the second thoracic vertebra? Clin Neurol Neurosurg 2017;163:156–162

18. Chan CYW, Chiu CK, Ler XY, et al. Upper instrumented vertebrae (UIV) tilt angle is an important postoperative radiological parameter that correlates with postoperative neck and medial shoulder imbalance. Spine 2018;43(19):E1143–E1151

19. Moorthy V, Goh GS, Guo C-M, Tan S-B, Chen JL-T, Soh RCC. Risk factors of postoperative shoulder imbalance in adolescent idiopathic scoliosis: the role of sagittal spinopelvic parameters and upper instrumented vertebrae selection. Clin Spine Surg 2022;35(1):E137–E142

20. Yuan S, Fan N, Hai Y, Wu Q, Du P, Zang L. What is the impact of scoliotic correction on postoperative shoulder imbalance in severe and rigid scoliosis. BMC Musculoskelet Disord 2021;22(1):868

21. Lehman RA Jr, Lenke LG, Helgeson MD, Eckel TT, Keeler KA. Do intraoperative radiographs in scoliosis surgery reflect radiographic result? Clin Orthop Relat Res 2010;468(3): 679–686

Andrea Redaelli and Claudio Lamartina

Introduction

Coronal and sagittal malalignment are the hallmark of adult deformity. Moreover, in the last decades, the number of deformity cases after previous fusion is dramatically increasing because of the aging population and the spreading of spine surgery. Coronal malalignment (CM) consists in the C7 plumbline lateral displacement of more than 4 cm from the central sacral vertical line (CSVL). It can result from trauma, infection, tumor, neurological disease, or degenerative conditions, but it can also derive from extra-spinal conditions like anatomical limb length discrepancy. Many patients poorly tolerate CM, especially when the spine is fused as a result of diseases or previous fixation or when both coronal and sagittal malalignment are present. However, the correlation with quality of life has been investigated for coronal deformity to a lower extent than for sagittal deformity. The etiology of CM determines its treatment. For example, in case of Pisa syndrome caused by Parkinson's disease or other neurodegenerative disorders, the stooped posture is a flexible and reversible condition that often improves with proper pharmacological treatment. On the other hand, limb lenght discrepancy may also lead to CM that is not caused by spinal disease and thus can be solved with limb surgery or use of orthosis. On the contrary, in case of spinal diseases or previous surgeries, CM is a stiff deformity that alters the spine in both standing and lying position and often requires surgery. The surgical treatment of CM is typically challenging, mainly in the presence of associated sagittal imbalance or previous failed surgery. Obeid and coauthors proposed a treatment-oriented classification that divides CM in two patterns[3]:

- Concave CM (type 1): coronal C7 plumbline falling at the side of the concavity of the main coronal curve
- Convex CM (type 2): coronal C7 plumbline falling at the side of the convexity of the main coronal curve

Moreover, the stiffness of the main coronal curve and the mobility of the lumbosacral junction are factors that potentially influence the surgical strategy.

Definition of the Technique and Indications

Kickstand (KR) and tie rod (TR) are techniques to address CM in deformity cases based on the use of an additional rod connecting the main spinal instrumentation with an independent iliac screw. TR and KR are innovative and useful tools to fine tune the spinal correction and reinforce the instrumentation, preventing hardware failure and pseudoarthrosis. However, considering the stiffness of adult deformities, it is unlikely to obtain the final correction relying only upon these two techniques. As a matter of fact, the major correction is achieved through posterior column releases such as arthrectomies, multiple posterior column osteotomies (PCOs), or more aggressive three-column osteotomies (PSO). In addition, anterior corrective procedures such as anterior lumbar interbody fusion (ALIF) or multiple lateral lumbar interbody fusion (LLIF) can sometimes be considered as alternatives to osteotomies in order to reduce the bleeding and avoid direct manipulation of neural elements.

The essential conditions to apply KR and TR are:

- Fusion to the ilium.
- One point of mobility in the lumbar spine (where to apply compression or distraction). This spinal mobility can be already present (i.e., in primary cases) or can result from a surgical release (i.e., osteotomy or anterior release in revision cases).

KR acts in distraction on the concave side of coronal imbalance, while TR works on the convex side, pulling the spine toward the midline. Compression and distraction on the satellite rods determine correction of the coronal deformity and induce modifications in the sagittal plane. Since the axis of the supplementary rod is posterior to the spinal axis, the compression on that rod (TR technique) causes an increase in the lumbar lordosis. In contrast, the distraction on supplementary rod (KR technique) tends to provoke a flat spine, similar to what happened in the past with Harrington rod. These facts imply the importance of an accurate preoperative planning both in the coronal and sagittal planes, and the necessity to check the obtained results intraoperatively. The TR technique is particularly appropriate for patients with CM and hypolordosis, whereas KR technique is more indicated for patients with previous overcorrection in the lumbar spine. A combination of the two techniques can also be beneficial, taking into account the effect of the interplay of compression and distraction in the sagittal plane. In case of hypolordosis the compressive maneuver is applied first, while the distraction is applied first in case of hyperlordosis. Whenever CM is not associated with sagittal deformity, it is crucial to not alter the correct degrees of lumbar lordosis. In this situation, the TR and KR techniques act in a complementary way in correcting the coronal deformity, while their effects on sagittal alignment are reciprocally neutralized. Finally, when the use of additional rods (KR and TR) is not sufficient to address the deformity, it is possible to fine tune the correction through compression or distraction either at the osteotomy level or between the previously released pedicle screws.

Surgical Technique

Preoperative planning is fundamental to assess the deformity of coronal and sagittal planes accurately. In case of both primary surgery and revision, the correction can be achieved with either anterior or posterior techniques according to the surgeon's evaluation and experience. As mentioned above, in patients with insufficient lumbar lordosis the TR technique is preferred while in those with excessive lumbar lordosis the KR technique is more appropriate.

Both techniques are performed with the patients under general anesthesia in the prone position. First, the spine and the iliac crest are exposed via a standard posterior approach and pedicle and two iliac screws are inserted, if not already present (**Fig. 26.1a**). Second, a third iliac screw is added, and an open domino connector is positioned at the thoracolumbar junction level (**Fig. 26.1b**). Once all the instrumentation has been placed, facet joint arthrectomies, PCOs or three-column osteotomy (3CO) can be performed in order to reach the targeted correction and a sufficient spinal release. Then the additional iliac screw and the domino connector are connected through an accessory rod (**Fig. 26.1c**). The accessory rod is distally locked and distractive (kickstand) (**Fig. 26.1d**) or compressive (tie) (**Fig. 26.2**) maneuvers are applied. Once the correction is achieved, the additional rod is definitely locked. It is worthwhile to note that the corrective maneuvers can be performed by distraction or compression on such accessory rod, which provides an advantageous lever arm due to its position relative to the spine. During corrective maneuvers, it is essential to keep the pedicle screws loose in the lower part of the instrumentation. The coronal and sagittal correction is finally verified through radiographic control, with the help of a 90-degree, cross-shaped tool placed on the superior border of the iliac crests and centered on S1 (**Fig. 26.3**). Such a tool allows to evaluate the extent of the C7 spinous process coronal displacement. All the instrumentation is definitely locked when the ideal

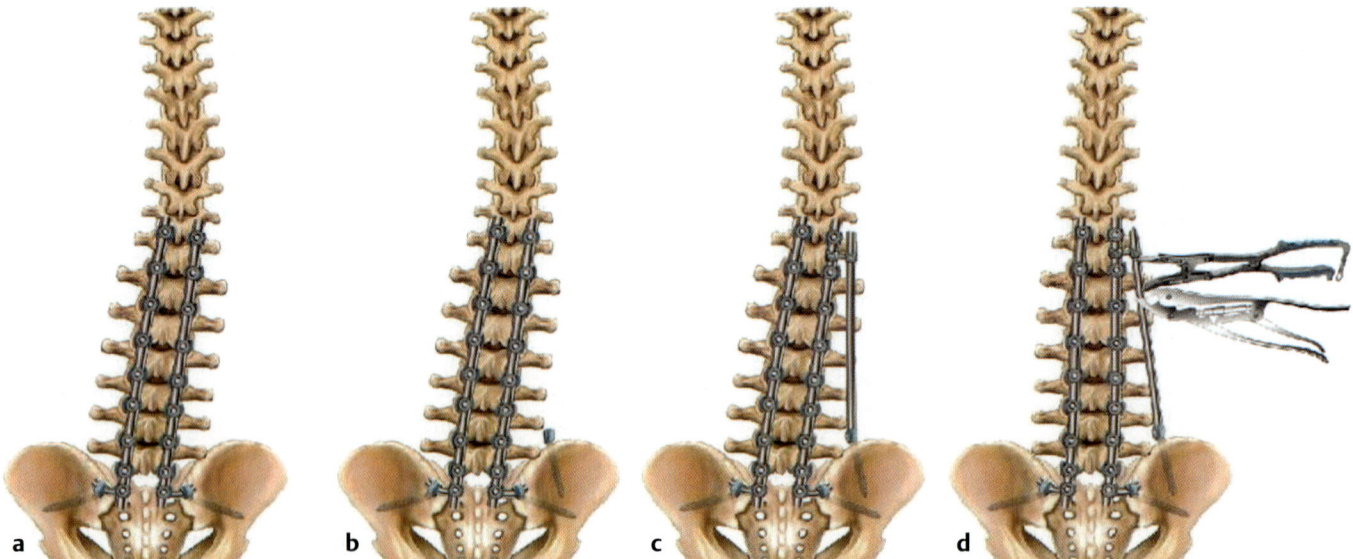

Fig. 26.1 Kickstand rod technique. Placement of the pedicle screws and iliac screws **(a)**. Placement of the extra-pelvic screw on concave side **(b)**. Placement of the kickstand rod between the extra-pelvic screw and corresponding side rod of the pedicle screws **(c)**. Release of the set screws and distraction on the kickstand rod to achieve correction **(d)**.

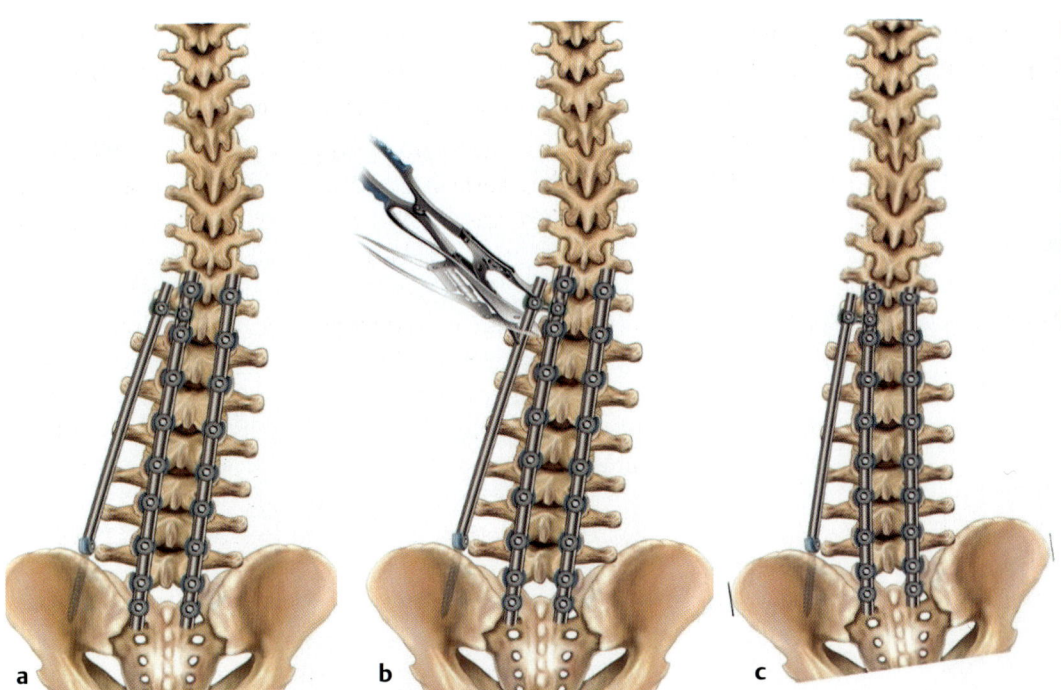

Fig. 26.2 Tie rod technique. Placement of the extra-pelvic screw on convex side **(a)**. Placement of the tie rod between the extra-pelvic screw and corresponding side rod of the pedicle screws **(b)**. Release of the set screws and compression on the tie rod to achieve correction **(c)**.

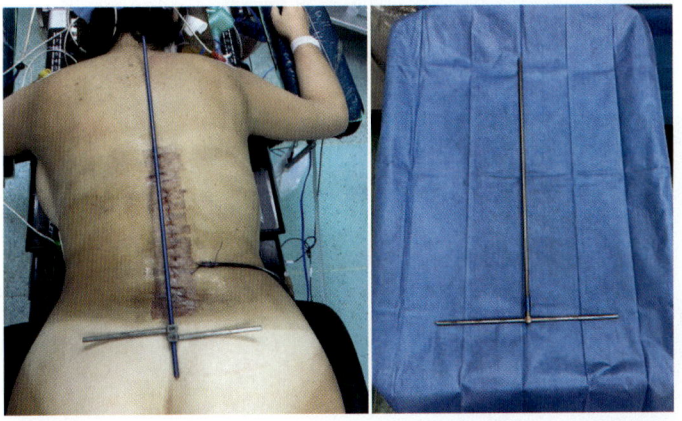

Fig. 26.3 A cross-shaped tool made with titanium rods is used to assess the coronal alignment preoperatively. This was a case of early postoperative coronal malalignment for which the patient underwent immediate revision with a tie rod. A similar intraopertive measurement is then performed to confirm the final alignment after the correction.

correction is obtained. Postoperative care does not require the use of braces and reckons during early mobilization of the patient.

Case Example: Tie Rod Technique

The patient is a 64-year-old woman (160 cm, 58 kg) (**Fig. 26.4**). She suffered a severe low back pain, and the preoperative radiographic evaluation showed a sagittal (>50 mm) and coronal (40 mm) malalignment toward the concave side of the curve. The patient already had a

previous L2–L5 fusion for degenerative disc disease and later underwent a T10–ilium fusion with L5–S1 ALIF and L4–L5 extreme lateral interbody fusion (LLIF) for sagittal deformity. Because of the residual CM, a revision with a TR was performed on the convex side. The coronal C7 plumbline improved from 40 mm preoperatively to 6 mm postoperatively. Lumbar lordosis increased from 54 to 63 degrees thanks to compression on the TR.

Case Example: Kickstand Rod Technique

The patient is a 68-year-old woman (165 cm, 73 kg) with four previous surgeries (**Fig. 26.5**). In particular, she underwent: an L4–L5 fusion; a cranial extension to L3 for proximal junctional kyphosis; an L2–L3 lateral interbody fusion together with an L1–L4 posterior fusion; and, finally, a cranial and caudal extension from T10 to ilium with L5–S1 ALIF for sagittal imbalance. Because of the residual CM toward the convexity, a revision with a kickstand rod is performed on the convex side. In addition, the right L5 screw is removed because of a radiculopathy. Coronal alignment improved from 44 mm preoperatively to 12 mm postoperatively. The lumbar lordosis decreased from 58 to 55 degrees with no significant modification in the sagittal profile.

Case Example: Combination of the Kickstand and Tie Rod Techniques

The patient is a 68-year-old woman (159 cm, 75 kg) with three previous surgeries (**Fig. 26.6**). She underwent a

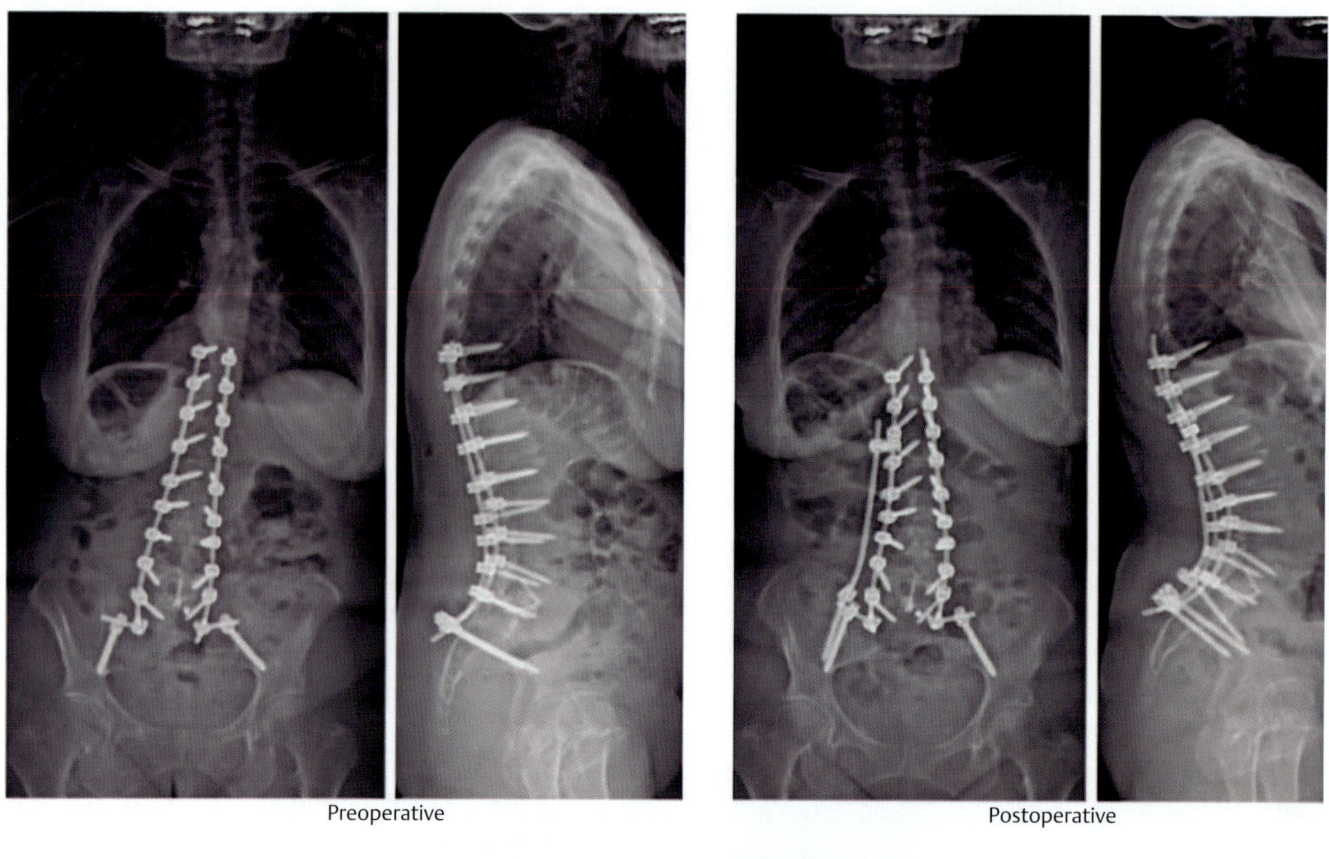

Preoperative

Postoperative

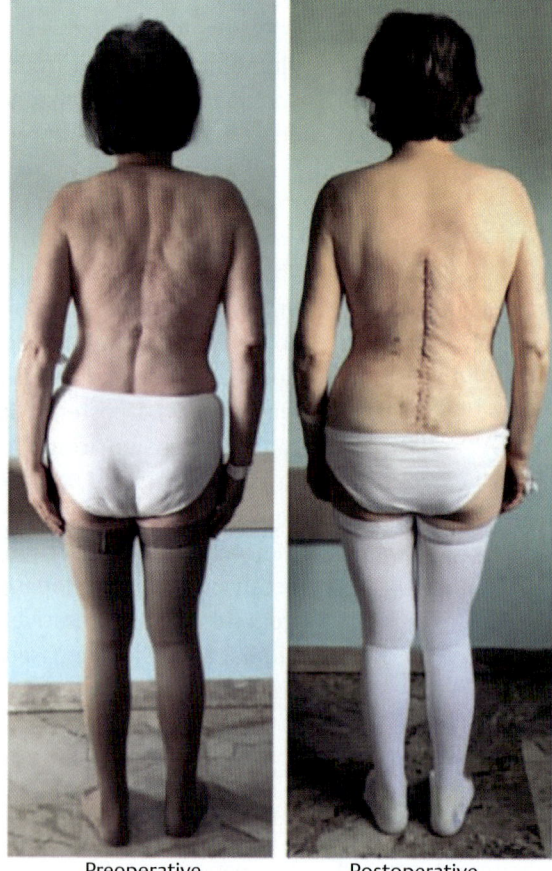

Preoperative   Postoperative

Fig. 26.4 A case of concave (type 1) coronal malalignment (CM) corrected with the tie rod.

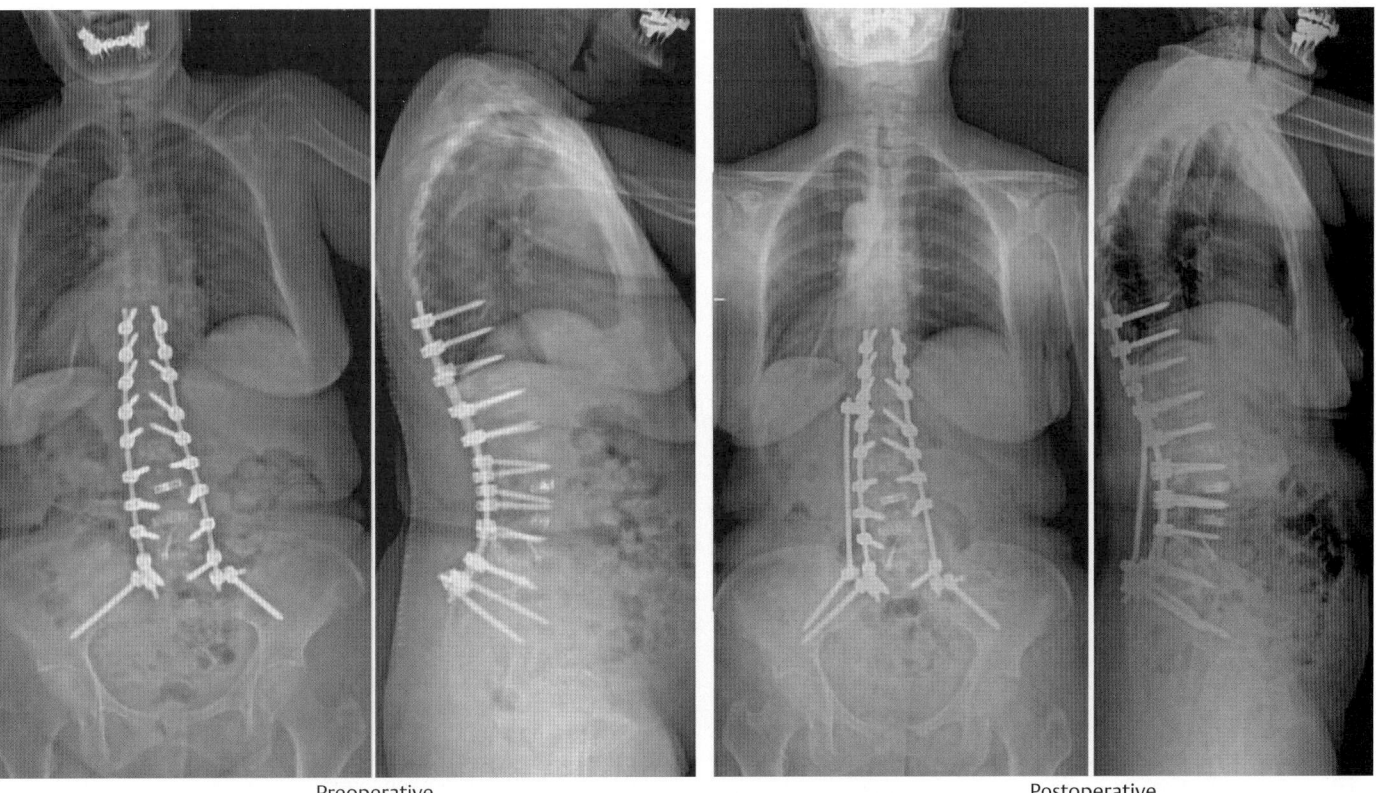

Preoperative   Postoperative

Fig. 26.5 A case of convex (type 2) coronal malalignment corrected with the kickstand rod.

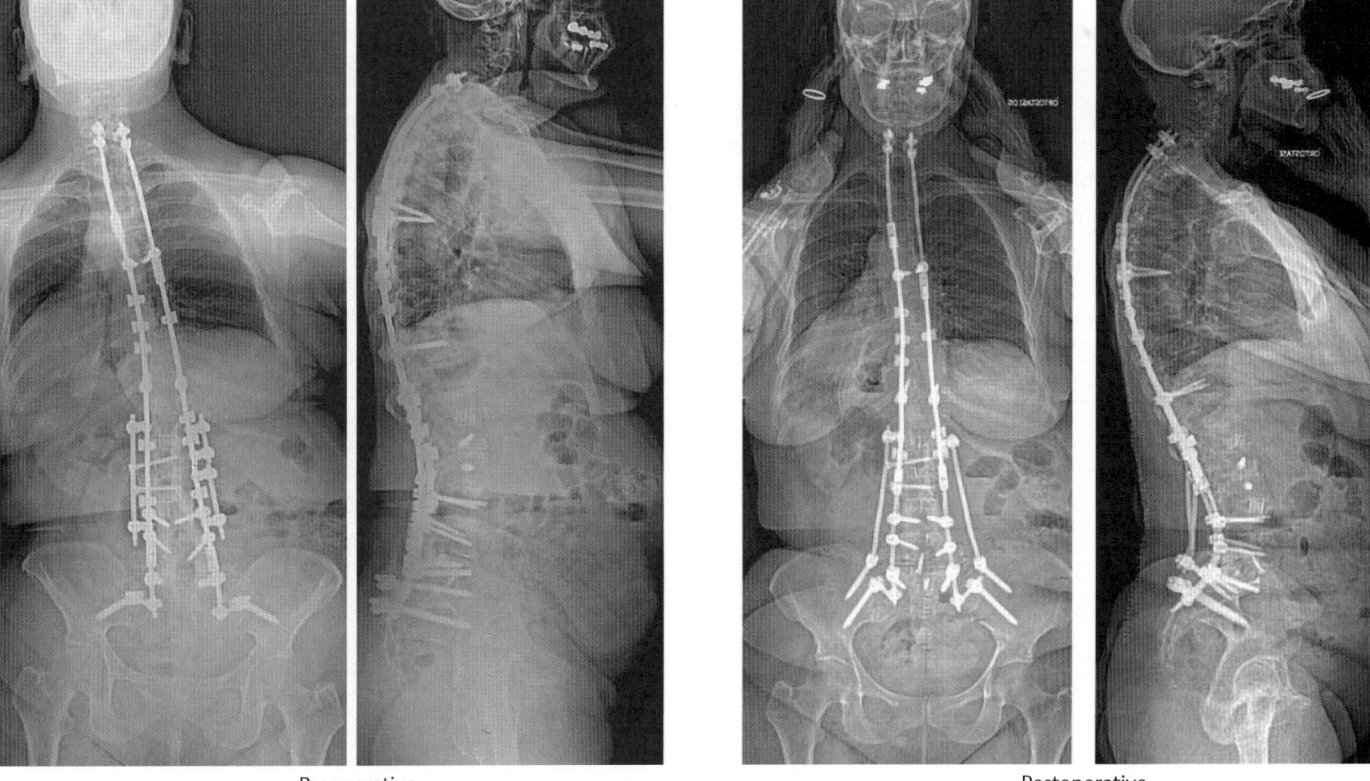

Preoperative   Postoperative

Fig. 26.6 A case of convex (type 2) coronal malalignment treated with both kickstand and tie rod techniques.

primary T2–L5 fusion and, given subsequent surgical site infection and proximal adjacent segment disease, a revision with extension to C7 and ilium was performed. Then she underwent an L1–L5 lateral interbody fusion together with the insertion of two supplementary rods due to pseudoarthrosis and hardware failure. She still suffered back pain and the preoperative radiographic evaluation showed a severe coronal and sagittal deformity on the convex side (76 mm) and rod breakage. The patient underwent an L5–S1 ALIF and a posterior revision with simultaneous KR (on the convexity) and TR (on the concavity) techniques. The two methods acted complementarily to correct the coronal deformity. C7–PL and lumbar lordosis improved from, respectively, 76 mm and 38 degrees preoperatively to, respectively, 24 mm and 55 degrees postoperatively.

Key Points

- KR and TR techniques are useful to correct coronal deformity.

- Both techniques require iliac screws. Thus, they are not suitable in case the pelvis is not included in the fusion area.

- Compression and distraction maneuvers performed in the lumbar area always determine modifications in the sagittal plane.

- In adult deformity, the amount of correction ideally needed typically exceeds the one that these techniques are able to provide. Thus, posterior osteotomies or aggressive anterior releases must be considered in the surgical plan.

- Additional TR and KR provide superior biomechanical performance in terms of construct stiffness and rod stress reduction, especially when they lie in a plane different from that of the main instrumentation. This helps to reduce the risk of hardware failure.

References

1. Redaelli A, Langella F, Dziubak M, et al. Useful and innovative methods for the treatment of postoperative coronal malalignment in adult scoliosis: the "kickstand rod" and "tie rod" procedures. Eur Spine J 2020;29(4):849–859
2. Makhni MC, Cerpa M, Lin JD, Park PJ, Lenke LG. The "Kickstand Rod" technique for correction of coronal imbalance in patients with adult spinal deformity: theory and technical considerations. J Spine Surg 2018;4(4):798–802
3. Obeid I, Berjano P, Lamartina C, Chopin D, Boissière L, Bourghli A. Classification of coronal imbalance in adult scoliosis and spine deformity: a treatment-oriented guideline. Eur Spine J 2019;28(1):94–113
4. Redaelli A, Pun A, Aebi M. The problems associated with revision surgery. Eur Spine J 2020;29(Suppl 1):2–5
5. Redaelli A, Berjano P, Aebi M. Focal disorders of the spine with compensatory deformities: how to define them. Eur Spine J 2018;27(Suppl 1): 59–69
6. Berjano P, Zanirato A, Langella F, et al. Anterior lumbar interbody fusion (ALIF) L5-S1 with overpowering of posterior lumbosacral instrumentation and fusion mass: a reliable solution in revision spine surgery. Eur Spine J 2021; 30(8):2323–2332
7. Berjano P, Xu M, Damilano M, et al. Supplementary delta-rod configurations provide superior stiffness and reduced rod stress compared to traditional multiple-rod configurations after pedicle subtraction osteotomy: a finite element study. Eur Spine J 2019;28(9):2198–2207
8. Cecchinato R, Berjano P, Aguirre MF, Lamartina C. Asymmetrical pedicle subtraction osteotomy in the lumbar spine in combined coronal and sagittal imbalance. Eur Spine J 2015;24(Suppl 1):S66–S71
9. Berjano P, Bassani R, Casero G, Sinigaglia A, Cecchinato R, Lamartina C. Failures and revisions in surgery for sagittal imbalance: analysis of factors influencing failure. Eur Spine J 2013;22(Suppl 6):S853–S858
10. Lamartina C, Berjano P. Classification of sagittal imbalance based on spinal alignment and compensatory mechanisms. Eur Spine J 2014; 23(6):1177–1189
11. Berjano P, Lamartina C. Far lateral approaches (XLIF) in adult scoliosis. Eur Spine J 2013; 22(Suppl 2):S242–S253

27 Translation Maneuver for Spinal Deformities

D. Güçlühan Güçlü and Onur Yaman

Introduction

Deformity treatment aims to correct the deformity as much as possible, which should be achieved mainly to maintain the corrected state of the spine by applying fusion along the curvature and to obtain a balanced spine on a flat pelvis, with the head in the midline that is accompanied by physiological sagittal contours. The basic procedure is the correction maneuver that should be performed on implants that were placed in order to allow the spine to take its final shape. Since using Harrington rod instrumentation for correction in 1960, scoliosis surgery has changed dramatically.[1] Harrington started the procedure by applying distraction force on the concave side as a corrective maneuver with distraction rod system developed by him. In the following years, compression was also used on the convex side by adding another rod to the convex side.[2]

In the early 1970s, Eduardo Luque, a Mexican surgeon, developed a new system called "segmental spinal instrumentation" (SSI), which consisted of "L"-shaped rods that were connected to accompany sublaminar wires placed at each level.[3]

Luque passed two sublaminar steel wires through each vertebral level, attached to the rods which were pre-bent according to the sagittal contours, and tightened by retracting through both the concave and convex areas as the first application of the translation maneuver.[4]

It was shown that this translation obtains higher correction rates in scoliotic curves compared to the Harrington rod system, and it was unquestionably superior in reconstructing sagittal contours.

In the following years, hook pedicle screws were implemented to create stronger stabilization systems and provide more appropriate corrections in deformity surgery.

Wiring and hook construct allowed for deformity correction but were inadequate for rotational correction because of the lack of torque necessary for triplanar correction.[5] The pedicle screw crosses the three columns of the spine from posterior to anterior, providing the strongest possible segmental fixation, thus allowing segmental manipulation in three dimensions for correction.[6]

The strength of the pedicle screw allows for enough torque to be applied to the spine in all three planes as it is realigned. In addition, the distribution of the force to many segments and the reduction of the load on each segment is provided with pedicle screws.[7]

Definition of the Technique

Translation is the movement of the spine segment laterally for the coronal plane and anteriorly or posteriorly for the sagittal plane. The primary mechanism of translation is based on the adduction of the spine with the anchor toward the rod. Laterally deviated spinal segments are gradually retracted to the midline and fixed in the rod. The translation maneuver can be used alone or as part of the correction process. There are also pedicle screw systems that were used only for translation.

Translation maneuver can be performed with various anchors, including standard pedicle screws or sublaminar wires and bands. In addition, multiaxial reduction screws or multiaxial screws with reduction towers have been used recently. Reduction screws placed in the apical and periapical region of the deformity facilitate the placement of the rod, the correction of the deformity, and the use of rod reduction instruments when necessary (**Figs. 27.1** and **27.2**).

A concave rod is measured and cut to a length. The rod is then bent into the targeted sagittal contour with increased sagittal alignment. First, the sagittal-contoured rod is loosely placed on the proximal screws (**Fig. 27.3**).

To protect the sagittal contour, the pre-bent rod is placed on the distal pedicle screws without rotation in the coronal plane. The distal set screws are placed and locked simultaneously, while the proximal screws are left loose because the spine needs to lengthen while being corrected.[8]

İnstrumented vertebrae are pulled toward the rod using various instruments such as the "persuader" or the reduction towers. If we use the reduction towers, we need to connect them to the multiaxial pedicle screws at the apical and periapical regions of the curve. In the next step, the rod is inserted into the screws for the following segments (**Fig. 27.4**).

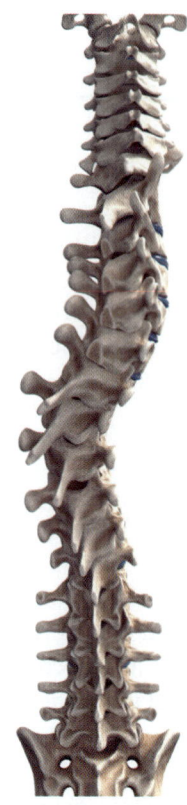

Fig. 27.1   A double curve scoliosis.

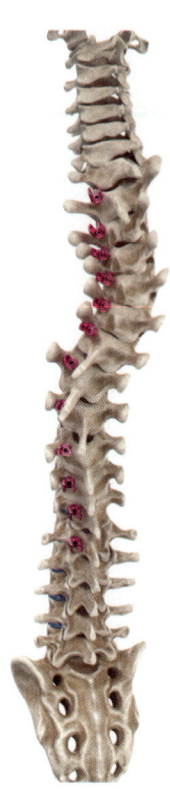

Fig. 27.2   Reduction screws placed in the apical and periapical region of the deformity to facilitate the placement of the rod.

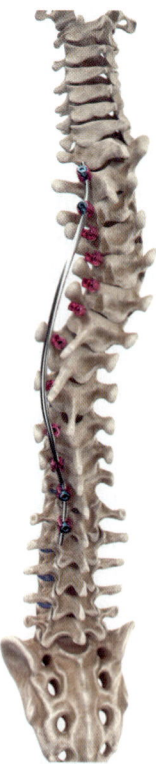

Fig. 27.3   A concave rod is measured and cut to a length. It is then bent into the targeted sagittal contour with increased sagittal alignment. The sagittal-contoured rod is loosely placed on the proximal screws.

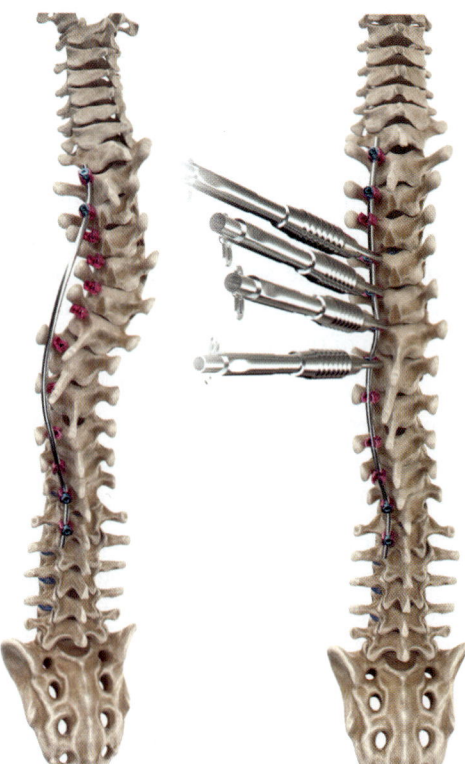

Fig. 27.4   By using the reduction towers, the rod is connected to the multiaxial pedicle screws at the apical and periapical regions of the curve. Then the rod is inserted into the screws for the following segments by pulling the curved spine to a corrected position.

When the rod is in proper coronal and sagittal orientation, starting from the vertebra closer to the rod, far from the apex, the reduction screws are slowly tightened, and the spine is pulled toward the rod[9] (**Fig. 27.5**).

The scoliosis is corrected while the apex of the deformity is retracted to the midline in the coronal plane. At the same time, the correction is provided in the coronal, sagittal, and axial planes as the rotated apical vertebrae are pulled posteromedially.

In the sagittal plane, kyphosis is restored by providing posterior translation. This technique also provides a gradual and slow correction by allowing reduction forces to be distributed over each segment of the deformity. Then the convex rod is placed. Distraction and compression are performed as needed to provide coronal and sagittal plane corrections. Distraction is applied on the concave side to restore the kyphosis further, while compression is used on the convex area for overall construct stability and to improve correction. After this correction, the set screws are locked. In situ rod bending is beneficial in fine adjustment correction in both the sagittal and coronal planes. This technique is beneficial for restoring the rod's lost contour (**Fig. 27.6**). If a significant amount of the sagittal contour is

lost during the translation maneuver, the concave rod can be removed and replaced with a newly bent rod to gain further correction after the convex rod has been placed and locked into position.

The most significant advantage of the translation system is that it spreads the corrective power to the segments and uses the viscoelastic creep feature of the tissues during slow processing.[10]

Before ending the surgery after the correction, a control radiograph showing the entire spine should be taken in the prone position. It should be checked that adequate correction is provided, and that there is no global imbalance or shoulder and pelvis asymmetry.

Indications

The correction technique to be chosen for the correction of the deformity may vary depending on the type, flexibility, and size of the curvature, the type of fixation technique selected, the characteristics of the implants to be used, and the reduction maneuver. Determination of the flexibility of the curvature during the preoperative evaluation is one of the

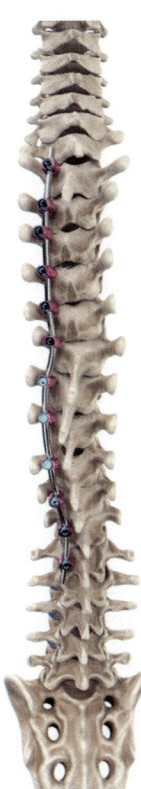

Fig. 27.5 When the rod is in proper coronal and sagittal orientation, starting from the vertebra closer to the rod, far from the apex, the reduction screws are slowly tightened, and the spine is pulled toward the rod.

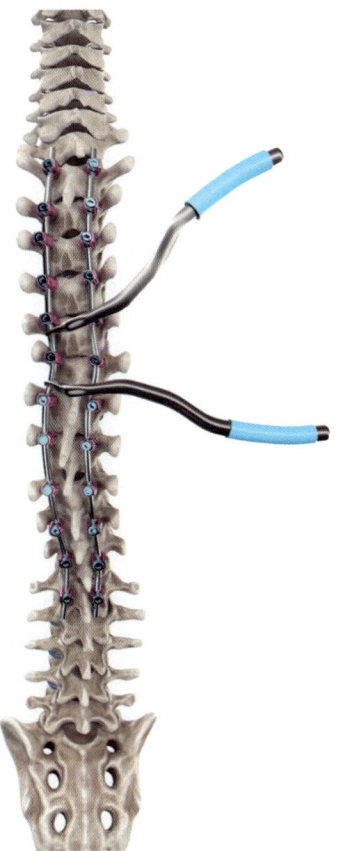

Fig. 27.6 In situ rod bending can be used for fine adjustment correction in both the sagittal and coronal planes.

essential factors in determining the surgical and correction technique to be chosen. Translation maneuver is indicated in both coronal and sagittal plane deformities. The translation maneuver alone is very effective, especially in correcting thoracic curves. This technique is essentially indicated for flexible curves and fixed curves may not reduce unless release procedures are performed. Successful correction of the deformity is possible with adequate spinal release and the skill and experience of the surgeon who applies the technique. If successful correction of the deformity cannot be achieved with a single method, a combination of different correction techniques may be necessary.

Complication Avoidance

- During translation and correction of the curve, spinal cord deficits may occur while the vascular and neural elements are pulled. If there is a spinal cord trauma, it may lead to ischemia of the spinal cord. To avoid such an injury neurophysiological monitoring should be used. Neuromonitoring, including motor-evoked potentials (MEPs) and somatosensory-evoked potentials (SSEPs), allows us for early alert.

- In the course of the correction maneuver, pay attention to the screw–bone interface. The surgeon should stop if there is evidence of a screw pullout.

- Bone quality and stiffness of the curvature are important because bone fractures or anchoring screw pullouts may occur in cases with rigid curves and those with low bone quality.

- Another complication is that after the convex rod has been placed and locked into position if there is a considerable decrement of the sagittal contour of the concave rod during the translation maneuver, then we will replace it with a newly bent rod to gain further correction.

Efficiency/Strength of the Technique

Delorme et al reported no difference in the three planes when the two instrumentation techniques, namely, rod derotation and posteromedial translation (PMT), were compared.[11,12]

However, Muschik et al showed more significant correction of the thoracic curve with rod rotation. They reported that translation was more beneficial for overall spinal balance.[5]

In a study on 126 patients with adolescent idiopathic scoliosis (AIS), Crandall and Revella showed better deformity correction by translation than rod derotation technique.[13]

Pesenti et al reported better sagittal restoration using PMT compared to cantilever or in situ bending.[14]

Clement et al pointed out that translation provides better correction of thoracic kyphosis than sequential approximation by cantilever in patients with preoperative hypokyphosis.[15]

Furthermore, translation is defined as a simple and effective method to achieve sagittal correction of thoracic hypokyphosis by Clement et al.[16]

In 2022, Pesenti et al compared four correction techniques (in situ bending, rod derotation, cantilever, and PMT) and stated that PMT allowed for a better thoracal kyphosis restoration when compared to the in situ bending, rod derotation, and cantilever techniques. Also, all methods had the same ability to correct spinal deformity in the coronal plane.[17]

As a result, especially in the correction of deformities of hypokyphotic patients for restoration of thoracic kyphosis, the primary corrective maneuver is the translation maneuver, while other techniques should be used as accessory techniques.

Tips and Tricks

- Before starting the correction procedure, if necessary, releasing of the soft tissue (resection of the interspinous ligament, ligamentum flavum, and facet capsules) and osteotomy should be performed to ensure adequate flexibility.

- Rod reduction instruments and multiaxial reduction screws are placed in the apical and periapical areas to facilitate rod insertion and correction of the deformity.

- To avoid pullout, the thickest and longest screw that can be applied should be preferred.

- The concave rod is overbent in the sagittal plane. However, the convex rod is underbent. Therefore, when the screw rod connection is provided, the concave side of the vertebra is pulled posteriorly. In contrast, the convex side is pushed anteriorly to correct the axial plane, thus reducing rib prominence.

- For more effective correction, cobalt-chromium (CoCr) or stainless steel (SS) rods with a more rigid structure than titanium (Ti) can be preferred.

Key Points

- The objective of the translation maneuver is to pull back the vertebra toward the rods.

- Translation maneuver provides a gradual and slow correction while allowing the reduction forces to be distributed over each segment of the deformity.

- Translation of apical vertebral segments to posteriorly located rod also contributes to the correction of thoracic kyphosis.

- Especially in the correction of deformities of hypokyphotic patients for restoration of thoracic kyphosis, the primary corrective maneuver is the translation maneuver, while other techniques should be used as accessory techniques.

References

1. Green NE. The role of Harrington rods and Wisconsin wires in idiopathic scoliosis. In: Bridwell KH, DeWald RL, eds. The Textbook of Spinal Surgery. 2nd ed. Lippincott – Raven Publishers; 1997:469–488

2. Renshaw TS. The role of Harrington instrumentation and posterior spine fusion in the management of adolescent idiopathic scoliosis. Orthop Clin North Am 1988;19(2): 257–267

3. Luque ER. Segmental spinal instrumentation for correction of scoliosis. Clin Orthop Relat Res 1982;(163):192–198

4. Luque ER. Segmental Spinal Instrumentation. Thorofare, New Jersey: Slack; 1984

5. Muschik M, Schlenzka D, Robinson PN, Kupferschmidt C. Dorsal instrumentation for idiopathic adolescent thoracic scoliosis: rod rotation versus translation. Eur Spine J 1999;8(2):93–99

6. Liljenqvist U, Lepsien U, Hackenberg L, Niemeyer T, Halm H. Comparative analysis of pedicle screw and hook instrumentation in posterior correction and fusion of idiopathic thoracic scoliosis. Eur Spine J 2002;11(4):336–343

7. Chi JH, Lee R, Mummaneni PV. Concepts of surgical correction-segmental derotation and translation techniques. Neurosurg Clin N Am 2007;18(2):325–328

8. Miller DJ, Cahill PJ, Vitale MG, Shah SA. Posterior correction techniques for adolescent idiopathic scoliosis. J Am Acad Orthop Surg 2020;28(9):e363–e373

9. Cordell DD, Lenke LG, Gupta MC. Posterior spinal deformity correction techniques. In: Bridwell KH, Gupta M, eds. Bridwell and Dewald's Textbook of Spinal Surgery. Lippincott Williams & Wilkins; 2019:2618–2670

10. Shah SA. Posterior correction techniques in late-onset scoliosis. In: Newton PO, O'Brien MF, Shufflebarger HL, Betz RR, Dickson RA, Harms J, eds. Idiopathic Scoliosis: The Harms Study Group Treatment Guide. New York, NY: Thieme Medical Publishers; 2011:165–178

11. Delorme S, Labelle H, Aubin CÉ, et al. Intraoperative comparison of two instrumentation techniques for the correction of adolescent idiopathic scoliosis. Rod rotation and translation. Spine 1999;24(19):2011–2017, discussion 2018

12. Delorme S, Labelle H, Aubin CÉ, et al. A three-dimensional radiographic comparison of Cotrel-Dubousset and Colorado instrumentations for the correction of idiopathic scoliosis. Spine 2000;25(2):205–210

13. Crandall D, Revella J. Translational vs. derotational correction of adult scoliosis: a comparison of clinical and radiographic outcomes: E-poster# LWW 33. Spine J Meet 2009;10:177–178

14. Pesenti S, Lafage R, Henry B, et al. Deformity correction in thoracic adolescent idiopathic scoliosis. Bone Joint J 2020;102-B(3):376–382

15. Clement JL, Chau E, Kimkpe C, Vallade MJ. Restoration of thoracic kyphosis by posterior instrumentation in adolescent idiopathic scoliosis: comparative radiographic analysis of two methods of reduction. Spine 2008;33(14):1579–1587

16. Clement JL, Chau E, Geoffray A, Suisse G. Restoration of thoracic kyphosis by simultaneous translation on two rods for adolescent idiopathic scoliosis. Eur Spine J 2014;23(4, Suppl 4):S438–S445

17. Pesenti S, Clément JL, Ilharreborde B, et al. Comparison of four correction techniques for posterior spinal fusion in adolescent idiopathic scoliosis. Eur Spine J 2022;31(4):1028–1035

Ülkün Ünlü Ünsal, Murat Baloğlu, and Çağrı Canbolat

Introduction

Idiopathic scoliosis is a complex three-dimensional deformity in the coronal, sagittal, and transverse planes. In adolescent idiopathic scoliosis (AIS), spinal derotation appears to be the most difficult part of the surgery, so there are many techniques and developments which have been made to improve this maneuver. First reported by Paul Harrington in 1962, surgical correction of AIS has been in widespread use for over two decades.[1] It was initially considered to apply distraction forces only, so it did not have any effect on spinal derotation and poor thoracic hump correction. Cotrel and Dubousset (CD) introduced the method of intraoperative curve derotation correction by using multihook segmental instrumentation in 1988. This maneuver was called single concave rod derotation. After popularization of pedicle screws, the CD technique with hook systems was modified with "segmental pedicle screw," recognized as a gold standard in posterior scoliosis surgery.[2–7] The correction of the spinal deformity can be achieved by pedicle screw fixation and modern corrective techniques. Thus, in typical thoracic AIS cases, optimal coronal correction, restoration of normal thoracic kyphosis, and realignment of thoracic torsion can be done by lifting the thoracic rib concavity out of the chest and reducing the convex rib deformity without the need for thoracoplasty.

A single method cannot be used for the surgical correction of scoliosis. Meticulous preoperative planning to maximize the effectiveness of implants and intraoperative inspection of the degree of correction are crucial for a successful operation. Also, the curve type, spinal flexibility/rigidity, the type of the implant materials, the type of vertebral fixation, and anticipation of the correction techniques should be considered (**Fig. 28.1**). The degree of possible or desired correction should be decided with respect to both coronal and sagittal plane flexibility. Coronal flexibility can easily be recognized on bending or traction X-ray; however, evaluation of sagittal flexibility, particularly thoracic lordosis, has been limited.

Posterior-only techniques are often inadequate in correction of hypokyphotic or lordotic thoracic deformities. Pre-operative planning should be done to understand whether the spine is flexible or rigid. It is possible to achieve a good response to all correction maneuvers made in flexible spines. However, rigid spines require appropriate mobilization with a combination of techniques.

Definition of the Technique

The derotation maneuver technique is used to rotate the spine to its normal curvature by placing the pedicle screws and fixing a prebent rod to these screws and then rotating it along the curvature (**Figs. 28.2** and **28.3**). Some of these derotation maneuvers are concave rod derotation, convex rod derotation, and simultaneous double rod derotation techniques.[8–10]

For a typical lordotic thoracic curve in AIS, the traditional "derotation" maneuver of CD can be used.[11] A prebent rod for the coronal plane deformity of the curve is placed in the screws on the concave side of the deformity. The screw nuts should be engaged within the screw head without tightening. After the first rod is rotated into its intended position, the second rod is located. With this maneuver, the lateral deviation theoretically converts into deviation in the sagittal plane. Since the thoracic curvatures mostly tend to be hypokyphotic, this maneuver can both correct coronal plane deformity and restore thoracic kyphosis.

Effectiveness of derotation in CD technique has been emphasized by many authors. There are two main forces stimulated by the rod derotation. First, the vector of "rod derotation" is routed posteriorly and medially, which corrects both coronal and sagittal plane deformities. However, the use of this maneuver in correction of transverse plane deformities is still debatable.[12] Pollock et al reported 30 degrees of spinal derotation in their series of 14 patients by using this method.[13] Lenke et al showed 11 degrees of spinal derotation.[6] Stokes et al noted that after 90 degrees of rod rotation the apical vertebra derotated 50 degrees toward the sagittal plane; however, the apical vertebra rotation (AVR) worsened by 8 degrees.[14] On the other hand, there are authors who insist that CD does not have any effect on spinal rotation.[15–19] Biomechanical simulation studies showed that during rod rotation there is no spinal derotation and AVR increases paradoxically.[20] In 2004, Lee et al reported the direct vertebral rotation (DVR) technique as a new method for rotational malalignment in AIS.[12]

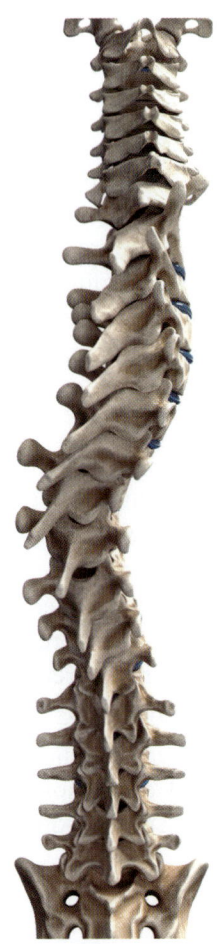

Fig. 28.1   Schematic illustration of the curve of spine.

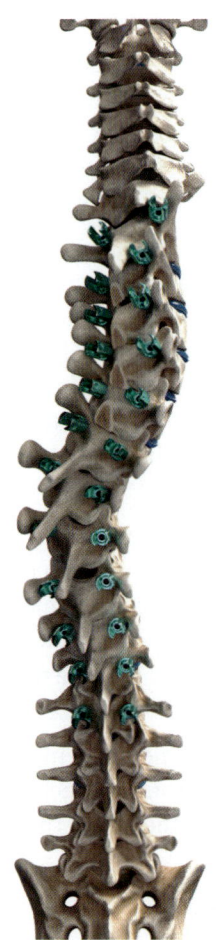

Fig. 28.2   Placement of the pedicle screws.

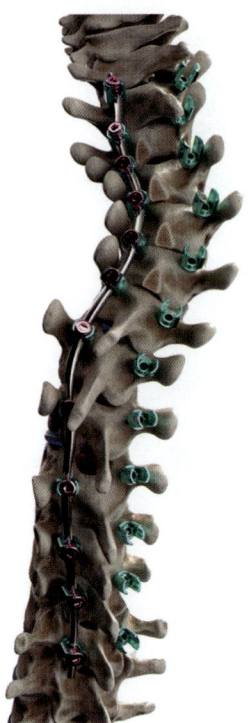

Fig. 28.3   Fixing a prebent rod to the screws on the concave side.

Both anterior and posterior approaches are recommended for the surgical correction of AIS via the DVR and single rod derotation (SRD) techniques. DVR may achieve curve correction and vertebral body rotation; however, it is a difficult technique. SRD might achieve curve correction in the coronal view, but it is not adequate for vertebral body rotation.

SRD is known to perform three-dimensional deformity correction in AIS.[3,6,13,21] Currently, SRD is a commonly used technique for curve correction in AIS. However, its effect on rotation correction is questionable. Some reports claim that SRD may achieve coronal and sagittal correction; however, the results for rotational correction are inadequate.[6,12] Other reports stated that with this maneuver about 20 to 40% maximum rotational correction can be obtained.[13,22]

In some reports, DVR is proven to be more successful in rotational and coronal correction than SRD. However, in these studies, no differences were reported in correction of clinical rib hump or patients' evaluation between the DVR and SRD groups.[12,23] Further correction of axial rotation does not confer better correction of patient's physical appearance. Although DVR may lead to further correction of the rotational angle than SRD, there was no significant difference in body image including the thoracic hump or satisfaction of patients. Pushing the thoracic hump down to correct it and rotational deformity during DVR can be challenging for both the surgeon and patients. SRD is technically easier compared to DVR and is a good option to correct AIS.

Thoracic hump, which might be caused by vertebral rotation in the axial plane, can create a distorted physical appearance. Thoracic hump is the second most common reason for surgical interventions for spinal deformity, and it is a significant measure in evaluating the success of the surgery.[24] However, the correlation between radiographic rotation correction and thoracic hump correction has not been clearly demonstrated.

A strong correlation between the preoperative AVR on computed tomography (CT) and the clinical thoracic hump has been reported.[25] However, some researchers suggest there is no correlation between AVR and trunk rotation on CT. Moreover, it is reported that the most rotated vertebra is not always associated with the apex of rib deformity.[26]

In the study of Delorme et al, in which they compared translation and rod derotation technique, they stated no technique is superior to the other. The choice of the surgical technique to correct the scoliotic deformities, whether using rod derotation, translation, or using both techniques, should be decided based on the surgeon's personal preference.[27]

Derotation of the prebent rod converts the scoliosis into kyphosis (**Fig. 28.4**). As a result, the sagittal alignment is restored, which is the basic step to correct the deformity in scoliosis surgery. However, there are other techniques that the surgeon may choose according to the circumstances or personal preferences. One of these techniques is concave derotation maneuver, which is until now performed primarily to avoid worsening of vertebral rotation and thoracic hump.[28,29]

There are also studies comparing the outcomes of convex and concave derotation techniques (**Fig. 28.5**). In the study of Anekstein et al, a convex-based rod derotation correction technique has been discussed. They reported that posterior correction and fusion using all-pedicle-screw constructs carried out using the convex rod derotation maneuver offers similar major and minor curve correction when compared to concave rod reduction techniques.[9,30]

Furthermore, in the study of Zifang et al, they compared convex and concave rod derotation techniques, and they stated that convex-rod derotation using pedicle-screw

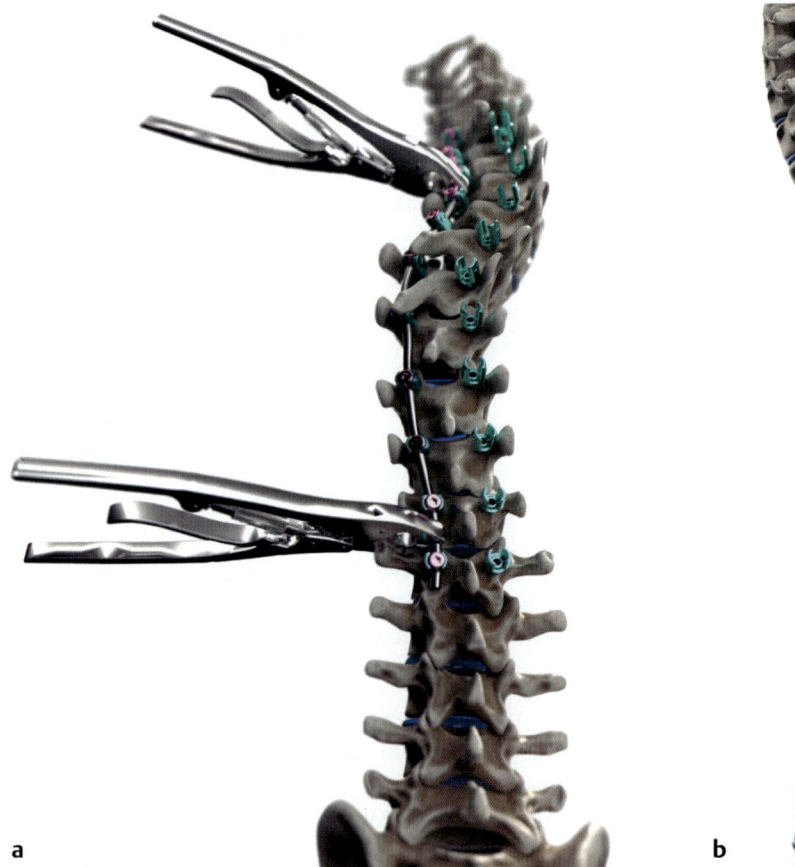
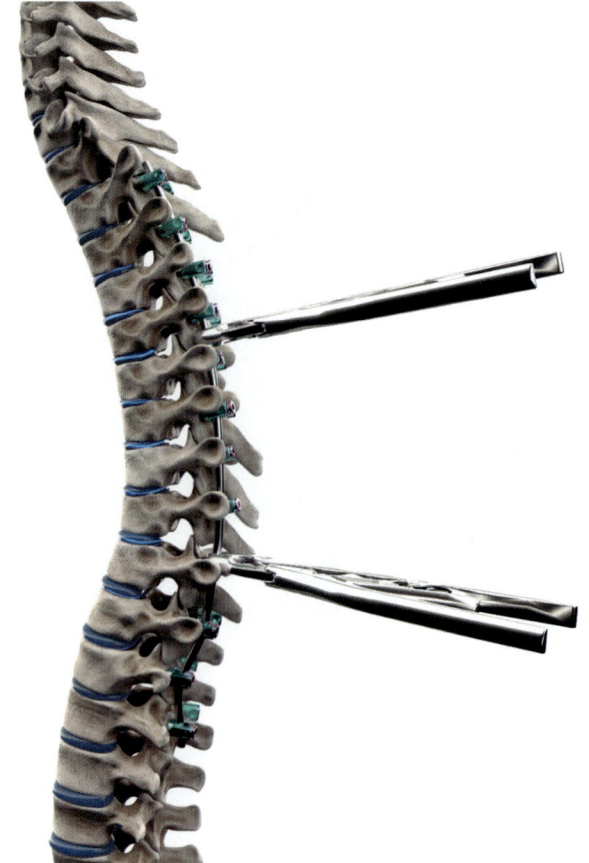

a   b

Fig. 28.4 Schematic illustration showing rotation of the spine along the curvature with rod holder: **(a)** Coronal view and **(b)** sagittal view.

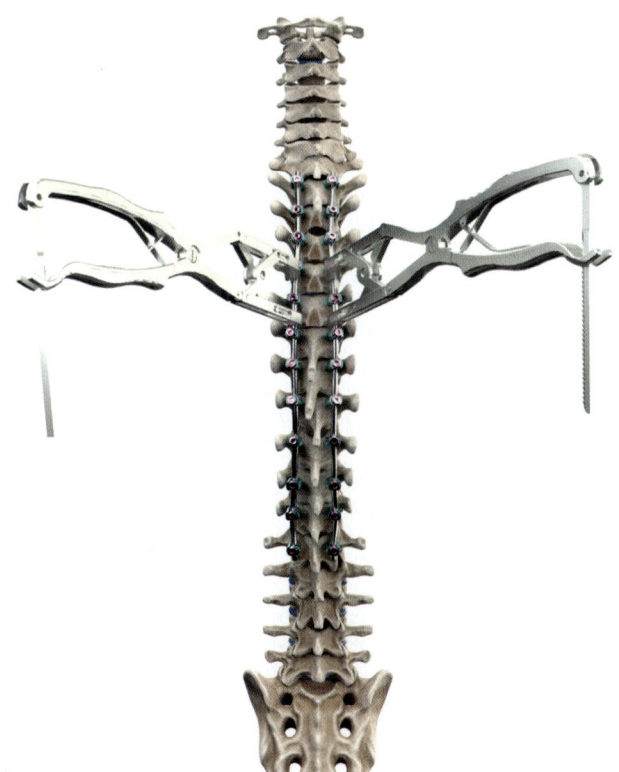

Fig. 28.5 Compression and distraction as the final adjustment after the curve is corrected with rod derotation.

instrumentation can provide a little better major curve correction without loss of thoracic kyphosis when combined with proper corrective techniques. Theoretically, this technique comes with benefits of reduced neurovascular damage due to a relatively lower risk of pedicle-screw misplacement.[31]

Kaliya-Perumal et al compared the efficacy of both the techniques in a study of 88 patients; they stated there was no worsening of AVR after correction of curves by these two maneuvers. They propounded the reason for this was that their patients had a relatively lower degree of spinal curvature deformity. Moreover, they suggested both these maneuvers are equally efficient in offering continuous correction in select cases.[32]

The authors suggest convex derotation is superior to concave derotation for the following reason: smaller pedicle width with higher cortical penetration on the concave side may lead to deviation toward convex derotation.[9,33] It is considered that even a minor injury to the medial cortex on the concave side may pose a potential risk of injury to neural structures and vascular structures outside the spinal canal, such as the aorta, due to the spinal cord's course on the concave side.[9,34] These parameters reveal that a medial pedicle impingement on the convex side is safer than on the concave side, particularly at the apex of the curve.[34] After easily locating the prebent rod, manipulation can

be done without overloading because the convex side has larger pedicle width and the distance between each other is bigger than concave side.[9]

It is debated that reversing this concept, which means convex rod derotation, is equally effective when compared to concave rod derotation.[9,29,35]

Simultaneous double rod derotation maneuver is also considered to be equally effective in reducing the curve, but the superiority of it over other techniques is yet to be proven.[10]

Tips and Tricks

- Adequate reduction of the rib hump is achieved after the SRD maneuver.

- There is no difference between DVR and SRD in terms of correction of clinical thoracic hump. More correction of axial rotation does not mean better correction of one's body image. Furthermore, pushing the thoracic hump down during DVR can be challenging for the surgeon and patients.

- Several studies demonstrated that pedicle wall perforation and dural injuries are observed with a higher incidence of screws placed on the concave side, especially in thoracic curvatures, since the pedicle diameter is thin on the concave side and the spinal cord follows the shortest course. On the other hand, concave derotation maneuver is still one of best options to avoid worsening of vertebral rotation and rib hump, which may occur if the convex side is initially rotated.

- The authors believe that SRD technique can provide an adequate and satisfactory correction in AIS.

Key Points

- Many techniques are available to correct a scoliotic spine. Depending on the type of deformity, the surgeon's preference, and the materials of the implants changing in accordance with technological developments, multiple methods can be selected. Depending on his/her experience, the surgeon can develop a combination of these many techniques, which leads to satisfactory results.

- The authors believe that SRD with pedicle screw instrumentation can successfully correct axial rotation without complications.

- This is more appropriate than DVR. Single rod rotation can be a good option in correcting the deformed curve of AIS.

References

1. Harrington PR. Treatment of scoliosis. Correction and internal fixation by spine instrumentation. J Bone Joint Surg Am 1962;44-A:591–610

2. Aaro S, Dahlborn M. The effect of Harrington instrumentation on the longitudinal axis rotation of the apical vertebra and on the spinal and rib-cage deformity in idiopathic scoliosis studied by computer tomography. Spine 1982;7(5):456–462

3. Cotrel Y, Dubousset J, Guillaumat M. New universal instrumentation in spinal surgery. Clin Orthop Relat Res 1988;227(227):10–23

4. Delorme S, Labelle H, Aubin CE, et al. A three-dimensional radiographic comparison of Cotrel-Dubousset and Colorado instrumentations for the correction of idiopathic scoliosis. Spine 2000;25(2):205–210

5. Muschik M, Schlenzka D, Robinson PN, Kupferschmidt C. Dorsal instrumentation for idiopathic adolescent thoracic scoliosis: rod rotation versus translation. Eur Spine J 1999;8(2):93–99

6. Lenke LG, Bridwell KH, Baldus C, Blanke K, Schoenecker PL. Cotrel-Dubousset instrumentation for adolescent idiopathic scoliosis. J Bone Joint Surg Am 1992;74(7):1056–1067

7. Wang JC, Sandhu HS, Yu WD, Minchew JT, Delamarter RB. MR parameters for imaging titanium spinal instrumentation. J Spinal Disord 1997;10(1):27–32

8. Kim JY, Song K, Kim KH, Rim DC, Yoon SH. Usefulness of simple rod rotation to correct curve of adolescent idiopathic scoliosis. J Korean Neurosurg Soc 2015;58(6):534–538

9. Anekstein Y, Mirovsky Y, Arnabitsky V, Gelfer Y, Zaltz I, Smorgick Y. Reversing the concept: correction of adolescent idiopathic scoliosis using the convex rod de-rotation maneuver. Eur Spine J 2012;21(10):1942–1949

10. Ito M, Abumi K, Kotani Y, et al. Simultaneous double-rod rotation technique in posterior instrumentation surgery for correction of adolescent idiopathic scoliosis. J Neurosurg Spine 2010;12(3):293–300

11. Dubousset J, Cotrel Y. Application technique of Cotrel-Dubousset instrumentation for scoliosis deformities. Clin Orthop Relat Res 1991;(264):103–110

12. Lee SM, Suk SI, Chung ER. Direct vertebral rotation: a new technique of three-dimensional deformity correction with segmental pedicle screw fixation in adolescent idiopathic scoliosis. Spine 2004;29(3):343–349

13. Pollock FE, Pollock FE Jr. Idiopathic scoliosis: correction of lateral and rotational deformities using the Cotrel-Dubousset spinal instrumentation system. South Med J 1990;83(2):161–165

14. Gardner-Morse M, Stokes IA. Three-dimensional simulations of the scoliosis derotation maneuver with Cotrel-Dubousset instrumentation. J Biomech 1994;27(2):177–181

15. Krismer M, Bauer R, Sterzinger W. Scoliosis correction by Cotrel-Dubousset instrumentation. The effect of derotation and three dimensional correction. Spine 1992;17(8, Suppl):S263–S269

16. Gray J, Smith B, Ashley R, et al. Derotational analysis of Cotrel-Dubousset instrumentation in idiopathic scoliosis. Spine 1992;17(11):391–393

17. Labelle H, Dansereau J, Bellefleur C, et al. Comparison between preoperative and postoperative three-dimensional reconstructions of idiopathic scoliosis with the Cotrel-Dubousset procedure. Spine 1995;20(23):2487–2492

18. Ghanem IB, Hagnere F, Dubousset JF, Watier B, Skalli W, Lavaste F. Intraoperative optoelectronic analysis of three-dimensional vertebral displacement after Cotrel-Dubousset rod rotation. A preliminary report. Spine 1997;22(16):1913–1921

19. Labelle H, Dansereau J, Bellefleur C, de Guise J, Rivard CH, Poitras B. Peroperative three-dimensional correction of idiopathic scoliosis with the Cotrel-Dubousset procedure. Spine 1995;20(12):1406–1409

20. Stokes IA, Bigalow LC, Moreland MS. Three-dimensional spinal curvature in idiopathic scoliosis. J Orthop Res 1987;5(1):102–113

21. Suk SI, Lee CK, Kim WJ, Chung YJ, Park YB. Segmental pedicle screw fixation in the treatment of thoracic idiopathic scoliosis. Spine 1995;20(12):1399–1405

22. Ecker ML, Betz RR, Trent PS, et al. Computer tomography evaluation of Cotrel-Dubousset instrumentation in idiopathic scoliosis. Spine 1988;13(10):1141–1144

23. Tang X, Zhao J, Zhang Y. Radiographic, clinical, and patients' assessment of segmental direct vertebral body derotation versus simple rod derotation in main thoracic adolescent idiopathic scoliosis: a prospective, comparative cohort study. Eur Spine J 2015;24(2):298–305

24. Pratt RK, Burwell RG, Cole AA, Webb JK. Patient and parental perception of adolescent idiopathic scoliosis before and after surgery in comparison with surface and radiographic measurements. Spine 2002;27(14):1543–1550, discussion 1551–1552

25. Carlson BB, Burton DC, Asher MA. Comparison of trunk and spine deformity in adolescent idiopathic scoliosis. Scoliosis 2013;8(1):2

26. Erkula G, Sponseller PD, Kiter AE. Rib deformity in scoliosis. Eur Spine J 2003;12(3):281–287

27. Delorme S, Labelle H, Aubin CE, et al. Intraoperative comparison of two instrumentation techniques for the correction of adolescent idiopathic scoliosis. Rod rotation and translation. Spine 1999;24(19):2011–2017, discussion 2018

28. Suk SI. Pedicle screw instrumentation for adolescent idiopathic scoliosis: the insertion technique, the fusion levels and direct vertebral rotation. Clin Orthop Surg 2011;3(2):89–100

29. Terai H, Toyoda H, Suzuki A, et al. A new corrective technique for adolescent idiopathic scoliosis: convex manipulation using 6.35 mm diameter pure titanium rod followed by concave fixation using 6.35 mm diameter titanium alloy. Scoliosis 2015;10(Suppl 2):S14

30. Wu X, Yang S, Xu W, et al. Comparative intermediate and long-term results of pedicle screw and hook instrumentation in posterior correction and fusion of idiopathic thoracic scoliosis. J Spinal Disord Tech 2010;23(7):467–473

31. Zifang H, Hengwei F, Yaolong D, et al. Convex-rod derotation maneuver on Lenke Type I adolescent idiopathic scoliosis. Neurosurgery 2017;81(5):844–851

32. Kaliya-Perumal AK, Yeh YC, Niu CC, Chen LH, Chen WJ, Lai PL. Is convex derotation equally effective as concave derotation for achieving adequate correction of selective Lenke's Type-1 scoliosis? Indian J Orthop 2018;52(4):363–368

33. Smorgick Y, Millgram MA, Anekstein Y, Floman Y, Mirovsky Y. Accuracy and safety of thoracic pedicle screw placement in spinal deformities. J Spinal Disord Tech 2005;18(6):522–526

34. Wang S, Qiu Y, Liu W, et al. The potential risk of spinal cord injury from pedicle screw at the apex of adolescent idiopathic thoracic scoliosis: magnetic resonance imaging evaluation. BMC Musculoskelet Disord 2015;16:310

35. Uçar BY. A new corrective technique for adolescent idiopathic scoliosis (Ucar's convex rod rotation). J Craniovertebr Junction Spine 2014;5(3):114–117

29 Double-Rod Derotation Technique for Adolescent Idiopathic Scoliosis

İdris Avcı and Salim Şentürk

Introduction

The term "scoliosis" is defined as a three-dimensional deformity of the spine and derives from the ancient Greek word "skolios" meaning crooked or curved. Adolescent idiopathic scoliosis (AIS) is the most common type and is seen in skeletally immature children between 10 and 18 years of age characterized by a lateral deviation of at least 10 degrees, usually combined with a rotation of the vertebrae and most often reduced kyphosis in thoracic curves. The overall prevalence of AIS is estimated as 0.47 to 5.2% in the current literature.[1] There is no known cause for AIS. Potential reasons are believed to be a multifactorial combination of genetic, hormonal, and environmental external factors causing asymmetric spine growth. Most adolescents with AIS do not show any medical conditions except the spinal deformity although a positive family history could be identified in 30% of all cases.[2] Diagnosis is made by plain and bending X-rays. A vertical line is drawn from the center of the mandibula or the C7 plumb line to the central vertical line. Any shift from this line with a Cobb angle of above 10 degrees is diagnosed as scoliosis (**Fig. 29.1**). Most cases are mild, and do not show any kind of symptoms. Observation for a 6 to 12 months period is advised for curves between 10 and 25 degrees until skeletal maturity is reached. For curves between 25 and 45 degrees, bracing for 16 to 23 hours per day is advised. Although it does not correct the scoliosis, it is shown to slow down curve progression in most of the patients.

In more severe cases, especially in curvatures above 40 degrees, which account for 0.3% of all patients with AIS, the deformation becomes more obvious cosmetically and psychological distress increases; walking difficulties, neuromuscular deficits due to stenosis of the spinal canal, or cardiopulmonary problems secondary to depressed thoracic cavity can occur and surgery is indicated.[3] As there are anterior and anterolateral approaches for surgical treatment for AIS, posterior instrumentation is the gold standard. In 1962, Paul Harrington was one of the first surgeons to treat AIS patients with posterior fixation (mostly with hook systems) and distraction. Although this technique was used over two decades, follow-up results were not very satisfactory, as it did not provide adequate correction of the coronal alignment and did show any effect on decreasing the rib hump.[4]

So, various derotation maneuvers after classic posterior transpedicular instrumentation surgery have been developed through the years. In the 1980s, Cotrel and Dubousset introduced the multi-hook segmental instrumentation technique which was later modified into pedicle screw constructs and single rod maneuvers in which the rod was pulled toward the concavity which became the gold standard for a while as the "single concave rod rotation" (SCRR).[5] Later, biomechanical studies revealed that SCRR has limited impact on vertebral derotation, and additionally cause apical vertebra rotation.[6] As most previous approaches were indirect and inaccurate, Lee et al reported the direct vertebral rotation (DVR) technique, in which direct rotational force is applied on the apical vertebra on the opposite side

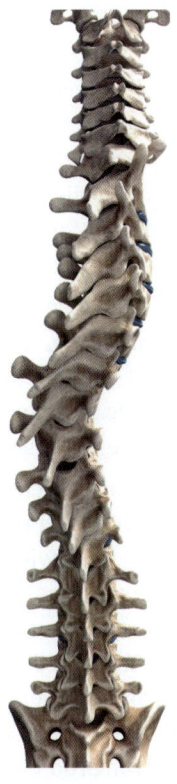

Fig. 29.1 Three-dimensional model illustration of spine showing scoliosis.

before the rod insertion. This can also be modified to single rod rotation maneuvers either on the convex or the concave side.[7] Although the DVR maneuver provides favorable outcomes in the form of sufficient alignment, it may not be suitable for excessive, double or triple curves (Lenke 2–5).[8] More recently, a dual/double- rod derotation technique (DRD) has been introduced; the authors mainly will focus on this technique in this chapter. In DRD, simultaneous rod application and derotation can improve the correction in the frontal and sagittal planes. Furthermore, by using pre-bent rods in which less kyphosis on the convex side and overbending on the level of the apical vertebrae on the concave side are applied, axial plane reduction can be achieved.

Definition of the Technique and Indications

- The surgery is performed under general anesthesia. Neuromonitoring probes are placed and each change in motor- or sensory-evoked potential (MEP, SEP) must be noted during each step of the surgery. Deep muscle relaxants should be avoided as they may interfere with neuromonitoring results. The patient is then put in prone position with padding under the axilla and inguinal area to overcome any neural or vascular injury. Under the fluoroscopic C-arm the surgical area is marked, cleansed, and draped sterile.

- A midline skin incision is made in concordance to the level of the instrumentation planned. Cutaneous and subcutaneous cuts are made with monopolar cautery. Paravertebral muscles are dissected and retracted and posterior elements in the form of spinous processes, laminae, and facets are visualized.

- Under fluoroscopic guidance polyaxial screws are inserted transpedicularly (**Fig. 29.2**). As each case is unique, the amount of laminectomy and the type of osteotomy (Ponte, pedicle subtraction osteotomy etc.), if any, depend on each patient individually.

- Pre-bent titanium rods are placed on the concave and convex sides of the deformity (**Fig. 29.3**). It is important that the rods should be bent with less kyphosis on the convex side, whereas overbending should be achieved on the apical vertebrae on the concave side. The screw nuts are put but not tightened closely to allow some movement. The surgeon and the assistant then move to the concave side. As the assistant on the concave side holds the rod with a strong rod holder, the surgeon pulls the rod of the convex side to the midline. MEP and SEP

must be monitored closely as this is the step where the risk of major neural injury is the largest. When the optimal alignment is reached the screw nuts are tightened and torqued.

- After hemostasis and insertion of drains, the wound is closed in anatomical fashion and the surgery is finished.

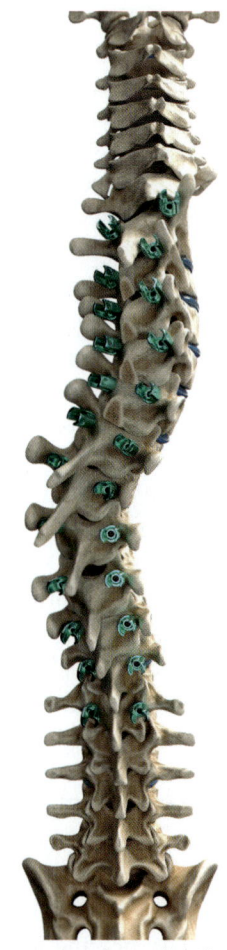

Fig. 29.2 Three-dimensional model illustration of spine after polyaxial pedicle screws are placed.

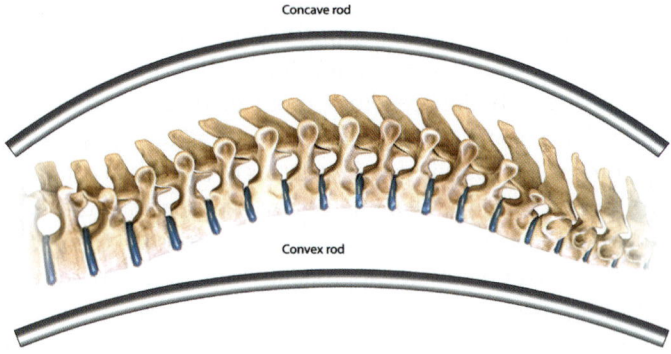

Fig. 29.3 Illustration of the rods bent in concave and convex sides.

Which Patients Are Suitable for the Dual-Rod Derotation Technique?

Every case must be evaluated individually. In general, most skeletally mature patients with a Cobb angle above 40 degrees are candidates for surgery. Secondary causes for the scoliosis need to be excluded before making the decision. Although anterior, anterolateral, and combined approaches are available, the gold standard to date is posterior instrumentation surgery, as most spinal surgeons are familiar with posterior approaches to the spine and its anatomy. The risk of major hemorrhage, and visceral and cardiopulmonary injury are less compared to the other approaches and show better final outcomes in spinal alignment postoperatively. To summarize, every patient with AIS who is suitable for posterior surgery is also suitable for the DRD technique (**Figs. 29.4** and **29.5**).

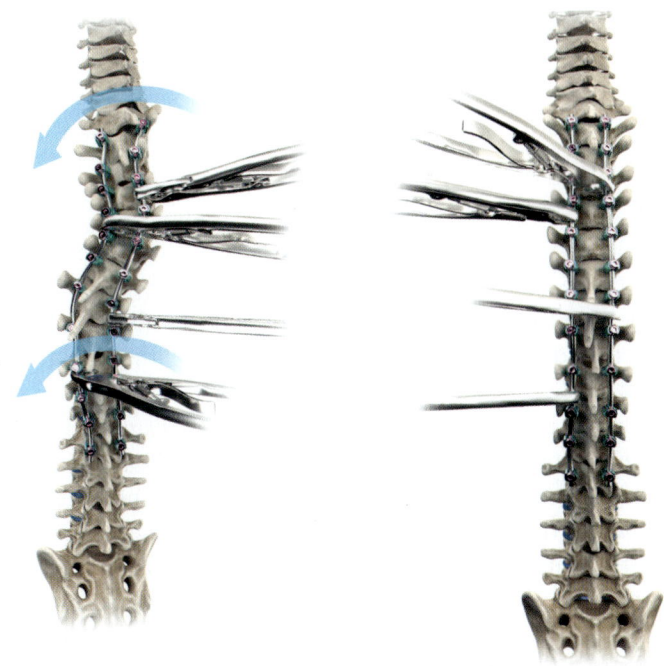

Fig. 29.4 Illustration of the double-rod derotation.

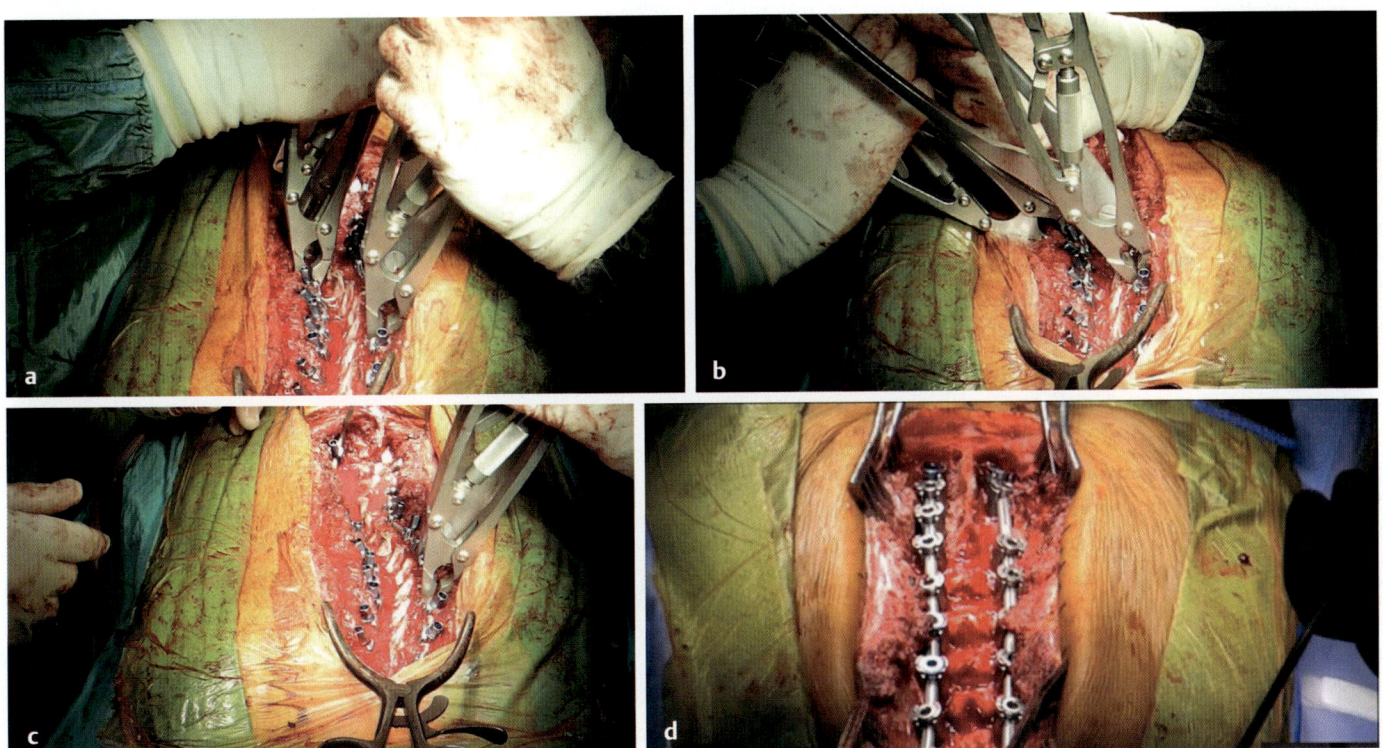

Fig. 29.5 (a–d) Steps of double-rod derotation during surgery.

Advantages and Disadvantages of the Dual-Rod Derotation Technique Compared to Other Posterior Instrumentation Techniques

Studies have shown that simple posterior instrumentation and distraction introduced by Harrington is not enough to achieve sufficient coronal alignment and did not have any effect in decreasing the rib hump.[4] Despite the fact that SCRR by Cotrel and Dubousset show better postoperative correction of the curvatures, the drawback of causing apical vertebra rotation and thoracic hypokyphosis makes it not an ideal option for treatment.[6] To date, DVR either with or without single rod rotation and DRD is considered as the most favorable technique in posterior instrumentation surgery for correction of AIS. Both show excellent results in postoperative spinal alignment. Both result in better coronal balance and decreased rib hump after surgery. In 2016, Pankowski et al compared surgical outcomes of 38 patients with AIS who were treated with either DVR or SCRR. The DVR patients showed a lesser deviation of the C7 plumb line, lesser apical vertebrae rotation, and decreased rib hump in comparison to those who underwent SCRR.[9] Okkaoğlu et al published their surgical outcomes of DRD in 23 AIS patients who showed excellent improvement of coronal alignment in Cobb angle, decreased thoracic lordosis, and increased thoracic kyphosis.[10] Although, both DVR and DRD are good choices for surgical treatment in patients with AIS, with DRD most favorable outcomes can be achieved in patients with excessive curvatures and/or double or triple curvatures (Lenke 2–5).[8] In DVR the applicable force for correction is limited. Without using rods as additional instruments the manual pull and push movements of the surgical team may not be enough especially when the vertebrae are continuously fixated which restrict action. Too harsh maneuvers can result in screw pullouts or iatrogenic fractures of vertebral elements. Using single rods can also be more challenging than two rods while doing these actions. The advantage of the DRD maneuver is that with the correct amount of posterior decompression like laminectomies or osteotomies depending on the severity of the case, coronal and sagittal alignment can be achieved by simple physical force without any other tools than screws and rods and a rod holder. Results and degree of correction can be seen instantly while derotating. The use of neuromonitoring during this step is crucial. But there are also pitfalls. The amount of correction despite the area of decompression or osteotomies is limited. Curves greater than 110 degrees are very difficult to correct by posterior-only techniques and need further anterior or lateral approaches. Compared to open anterior or thoracoscopic surgery more levels of instrumentation are necessary. Especially in skeletally immature patients, higher levels of fusion lead to decreased flexibility and limited spinal range of motion. In patients who are still in their growth period, early fusion can lead to further asymmetric spinal growth which can again result in iatrogenic deformities.[11] But this can be overcome using tube or magnetic rods which tend to expand as the patient grows.

Key Points

- AIS is the most common type of scoliosis characterized by three-dimensional deformity of the spine with a lateral deviation of at least 10 degrees in children aged between 10 and 18 years.

- Although in mild cases clinical observation, physical therapy, and bracing show satisfactory results, in symptomatic patients with a Cobb angle above 40 degrees surgery is inevitable.

- Posterior instrumentation remains the gold standard for surgery in AIS.

- In the DRD technique pre-bent rods are placed on the concave and convex sides in which the rods should be bent with less kyphosis on the convex side, whereas overbending should be achieved on the apical vertebrae on the concave side. The screw nuts are not tightened closely to allow some movement. As the assistant on the concave side holds the rod with a strong rod holder, the surgeon pulls the rod of the convex side to the midline using neuromonitoring. When the optimal alignment is reached the screw nuts are tightened and torqued.

- The advantage of the DRD maneuver is that with the correct amount of posterior decompression like laminectomies or osteotomies depending on the severity of the case, coronal and sagittal alignment can be achieved by simple physical force without any other tools than screws and rods and a rod holder and results and degree of correction can be seen instantly while derotating.

Conclusion

Posterior transpedicular fixation is the gold standard in AIS patients with a Cobb angle above 45 degrees. Recent data show that direct vertebral rotation and DRD have the most favorable outcomes. DRD is a modification of the classic posterior transpedicular approach in which, depending on the severity of the case, with the correct number of laminectomies or/and osteotomies, coronal and sagittal alignment can be achieved just by screws, rods, rod holders, and physical force.

References

1. Konieczny MR, Senyurt H, Krauspe R. Epidemiology of adolescent idiopathic scoliosis. J Child Orthop 2013;7(1):3–9
2. Kikanloo SR, Tarpada SP, Cho W. Etiology of adolescent idiopathic scoliosis: a literature review. Asian Spine J 2019;13(3):519–526
3. Horne JP, Flannery R, Usman S. Adolescent idiopathic scoliosis: diagnosis and management. Am Fam Physician 2014;89(3):193–198
4. Aaro S, Dahlborn M. The effect of Harrington instrumentation on the longitudinal axis rotation of the apical vertebra and on the spinal and rib-cage deformity in idiopathic scoliosis studied by computer tomography. Spine 1982;7(5):456–462
5. Cotrel Y, Dubousset J, Guillaumat M. New universal instrumentation in spinal surgery. Clin Orthop Relat Res 1988; 227(227):10–23
6. Stokes IA, Bigalow LC, Moreland MS. Three-dimensional spinal curvature in idiopathic scoliosis. J Orthop Res 1987;5(1): 102–113
7. Lee SM, Suk SI, Chung ER. Direct vertebral rotation: a new technique of three-dimensional deformity correction with segmental pedicle screw fixation in adolescent idiopathic scoliosis. Spine 2004;29(3):343–349
8. Giacomini S, Di Silvestre M, Lolli F, et al. Is there a better derotation manoeuvre in posterior correction of thoracic adolescent idiopathic scoliosis? Scoliosis 2015;10(Suppl 1): O69
9. Pankowski R, Roclawski M, Ceynowa M, Mikulicz M, Mazurek T, Kloc W. Direct vertebral rotation versus single concave rod rotation: low-dose intraoperative computed tomography evaluation of spine derotation in adolescent idiopathic scoliosis surgery. Spine 2016;41(10):864–871
10. Okkaoğlu MC, Evren AT, Demirkale İ, Yaradılmış YU, Altay M. The effect of simultaneous dual-rod derotation technique on thoracal kyphosis in patients with adolescent idiopathic scoliosis. Turk J Clin Lab 2022;1:71–75
11. Sud A, Tsirikos AI. Current concepts and controversies on adolescent idiopathic scoliosis: Part II. Indian J Orthop 2013;47(3):219–229

30 Direct Vertebral Segmental Derotation for Adolescent Idiopathic Scoliosis

Ender Ofluoğlu and Mehmet Zileli

Introduction

Idiopathic scoliosis is a deformity that affects the spinal column in all dimensions. In addition to the deviation in the coronal plane, thoracic hypokyphosis in the sagittal plane and intravertebral/intervertebral rotation in the transverse plane are also seen.[1] Correction of scoliosis by using thoracic pedicle screw constructs was first described in 1999 by Suk et al.[2] Then the standard surgery for adolescent idiopathic scoliosis (AIS) became posterior correction using pedicle screws.[3] Pedicle screws provided a very strong fixation and helped in improved correction of the scoliotic curves. However, rib hump reduction and reduction of the apical rotation were limited. The enhanced instrumentation techniques and ability to apply corrective rotational forces have provided significant correction of axial rotation. Two methods can achieve derotation of the spine: Derotation of the whole thoracic curvature (en-bloc vertebral derotation) or derotation at each segment (direct segmental derotation).

Definition of the Technique

The concept of direct vertebral segmental derotation (DVSD) involves applying posterior rotational forces in the opposite direction of the deformity. Pedicle screws extend from posterior to anterior and attach to all three vertebral columns. They then transmit the forces applied from the posterior to the anterior. The rotational deformity can be corrected by sharing the rotational force with the whole vertebral body. Long screw derotators on each curve side help apply torque on the pedicle screws. Direct vertebral rotation (DVR) can correct intervertebral rotation and whole scoliosis. Its direction must be opposite to the vertebral rotation. In case there is a right thoracic curve, a clockwise rotation of the apical vertebrae should be applied. In general, the DVR direction must be opposite to the rotational deformity. It should also be counterclockwise in the transverse plane. However, the direction of DVR on the lower instrumented vertebral screws must be in accordance with the compensatory lumbar curve. At this level, the surgeons must avoid the application of compression or distraction. Such compression or distraction may cause complications like flat back deformity.[1]

Indications

The rib hump is a result of the axial rotation of a scoliotic curve, and it is the patient's main reason for cosmetic dissatisfaction.[4–6] One of the main goals of deformity surgery in scoliosis is decreasing rib prominence. The more apical vertebral rotation is, the more correction of the rib hump.[7] Harrington rods cannot provide apical derotation. Weatherley et al evaluated changes after Harrington distraction and posterior fusion and reported rib prominences had worsened 1 year after surgery in 36% of their patients.[8] Apical derotation can be better provided by pedicle screw instrumentations, although it ranged from 9 to 40% of apical rotational correction.[9] Another option to improve cosmetic correction is to use thoracoplasty in addition to fixation.[10] Exposure of the ribs by a more lateral incision and resection of four to six prominent ribs help to reduce the rib hump asymmetry quite efficiently. Pedicle screw instrumentation plus thoracoplasty can reduce rib prominence by 71%; however, it is only 17% by scoliosis correction.[11]

Using DVSD with pedicle screw constructs can significantly correct apical rotation. Min et al used thoracoplasty whose inclinometer exceeded 15 degrees preoperatively; they reported 44% rib prominence improvement with thoracoplasty, while improvement was 37% without thoracoplasty.[12] Similar results of best correction by using DVBD and thoracoplasty have also been reported by Suk et al.[9]

Surgical Procedure

- The pedicle screws are inserted at each segment on the thoracic concave side and at every second or third on the thoracic convex side of the curves.

- Counterclockwise rotation of the contoured rod on the concave side is carried out without any compression or distraction (DVSD) (**Fig. 30.1**).
- Screw derotators[4–6,9,12] are inserted onto the pedicle screws both on the concave and convex sides (**Figs. 30.2** and **30.3**).

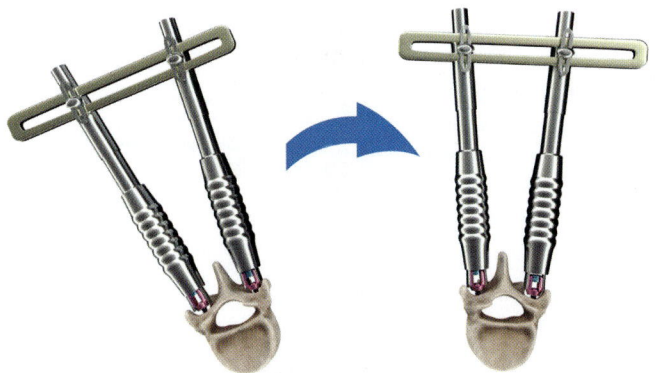

Fig. 30.1 The pre-contoured rod is rotated on the correction sides (counterclockwise) without any compression or distraction.

- Screw derotators must be rotated in the opposite direction (clockwise) of the rod derotation (**Figs. 30.4** and **30.5**).
- The lowermost pedicle screw(s) must be rotated depending on the unfused lumbar curve (**Figs. 30.2** and **30.3**).
- The concave rod is locked in the corrected position; another contoured rod is placed on the convex side and locked in place.
- Two cross-links may be placed to connect the rods. In the end, bone grafts are placed to provide posterior fusion.

Complication Avoidance

The vertebral derotation maneuver decreases thoracic kyphosis since it elongates the anterior column of the thoracic spine by shifting the convex wall and the anterior wall in the ventral direction. Suppose a hypokyphotic spine has occurred after completing en-bloc and segmental

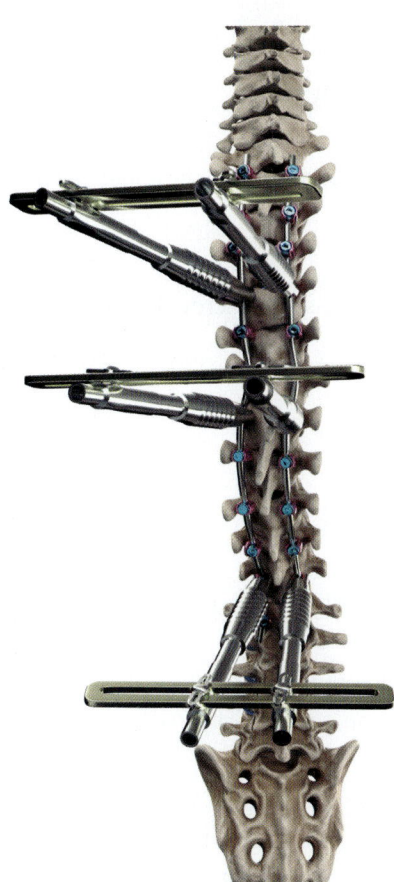

Fig. 30.2 Four to eight screw derotators inserted into the pedicle screws of the juxta-apical vertebrae on the concave and convex sides.

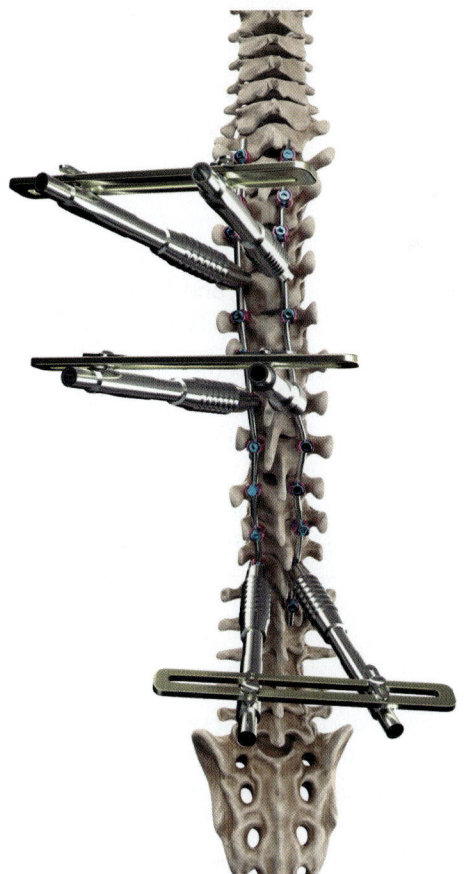

Fig. 30.3 Depending on the unfused lumbar curve, the lowermost pedicle screw(s) are rotated first. Turning the screw derotators on the caudal end starts correction.

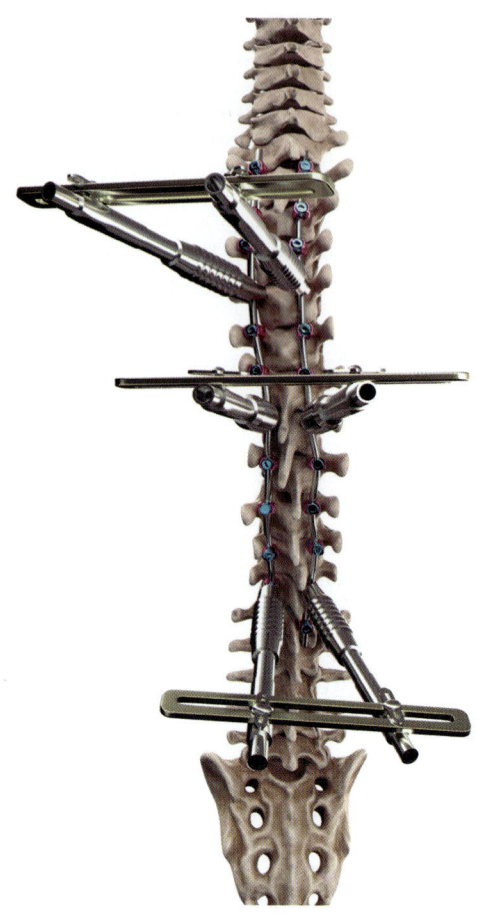

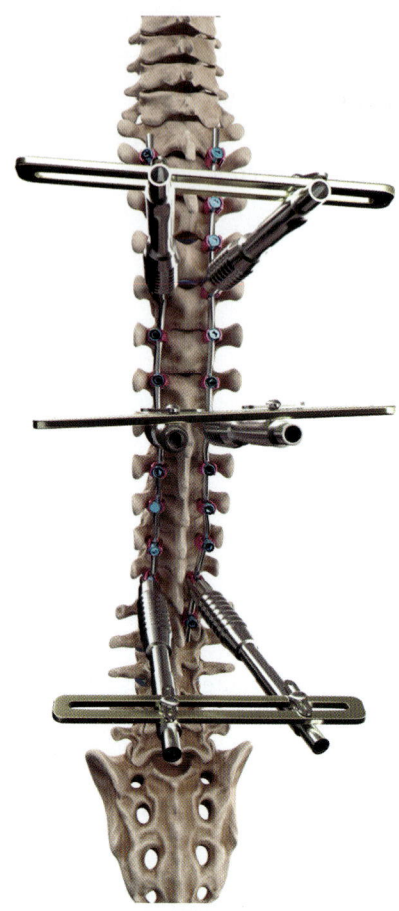

Fig. 30.4 Then the medial screw derotators join the rotation and correction.

Fig. 30.5 After cranial end rod derotation, a total reduction is achieved. Two cross-links should better be added to connect the two rods.

derotations. In that case, hypokyphosis should be reduced by trying to give kyphosis to the rods with in-situ benders.

Another complication is pedicular screw breakage of the medial wall of the pedicle. It can cause spinal cord compression during the derotation maneuver. To prevent this, place pedicle screws on all segmental vertebrae, especially in the apical vertebrae, and ensure load sharing while not taking risks and screwing in suspicious pedicles.

Tips and Tricks

Any possible level of pedicle screws, especially in the apical vertebrae, is one of the essential points for a direct segmental and en-bloc derotation maneuver. To perform these maneuvers, unique tubular systems are needed to hold the screw heads of the pedicle screws. While multiple derotation tubes are needed for the en-bloc derotation

maneuver, only two set-screw screwdrivers can work in segmental derotation.

Key Points

- Full pedicular screwing of scoliosis, predominantly apical rotated vertebras.

- Tubular derotation system compatible with pedicular screws is needed.

- Rod derotation should be applied first, then direct en-bloc vertebral derotation, and finally, segmental derotation should be applied.

- After the derotational maneuver is finished, the thoracic spines should be evaluated for hypokyphosis; if a hypokyphotic spine has occurred, kyphosis should be re-established with rod benders in situ.

References

1. Lee SM, Suk SI, Chung ER. Direct vertebral rotation: a new technique of three-dimensional deformity correction with segmental pedicle screw fixation in adolescent idiopathic scoliosis. Spine 2004;29(3):343–349
2. Suk SI, Kim WJ, Kim JH, Lee SM. Restoration of thoracic kyphosis in the hypokyphotic spine: a comparison between multiple-hook and segmental pedicle screw fixation in adolescent idiopathic scoliosis. J Spinal Disord 1999;12(6):489–495
3. Kim YJ, Lenke LG, Kim J, et al. Comparative analysis of pedicle screw versus hybrid instrumentation in posterior spinal fusion of adolescent idiopathic scoliosis. Spine 2006;31(3):291–298
4. Aaro S, Dahlborn M. The effect of Harrington instrumentation on the longitudinal axis rotation of the apical vertebra and on the spinal and rib-cage deformity in idiopathic scoliosis studied by computer tomography. Spine 1982;7(5):456–462
5. Geissele AE, Ogilvie JW, Cohen M, Bradford DS. Thoracoplasty for the treatment of rib prominence in thoracic scoliosis. Spine (Phila Pa 1976). 1994;19(14):1636–1642
6. Theologis TN, Jefferson RJ, Simpson AH, Turner-Smith AR, Fairbank JC. Quantifying the cosmetic defect of adolescent idiopathic scoliosis. Spine 1993;18(7):909–912
7. Thulbourne T, Gillespie R. The rib hump in idiopathic scoliosis. Measurement, analysis and response to treatment. J Bone Joint Surg Br 1976;58(1):64–71
8. Weatherley CR, Draycott V, O'Brien JF, et al. The rib deformity in adolescent idiopathic scoliosis. A prospective study to evaluate changes after Harrington distraction and posterior fusion. J Bone Joint Surg Br 1987;69(2):179–182
9. Suk SI, Lee CK, Kim WJ, Chung YJ, Park YB. Segmental pedicle screw fixation in the treatment of thoracic idiopathic scoliosis. Spine 1995;20(12):1399–1405
10. Glassman SD, Bridwell K, Dimar JR, Horton W, Berven S, Schwab F. The impact of positive sagittal balance in adult spinal deformity. Spine 2005;30(18):2024–2029
11. Harvey CJ Jr, Betz RR, Clements DH, Huss GK, Clancy M. Are there indications for partial rib resection in patients with adolescent idiopathic scoliosis treated with Cotrel-Dubousset instrumentation? Spine 1993;18(12):1593–1598
12. Min K, Waelchli B, Hahn F. Primary thoracoplasty and pedicle screw instrumentation in thoracic idiopathic scoliosis. Eur Spine J 2005;14(8):777–782

Yunus Emre Özdemir, Çağlar Yılgör, and Ahmet Alanay

Introduction

Scoliosis is the most common spinal deformity in children, and spinal fusion surgery is the gold standard treatment for children with severe scoliosis. Although spinal fusion has good long-term results in terms of deformity correction, it also brings some problems, such as growth arrest and permanent limitation of spinal motion.[1] Fusion may further cause adjacent segment degeneration in the long-term follow-up.[2] These consequences of fusion surgery have led to search for nonfusion solutions which can preserve spinal motion and intervertebral disc health, while correcting the deformity. Vertebral body tethering (VBT) is an important step toward this direction.

There is still a paucity of data; thus, the clinical value of VBT remains unclear. A better understanding of ideal bone age, ideal curve location and size, and optimal timing for VBT is needed to identify the patients for whom this procedure is likely to be successful. Nonetheless, as of today, VBT has become an alternative to fusion surgery, as a surgical growth modulation technique, in a select group of patients who exceed the limit for brace treatment. It has been about a decade now that VBT has been applied more routinely, and in this chapter, we will discuss current literature blended with our own clinical experience.

Definition of the Technique

VBT is the application of vertebral body screws on the convexity and the attachment of a polyethylene tether that is then tightened. The main purpose of tethering is to maintain a more normal spinal contour while preserving motion. The working principle of this technique is based on the Hueter-Volkmann law which states that the growth plates under pressure grow slower than those which are not.[3] VBT aims to compress the growth plates on the convex side to inhibit vertebral body growth, while distracting the growth plates on the concave side to stimulate vertebral body growth. The remaining growth potential of the child will urge more growth on the concavity, thereby lessening or reversing the deformity and this is the reason why this technique is a viable alternative to fusion in skeletally immature patients (**Fig. 31.1**).

Biomechanical studies of tethering were first demonstrated in porcine[4] and goat[5] models. Then, in 2010, Crawford and Lenke reported the first case treated with VBT at the age of 8 with a 40-degree right thoracic curve.[6] It became more popular in the following years as the first published case series by Samdani et al had encouraging results.[7,8]

Surgical Technique

The child is placed in a lateral decubitus position with the convexity of the curve facing up. Intraoperative neuro-monitoring is used to monitor spinal cord function during surgery. A double lumen endotracheal tube is used for selective lung deflation which allows easier access to the thoracic vertebral bodies during surgery.

Approach to the thoracic cavity can be gained by three different methods: (1) Thoracoscopic, where the entire surgery is visualized via a camera and performed through ports using a monitor. (2) Video-assisted open thoracotomy, where a thoracic cage retractor is in place (regardless of the size of the incision) and the surgery, at least in part, is accompanied by a camera and a monitor. Some implants (i.e., cranial or more caudal ones) might or might not be placed using ports. (3) Open thoracotomy, where a thoracic cage retractor is in place (regardless of the size of the incision) and no camera or monitor is used throughout the surgery. Thoracic cavity anatomical structures are seen through direct vision. Some implants might or might not be placed using ports.

Abovementioned three approaches allow instrumentation down to L1, and occasionally to L2. A retroperitoneal approach is usually required for instrumentation to or below L2.[9]

Vertebral bodies planned to be instrumented are marked under fluoroscopy guidance. Along the length of the curve, the pleura is dissected off the lateral aspect of the vertebral bodies anterior to the rib heads. Since the implantation is done at the mid-corpus level, segmental vessels are dissected, and either coagulated or preserved depending on the case and surgeon's preference. Care must be taken to protect the intervertebral discs.

The screws are inserted anterior to the rib head and directed toward the concavity across the anterolateral aspect

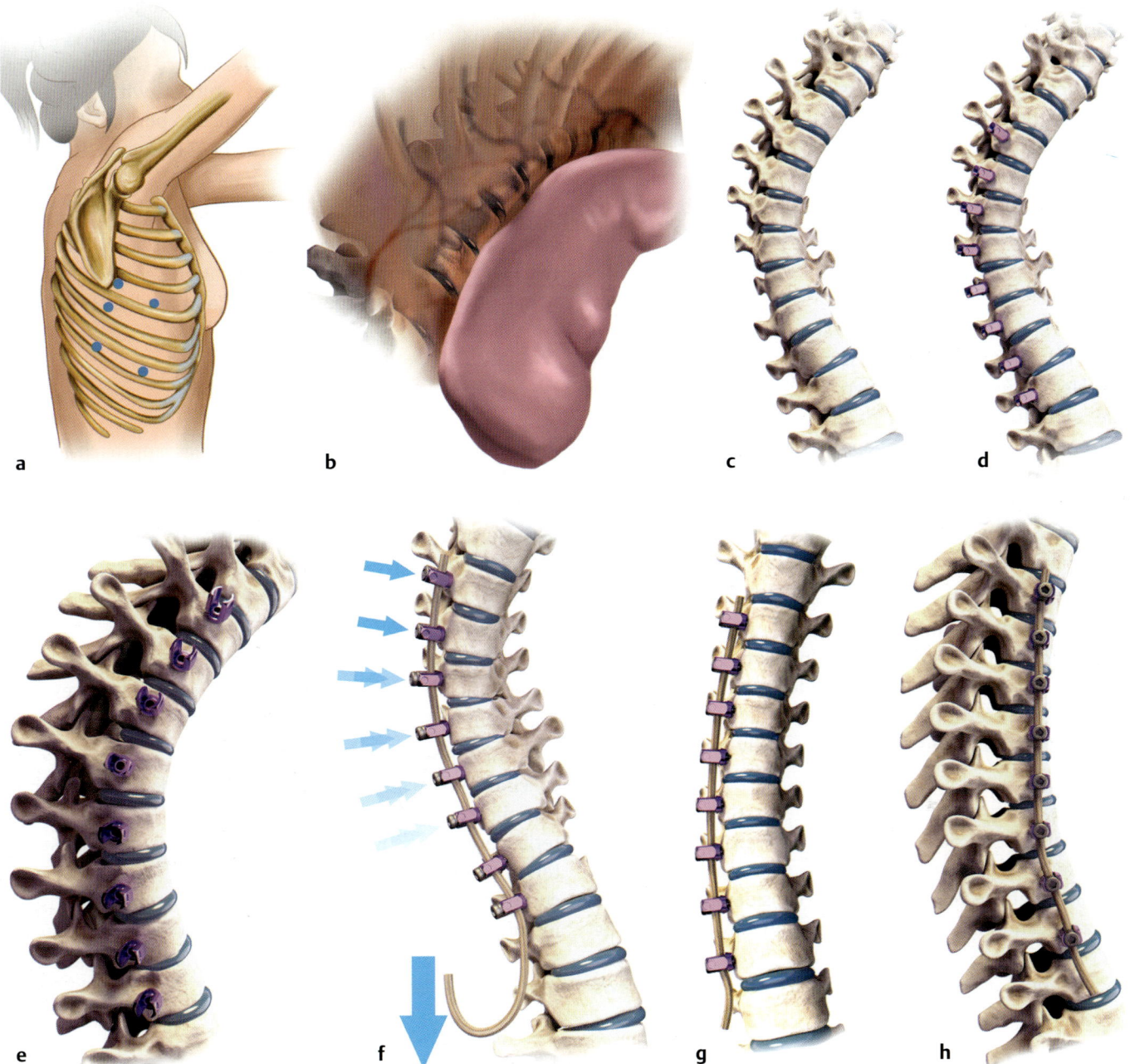

Fig. 31.1 Schematic view of surgical steps. In lateral decubitus position, the thoracoscopy portals are opened **(a)**. Lung is deflated and spinal column is observed after lung retraction **(b)**. On the convex side of the curvature **(c)**, vertebral body screws are placed **(d, e)**. Tether is placed onto the screw heads **(f)**. The curve is reduced by tightening the tether **(g, h)**.

of the vertebral body. The polyethylene tether is then placed starting from the most cranial end. Each nut is tightened one by one while achieving correction through both tensioning of the tether and translation of the spine. However, there is no consensus on the amount of the tension force to be applied to each segment.[9] Surgeons usually prefer to tighten to a magnitude that will make the end plates parallel to each other at the apical levels and tighten less in the cranial and caudal ends of the construct to avoid overcorrection.

Before the wound is closed, the thoracic cavity should be irrigated, and a meticulous hemostasis should be performed. The lung is re-inflated, and a chest tube drain is placed.

Indications

The indications for VBT are still uncertain. Perhaps the most important factor to consider for a growth modulation technique is the child's remaining growth potential. Unfortunately, there is no precise method to determine that, and we tend to use scales and classifications such as Risser scale[10] and Sanders classification,[11] and depend on family history, height of the parents, height of the child, and secondary sex characteristics and menarche status. There is no definite limit on age. Main concerns with early applications of this procedure are that the current instruments may not be suitable for younger children with smaller vertebral bodies, and that this powerful technique can lead to overcorrection.

In 2019, VBT got U.S. Food and Drug Administration (FDA) Humanitarian Device Exemption (HDE) approval for skeletally immature (Sanders score of 2 to 5 and Risser scale of 0 to 4) scoliosis patients that require surgical treatment for progressive idiopathic scoliosis. The approval comprised thoracic and lumbar curves of 30 to 65 degrees in magnitude (in practice it is applied as 40 to 65 degrees) for patients who failed bracing or were intolerant to brace wear. Contraindications were listed as a T-score of −1.5 or less, and previous surgery at the spinal levels of planned VBT.[12]

More recent Conformité Européen approval pointed toward very similar indications for patients whose osseous structure is dimensionally adequate to accommodate screw fixation, as determined by radiographic imaging. One difference was that this approval was only for Lenke type 1 curves.

The flexibility of the curve also needs to be evaluated. In general, at least 50% flexibility is desired. Although rare in adolescent idiopathic scoliosis (AIS), hyperkyphosis measuring above 40 degrees is considered a relative contraindication in order to avoid potential hyperkyphosing effect of anterior surgery.[8] As most of the AIS patients are hypokyphotic, a more anterior placement of the screws

has been suggested to increase initial and growth-related kyphosing effect. However, there is no evidence, yet, that kyphosis can be restored by VBT. **Table 31.1** summarizes kyphosis restoration results of studies with >2 years follow-up. It is the authors' preference to perform fusion to restore kyphosis in patients with T2–T12 kyphosis of less than 10 degrees.

Regarding axial rotation, there is not yet any threshold which may affect the decision-making for VBT. However, there is a common consensus that patients with hump size of more than 20 degrees may not be good candidates for VBT.

Complication Avoidance

As in other thoracic surgeries, VBT has approach-related complications such as pleural effusion, atelectasis, pneumothorax, and chylothorax. It might be a good option to perform these surgeries together with a thoracic surgeon in order to both avoid lung complications and speed up the learning curve. Early postoperative pulmonary rehabilitation is also essential to improve lung function.

In order to prevent pressure ulcers and nerve injuries to the brachial plexus, and ulnar and peroneal nerves, it is important to place soft gels during the surgical positioning.[17]

Tether breakage and overcorrection are considered specific complications for this surgery. The most common complication affecting VBT patients was reported to be tether breakage.[18] But, it is not always easy to demonstrate tether breakage with plain radiography. An increase in curve magnitude should arouse suspicion, and an increase in coronal angulation of >5 degrees between two adjacent screws suggests tether breakage.[13] In one study, it was reported that breakages occurred most frequently between

Table 31.1 Summary of the literature with >2 years follow-up regarding kyphosis restoration

	Number of patients	Age (mean, range)	Sanders score (mean, range)	Risser score (mean, range)	Preop kyphosis*, (mean ± SD, range)	First Erect kyphosis* (mean ± SD, range)	Last follow-up kyphosis* (mean ± SD, range)
Samdani et al[7]	11	12 (9–14)	3.4 (2–3)	0.6	20.8 ± 13.3 (1.7–46.0)	13.5 ± 8.7 (0.2–30.0)	21.6 ± 12.7 (4.9–37.6)
Newton et al[13]	17	11 (9–14)	2.5 (2–3)	0	25 ± 13 (9–54)	22 ± 14 (1–62)	22 ± 10 (11–43)
Newton et al[14]	23	12 (9–15)	2.5 (2–3)	0 (0–1)	25 ± 12 (6–54)	23 ± 12 (8–62)	19 ± 13 (22–52)
Miyanji et al[15]	112	13 (8–17)	-	0.5 (0–3)	18.6 ± 11.4 (−8–47)	18.8 ± 11.8 (−12–45)	21.4 ± 13.0 (−14–66)
Baroncini et al[16]	86	13	≤7	1.7 (0–4)	28.3 ± 13.8	-	33 ± 13

Abbreviation: SD, standard deviation.
Note: *Kyphosis reported between T5 and T12 in Samdani et al and Miyanji et al studies, between T2 and T12 in Newton et al studies, and between T1 and T12 in Baroncini et al study.

T9 and T12 and were detected at an average of 32.5 months after surgery.[19] Meyers et al reported large curve magnitude and limited flexibility as main preoperative risk factors and a large residual curve as postoperative risk factor.[20] If breakage occurs when the patient reaches skeletal maturity, revision surgery may not be necessary. To avoid breakage, double-row technique has been described, although the evidence for its effectiveness is limited. Perhaps, improved material and design will reduce the risk of these complications in the future.

Overcorrection has been reported as the second most common complication and the most common reason for reoperation.[18] Although remaining growth potential is indispensable for this surgery, the risk of overcorrection is high when applied too early. Wong et al[21] recommended that it should not be used in patients with open triradiate cartilage. Adjustment of initial correction is another strategy for avoiding this complication, but there is no consensus for the degree of surgical correction. We previously published a set of recommendations in an attempt to balance expected growth-dependent correction and index surgical correction.[22] **Table 31.2** summarizes an updated version of these recommendations. Although there is not enough evidence, temporary brace treatment affecting in the same or opposite direction of the tether may also help adjust final correction in some patients.

Tips and Tricks

- Patient positioning with dedicated pads is a key factor affecting kyphosis restoration and derotation.
- Relatively small curves, around 40 degrees, should be chosen as initial cases.
- During tether placement, zero tensioning of the cranial-most two screws, and using this foundation for the rest of tensioning helps prevent plowing of the cranial-most screw.
- External translation and derotation maneuvers applied to the screws using T-handles should precede correction gained by tether tensioning.
- Maximum positive tensioning should be applied to apical screws, while zero or negative tensioning should be applied to the caudal end of the construct around the thoracolumbar junction.
- Surgeons should be aware that there will be approximately 10 degrees of increase in the curve size in the first erect radiograph compared to intra-postoperative fluoroscopic images. This initial "slacking" will depend on the magnitude of compression as well as the presence of single versus dual rows of tethers.

Table 31.2 Authors' recommendations regarding patient selection and decision on the magnitude of surgical correction for patients in different Sanders skeletal maturity stages

Sanders stage	Recommendation	Rationale
1	With its current way of application, growth modulation should be avoided	Overcorrection, related mechanical complications, and reoperation might be inevitable
2	Either achieve less correction on the table and have >30 degrees Cobb angle postoperatively or Postpone surgery until later stages of Sanders 2 (i.e., closed triradiate cartilage) or Sanders 3	With the capability of growing more than 10 cm and achieving more than 30 degrees of correction, they might be prone to overcorrection and implant-related complications Intentional undercorrection might lead to ineffectiveness in growth modulation and result in progression of deformity Postponing surgery while trying to control the curves via bracing and exercises might be logical
3	Probably best candidates	Based on the amount of correction achieved and observation of less likelihood of overcorrection and mechanical complications, they are considered to grow enough to release the stresses on the tether, while reaching maturity before overcorrection occurs Correction to 15 degrees on the first erect images might be a good goal to aim for
4–5	Probably good candidates, however longer follow-up is warranted for stronger evidence on long-term tether survival	With the remaining growth of 3 to 5 cm on average and curve modulation of up to approximately 10 degrees, near-full correction on the table might be a logical goal Follow-up correction might be enough to release the tension on the tether
6–7	Longer follow-up is warranted for long-term tether integrity	They generally display a stable follow-up for at least 2 years Minimal growth potential suggests that the tether would be still under the tension that was loaded during the surgery

Key Points

- Estimation of the remaining growth potential is a key factor regarding the success of VBT surgery. One should not count on a single parameter, but depend on skeletal markers as well as clinical features in determining the remaining growth.

- Since it is a motion-preserving surgery, the health of the intervertebral discs is important for longevity of the construct and great care should be taken not to damage the intervertebral discs during the surgery.

- Patient positioning using dedicated pads is key in kyphosis restoration and derotation.

- Co-performing the surgery with a thoracic surgeon might help in avoiding lung complications, especially in the early part of the learning curve.

References

1. Kepler CK, Meredith DS, Green DW, Widmann RF. Long-term outcomes after posterior spine fusion for adolescent idiopathic scoliosis. Curr Opin Pediatr 2012;24(1):68–75

2. Hilibrand AS, Robbins M. Adjacent segment degeneration and adjacent segment disease: the consequences of spinal fusion? Spine J 2004;4(6, Suppl):190S–194S

3. Mehlman CT, Araghi A, Roy DR. Hyphenated history: the Hueter-Volkmann law. Am J Orthop 1997;26(11):798–800

4. Newton PO, Farnsworth CL, Upasani VV, Chambers RC, Varley E, Tsutsui S. Effects of intraoperative tensioning of an anterolateral spinal tether on spinal growth modulation in a porcine model. Spine 2011;36(2):109–117

5. Braun JT, Ogilvie JW, Akyuz E, Brodke DS, Bachus KN. Creation of an experimental idiopathic-type scoliosis in an immature goat model using a flexible posterior asymmetric tether. Spine 2006;31(13):1410–1414

6. Crawford CH III, Lenke LG. Growth modulation by means of anterior tethering resulting in progressive correction of juvenile idiopathic scoliosis: a case report. J Bone Joint Surg Am 2010;92(1):202–209

7. Samdani AF, Ames RJ, Kimball JS, et al. Anterior vertebral body tethering for idiopathic scoliosis: two-year results. Spine 2014;39(20): 1688–1693

8. Samdani AF, Ames RJ, Kimball JS, et al. Anterior vertebral body tethering for immature adolescent idiopathic scoliosis: one-year results on the first 32 patients. Eur Spine J 2015;24(7): 1533–1539

9. Bizzoca D, Piazzolla A, Moretti L, Vicenti G, Moretti B, Solarino G. Anterior vertebral body tethering for idiopathic scoliosis in growing children: a systematic review. World J Orthop 2022;13(5):481–493

10. Risser JC. The Iliac apophysis; an invaluable sign in the management of scoliosis. Clin Orthop 1958;11(11):111–119

11. Sanders JO, Khoury JG, Kishan S, et al. Predicting scoliosis progression from skeletal maturity: a simplified classification during adolescence. J Bone Joint Surg Am 2008;90(3):540–553

12. Samdani AF, Pahys JM, Ames RJ, et al. Prospective follow-up report on anterior vertebral body tethering for idiopathic scoliosis: interim results from an FDA IDE study. J Bone Joint Surg Am 2021;103(17):1611–1619

13. Newton PO, Kluck DG, Saito W, Yaszay B, Bartley CE, Bastrom TP. Anterior spinal growth tethering for skeletally immature patients with scoliosis: a retrospective look two to four years postoperatively. J Bone Joint Surg Am 2018;100(19): 1691–1697

14. Newton PO, Bartley CE, Bastrom TP, Kluck DG, Saito W, Yaszay B. Anterior spinal growth modulation in skeletally immature patients with idiopathic scoliosis: a comparison with posterior spinal fusion at 2 to 5 years postoperatively. J Bone Joint Surg Am 2020; 102(9):769–777

15. Miyanji F, Fields MW, Murphy J, et al; Pediatric Spine Study Group (PSSG). Shoulder balance in patients with Lenke type 1 and 2 idiopathic scoliosis appears satisfactory at 2 years following anterior vertebral body tethering of the spine. Spine Deform 2021;9(6):1591–1599

16. Baroncini A, Courvoisier A, Berjano P, et al. The effects of vertebral body tethering on sagittal parameters: evaluations from a 2-year follow-up. Eur Spine J 2022;31(4):1060–1066

17. Parent S, Shen J. Anterior vertebral body growth-modulation tethering in idiopathic scoliosis: surgical technique. J Am Acad Orthop Surg 2020;28(17):693–699

18. Shin M, Arguelles GR, Cahill PJ, Flynn JM, Baldwin KD, Anari JB. Complications, reoperations, and mid-term outcomes following anterior vertebral body tethering versus posterior spinal fusion: a meta-analysis. JBJS Open Access 2021;6(2):e21.00002

19. Miyanji F, Pawelek J, Nasto LA, Rushton P, Simmonds A, Parent S. Safety and efficacy of anterior vertebral body tethering in the treatment of idiopathic scoliosis. Bone Joint J 2020; 102-B(12):1703–1708

20. Meyers J, Eaker L, von Treuheim TDP, Dolgovpolov S, Lonner B. Early operative morbidity in 184 cases of anterior vertebral body tethering. Sci Rep 2021;11(1):23049

21. Wong HK, Ruiz JNM, Newton PO, Gabriel Liu KP. Non-fusion surgical correction of thoracic idiopathic scoliosis using a novel, braided vertebral body tethering device: minimum follow-up of 4 years. JBJS Open Access 2019; 4(4):e0026

22. Alanay A, Yucekul A, Abul K, et al. Thoracoscopic vertebral body tethering for adolescent idiopathic scoliosis: follow-up curve behavior according to Sanders skeletal maturity staging. Spine 2020;45(22):E1483–E1492

32 Less Invasive Instrumentation and Correction in Pediatric Deformity

Bronek Boszczyk and Areena D'Souza

Introduction

Instrumenting the spine in children with spinal deformity has become a common practice. Nevertheless, challenges remain especially with younger children who have significant growth remaining. Although stabilization and deformity correction are necessary, early fusion needs to be avoided. The best method of avoiding unwanted fusion is least possible periosteal exposure. In the lumbar spine, muscle splitting techniques have been popularized over the last decades. However, these have found little attention in the thoracic spine. With correct anatomical techniques, it is possible to instrument the thoracic spine utilizing muscle splitting techniques while minimizing the impact on the osseous structures.

Indications

Indications for muscle splitting approaches include posterior spinal instrumentation for growth modulation and a temporary instrumentation of spinal levels. In these cases blood loss needs to be minimized due to overall comorbidities.

Definition of the Technique

Positioning and anesthetic preparation for the thoracic muscle splitting technique are the same as for conventional instrumentation. Patients are placed prone under general anesthesia. Standard draping is employed. Use of a radiolucent table is advisable if instrumentation is to be confirmed under fluoroscopic imaging. A standard midline incision is performed. However, the next step differs from conventional exposure. The trapezius muscle in children is often very thin and attaches to the midline of the spinous process. This is gently incised at the medial border and reflected laterally without disrupting the actual paravertebral muscle (**Fig. 32.1a, b**). Once the trapezius muscle is lifted, the exposure of the erector spinae paravertebral muscle group is easily accomplished (**Fig. 32.1c**). The medial and lateral tracts are separated by natural clefts between the muscle groups.

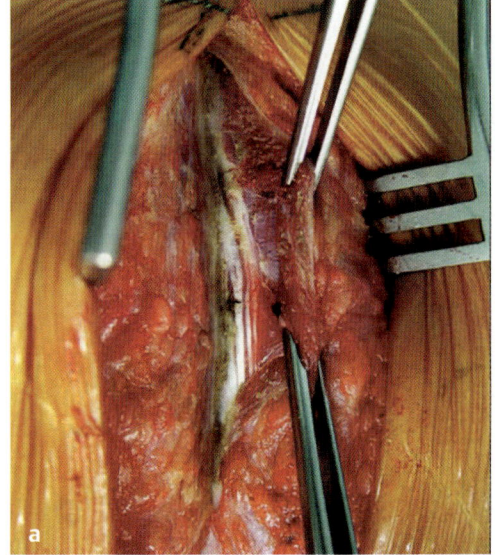 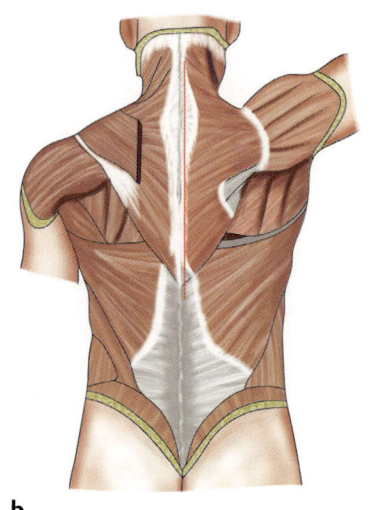 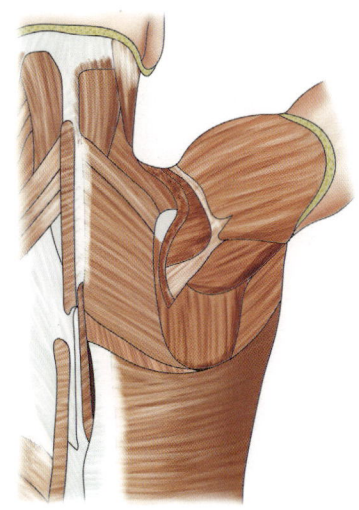

Fig. 32.1 Detachment of trapezius muscle and anatomical layers. **(a)** The trapezius muscle in children is very thin. Here it is detached from the midline on the right and held with forceps. The rhomboid attachments are often sectioned with the trapezius. However, care is taken not to detach deeper muscle layers. **(b)** Overview of trapezius muscle. **(c)** Trapezius muscle reflected, exposing rhomboid muscle and deep to this, the erector spinae group.

These can be palpated digitally with gentle pressure. These clefts are usually found exactly over the transverse process in the projection of the pedicle entry site. A groove can typically be felt with a finger and using gentle dissecting techniques. Splitting the medial and lateral paravertebral muscle groups allows exposure of the tip of the transverse process. This can be followed to the pedicle entry site (**Fig. 32.2**). Retraction is minimal and the actual lamina and intervertebral joints are not exposed. With practice, the exposure of the transverse process can also be kept to a minimum. As this approach leads directly onto the pedicle entry site in the junction between the transverse process and lamina, very little soft tissue resistance is encountered and placing medially directed pedicle screws is comparatively easy (**Fig. 32.3a, b**). The screws themselves are placed in the conventional technique as per the preference of the surgeon. This technique does not lend itself well to navigation as the spinous process itself is not dissected for any attachment; the surgeon needs to rely on anatomical landmarks and interoperative fluoroscopy. Due to the muscle splitting nature, blood loss is minimal and for a bilateral split approach of the entire thoracic spine, typically blood loss is less than 200 mL. Through this approach it is possible to not only place conventional screw and rod systems but also growing rod systems such as magnetic devices. It is technically somewhat challenging to add crosslinks. However, this can be accomplished with

a little practice. Drains are typically not utilized as bleeding is minimal. When closing the wound, particular care needs to be taken to resuture the trapezius muscle to the midline. Postoperatively, patients can mobilize freely. However, for the first 6 to 8 weeks, it is recommended that patients do not lift or carry heavy objects to avoid detaching the trapezius muscle, which in principle does not differ from other thoracic spinal procedures. Obviously, the muscle split in the thoracic spine can be extended down to the lumbar spine as required, whereby at the thoracolumbar junction, it is necessary to detach muscle bundles crossing the muscle split or alternatively to undermine these for passing the implant systems.

Complication Avoidance

Avoid dissecting too far lateral as this will lead to exposure of the ribs which is too lateral for conventional pedicle screw insertion (unless a far lateral approach is desired for "in-out-in" placement). Bleeding is usually not extensive; however, multiple small vessels are encountered in the cleft between the muscles so that careful use of bipolar cautery is advised. Care needs to be taken not to open the facet joint during exposure to avoid auto-fusion. Ensure trapezius muscle is reattached to avoid muscle retraction.

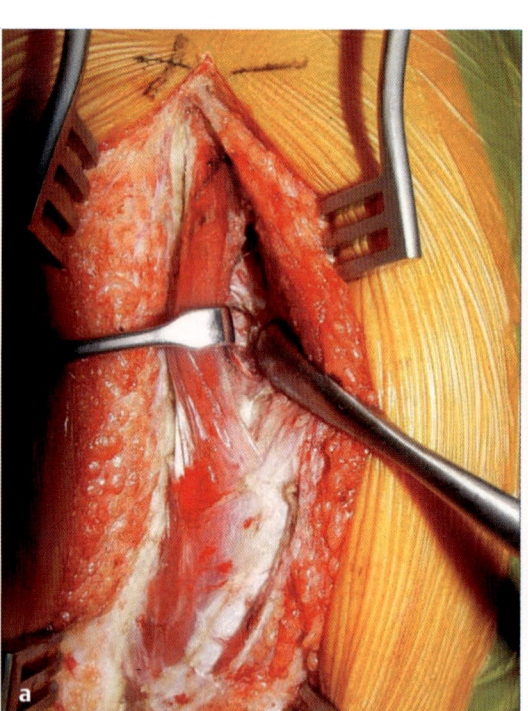
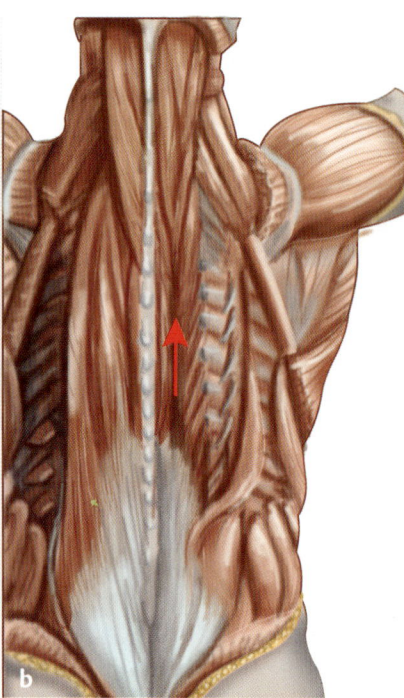

Fig. 32.2 **(a, b)** Muscle splitting approach through erector spinae. Gentle dissection between the medial (spinalis thoracis) and lateral (longissimus thoracis) tracts of erector spinae (arrows in cleft between muscles) exposes the tip of the transverse process.

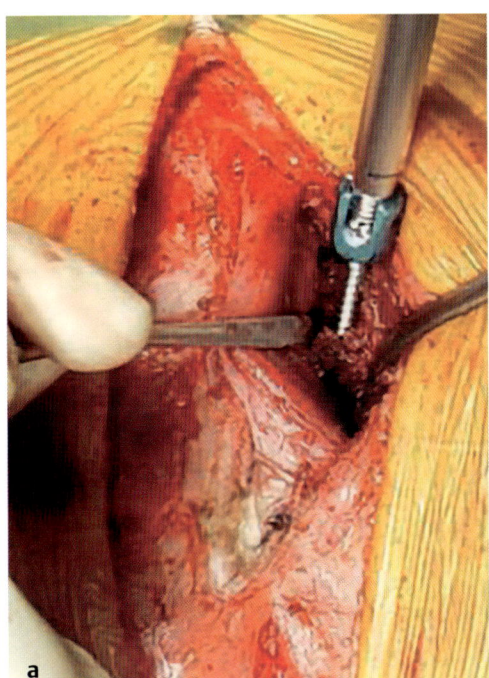 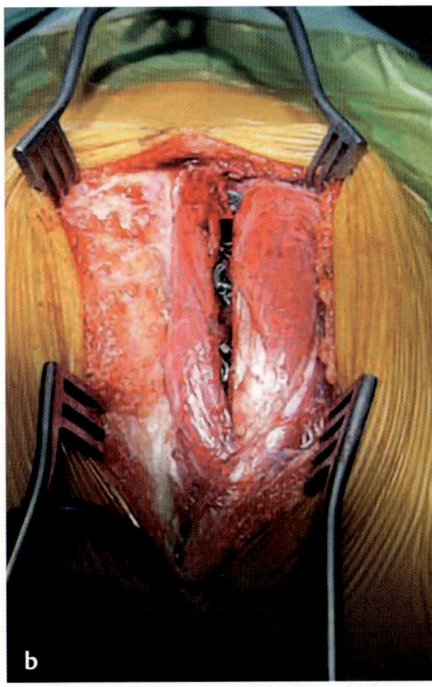

Fig. 32.3 Completed instrumentation. **(a)** Insertion of pedicle screw with minimal exposure of bone. Convergence is easy to achieve. **(b)** Completed screw insertion on the right side with muscle coverage.

Tips and Tricks

- Palpate for the tip of the transverse process while exposing through the muscle cleft.
- Use anteroposterior (AP) fluoroscopy to verify screw entry site and trajectory.
- Infiltrate erector spinae with local anesthetic.

Key Points

- Muscle splitting thoracic exposure allows convergent pedicle screw placement with minimal periosteal exposure.
- Blood loss is minimal with muscle splitting exposure.
- Soft tissue coverage is excellent as muscle remains perfused.

Part VI

Special Topics

Sedat Dalbayrak and Ahmet Öğrenci

Introduction

High-grade spondylolisthesis is an uncommon disorder of the spine and is defined as slippage of greater than 50% of vertebra and Meyerding grade III or higher.[1] It is seen in approximately 1% of all spinal spondylolisthesis cases. Surgical reduction of spondylolisthesis can be challenging. But if it is achieved, spondylolisthesis reduction restores spinopelvic parameters and sagittal balance. However, the role of surgical reduction in high-grade spondylolisthesis is still controversial because of some problems such as its potential complications, including neurologic deficits and implant failure.[2] However, it is accepted that correction with reduction provides a more significant clinical and radiological improvement.[3]

Although some authors state that anterior approaches such as anterior lumbar interbody fusion (ALIF) are better options with fewer complications and provide more lordosis, posterior approaches are preferred.[4,5]

In the posterior approaches, technical difficulties arise regarding whether reduction should be performed or not. Therefore, this chapter will describe the posterior approach with reduction technique and interbody cage application.

Definition of the Technique

A standard posterior midline lumbosacral approach is used from L4–sacrum (S1). First, the muscles and fascia are stripped laterally on both sides. Then the level is determined by fluoroscopy. Afterward, a total laminectomy is performed at the L5 level. The purpose of applying total laminectomy is to decompress the roots and dura, protect them from neural damage during reduction, and facilitate the reduction. In addition, the reduction will be more straightforward by removing the posterior tension band. Then L5 and S1 roots are completely decompressed bilaterally with the aid of a microscope.

After this stage, the bone dome (S1 posterior superior part) that may interfere with the reduction should be broken off and removed with an osteotome. This action will facilitate the reduction and open up posterior disc space to apply a suitable thickness interbody cage for the L5–S1 level **(Fig. 33.1)**.

Afterward, bilateral transpedicular screwing is applied to L4, L5, and S1 levels. Pedicle screws to the L4 level should be used to support the reduction. After reduction, in the last step, L4 pedicle screws can be removed one-sidedly step by step, and the system can be locked with L5–S1 screws. Still, we recommend applying permanent L4 screws to aaoid reduction loss.

While applying the pedicle screw, the most challenging part is the L5 screws. Because the L5 corpus is settled anteriorly, it may be challenging to reach the pedicle, and screwing may fail. However, it should not be forgotten that this is a fundamental level. Spondylolisthesis screws (reduction screws) should be as long and thick as possible and length size. First, it would be wise to use a thinner screw and check whether it is placed correctly.

After completing the placement under fluoroscopy, bilaterally appropriate lordotic rods are placed. Afterward, while placing the nuts with the help of a spondylolisthesis screw, distraction is applied with the distractor between L5 and S1 at the same time. Then the system is temporarily locked, and diskectomy is performed between L5 and S1. A wide interbody cage should then be applied to the L5–S1 disc space. We recommend preferring titanium cages. Then the system is loosened, and the deflection to the operating table is performed to gain lordosis to the patient. Finally, the system is locked again and is finalized **(Fig. 33.1)**.

We recommend at least one more segment screwing (S2 or S2 alar–iliac) in addition to the single level (S1) below the L5–S1 level **(Fig. 33.2)**. This will reduce pseudoarthrosis and screw loosening.

Indications

Indications of surgery for high-grade lumbar listhesis are as follows:

- Chronic low back pain resistant to conservative methods
- Resistant radicular pain with conservative methods

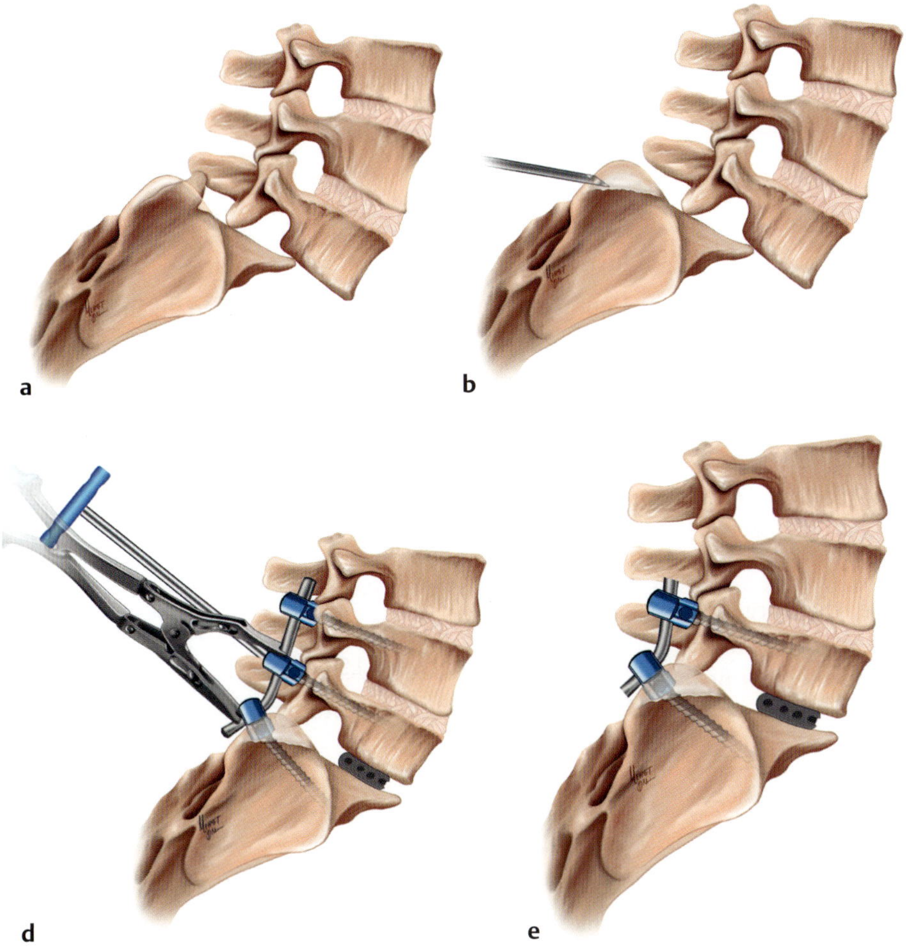

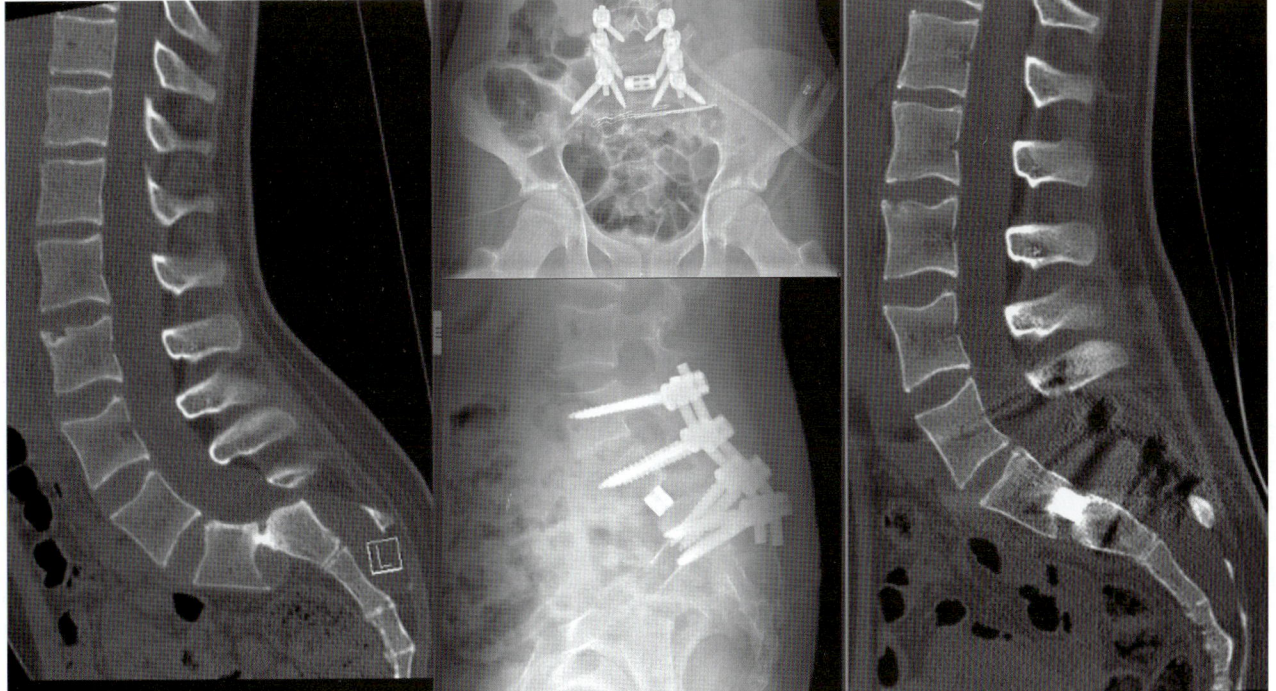

Fig. 33.1 Demonstration of the technique. After removing the superior posterior dome of the sacrum **(a, b)**, a reduction screw was placed in L5 **(c)** together with an L4 screw **(d)**, and distraction with reduction simultaneously was performed after transforaminal lumbar interbody fusion (TLIF) application. The L4 screw may be transitory or permanent **(e)**.

Fig. 33.2 An illustrative case. A 13-year-old female patient has been admitted with chronic pain in both legs and low back pain. Radiological examination revealed a high-grade listhesis at L5–S1. She was treated with L4–S2 alar screw fixation with reduction and interbody fusion.

- Postural disorder due to impaired spinopelvic parameters and insufficient compensatory mechanisms[6,7]
- No fusion in radiological examinations
- Suitable bone structure for instrumentation (especially sacrum and L5 pedicle structure)

Complication Avoidance

Complications are relatively higher in this operation compared to other spinal surgeries.[8,9] Therefore, every stage of surgical treatment should be controlled.

Neural complications may arise from long operation time, bleeding, and instrumentation failure. We recommend neural decompression first during surgery to avoid distraction of roots.

When applying screws to the L5 pedicle, the surgeon should ensure it is on the pedicle and in the correct route. L5 screws are the most essential screws, and there is no alternative for reduction.

Consideration should be given to neural damage during fracture of the bone dome with the osteotome. In addition, care should be taken not to perform excessive bone removal during dome resection. Otherwise, it may cause insufficient bone tissue in the sacrum or S1 pedicle fractures.

If there is a pull-out movement in the L5 screws during reduction, the reduction should be terminated as it is, and the cage should be applied and stabilized without forcing for reduction.

After correction with reduction, the spinal roots can be stretched and should be checked again.[10]

If a problem develops during the reduction phase, in situ fusion without reduction can be considered as another option. In the literature, both positive and negative aspects of performing in situ fusion such as transdiskal–transvertebral have been mentioned a lot.[11–14] While some publications have stated more bleeding and neural injury, there are also publications stating the opposite in treating in situ fusion. Therefore, if the reduction is possible, it should be performed. Otherwise, stabilization and decompression (in situ fusion) should be considered. Even if the reduction is achieved, in addition to posterior stabilization, a transdiskal (from S1 to L5 vertebra) screw can be added to the system.

The dura is usually thinner due to stretching in these patients, and careful decompression should be performed due to the risk of dural damage. In addition, if cerebrospinal fluid leakage occurs after a dural injury, bleeding from epidural veins will increase and it will be challenging.

Tips and Tricks

- Radiological evaluation before surgery, especially for fusion
- Neural decompression before reduction during surgery
- Continue fluoroscopy if necessary while applying L5 screws
- Deflection from the table after application of interbody cage for lordosis gain
- Rechecking the roots and dura for decompression in the last stage of the operation
- Application of as wide cage as possible
- In addition to interbody fusion, posterolateral fusion with autograft between L5 and S1
- Use a rigid brace in the postoperative period

Key Points

- Correction with reduction in high-grade listhesis gives better clinical and radiological results.
- L5 screws are critical in the reduction stage.
- The S1 posterior superior dome structure should be removed to avoid an obstacle to reduction and allow wide cage application.
- Nerve decompression should be performed before the reduction phase and checked after reduction.
- Before the final locking of the system, deflection of the operation table should be performed to gain lordosis.
- In addition to reduction, a transdiskal screw can be added.

References

1. Meyerding HW. Spondylolisthesis. Surg Gynecol Obstet 1932;54:371–377
2. Molinari RW, Bridwell KH, Lenke LG, Ungacta FF, Riew KD. Complications in the surgical treatment of pediatric high-grade, isthmic dysplastic spondylolisthesis. A comparison of three surgical approaches. Spine 1999;24(16): 1701–1711
3. Labelle H, Mac-Thiong JM, Roussouly P. Spino-pelvic sagittal balance of spondylolisthesis: a review and classification. Eur Spine J 2011; 20(Suppl 5):641–646

4. Lee SH, Choi WG, Lim SR, Kang HY, Shin SW. Minimally invasive anterior lumbar interbody fusion followed by percutaneous pedicle screw fixation for isthmic spondylolisthesis. Spine J 2004;4(6):644–649

5. Ishihara H, Osada R, Kanamori M, et al. Minimum 10-year follow-up study of anterior lumbar interbody fusion for isthmic spondylolisthesis. J Spinal Disord 2001;14(2):91–99

6. Li Y, Hresko MT. Radiographic analysis of spondylolisthesis and sagittal spinopelvic deformity. J Am Acad Orthop Surg 2012;20(4): 194–205

7. Martikos K, Greggi T, Faldini C. High grade isthmic spondylolisthesis; can reduction always re-align the unbalanced pelvis? BMC Musculoskelet Disord 2019;20(1):499

8. Boos N, Marchesi D, Zuber K, Aebi M. Treatment of severe spondylolisthesis by reduction and pedicular fixation. A 4-6-year follow-up study. Spine 1993;18(12):1655–1661

9. Gandhoke GS, Kasliwal MK, Smith JS, et al. A multicenter evaluation of clinical and radiographic outcomes following high-grade spondylolisthesis reduction and fusion. Clin Spine Surg 2017;30(4):E363–E369

10. Petraco DM, Spivak JM, Cappadona JG, Kummer FJ, Neuwirth MG. An anatomic evaluation of L5 nerve stretch in spondylolisthesis reduction. Spine 1996;21(10):1133–1138, discussion 1139

11. Lak AM, Abunimer AM, Devi S, et al. Reduction versus in situ fusion for adult high-grade spondylolisthesis: a systematic review and meta-analysis. World Neurosurg 2020;138: 512–520.e2

12. François J, Lauweryns P, Fabry G. Treatment of high-grade spondylolisthesis by posterior lumbosacral transfixation with transdiscal screws: surgical technique and preliminary results in four cases. Acta Orthop Belg 2005; 71(3):334–341

13. Muschik M, Zippel H, Perka C. Surgical management of severe spondylolisthesis in children and adolescents. Anterior fusion in situ versus anterior spondylodesis with posterior transpedicular instrumentation and reduction. Spine 1997; 22(17):2036–2042, discussion 2043

14. Poussa M, Schlenzka D, Seitsalo S, Ylikoski M, Hurri H, Osterman K. Surgical treatment of severe isthmic spondylolisthesis in adolescents. Reduction or fusion in situ. Spine 1993;18(7): 894–901

Assaker Jordan, Pierre Haettel, Henri-Arthur Leroy, Benoit Derre, and Richard Assaker

Introduction

Adult spinal deformity (ASD) is defined as a Cobb angle higher than 10 degrees. ASD occurs as a "de novo" deformity, an age-related asymmetrical diskopathies, or an increased deformity on pre-existing idiopathic scoliosis or induced iatrogenically. The prevalence of ASD in the population over 60 years of age is estimated at 68%[1] and progresses concomitantly with aging. ASD affects the spinal balance with an anterior shift of the trunk outside the Dubousset's "cone of economy." This positive sagittal imbalance is correlated to increasing disability.[2-4] ASD is one of the most frequent indications for surgery in a population over 65 years old.[5-10] Fusion with multilevel pedicle screw-based instrumentation has become the standard of care for patients with positive imbalance associated with disability.[11-26] Despite the increasing surgery rate in this population, debates are still ongoing on decision-making and technical challenges owing to the perioperative morbidities associated with surgical correction of these deformities.[27-30] The rate of surgical complication in patients is about 40%.[31-33] Conventional fusion techniques are performed in an open posterior midline approach exposing these elderly patients to significant blood loss, prolonged operating time, wound breakdown, and infection.[34] An alternative to open surgery is minimal invasive accesses that reduce access-related trauma, blood loss, and infections.[26,35-37]

Minimal invasive surgery (MIS) has gained popularity in various degenerative spine pathologies. It reduces trauma to the surrounding muscle and is associated with less postoperative pain and better postoperative comfort.[38-41] The benefits of MIS over traditional open surgery are the decrease of blood loss, drop in infection rate,[36,38,41,42] and consequently, reduction of perioperative morbidities. Current MIS technologies have proven benefits and advantages in several spinal disorders, but their adoption in deformity surgery is still questionable. The main limitations of MIS in deformity surgery are achieving the appropriate sagittal and coronal alignment, ensuring a good fusion, and adequate decompression.

Advances in MIS technologies and better surgeon experience have made MIS options viable for spinal deformity correction.

Challenges of MIS in Deformity Correction

Decision-making in ASD relies on clinical symptoms, radiographic parameters, and the patient's comorbidities. Surgical strategies vary from simple and segmental decompression to multilevel and global realignment in both sagittal and coronal planes. The main objectives of ASD surgical treatment are to reduce pain and disability, arrest the progression of the deformity, restore "economic" sagittal balance, and improve function and cosmesis. Restoration of spinopelvic harmony is essential in surgical correction of ASD. Correlations between pelvic parameters and lumbar alignment are the basis for planning surgical correction (**Fig. 34.1**). Optimal correction might necessitate posterior shortening of the column through several types of osteotomies that are easier to achieve through open approaches[43-45] (**Fig. 34.2**).

The main challenges for MIS to achieve the principles of deformity correction are:

- **Suboptimal correction of the global balance and regional curves**: Multilevel osteotomies are not easy to obtain by MIS, and this would lead to suboptimal clinical outcomes and the risk of proximal junctional kyphosis (PJK) or proximal junctional failure (PJF).

- **Multilevel fusion**: A large surface and a large amount of graft material are challenging to address through minimal invasive accesses.

- A reliable and solid fixation to the pelvis.

Considering these limitations, MIS is viable in select candidates for surgical alignment correction.

Minimally Invasive Decompression

Decompression alone might be the appropriate option for patients with ASD presenting with leg pain and acceptable disability from back pain and malalignment. For example, leg pain might be due to mono-radiculopathy or neurogenic claudication from multilevel root compression. In such a situation, decompression is proposed to relieve the predominant pain and improve quality of

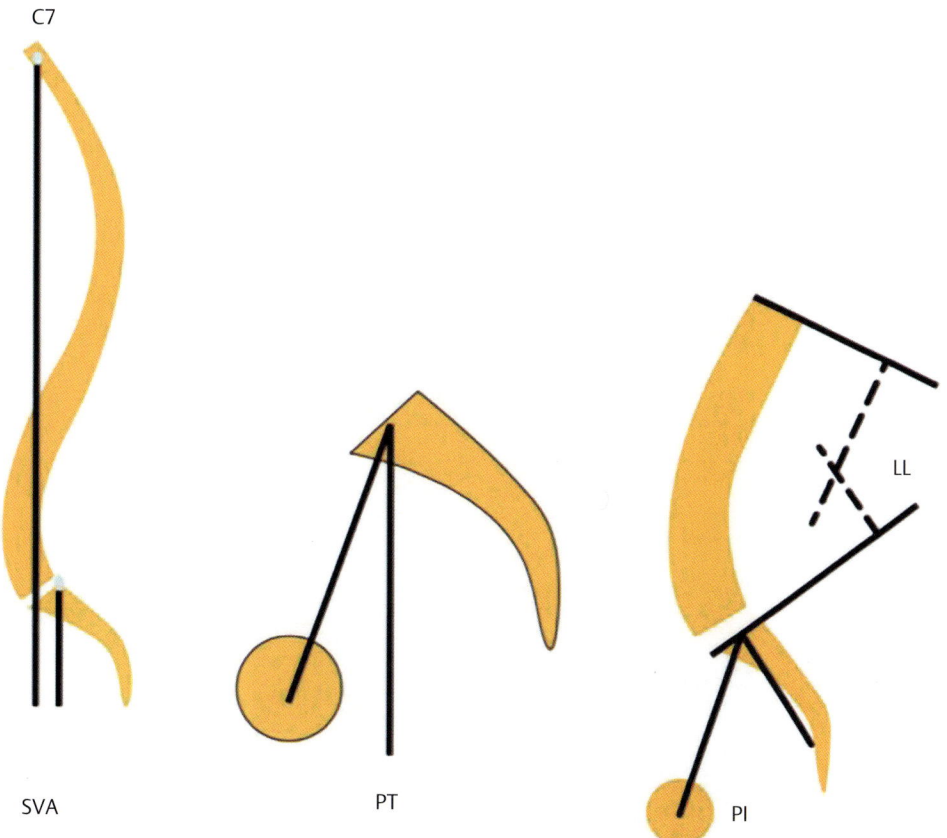

Fig. 34.1 Sagittal parameters used for surgical planning: sagittal vertical axis (SVA) <50 mm, pelvic tilt (PT) <20 degrees, pelvic incidence–lumbar lordosis (PI-LL) mismatch.

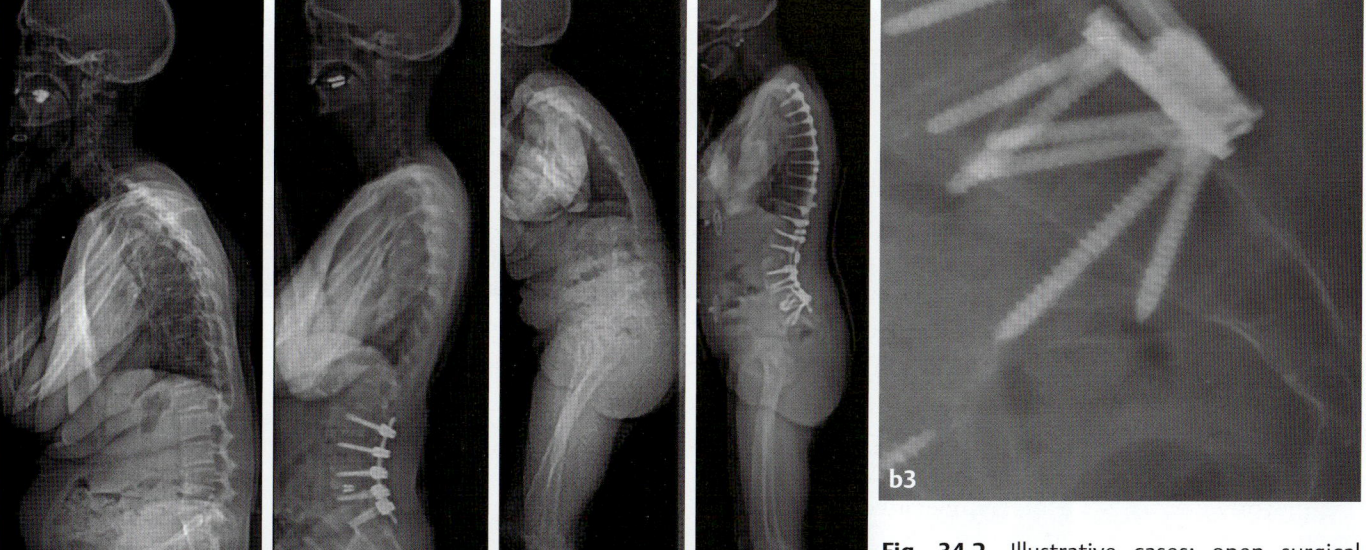

Fig. 34.2 Illustrative cases: open surgical treatment of adult spinal deformity (ASD). Case A: Lumbosacral realignment through Smith-Peterson osteotomy (SPO) and short construct. Case B: Thoraco-lumbo-sacral realignment through pedicle subtraction osteotomy (PSO), SPO, and sacro-pelvic multipoint fixation.

life (QoL).[46–48] This solution provides benefits without the risks of major surgery. The advantage of minimally invasive decompression compared to open decompression is clearly to avoid iatrogenic instabilities. Furthermore, by preserving muscle insertion, and ligamentous and bony structures, minimal invasive accesses limit postoperative instabilities in the highly fragile elderly patients. Minimally invasive techniques include tubular access (**Fig. 34.3**) and microscopic decompression or full endoscopic unilateral laminotomy with bilateral decompression (**Fig. 34.4**).

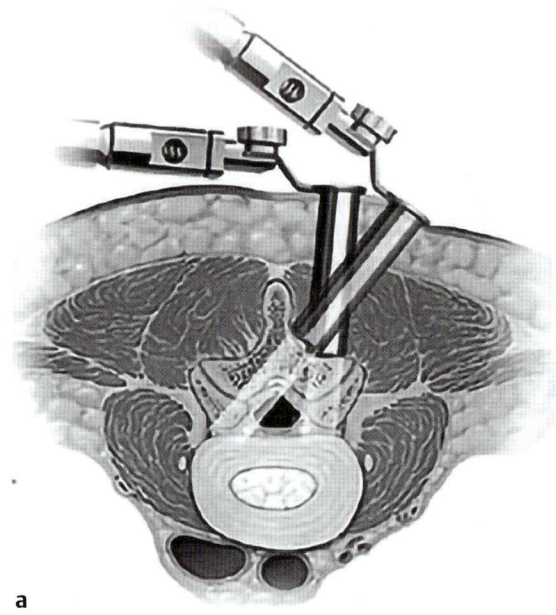

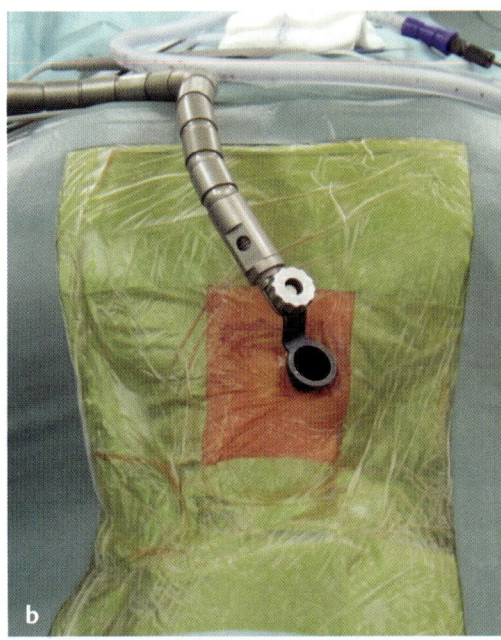

Fig. 34.3 (a, b) Tubular access for unilateral laminotomy with bilateral decompression.

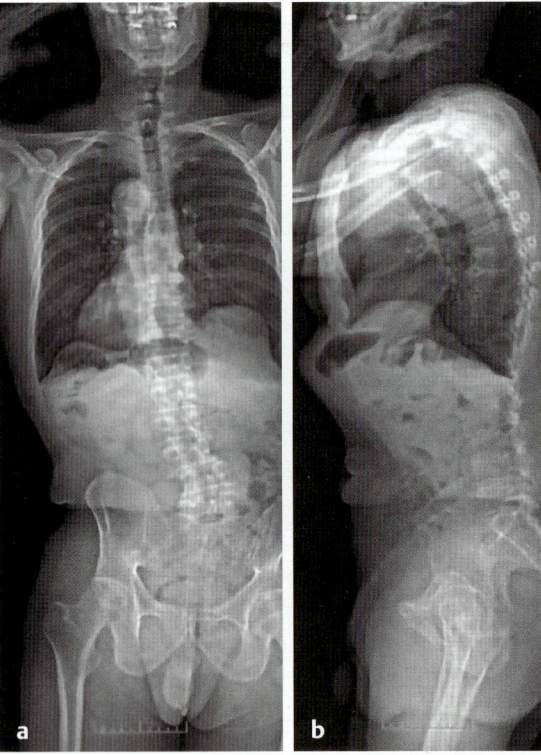

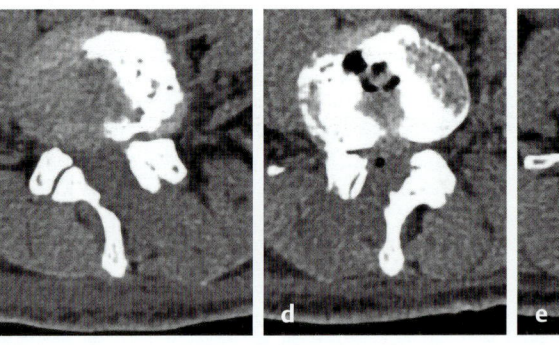
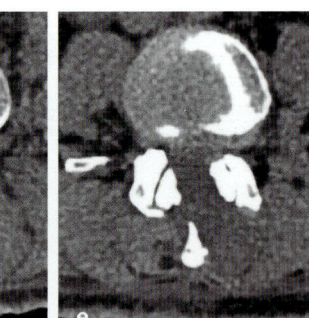

Fig. 34.4 (a–e) Illustrations showing a minimally invasive surgical decompression at three levels without addressing the deformity.

Percutaneous Screw and Rod Insertion

Placing pedicle screws percutaneously is a routine practice and has been adopted for several years. Generally, the placement of the pedicle screws is guided by K-wires introduced through a Jamshidi needle under fluoroscopy. Under an anteroposterior (AP) fluoroscopic view, the pedicle line and points of entry are identified. A Jamshidi needle is inserted in the index pedicle and checked on AP and lateral fluoroscopy (**Fig. 34.5**). A guide wire is then placed in the Jamshidi until half of the body of the vertebrae. The wire guides the cannulated tap, and cannulated screw is introduced and monitored by the fluoroscopy (**Fig. 34.6**). Percutaneous posterior instrumentation could be combined with anterior transpsoatic alignment in a nonrigid deformity (**Fig. 34.7**).

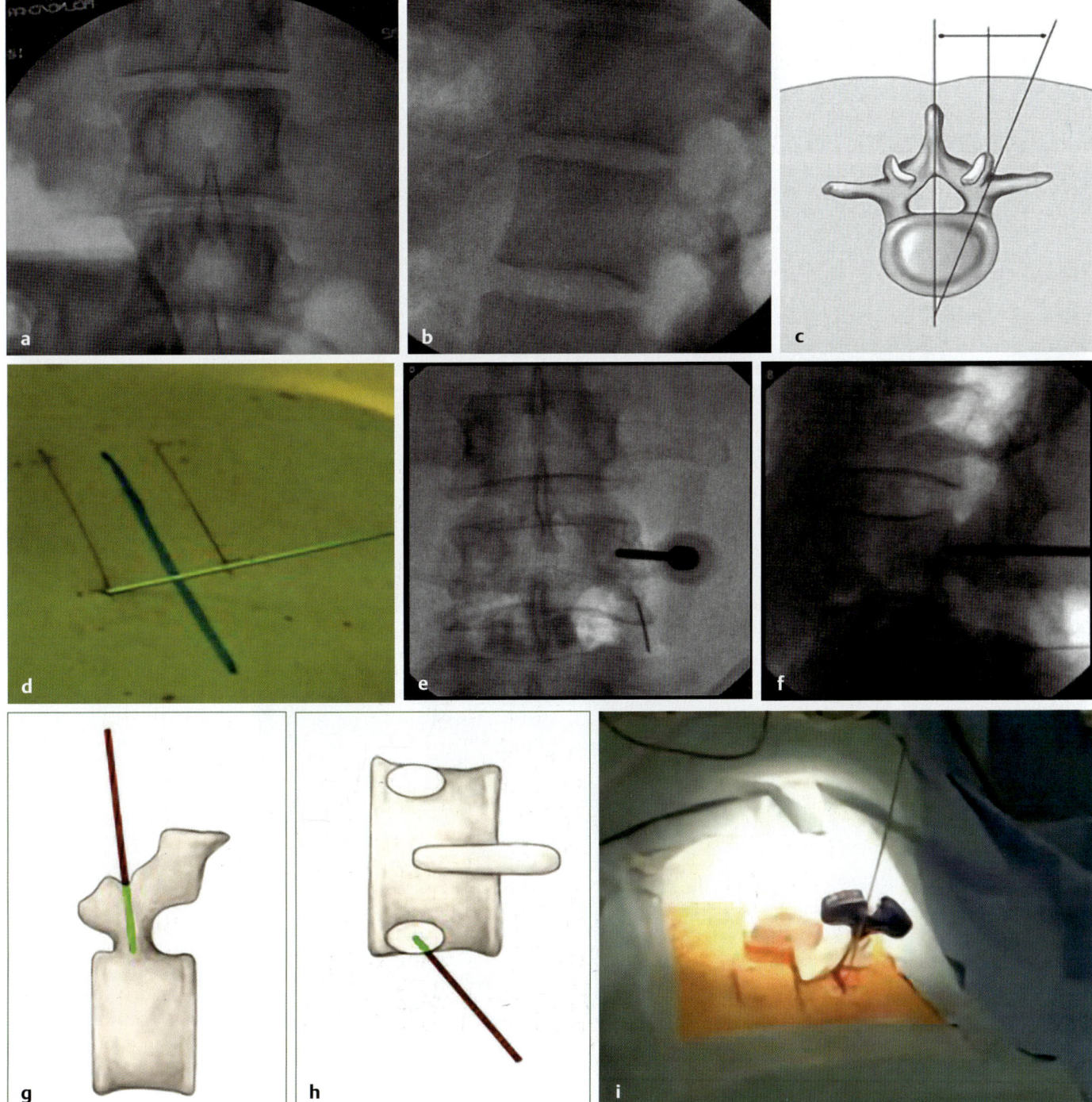

Fig. 34.5   (a–i) Technical preparation for percutaneous screw placement.

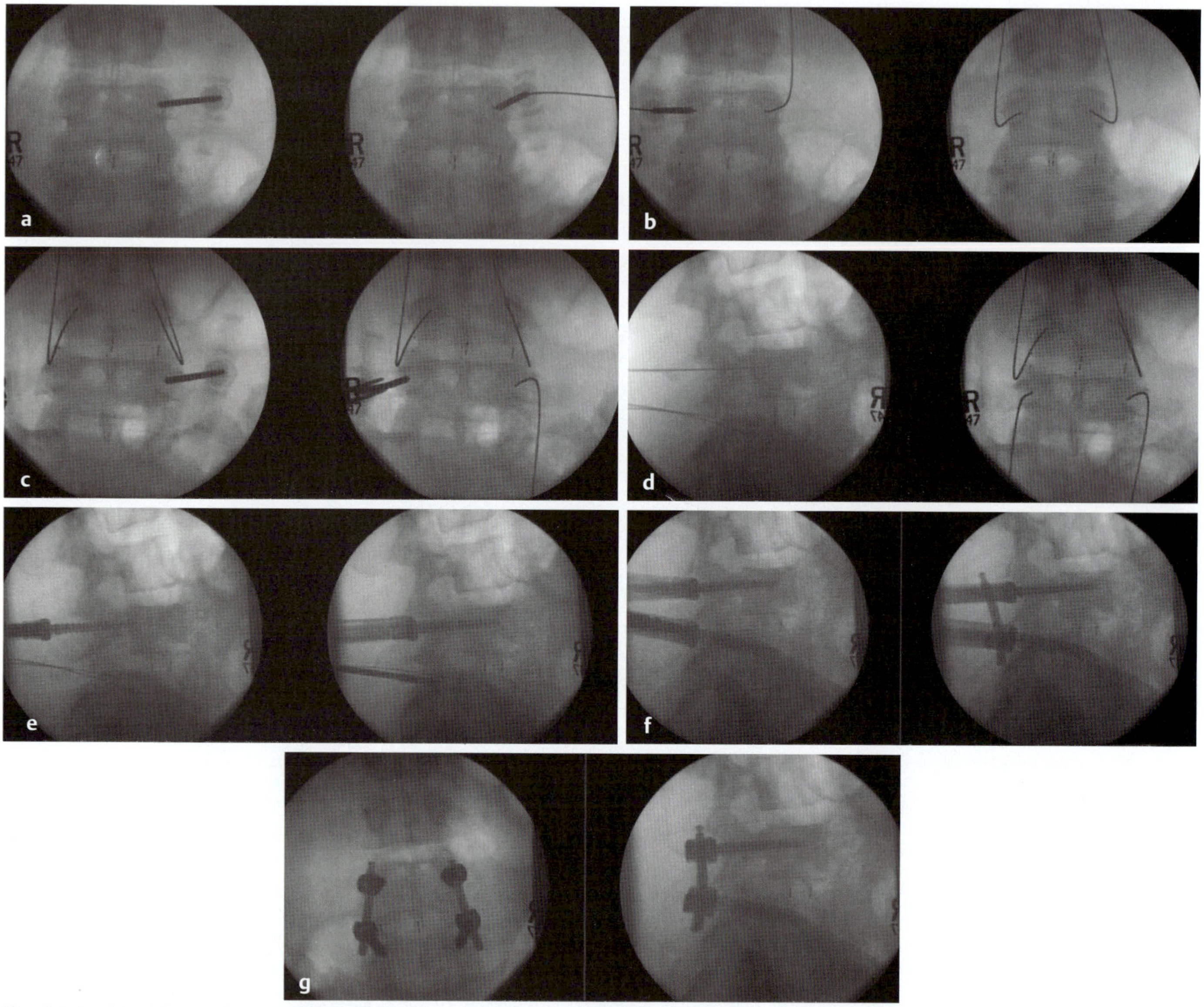

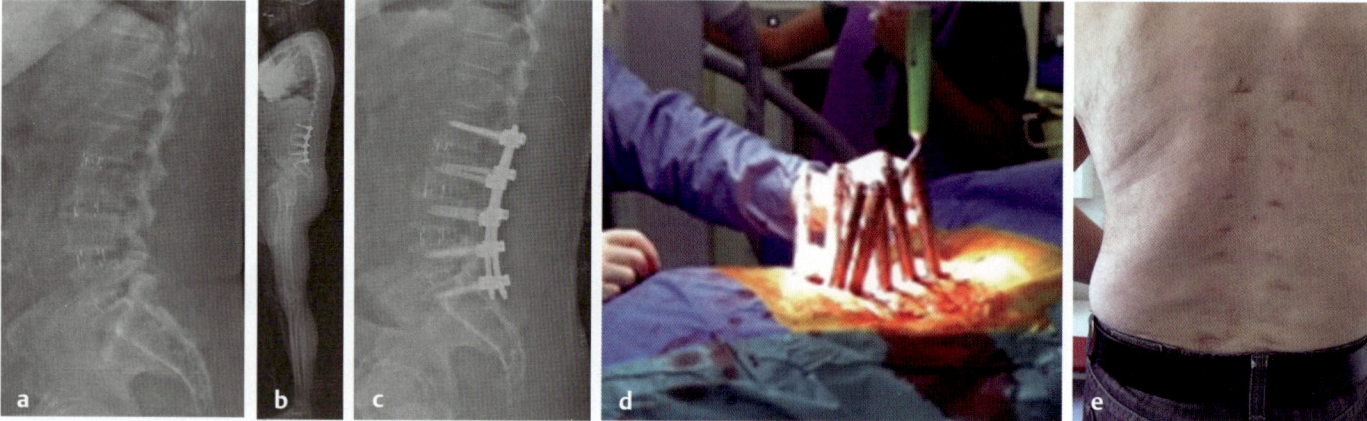

Fig. 34.6 (a–g) Steps showing the screws and rod placement under fluoroscopy.

Fig. 34.7 (a–e) Illustrative case showing a minimally invasive correction of adult spinal deformity (ASD): anterior interbody alignment followed by percutaneous screw and rod fixation.

Minimally Invasive Fusion Techniques

Surgery in ASD must be combined with bone fusion to maintain the correction durably. Because of incomplete visibility, MIS access does not allow exposure of posterior bony elements for grafting. Despite this limitation, surgical techniques to ensure fusion in MIS continue to be refined and evolve over time. There are three technical options to fuse in MIS access.

Tubular Access to the Facet Complex for Decortication and Grafting

The levels to be fused are predetermined preoperatively, always combined with percutaneous screws. The guide wires are placed first; then a tubular exposure of the facets is performed. The access is transmuscular by sequential dilators and creates a 14 mm tubular corridor. Next, a Bovie is used to clear the soft tissue and clearly expose the joint. Next, the facet complex is drilled using a high-speed drill combined with irrigation. Finally, the bone graft is placed over the drilled area and around the facet joint.

Interbody Fusion Through Tubular Foraminal Access (TLIF)

Multilevel TILF is also an option but time-consuming. Performing facetectomies, diskectomies, and cage insertion through tubular access is popular and well-defined but arduous in multilevel fusion.

Lateral Lumbar Interbody Fusion (LLIF) Through Transpsoas or Anterior to Psoas Access

Transpsoatic or anterior to psoas accesses have the advantages of direct access to the disc, better preparation of the fusion site, insertion of a large footprint implant, and partial correction of the alignment. It could be the first step of the surgical plan followed by posterior percutaneous pedicle screws or posterior open instrumentation (if osteotomies are needed) or the second step after posterior alignment to restore good structural support to the anterior column (**Fig. 34.8**).

Minimally Invasive Osteotomies

Rigid deformity might need osteotomies to different levels to destabilize and be able to realign. Planning the type and levels of osteotomies is usually done before surgery. Simulation software could help determine the correct angle according to planned osteotomy. One major limitation of MIS is exposure for comfortable osteotomy, which is the cause of under-correction.

A significant advancement has been made in the understanding and techniques of osteotomies to reach an optimal alignment. The question is the feasibility of these osteotomies concerning MIS principles.

Combining percutaneous screws to grade 1 or 2 osteotomies is possible but could be arduous and time-consuming according to the number of levels addressed. However, in case of focal kyphosis, a grade 3 or 4 is possible by mini-open access at the index level, and reconstruction is performed by MIS techniques (**Fig. 34.9**).

Sacro-Pelvic Fixation

Since long constructs are needed to correct degenerative deformities, extending these constructs to the sacro-pelvic end raises many technical questions.[49] Lack of rigid sacral fixation, such as bilateral S1 screws, anterior interbody fusion, or extension to the ileum, has been associated with a significantly increased risk of pseudarthrosis and, thus, poor outcomes.

Many options have been proposed for load-sharing: S1 pedicle combined to alar screws, to the ileum, or S2-ileum with or without sacral plates associated or not to the anterior interbody fusion of the L5–S1 disc (**Figs. 34.10** and **34.11**).

In minimally invasive access, sacro-pelvic fixation must be planned to anticipate rod contouring and passage. S1 pedicle and an iliac screw placed percutaneously seem the most specific and viable combination for sacro-iliac fixation. This might be reinforced by an anterior interbody fusion to guarantee the fusion to the caudal end of the long construct.

Decision-Making and Surgical Strategy

Lenke et al published an algorithm to guide decision-making and surgical planning in ASD.[5] Six treatment levels are defined based on clinical findings and radiographical parameters (**Table 34.1**).[50] Mummaneni et al proposed a modified algorithm dedicated to the MIS approach and treatment of ASD (**Flowchart 34.1**). This algorithm, named MiSLAT, is divided into six levels according to the severity of the deformity and the surgical treatment.[51]

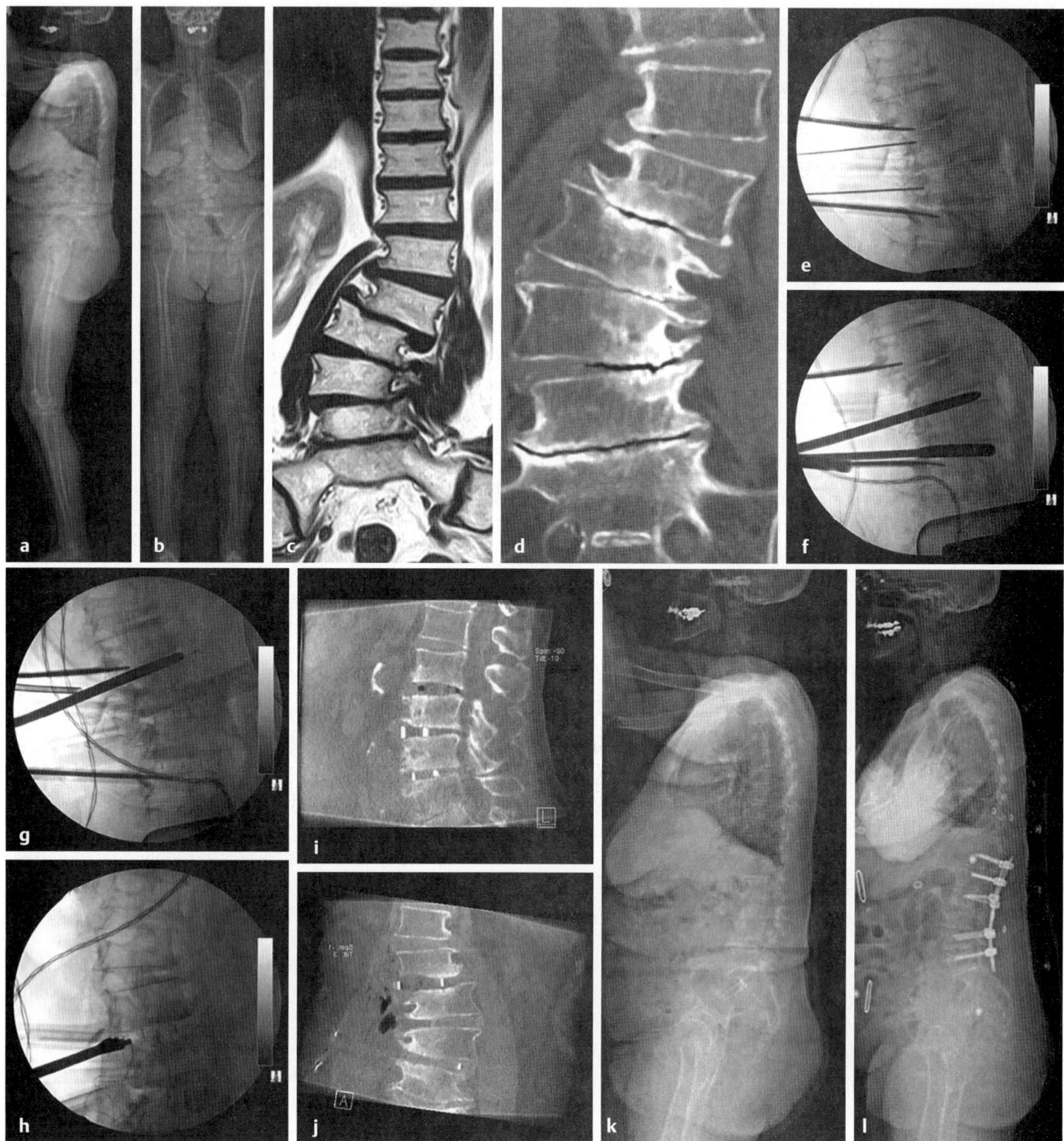

Fig. 34.8   (a–l) One-stage alignment correction combining anterior transpsoas access first, followed by percutaneous screws and rod stabilization.

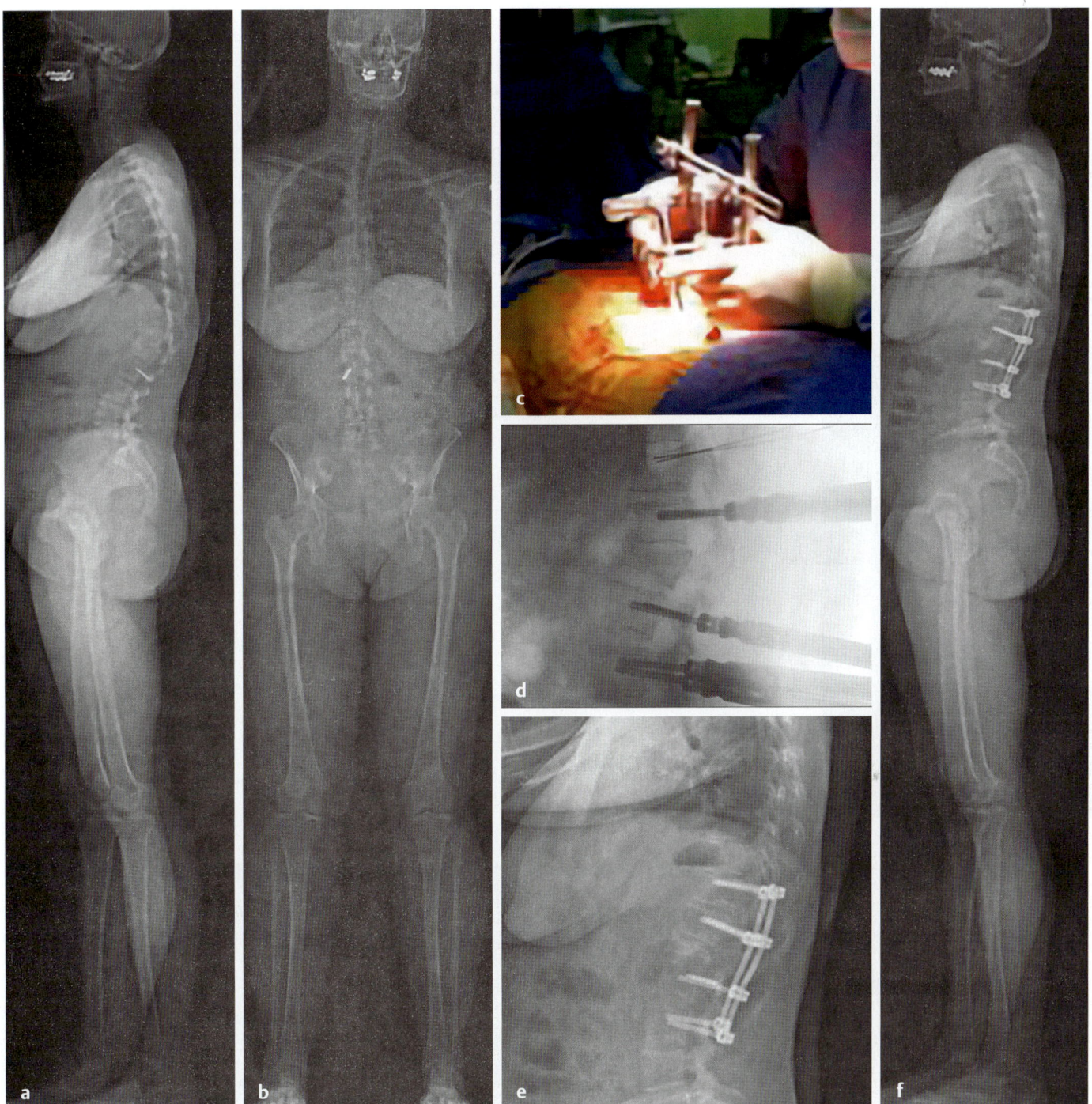

Fig. 34.9 **(a–f)** Pedicle subtraction osteotomy at L1 combined to percutaneous screws and rod realignment.

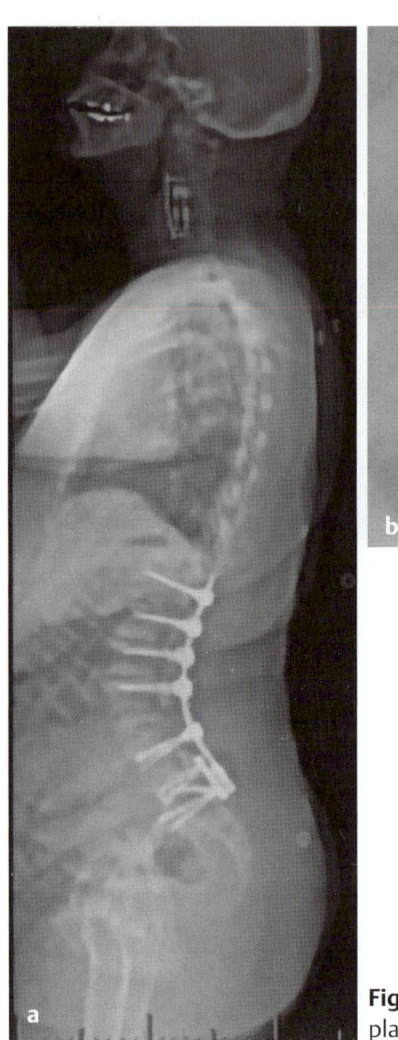

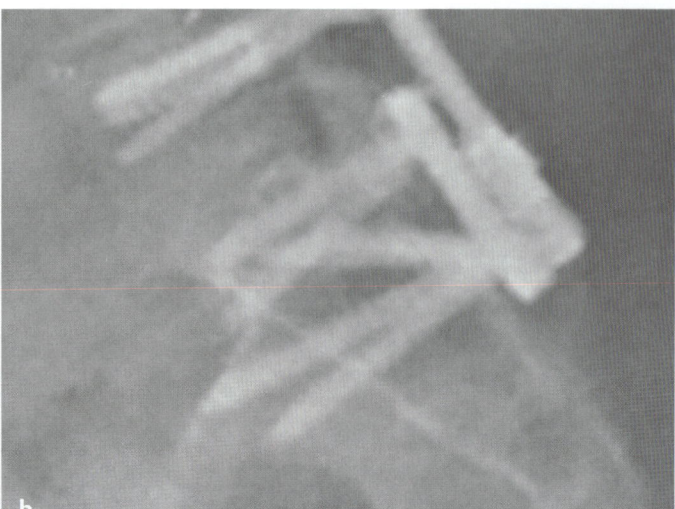

Fig. 34.10 (a–c) Multipoint fixation to the pelvis: S1 pedicle, alar and iliac screws with a sacral plate.

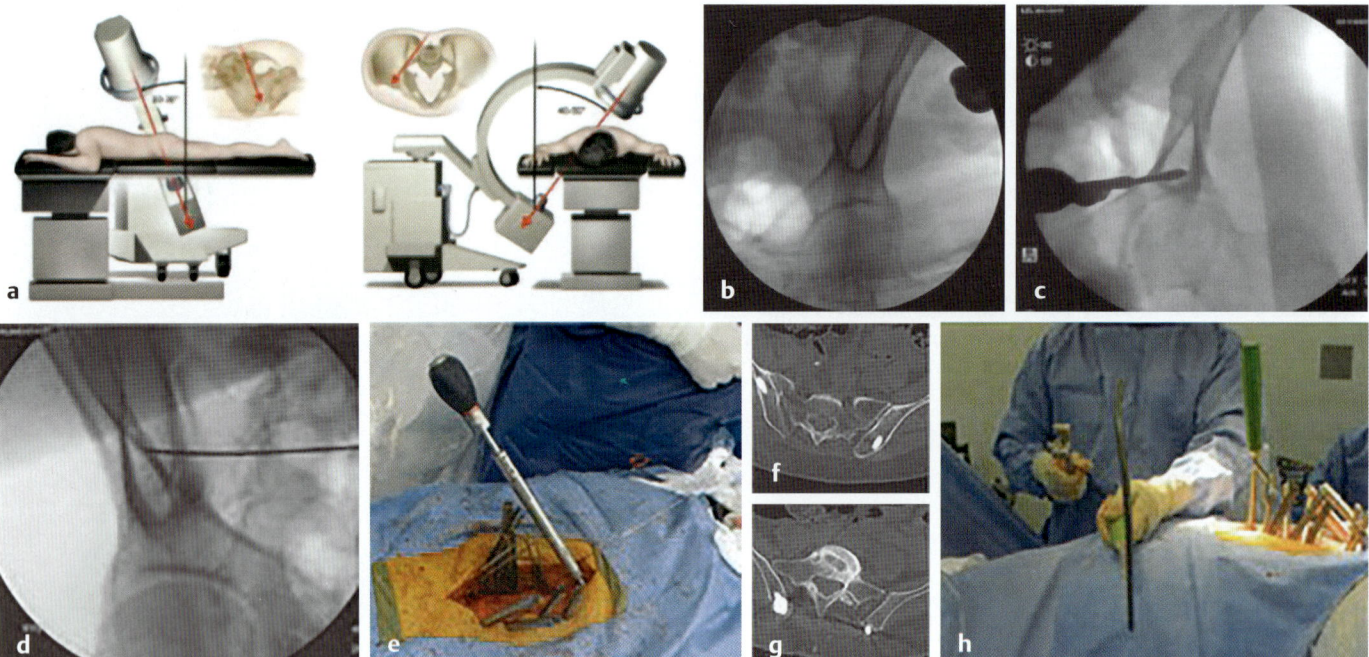

Fig. 34.11 (a–h) Percutaneous placement of an iliac screw.

Table 34.1 Grading of osteotomy techniques as described by Lenke

	Anatomical Resection	Description	Surgical Approach Modifiers
Grade 1	Partial facet joint	Resection of the inferior facet and joint capsule at a given spinal level	**A/P** (anterior soft tissue release combined with posterior resection) **P** (posterior approach only)
Grade 2	Complete facet joint	Both superior and inferior facets at a given spinal segment are resected with complete ligamentum flavum removal; other posterior elements of the vertebra including the lamina, and the spinous processes may also be resected	**A/P** (anterior soft tissue release combined with posterior resection) **P** (posterior approach only)
Grade 3	Pedicle/Partial body	Partial wedge resection of a segment of the posterior vertebral body and portion of the posterior vertebral elements with pedicles	**A** (anterior release) **P** (posterior approach only) **A/P** (both)
Grade 4	Pedicle/Partial body/Disc	Wider wedge resection through the vertebral body; includes a substantial portion of the posterior vertebral body, posterior elements with pedicles and includes rejection of at least a portion of one endplate with the adjacent intervertebral disc	**A** (anterior release) **P** (posterior approach only) **A/P** (both)
Grade 5	Complete vertebral and disc	Complete removal of a vertebra and both adjacent discs (rib resection in the thoracic region)	**A** (anterior release) **P** (posterior approach only) **A/P** (both)
Grade 6	Multiple vertebrae and disc	Resection of more than one entire vertebra and adjacent discs; Grade 5 resection and additional adjacent vertebral resection	**A** (anterior release) **P** (posterior approach only) **A/P** (both)

MiSLAT 1 to 4 could be addressed with MIS. MiSLAT 1 and 2 are qualified "small" surgery that consists of minimally invasive decompression alone or minimally invasive decompression and fusion at the index levels. MiSLAT 3 and 4 are considered as "medium" surgery and consists of minimally invasive decompression and alignment correction of the entire coronal Cobb of the curve. MiSLAT 5 and 6 are "big" surgery done in open access with osteotomies and extension of the fusion to the thoracic spine.

Spinal Navigation and Robotics in MIS for ASD

In minimal invasive access, targeting depends on imaging technologies. The most popular and easy to use remain the C-arm fluoroscopy. The disadvantages of C-arm fluoroscopy include radiation exposure, discomfort of wearing a protective apron, and need for a radiation technician to manipulate the C-arm unit. In the 1990s, image-guided navigation was introduced in brain surgery and later in spine surgery. The advantages of these computer-assisted intraoperative image guidance were precision,[52–59] comfort, and less radiation.[60] Three-dimensional fluoroscopy-based navigation using intraoperative images gained popularity and appears as the best imaging technology for guidance, especially in minimal access surgery where there is a lack of exposure to anatomical landmarks (**Figs. 34.12–34.14**).

The increasing interest in MIS in deformity surgery has fueled the need for navigation technologies and later for robotics[61] (**Fig. 34.15**). The Food and Drug Administration (FDA) cleared the first robot designed for spine surgery in 2004. As spine robots evolve, adoption in spine surgery increased, particularly for complex anatomy and deformity.

The current spinal robots are a "shared control" system, semi-active, designed to execute the preoperative planning done by the surgeon on a pre- or intraoperative CT scan. The surgeon is acting through the robotic end arm controlled by navigation (**Figs. 34.16** and **34.17**). Many publications report the adoption of these robotic platforms with evidence of increased accuracy, decreased radiation exposure, and better workflow and comfort.[61–67]

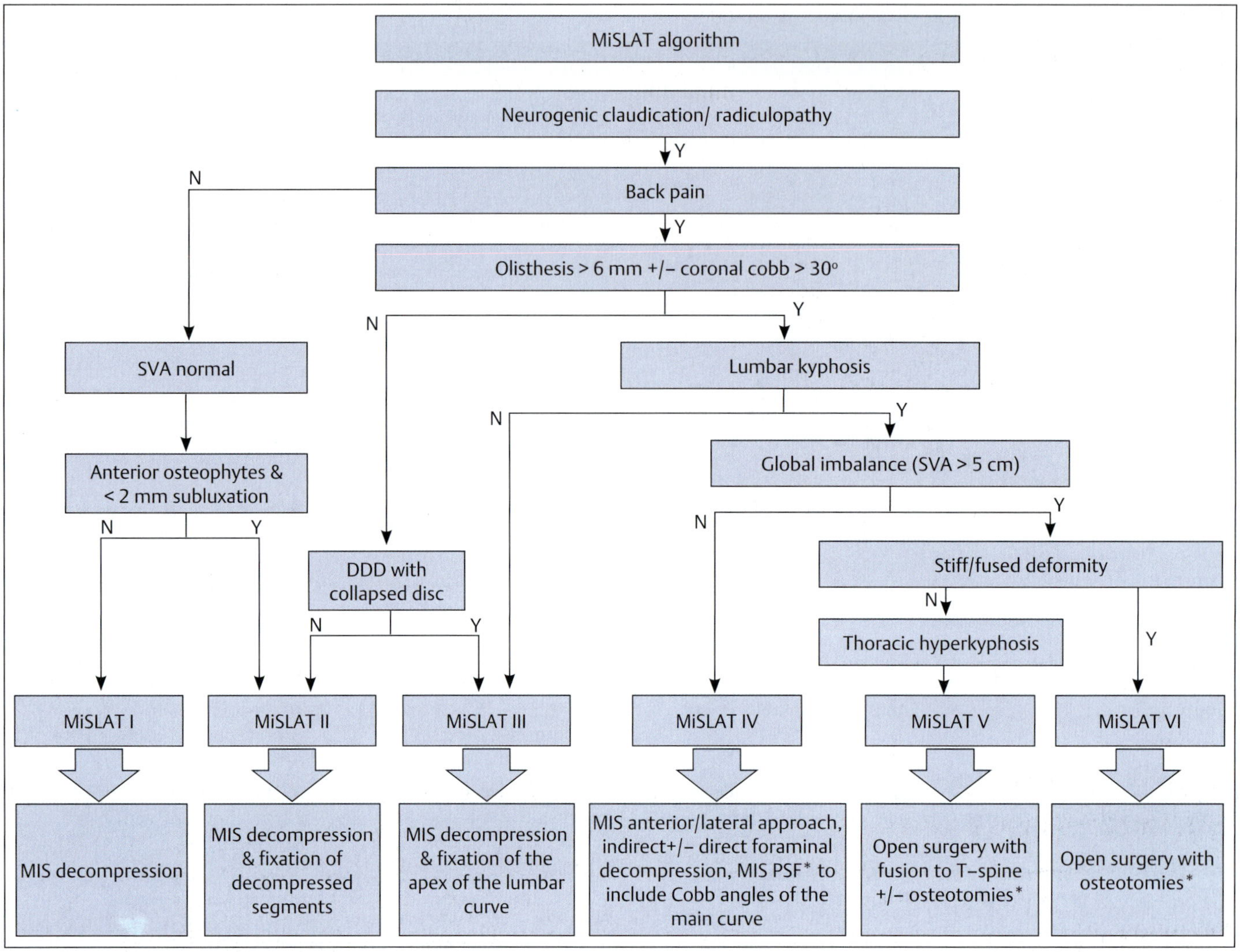

MiSLAT algorithm

Neurogenic claudication/ radiculopathy

↓Y

Back pain

N ←——— ↓Y

Olisthesis > 6 mm +/− coronal cobb > 30°

N ←——— ↓Y

SVA normal   Lumbar kyphosis

↓   N ←——— ↓Y

Anterior osteophytes & < 2 mm subluxation   Global imbalance (SVA > 5 cm)

N   Y   N ←——— ↓Y

DDD with collapsed disc   Stiff/fused deformity

N   Y   N ↓   Y

Thoracic hyperkyphosis

MiSLAT I	MiSLAT II	MiSLAT III	MiSLAT IV	MiSLAT V	MiSLAT VI
MIS decompression	MIS decompression & fixation of decompressed segments	MIS decompression & fixation of the apex of the lumbar curve	MIS anterior/lateral approach, indirect+/− direct foraminal decompression, MIS PSF* to include Cobb angles of the main curve	Open surgery with fusion to T−spine +/− osteotomies*	Open surgery with osteotomies*

Flowchart 34.1 MiSLAT algorithm.

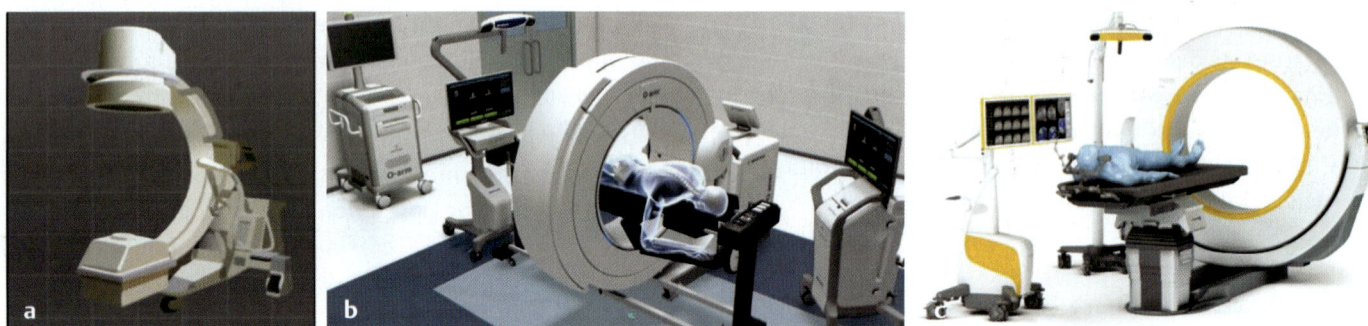

Fig. 34.12 Intraoperative imaging modalities: **(a)** Fluoroscopy, **(b)** cone-beam computed tomography (CT), and **(c)** fan-beam CT.

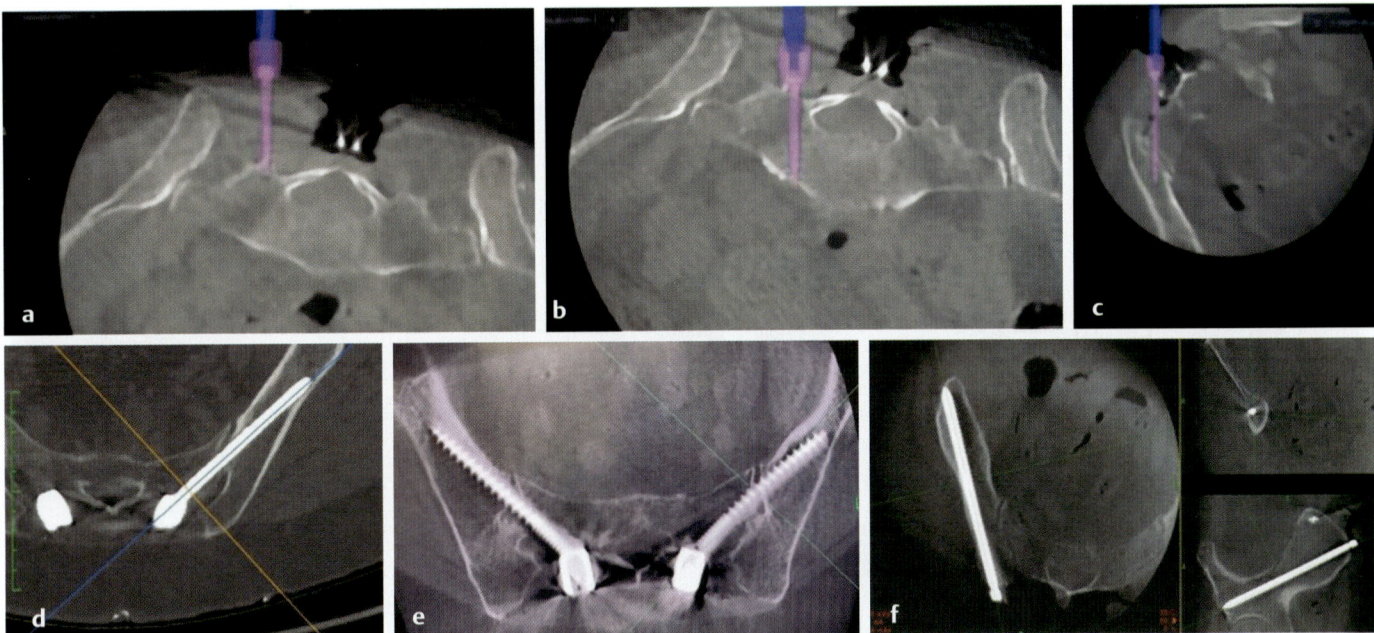

Fig. 34.13 (a–f) Spinal implants placed by navigation. Upper line shows virtual images and the lower line shows intraoperative control of implant's placement.

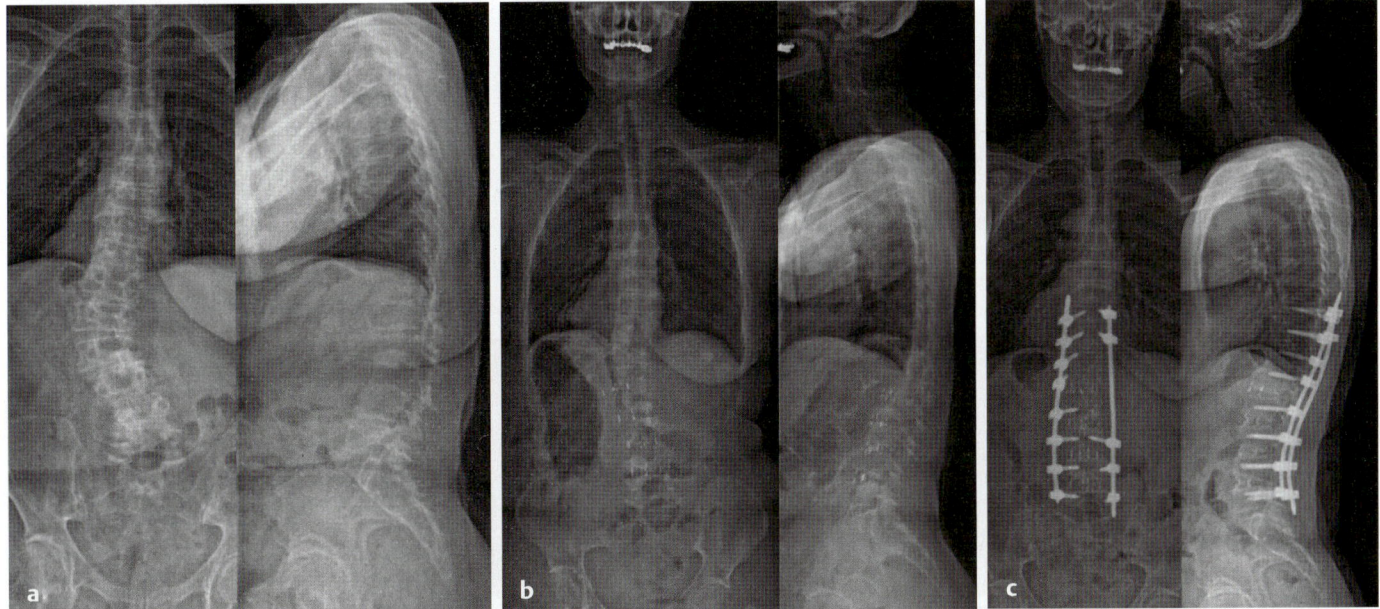

Fig. 34.14 (a–c) Case illustration of adult spinal deformity (ASD) **(a)** treated surgically by anterior realignment **(b)**, followed by percutaneous screw and rods instrumentation **(c)**.

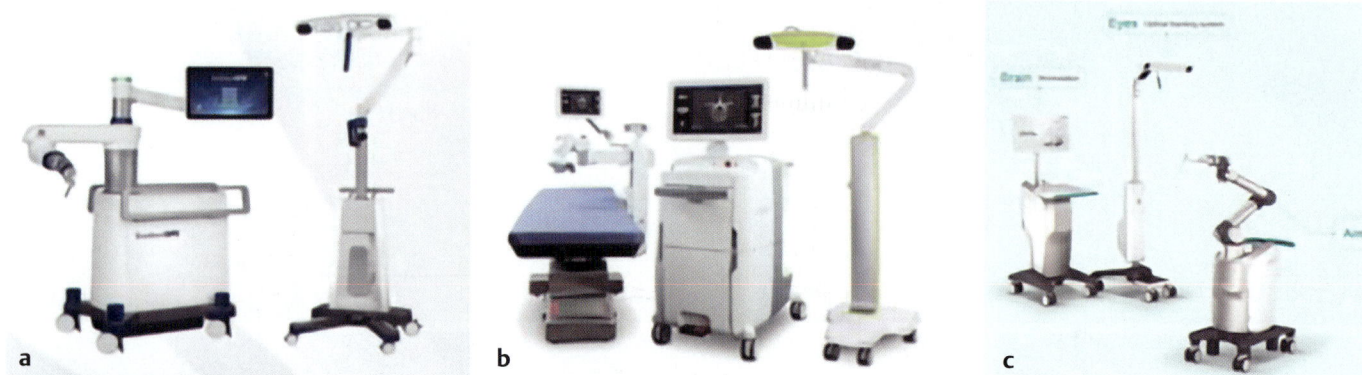

Fig. 34.15 **(a–c)** Robotics platforms: **(a)** Excelsius GPS, **(b)** MazorX stealth, and **(c)** Tinavi TiRobot.

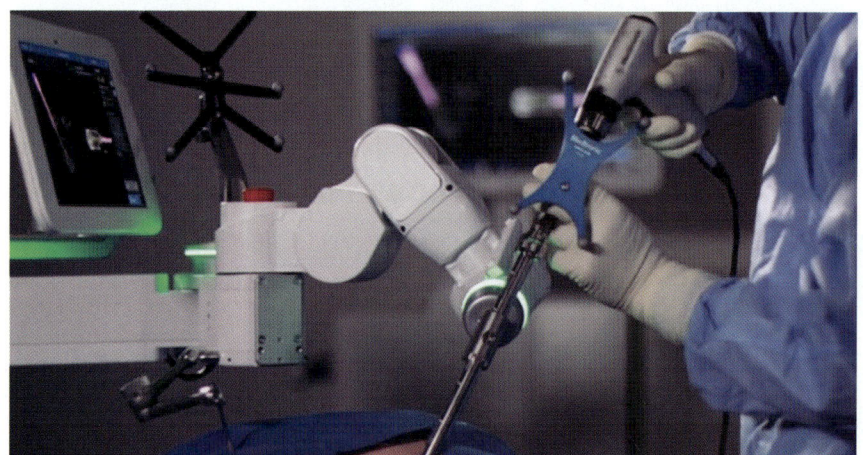

Fig. 34.16 Robotic end arm.

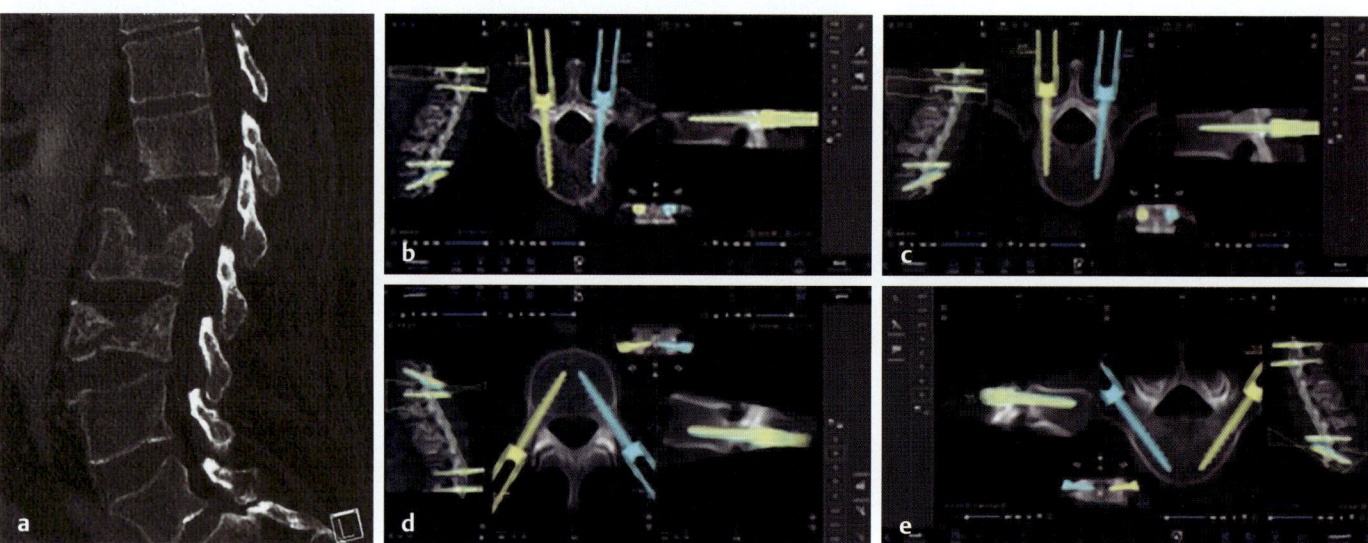

Fig. 34.17 Case illustration of a robotic minimally invasive thoracolumbar stabilization and alignment. **(a)** Preoperative computed tomography (CT) scan. **(b–e)** Planning screw placement at T10, T11, L4, and L5. *(Continued)*

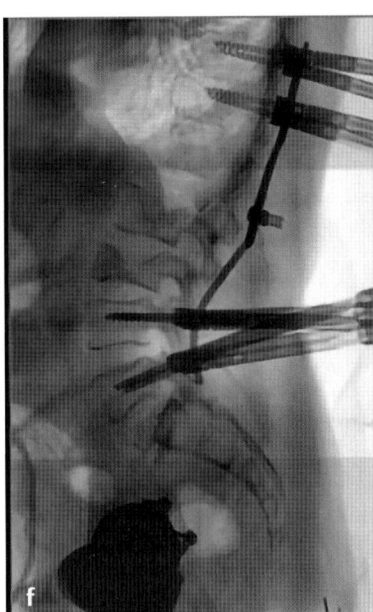
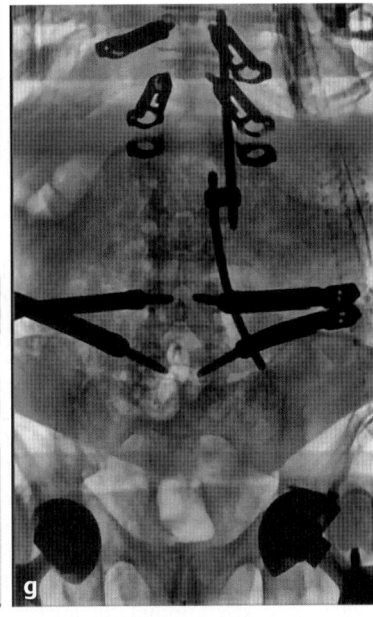

Fig. 34.17   *(Continued)* **(f, g)** Intraoperative control.

Conclusion

MIS in ASD is a viable option; clinical outcomes and radiographical results in select cases are better than in traditional open surgery. Faster recovery, better self-image, and better mental health scores are reported in patients with minimally invasive correction of the degenerative deformity. However, MIS has limitations that must be considered: the ability to optimally correct alignment in rigid and severe deformity is questionable. Decision-making is crucial, and depends on the severity of the deformity, the reducibility, and the type of instrumentation needed for surgical correction.

References

1. Behensky H, Giesinger K, Ogon M, et al. Multisurgeon assessment of coronal pattern classification systems for adolescent idiopathic scoliosis: reliability and error analysis. Spine 2002;27(7):762–767
2. Nash CL Jr, Moe JH. A study of vertebral rotation. J Bone Joint Surg Am 1969;51(2):223–229
3. Smith JS, Shaffrey CI, Kuntz C IV, Mummaneni PV. Classification systems for adolescent and adult scoliosis. Neurosurgery 2008;63(3, Suppl):16–24
4. Mummaneni PV, Ondra SL, Haid RW. Principles of spinal deformity: part II. Advances in the operative treatment of thoracolumbar deformity. Contemp Neurosurg 2002;24(20):1–10
5. Lenke LG, Betz RR, Harms J, et al. Adolescent idiopathic scoliosis: a new classification to determine extent of spinal arthrodesis. J Bone Joint Surg Am 2001;83(8):1169–1181
6. Cummings RJ, Loveless EA, Campbell J, Samelson S, Mazur JM. Interobserver reliability and intraobserver reproducibility of the system of King et al. for the classification of adolescent idiopathic scoliosis. J Bone Joint Surg Am 1998;80(8):1107–1111
7. Bernhardt M, Bridwell KH. Segmental analysis of the sagittal plane alignment of the normal thoracic and lumbar spines and thoracolumbar junction. Spine 1989;14(7):717–721
8. Bridwell KH, Betz R, Capelli AM, Huss G, Harvey C. Sagittal plane analysis in idiopathic scoliosis patients treated with Cotrel-Dubousset instrumentation. Spine 1990;15(9):921–926
9. Ogon M, Giesinger K, Behensky H, et al. Interobserver and intraobserver reliability of Lenke's new scoliosis classification system. Spine 2002;27(8):858–862
10. Richards BS, Sucato DJ, Konigsberg DE, Ouellet JA. Comparison of reliability between the Lenke and King classification systems for adolescent idiopathic scoliosis using radiographs that were not premeasured. Spine 2003;28(11):1148–1156, discussion 1156–1157
11. Ali RM, Boachie-Adjei O, Rawlins BA. Functional and radiographic outcomes after surgery for adult scoliosis using third-generation instrumentation techniques. Spine 2003;28(11):1163–1169, discussion 1169–1170
12. Bess RS, Lenke LG, Bridwell KH, Cheh G, Mandel S, Sides B. Comparison of thoracic pedicle screw to hook instrumentation for the treatment of adult spinal deformity. Spine 2007;32(5):555–561
13. Cho KJ, Suk SI, Park SR, et al. Risk factors of sagittal decompensation after long posterior instrumentation and fusion for degenerative lumbar scoliosis. Spine 2010;35(17):1595–1601
14. Lapp MA, Bridwell KH, Lenke LG, et al. Long-term complications in adult spinal deformity patients having combined surgery a comparison of primary to revision patients. Spine 2001;26(8):973–983
15. Cho KJ, Suk SI, Park SR, et al. Complications in posterior fusion and instrumentation for degenerative lumbar scoliosis. Spine 2007;32(20):2232–2237
16. Liu W, Chen XS, Jia LS, Song DW. The clinical features and surgical treatment of degenerative lumbar scoliosis: a review of 112 patients. Orthop Surg 2009;1(3):176–183
17. Cho KJ, Suk SI, Park SR, et al. Short fusion versus long fusion for degenerative lumbar scoliosis. Eur Spine J 2008;17(5):650–656

18. Isaacs RE, Hyde J, Goodrich JA, Rodgers WB, Phillips FM. A prospective, nonrandomized, multicenter evaluation of extreme lateral interbody fusion for the treatment of adult degenerative scoliosis: perioperative outcomes and complications. Spine 2010;35(26 Suppl):S322–S330

19. Khan SN, Hofer MA, Gupta MC. Lumbar degenerative scoliosis: outcomes of combined anterior and posterior pelvis surgery with minimum 2-year follow-up. Orthopedics 2009; 32(4):258

20. Kim YB, Lenke LG, Kim YJ, et al. The morbidity of an anterior thoracolumbar approach: adult spinal deformity patients with greater than five-year follow-up. Spine 2009;34(8):822–826

21. Kim YB, Lenke LG, Kim YJ, Kim YW, Bridwell KH, Stobbs G. Surgical treatment of adult scoliosis: is anterior apical release and fusion necessary for the lumbar curve? Spine 2008;33(10):1125–1132

22. Kostis JP, Hall BB. Spinal fusions to the sacrum in adults with scoliosis. Spine 1983;8(5):489–500

23. Peelle MW, Boachie-Adjei O, Charles G, Kanazawa Y, Mesfin A. Lumbar curve response to selective thoracic fusion in adult idiopathic scoliosis. Spine J 2008;8(6):897–903

24. Simmons ED Jr, Kowalski JM, Simmons EH. The results of surgical treatment for adult scoliosis. Spine 1993;18(6):718–724

25. Transfeldt EE, Topp R, Mehbod AA, Winter RB. Surgical outcomes of decompression, decompression with limited fusion, and decompression with full curve fusion for degenerative scoliosis with radiculopathy. Spine 2010;35(20):1872–1875

26. Wang MY, Mummaneni PV. Minimally invasive surgery for thoracolumbar spinal deformity: initial clinical experience with clinical and radiographic outcomes. Neurosurg Focus 2010;28(3):E9

27. Bess S, Line B, Fu KM, et al; International Spine Study Group. The health impact of symptomatic adult spinal deformity: comparison of deformity types to United States population norms and chronic diseases. Spine 2016;41(3):224–233

28. Ames CP, Scheer JK, Lafage V, et al. Adult spinal deformity: epidemiology, health impact, evaluation, and management. Spine Deform 2016;4(4):310–322

29. Anand N, Agrawal A, Burger EL, et al. The prevalence of the use of MIS techniques in the treatment of adult spinal deformity (ASD) amongst members of the Scoliosis Research Society (SRS) in 2016. Spine Deform 2019;7(2):319–324

30. Kanter AS, Tempel ZJ, Ozpinar A, Okonkwo DO. A review of minimally invasive procedures for the treatment of adult spinal deformity. Spine 2016;41(Suppl 8):S59–S65

31. Aebi M. The adult scoliosis. Eur Spine J 2005;14(10):925–948

32. Schwab F, Farcy JP, Bridwell K, et al. A clinical impact classification of scoliosis in the adult. Spine 2006;31(18):2109–2114

33. Schwab F, Ungar B, Blondel B, et al. Scoliosis Research Society-Schwab adult spinal deformity classification: a validation study. Spine 2012;37(12):1077–1082

34. Mummaneni P, Smith J, Shaffrey C, et al. Risk factors for major perioperative complications in adult spinal deformity surgery. In 79th AANS Annual Scientific Meeting. Denver, 2011

35. Chi JH, Dhall SS, Kanter AS, Mummaneni PV. The mini-open transpedicular thoracic discectomy: surgical technique and assessment. Neurosurg Focus 2008;25(2):E5

36. Dhall SS, Wang MY, Mummaneni PV. Clinical and radiographic comparison of mini-open transforaminal lumbar interbody fusion with open transforaminal lumbar interbody fusion in 42 patients with long-term follow-up. J Neurosurg Spine 2008;9(6):560–565

37. Mummaneni PV, Wang MY, Silva FE, Lenke LG, Amin BY, Tu TH. Minimally invasive evaluation and treatment for adult degenerative deformity using the MiSLAT algorithm. Scoliosis Research Society E-text; 2013. Available: http://etext.srs.org/book/

38. Anand N, Rosemann R, Khalsa B, Baron EM. Mid-term to long-term clinical and functional outcomes of minimally invasive correction and fusion for adults with scoliosis. Neurosurg Focus 2010;28(3):E6

39. Fessler RG, Khoo LT. Minimally invasive cervical microendoscopic foraminotomy: an initial clinical experience. Neurosurgery 2002;51(5, Suppl):S37–S45

40. Harrington JF, French P. Open versus minimally invasive lumbar microdiscectomy: comparison of operative times, length of hospital stay, narcotic use and complications. Minim Invasive Neurosurg 2008;51(1):30–35

41. Rahman M, Summers LE, Richter B, Mimran RI, Jacob RP. Comparison of techniques for decompressive lumbar laminectomy: the minimally invasive versus the "classic" open approach. Minim Invasive Neurosurg 2008;51(2):100–105

42. O'Toole JE, Eichholz KM, Fessler RG. Surgical site infection rates after minimally invasive spinal surgery. J Neurosurg Spine. 2009;11(4):471–476

43. Bridwell KH, Lewis SJ, Rinella A, Lenke LG, Baldus C, Blanke K. Pedicle subtraction osteotomy for the treatment of fixed sagittal imbalance. Surgical technique. J Bone Joint Surg Am 2004;86-A(Suppl 1):44–50

44. Berjano P, Aebi M. Pedicle subtraction osteotomies (PSO) in the lumbar spine for sagittal deformities. Eur Spine J 2015;24(Suppl 1):S49–S57

45. Bridwell KH. Decision making regarding Smith-Petersen vs. pedicle subtraction osteotomy vs. vertebral column resection for spinal deformity. Spine 2006;31(19, Suppl):S171–S178

46. Kelleher MO, Timlin M, Persaud O, Rampersaud YR. Success and failure of minimally invasive decompression for focal lumbar spinal stenosis in patients with and without deformity. Spine 2010;35(19):E981–E987

47. Matsumura A, Namikawa T, Terai H, et al. The influence of approach side on facet preservation in microscopic bilateral decompression via a unilateral approach for degenerative lumbar scoliosis. Clinical article. J Neurosurg Spine 2010;13(6):758–765

48. Yamada K, Matsuda H, Nabeta M, Habunaga H, Suzuki A, Nakamura H. Clinical outcomes of microscopic decompression for degenerative lumbar foraminal stenosis: a comparison between patients with and without degenerative lumbar scoliosis. Eur Spine J 2011;20(6):947–953

49. Bridwell KH. Selection of instrumentation and fusion levels for scoliosis: where to start and where to stop. Invited submission from the Joint Section Meeting on Disorders of the Spine and Peripheral Nerves, March 2004. J Neurosurg Spine 2004;1(1):1–8

50. Silva FE, Lenke LG. Adult degenerative scoliosis: evaluation and management. Neurosurg Focus 2010;28(3):E1

51. Mummaneni PV, Wang MY, Silva FE, Lenke LG, Amin BY, Tu TH. Minimally invasive evaluation and treatment for adult degenerative deformity using the MiSLAT algorithm. Scoliosis Research Society E-text; 2013.

52. Tian NF, Huang QS, Zhou P, et al. Pedicle screw insertion accuracy with different assisted methods: a systematic review and meta-analysis of comparative studies. Eur Spine J 2011;20(6):846–859

53. Assaker R, Reyns N, Vinchon M, Demondion X, Louis E. Transpedicular screw placement: image-guided versus lateral-

view fluoroscopy: in vitro simulation. Spine 2001;26(19): 2160–2164

54. Austin MS, Vaccaro AR, Brislin B, Nachwalter R, Hilibrand AS, Albert TJ. Image-guided spine surgery: a cadaver study comparing conventional open laminoforaminotomy and two image-guided techniques for pedicle screw placement in posterolateral fusion and nonfusion models. Spine 2002; 27(22):2503–2508

55. Nottmeier EW, Seemer W, Young PM. Placement of thoracolumbar pedicle screws using three-dimensional image guidance: experience in a large patient cohort. J Neurosurg Spine 2009;10(1):33–39

56. Shin BJ, James AR, Njoku IU, Härtl R. Pedicle screw navigation: a systematic review and meta-analysis of perforation risk for computer-navigated versus freehand insertion. J Neurosurg Spine 2012;17(2):113–122

57. Parker SL, McGirt MJ, Farber SH, et al. Accuracy of free-hand pedicle screws in the thoracic and lumbar spine: analysis of 6816 consecutive screws. Neurosurgery 2011;68(1):170–178, discussion 178

58. Rajasekaran S, Vidyadhara S, Ramesh P, Shetty AP. Randomized clinical study to compare the accuracy of navigated and non-navigated thoracic pedicle screws in deformity correction surgeries. Spine 2007;32(2):E56–E64

59. Richter M, Mattes T, Cakir B. Computer-assisted posterior instrumentation of the cervical and cervico-thoracic spine. Eur Spine J 2004;13(1):50–59

60. Nottmeier EW, Bowman C, Nelson KL. Surgeon radiation exposure in cone beam computed tomography-based, image-guided spinal surgery. Int J Med Robot 2012;8(2):196–200

61. Devito DP, Kaplan L, Dietl R, et al. Clinical acceptance and accuracy assessment of spinal implants guided with SpineAssist surgical robot: retrospective study. Spine 2010;35(24): 2109–2115

62. Lieberman IH, Hardenbrook MA, Wang JC, Guyer RD. Assessment of pedicle screw placement accuracy, procedure time, and radiation exposure using a miniature robotic guidance system. J Spinal Disord Tech 2012;25(5):241–248

63. Hu X, Ohnmeiss DD, Lieberman IH. Robotic-assisted pedicle screw placement: lessons learned from the first 102 patients. Eur Spine J 2013;22(3):661–666

64. Kantelhardt SR, Martinez R, Baerwinkel S, Burger R, Giese A, Rohde V. Perioperative course and accuracy of screw positioning in conventional, open robotic-guided and percutaneous robotic-guided, pedicle screw placement. Eur Spine J 2011;20(6):860–868

65. Martin BI, Mirza SK, Spina N, Spiker WR, Lawrence B, Brodke DS. Trends in lumbar fusion procedure rates and associated hospital costs for degenerative spinal diseases in the United States, 2004 to 2015. Spine 2019;44(5):369–376

66. Vo CD, Jiang B, Azad TD, Crawford NR, Bydon A, Theodore N. Robotic spine surgery: current state in minimally invasive surgery. Global Spine J 2020;10(2, Suppl):34S–40S

67. Jiang B, Azad TD, Cottrill E, et al. New spinal robotic technologies. Front Med 2019;13(6):723–729

35 Dynamic Stabilization for Spinal Deformities

Ali Fahir Özer and Göktuğ Akyoldaş

Introduction

One of the most challenging problems of spine surgery is a spinal deformity. The spine is a structure in which the nervous system is located. Starting from the lower part of the medulla at the base of the skull, it contains the spinal cord in its continuity to the L1 level. The remaining lumbar spine is filled with nerve fibers formed by the nerve roots coming out of the spinal cord and contains these fibers up to the end of the sacral spine. This structure has a natural curve of its own. Although it shows some minor changes from person to person, the cervical region is lordotic, the thoracic region is kyphotic, the lumbar region is lordotic, and the sacral region is kyphotic. These naturally occurring curves serve to dissipate the mechanical stress that occurs during the standing position and in motion.

It is essential to preserve the anatomical integrity of this structure in maintaining a healthy and high-quality human life. Unfortunately, various pathologies cause the integrity of this structure to deteriorate, and the quality of life deteriorates. Leaving traumas aside, pathologies develop slowly, and their early recognition is essential in their correction with more straightforward surgical or nonsurgical methods.

Spinal Deformities

Spinal deformities are mainly divided into coronal and sagittal plane deformities.

Coronal Plane Deformities (Scoliosis)

Scoliosis is defined as an abnormal C- or S-shaped curvature of the spine. The curve can occur on the left side or right side. In addition, abnormal curvature is usually evident when the patient is viewed from the front or the back. For years, the aim of scoliosis treatment has focused on the coronal curve. With advancements in knowledge surgeons developed methods to measure and classify abnormal curves. However, many classifications have been developed for scoliosis. Historically, the first modern classification was King's system. This classification system was named King

classification system, which defines five different types of thoracic scoliosis curves but considers only coronal plane X-rays in the assessment.

Scoliosis is recognized by surgeons as a complex, three-dimensional deformity that affects the balance of the spine in the coronal planes, and sagittal and axial planes. Coronal plane is the front and back of the body. Sagittal plane is the left and right sides of the body. Axial plane is the system we see when looking down from the top of the body.

As a member of a multicenter scoliosis working group in the early 1990s, Dr. Lenke began work on a new, comprehensive radiographic classification of adolescent idiopathic scoliosis (AIS). This is the most common form of scoliosis. In the beginning, all the three planes (coronal, sagittal, and axial) were included in the classification but were ultimately excluded from the classification due to the inconsistency and low reliability of the measurement assessment. Thus, a two-dimensional system called the Lenke classification was created in 2011 by Lenke et al. Although there are still some objections because it does not fully cover all types of scoliosis, such as adult scoliosis, it is the most widely accepted classification in use today.

The Lenke classification provides surgeons with a simple, accurate, and repeatable way to communicate about scoliosis with each other. The system is based on measurements from standard radiographs (X-rays). First, the surgeon evaluates the patient's X-rays in the anterior-posterior (AP), lateral, and lateral bending positions. Each scoliosis curve is then classified in three ways.

In this classification, the types of curves are divided according to the three regions of the spine: proximal thoracic, main thoracic, and thoracolumbar/lumbar structural or nonstructural.

A lumbar spine modifier based on the distance from the center of the lumbar spine to the midline and a sagittal thoracic modifier based on the amount of lateral curvature to the thoracic region were added to the classification in time.

One of the most critical steps in classification is lateral bending radiographs. With these radiographs, it is evaluated whether the deformity is relatively rigid or flexible (mobile). Therefore, the triad system puts together the curve type (1–6), lumbar modifier (A, B, C), and sagittal thoracic modifier (−, N, +) to create the entire classification. For instance, the most common type is the 1AN curve classification (**Fig. 35.1**).[1]

Since the Lenke classification causes problems in evaluating adult spinal deformity, Schwab and Scoliosis Research Society (SRS) developed a new classification for adult spinal deformity in 2012. In this classification, the coronal curve is divided into four types: (1) thoracic curve (curve type T)—apical Tp and above and Cobb angle >30 degrees; (2) thoracolumbar or lumbar curve (curve type L)—Cobb angle >30 degrees; (3) double curve (curve type D)—the patient has both lumbar and thoracic curves, and both are >30 degrees; (4) in the fourth type, the curve is low (slope type N), that is, the patient has a curve, but it is <30 degrees. In addition, there are sagittal modifiers. The first of these determinants is the difference between pelvic incidence and lumbar lordosis (PI − LL), the other is the distance of the sagittal vertebral axis (SVA) to the posterior sacrum, and the last determinant is pelvic tilt (PT). The standard and pathological values of sagittal modifiers are given in **Fig. 35.2** together with the classification.[2]

Sagittal Plane Deformity (Kyphosis)

The sagittal determinants in this classification provide us with crucial information to evaluate the patient's sagittal balance. As it is known, the development of deformity in the sagittal plane occurs as a result of increasing or decreasing natural curves of the spine. In normal human posture, the projection of the head falls into the pelvis. With the development of deformity in the sagittal plane, this balance is disturbed, but the human body tries to compensate for it. The most common pathologies that cause deformation in the sagittal plane are Scheuermann's kyphosis, loss of lordosis due to lumbar leaning, and the head being pushed forward due to the effect of thoracic kyphosis, gradually shifting forward in the pelvis. Lastly, among the most common causes, the increase in kyphosis due to osteoporotic fractures is accompanied by the deterioration of sagittal balance.

The evaluation of sagittal balance is as important as coronal deformity. If we look briefly at the main points in terms of sagittal balance, a person with both feet on the ground can stand with minimal effort. This corresponds

Curve Type				
Type	Proximal throcacic	Main thoracic	Thoracolumbar/lumbar	Description
1	Nonstructural	Structural (Major)	Nonstructural	Main thoracic (MT)
2	Structural	Structural (Major)	Nonstructural	Double thoracic (MT)
3	Nonstructural	Structural (Major)	Structural	Double Major (DM)
4	Structural	Structural (Major)	Structural (Major)	Triple Major (TM)
5	Nonstructural	Nonstructural	Structural (Major)	Thoracolumbar/lumbar (TL/L)
6	Nonstructural	Structural	Structural (Major)	Thoracolumbar/lumbar—main thoracic (TL/L-MT)

Structural Criteria (Minor Curves)	
Proximal Thoracic	Side bening cobb ≥ 25° T2-T5 kyphosis ≥ +25°
Main Thoracic	Side bening cobb ≥ 25° T10-L2 kyphosis ≥ +25°
Thoracolumbar/lumbar	Side bening cobb ≥ 25° T10-L2 kyphosis ≥ +25°

Location of apex (SRS definition)	
Curve	Apex
Thoracic	T2-T11/12 disc
Thoracolumbar	T12-L1
Thoracolumbar/Lumbar	L1/2 disc – L4

Thoracic sagittal Profile T5-T12	
- (hypo)	< 10°
N (normal)	10° - 40°
+ (hyper)	> 10°

Modifiers	
Lumbar spine modifiers	CSVL to lumbar apex
A	CSVL between pedicles
B	CSVL touches apical body(ies)
C	CSVL completely medial

Fig. 35.1   Lenke classification. CSVL, central sacral vertical line; SRS, Scoliosis Research Society. (Modified from Lenke et al.[1])

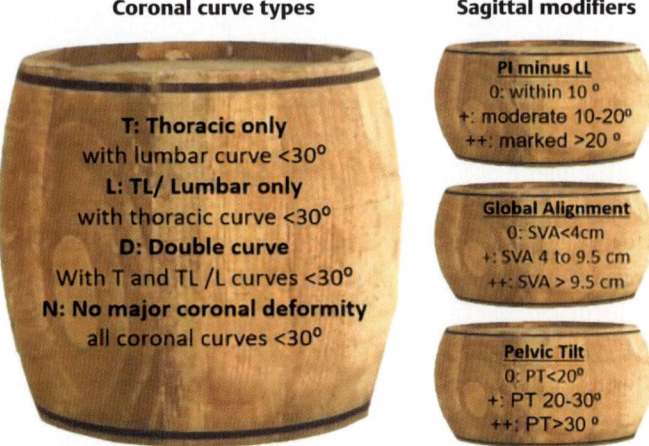

Fig. 35.2 Scoliosis Research Society (SRS)–Schwab classification. Main coronal curve and sagittal modifiers are seen. LL, lumbar lordosis; PI, pelvic incidence; SVA, sagittal vertebral axis.

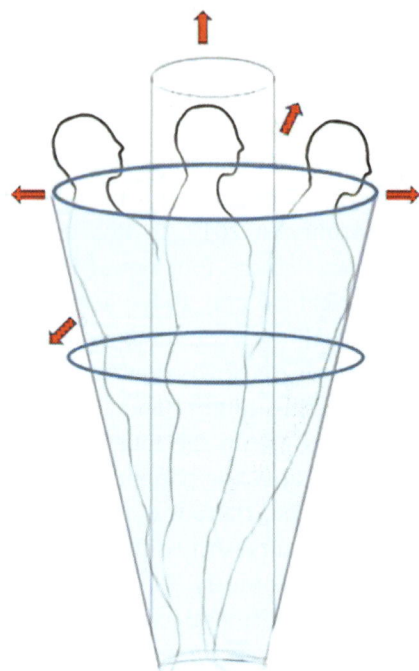

Fig. 35.3 The cone formed by the circle on which the person stands is the standing position with the least energy expenditure. If the person moves out of this cone, it will consume more energy.[3]

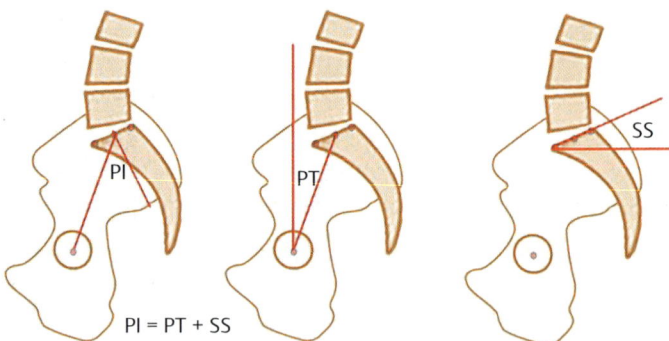

Fig. 35.4 Pelvic parameters. Definition of different pelvic angles: PI, pelvic incidence angle, PT, pelvic tilt, SS, sacral tilt. These last two parameters reflect the spatial orientation of the pelvis.

to a small circle around both feet. If the person goes out of this circle and draws wider circles with waist and head movements, he/she must spend energy on this. In other words, leaving the economic circle will have a cost. The disruption of the sagittal balance forces the person to pay this cost against his/her will. After people started standing and walking on two legs, their pelvis also expanded due to bipedalism. Especially as a result of the enlargement of the anterior and posterior diameter, the projection of the head increased the probability of staying in the pelvis.

Sagittal measurements of a person in standing position were defined based on the vertical line passing through the femoral head. In a person with normal alignment of the spine, the spine rises above the pelvis. However, for the spine to stand upright, some changes in the orientation of the pelvis occur. Thus, the deterioration of its relationship with the pelvis affects the standard curves of the entire spine (**Fig. 35.3**).[3]

Spinopelvic Parameters

Pelvic incidence (PI) is the first pelvic parameter to consider. PI corresponds to the angle between the line perpendicular to the midpoint of the line passing through the upper end plate of S1 and the line connecting it to the axis of the femoral heads, as described by Legaye et al[4] and Duval-Beaupère et al.[5] The characteristic of PI is that it remains constant from childhood to adolescence.

The sacral slope angle (SS) is defined as the angle between a line tangential to the upper S1 end plate and the horizontal line. A vertical pelvis will mean a low angle of sacral tilt, while a horizontal pelvis will have a high angle of sacral tilt (**Fig. 35.4**).

Pelvic tilt (PT) is defined as the angle between the line connecting the center of the vertical and sacral end plates to the axis of the femoral heads. These two angles are positional and related to pelvis orientation because the pelvis can rotate around the axis of the femoral head. This movement can be forward, anteversion (**Fig. 35.5a**), or backward retroversion (**Fig. 35.5b**). Therefore, the PT angle increases during pelvic retroversion.

There is a relationship between these three parameters[5] (**Fig. 35.4**): PI is equal to the arithmetic sum of sacral tilt and pelvic tilt (PI = PT + SS). This indicates that a patient with a high PI angle has a more significant potential for pelvic

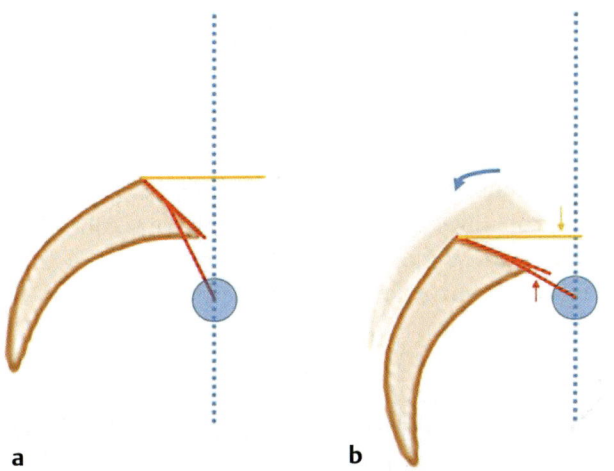

a   b

Fig. 35.5 **(a)** Normal pelvic version. **(b)** Pelvic tilt (PT) increases with more vertical sacrum and decrease in sacral tilt (SS) while the pelvic angle of incidence (PI) remains constant. This corresponds to retroversion of the pelvis.

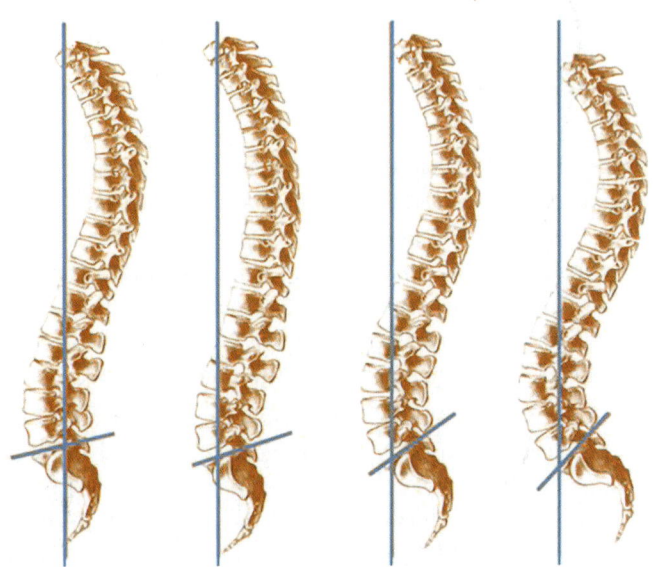

Fig. 35.6 Spine types according to Roussouly.

retroversion. This is one of the essential compensation mechanisms and is also crucial for the patient. Disruption of the spinopelvic relationship affects the entire spine. Let us start with the lumbar parameters.

There is a strong correlation between sacral slope and LL. The relationship between sacral slope and PI explains the relationship between PI and LL. For example, it is stated that there is a mathematical relationship between LL and PI. For instance, Schwab et al[6] suggested that PI=LL±9 degrees could be formulated. Similar mathematical calculations have been made. However, Roussouly et al,[7] in a prospective study of people without spinal pathologies, identified four types of vertebrae with different spinal and pelvic parameters, particularly in terms of a transition from LL to thoracic kyphosis (**Fig. 35.6**):

- Types 1 and 2 are characterized by a slight sacral slope (less than 35 degrees).

- Type 1 has a slightly lower lordosis curve with a lower lordosis apex (approximately L5). Therefore, the lordosis is short, and the kyphosis is thoracolumbar.

- Type 2 has a flattened lower arch with very little curvature. The back is straight.

- Type 3 corresponds to the lordotic apex at L4 and the mean sacral inclination is between 35 and 45 degrees. The lordosis is almost evenly distributed over the two arches. This is the most balanced type.

- Type 4 corresponds to a steep sacral slope (greater than 45 degrees) with a lordotic apex at the anterior-bottom corner of L3. The global lordosis angle (LL) is larger and contains more vertebrae than other types. Thoracic kyphosis is shorter.

Based on Roussouly's definition, adding the studies of Barrey et al[8] and later Le Huec and Hasegawa,[9] it is generally observed that lordosis angle tends to increase for PI below the mean value (50 degrees). In contrast, we can conclude that lordosis tends to be equal to incidence when the PI is approximately 50 degrees (LL=PI). In addition, when the incidence is above 65 degrees, the LL tends to be less than the PI. Therefore, the frequently used formula PI=LL+9 degrees is valid only for small PI angles. This leads to many estimation errors when the PI exceeds 50 degrees.[6,10]

The most critical measurement in the thoracic region is the thoracic kyphosis angle. We have already mentioned enough about how the lumbar region affects the thoracic region while describing the lumbar region above. Thoracic kyphosis is the angle between the lines tangent to the upper T1 end plate and the lower T12 end plate. The theoretical value of thoracic kyphosis has been shown to be equal to 0.75 times the global LL angle, L1 to S1 (9): T1T12 lordosis=0.75×L1S1 lordosis.

In addition, it is stated that the measurement of the thoracic kyphosis angle between T4 and T12 would be more appropriate for ease of measurement since the humeral heads are superimposed, and standard radiographs are often of poor quality. In a study involving 403 patients, the thoracic kyphosis angle (TC) was found to be 43.55 ± 6.44.[11]

It is one of the most affected areas in the cervical region. Although various parameters are used in the cervical region, three parameters are crucial for physicians[12]:

- High cervical angle O–C2 (occipital C2 vertebra): The angle between the McGregor line and the line passing tangentially from the lower C2 end plate. The McGregor line connects the posterior edge of the hard palate to the lower point of the occipital bone. The mean value of this angle is 15.81 degrees (±7.15 degrees), which is always lordotic, with a mean value between 20 and 39 years of age.

- C2–C7 angle: The angle between the tangential line passing through the C2 end plate and the divergent lines on the lower C7 end plate, ranging from kyphosis to lordosis in the normal population. It is ordinarily lordotic with an average value of 17.15 ± 12.33. It changes markedly with age. Angles of O–C2 and C2–C7 work in reverse: As one increases, the other decreases (**Fig. 35.7**).

- The C7 slope angle (slope) is a crucial parameter for statistically evaluating the cervical spine.[12] The median value is 20 degrees. Patients with a C7 curve greater than 20 degrees have a lordotic cervical spine (lordosis between C2 and C7). Conversely, patients with a C7 slope of less than 20 degrees have a neutral or kyphotic cervical spine between C2 and C7.

As a result, if pathology in the lumbar region cannot be corrected with compensation mechanisms, it will affect the thoracic region. However, since the thoracic spine is attached to the rib cage, we can observe a variety of deformities from kyphosis to hyperlordosis in the cervical area; hence, the cervical spine will be extensively affected and very mobile (**Fig. 35.8**).

As a result, there are four pathologies that we frequently encounter that cause the sagittal balance to deteriorate. Scheuermann's kyphosis is a flat lumbar deformity that occurs due to ankylosing spondylitis. LL disappears, increasing kyphotic deformity due to osteoporotic fractures and disappearance of LL due to degeneration.

The problem is solved with rigid instrumentation and fusion surgery in the first two of these. In osteoporotic fractures, we can treat some cases with dynamic stabilization systems, and fusion surgery may not be necessary in these cases.[13] However, in patients with a flat back, we can use dynamic stabilization in one or two levels in the first compensation levels, where the patient can control the deformity. With a more straightforward surgery, we can protect the patient from more severe deformity that will develop in the future.

Age-Related Problems and Compensation Mechanisms

Changes in the spine during aging occur in three anatomical structures, namely, spinal, pelvic, and lower extremities .Compensating mechanisms do not to deteriorate the spine's posture and enable looking ahead in the horizontal plane. Evaluating these data helps in planning more appropriate surgical management of patients. It should not be considered as a fusion surgery alone. Creating an image of the entire spine and measuring the spinopelvic parameters will help determine whether dynamic or fusion surgery or a hybrid surgery should be selected for the correction to be made during the surgery by integrating all these parameters. These parameters will also enable us to understand the complications involved in each types of surgery.

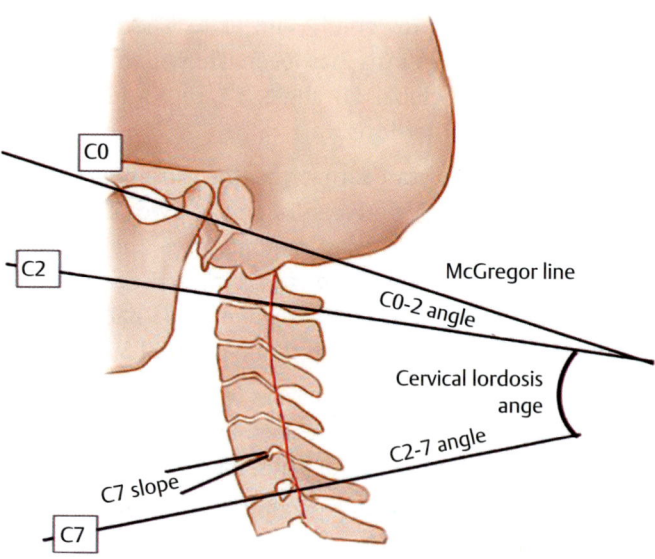

Fig. 35.7 C0–C2 angle, C7 slope angle, and cervical lordosis angle.

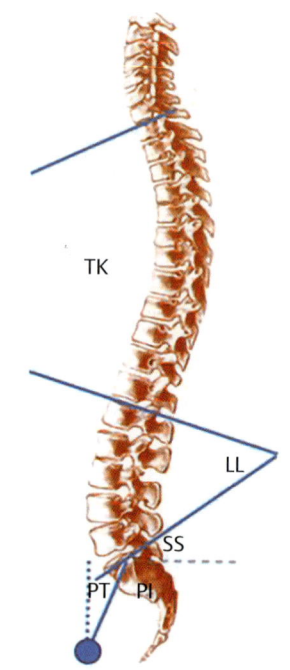

Fig. 35.8 Lordotic and kyphotic relationship of the pelvic, lumbar, thoracic, and cervical regions. LL, lumbar lordosis; PI, pelvic incidence; PT, pelvic tilt; SS, sacral slope; TK, thoracic kyphosis.

Osteoporotic fractures or degeneration and fusion of the lower lumbar spine occur together with an increase in segmental lordosis and elevation of the disc and anterior–posterior space in the adjacent spine. Spinous processes touch each other, and retrolisthesis develops. In the meantime, the patient tries to pull back the straightened waist by using the waist muscles. However, this does not provide long-term relief. Retroverting the pelvis increases the PT angle and tries to keep the spine upright. Thoracic kyphosis decreases but is limited, and cervical hyperlordosis develops. If all these mechanisms are insufficient, the patient attempts to maintain horizontal gaze by flexing the knee joints and extending the feet from the heel.

The Lenke-Silva,[14] Berjano-Lamartine,[15] and SRS-Schwab[16] classifications are essential for us to identify the deformity. The purpose of the classification is to define the deformity jointly and standardize the surgery. Those who make these classifications, and their practitioners are people dedicated to fusion surgery. However, with the current knowledge and technology, it has emerged that it is possible to operate some of the cases in this classification without requiring fusion (**Fig. 35.9**).

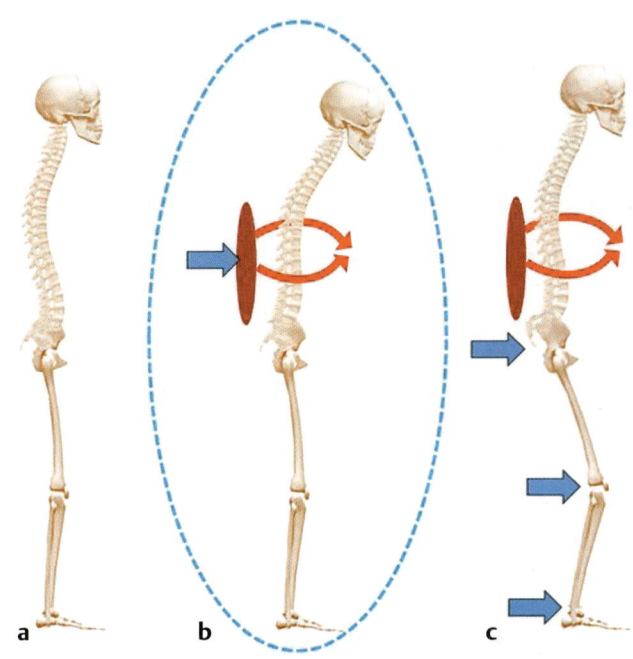

Fig. 35.9 Deformity stages. **(a)** Normal spine. **(b)** When the patient stands or walks for a long time, the trunk leans forward as the lumbar lordosis disappears. **(c)** If all these mechanisms are insufficient, the patient attempts to maintain horizontal gaze by flexing the knee joints and extending the feet from the heel.

Philosophy of Using Dynamic System in Deformity

The problem in deformity is to reveal whether the deformity is structural or nonstructural. If you correct the structural deformity, you do not need to intervene in the nonstructural deformity, and it will correct itself. In this, lateral bending radiographs are taken because lateral bending radiographs do not correct structural deformities. However, it is known that structural deformities are also mobile, especially in childhood and early adolescents. It has also been shown that most of the deformities that are considered structural in the early stages of adult deformity are not corrected by lateral bending radiographs but can be corrected when force is applied. To demonstrate this, methods such as lying down and standing X-rays and determining whether the deformity is mobile while lying under traction are used. Again, if there is an improvement in the radiographs taken by pressing the apex of the deformity, it indicates that the deformity is mobile (**Fig. 35.10**).

This knowledge shows that we can improve fusion surgery by maneuvering the instruments without deteriorating the anatomy. This is where dynamic systems considered. A mobile deformity can be corrected with mobile systems, without the necessity of rigid systems.

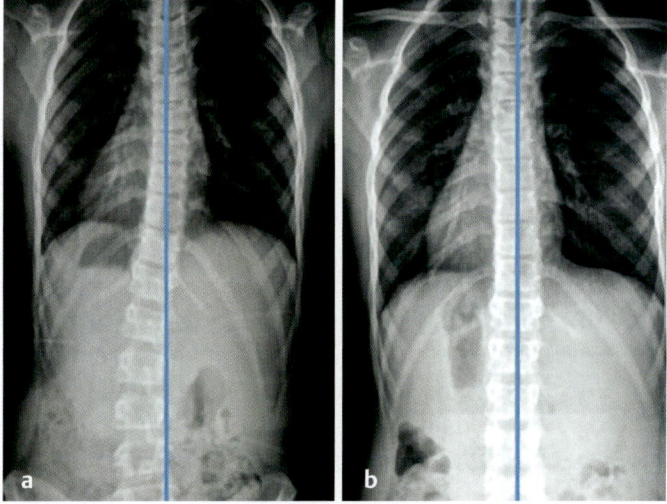

Fig. 35.10 Anteroposterior (AP) X-ray **(a)** before and **(b)** after traction.

Surgical Techniques

Vertebral Body Tethering

Vertebral body tethering was developed to allow directed growth for growing children with progressive scoliosis. During postoperative development, the deformity may

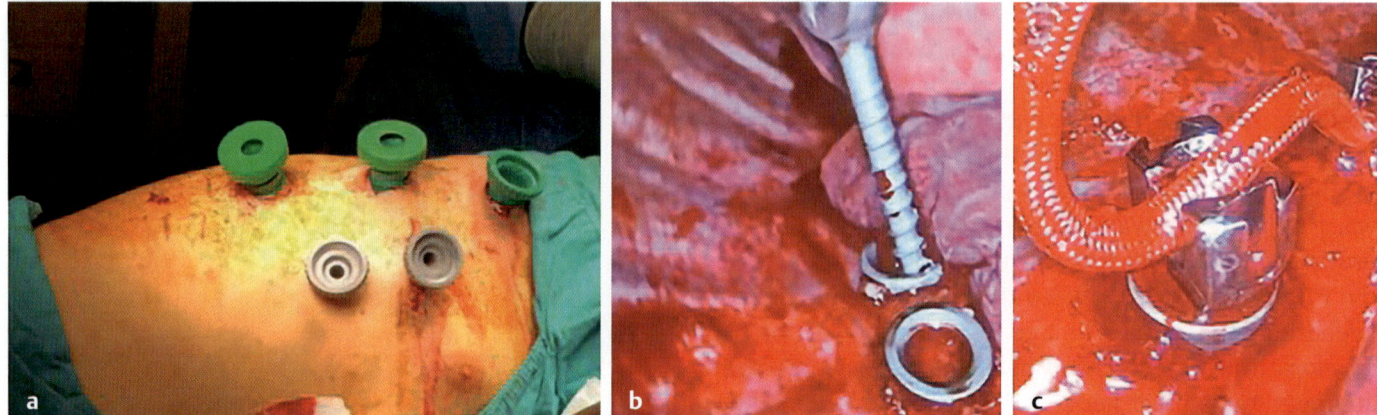

Fig. 35.11 **(a)** Opening the ports. **(b)** Video-assisted placement of the screws. **(c)** Fixing the screws to each other with rods.

gradually improve over time. This technique was inspired by the growth modulation techniques used in children's lower extremities, which have been commonly used for years—for example, the Zimmer spine approved by the FDA in 1919. It is a technique that connects the vertebral bodies at the apex of the curvature, allowing continuous growth without fusion and therefore preserving motion.

The procedure is designed for children with continued growth and idiopathic curvatures between 35 and 70 degrees. Children approaching skeletal maturity based on bone age film or iliac crest apophysis are not candidates for this procedure. The most typical age for tethering is 10 to 15 years old. In some cases, it may be considered in children under the age of 10 and even in late adolescence. Since it is a newly applied technique, its indications will increase with technical development. The goals of surgery include stabilization of the convex portion of the curve with fusion-free instrumentation, achieving modest correction in the operating room, and further modification of future growth and deformity. If the deformity is fully corrected during surgery in a patient with incomplete bone healing, the growing side bends the spine toward the opposite side, causing the development of a deformity toward the opposite side due to insufficient bone growth.

Surgical Technique

The procedure is performed under general anesthesia in the lateral decubitus position with the apex of the curve up. A double-lumen endotracheal tube should be used to allow the lung to shrink for imaging. Standard neurological monitoring is used in all cases.

Before the surgery, the vertebrae where the screws will be placed are marked with the C-arm at the apex, and the thorax is entered by opening the portals from the marked parts with video-assisted thoracoscopy. Three to five portal openings are usually sufficient (**Fig. 35.11a**). In addition to

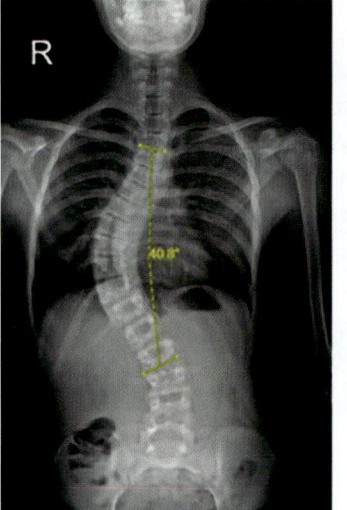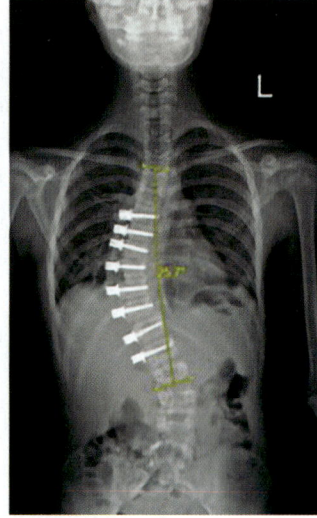

Fig. 35.12 Preoperative and postoperative radiograms.

fluoroscopic guidance, special screws developed by Zimmer are sent from these portals to the vertebral bodies from the side of the apex at each level, under camera imaging (**Fig. 35.11b**). This instrumentation is then screwed together with the flexible rod of the system and a tensioned clamping device controlled by the surgeon (**Figs. 35.11c** and **35.12**).

Postoperative tube use is not routine. This is because while the lungs are under positive pressure, the portals are rapidly closed.

Postoperative Care

If a chest tube is placed after the surgery, typically it takes 2 to 3 days of care in the hospital for the chest tube. Activity restrictions are only for 6 weeks, after which patients can resume all activities they can tolerate. After that, patients are followed at 6-month intervals to monitor radiographic changes as they grow. Complications are rare but may include pulmonary complications, screw failure, thread failure, overcorrection, and neurological damage.

Since this technique is in its infancy, no long-term studies are available yet. However, short- to medium-term data suggest that the procedure is safe and can provide satisfactory correction both in the operating room and over time, eliminating the need for fusion. Future studies are warranted as the use of this technique becomes more widespread.

Posterior Approach in Adult Scoliosis

Deformity develops in two ways in adult scoliosis. The patient has a nonsurgical deformity in younger years and progresses in menopause or andropause. Or, when the patient does not have any problems, the deformity develops gradually as part of the degenerative process that develops in women, especially after menopause. It is important to follow up with the patient as the deformity develops. At this stage, most of the deformities are mobile and should be treated immediately if the deformity progresses. At an advanced age, patients with progressive adult deformity who often have additional medical problems may have to undergo more painful surgeries. However, this can be prevented with a simple surgery at the beginning.

Surgery performed at an early stage has two essential advantages. The first is to correct the deformity to some extent, and the second and most important one is to stop the progression of the deformity, even if the improvement is not perfect. Trying to reach perfection during progression is not very important in this age group. It is enough to try to stay within acceptable parameters.

We applied this approach in adult scoliosis patients. In the development process of progressive deformities, besides the routine examinations, we take anterior–posterior spine X-rays lying down and standing. In this radiograph, if there is an improvement in the spine alignment in the lying anterior–posterior radiograph, we stabilize it with the posterior dynamic system. Here, we use both the Orthrus system that we defined and the Dynesys system defined by Zimmer spine.

Dynamic systems were first applied in scoliosis surgery by Di Silvestre et al[17] in 2010. In this paper, they reported positive results in the clinic using a dynamic stabilization system. They concluded that dynamic stabilization with pedicle screws is a safe procedure in addition to decompressive laminectomy in elderly patients with degenerative lumbar scoliosis. It maintained sufficient stability to prevent the progression of scoliosis and instability and allowed for an extensive laminectomy in cases of associated lumbar stenosis. Furthermore, this nonfusion stabilization technique was less aggressive than instrumental fusion and resulted in a statistically significant improvement in clinical outcome at final follow-up.

Di Silvestre et al later compared their scoliosis surgeries performed with the Dynesys system in 2014 with those performed with the rigid fusion system.[18] In this article, they stated that they achieved better results with rigid systems in correcting scoliosis. Still, shorter operation time and less undesirable effects were observed with the dynamic system, although less scoliosis correction was achieved with the dynamic system. More importantly, there was no difference between the fusion and dynamic systems at 5-year follow-up.

In 2013, Di Silvestre et al published mid-term results in a group of patients who did not undergo fusion.[19] They concluded that "In elderly patients with mild degenerative lumbar scoliosis without sagittal imbalance, pedicle screw with dynamic stabilization is an effective option with a low incidence of complications, curve stabilization over time, and satisfactory clinical results." In 2014, Lee et al stabilized 21 patients with lumbar stenosis and degenerative scoliosis with the Dynesys system and followed up for 2 years.[20] They concluded that the addition of nonfusion stabilization after decompressive surgery resulted in a safe and effective procedure for elderly patients with lumbar stenosis with mild to moderate scoliosis angle (<30 degrees). In addition, a statistically significant improvement in clinical outcome was achieved at the last follow-up evaluation, without any progression in degenerative scoliosis.

Surgical Technique

The patient is placed in the prone position under general anesthesia. Nerve roots are monitored by preoperative neuromonitoring. After making a midline skin incision, the fascia is opened on both sides, approximately 3 to 4 cm lateral to the midline, parallel to the midline. The transverse process is reached by blunt dissection between the medial multifidus and longissimus dorsi muscle. The lateral wall of the facet joint is found by following the transverse process. The hook of the retractors with a single blade and hook on the other side are attached to the facet joint, and the blade part and the muscle are retracted. In fact, there is often no need to use a retractor. After the lateral access path is found, the entry point is found with the help of a finger under the C-arm control, and the screws are inserted from the outside of the facet joint by the Wiltse method without damaging the facet joint (**Fig. 35.13**).[21–23]

If the Orthrus system is used, the convex side is compressed and the concave side is distracted, and the rods are placed. It is not correct to try to achieve the ideal spine

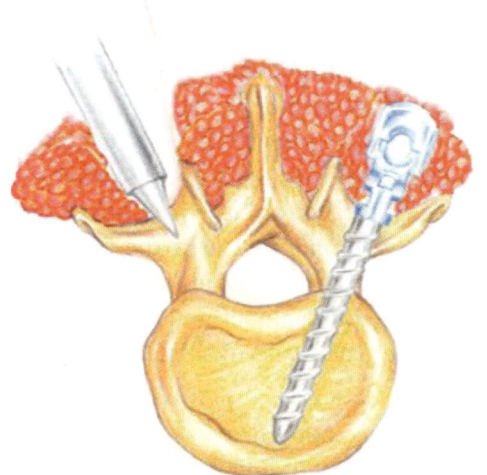

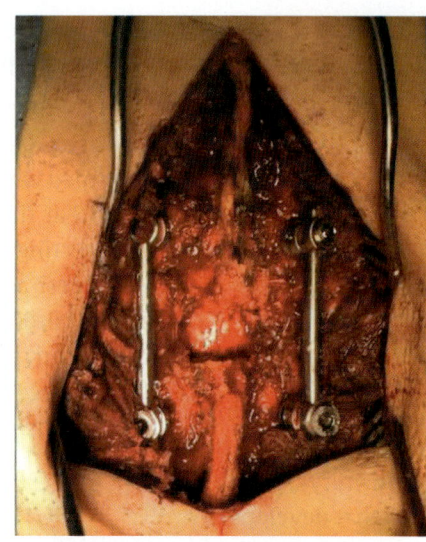

Fig. 35.13 Screws are inserted into the vertebrae by Wiltse method. If Dynesys system is used, each module is attached with a cord; if Orthrus system is used, each module is attached to each other with rods.

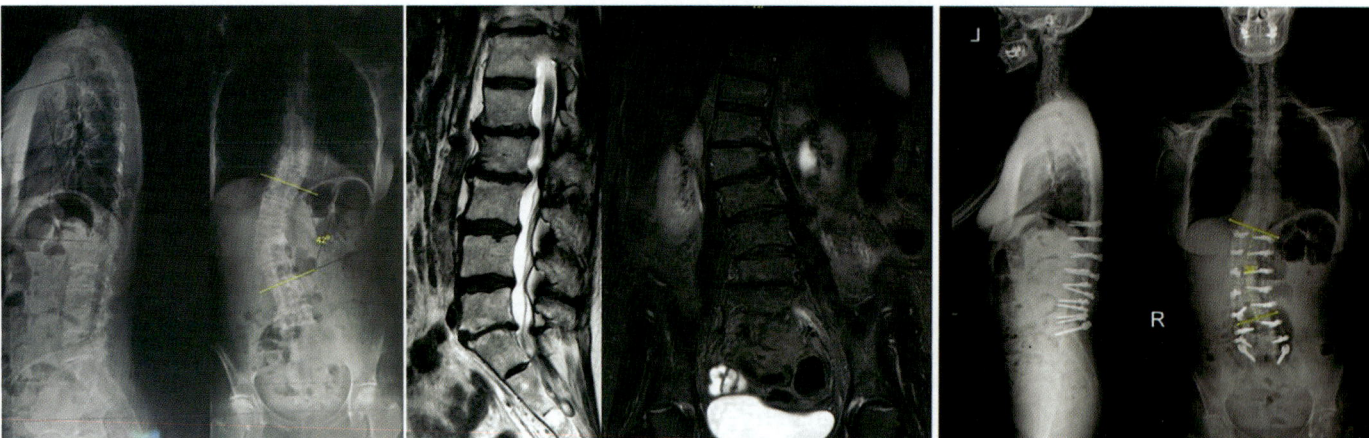

Fig. 35.14 A 61-year-old female patient complained of severe back pain. She has had scoliosis since she was a child and for the last 2 years, she has had severe back pain, especially while standing. Degenerated L1–L2 and L2–L3 discs is a possible source of pain. The patient is stabilized with the Orthrus system. Since the Orthrus system is a modular system, if there is a problem, only that level can be revised and there is no need to expose the whole system.

alignment in adult deformities. The deformity should be corrected as much as possible (**Fig. 35.14**).

If the Dynesys system is used, spacers are cut shorter than the distance between the screws on the apex side and the cord is attached to the screw under compression. The spacer and rise lengths on the concave side are kept long, and the cable is connected to the screws by distraction. Thus, the correction that occurs while lying down is obtained by forcing the system. In the Orthrus system, screw heads are compressed on the convex side and compressed on the concave side, and extra correction of the curve is attempted (**Fig. 35.15**).

These patients are of advanced age and generally have poor bone quality. During surgery, additional loads occur on the screws by distraction or compression. In this case, it causes loosening of the screws. In that case, it would be wiser to do the surgery both times under spinal anesthesia. Small holes are made in the skin in the first operation, and screws are inserted percutaneously. Wait for 4 to 6 months for the osteointegration of the screws. Care must be taken to ensure that the screw sides face each other and that the screw heights are the same. This is very important for easy application of the rod to be placed or the cord to be stretched later. The patient is discharged to wait for osteointegration for 4 to 6 months (). There is a similarity of dentists' policy for teeth implants to apply a two-stage surgery; placing the implant first, wait for osteointegration for some months, and place the prosthesis to allow compressive forces. The patient is then admitted to the hospital for the second surgery. Putting rods on the screws or stretching the cord after osteointegration makes the operation much more trouble-free. The possible complications that will occur after the procedure are avoided.

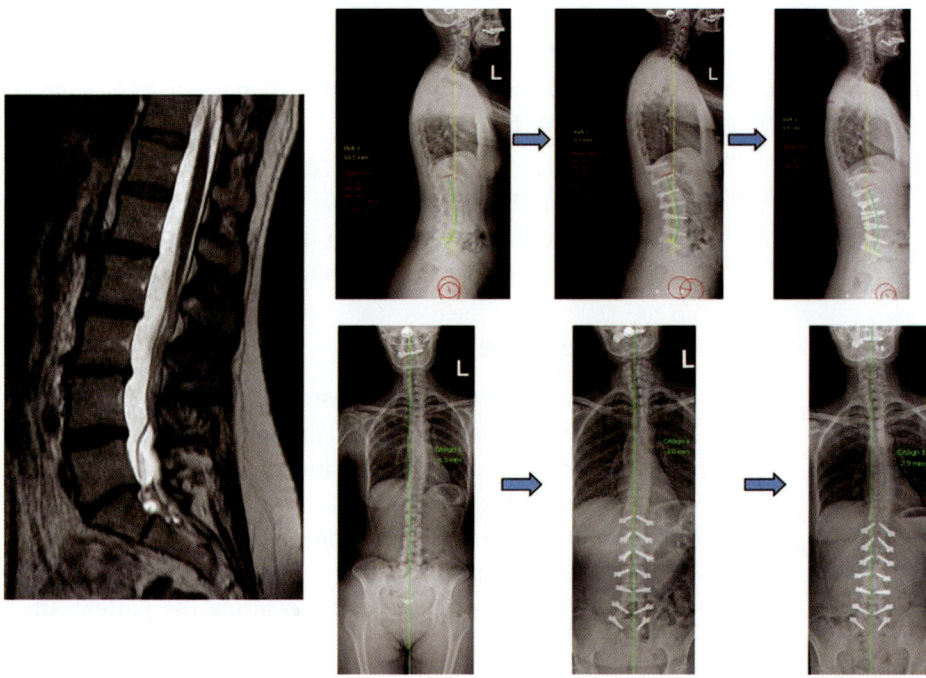

Fig. 35.15 A 47-year-old female patient had severe low back pain when standing for a long time and felt the need to bend forward. The patient is stabilized with the Dynesys system. After surgery, lordosis of the lumbar spine improved, along with sagittal and coronal balance.

Postoperative Care

It does not require any specialty. The patient is mobilized immediately after the surgery. If the surgery is performed in a single stage, the patient can be discharged after the drains placed in the muscle are removed; if it is performed in two stages, the patient can be discharged after the drains placed after the second surgery are removed. In these surgeries, there is no chain of possible complications awaiting the patient after fusion surgery for deformity.

It is sufficient to perform the first follow-up after 4 months and the other follow-ups once a year in a one-stage surgery. After the two-stage surgery, the first control can be done in the 2nd month; the next controls can be done once a year.

Posterior Approach in Adult Kyphotic Deformity

There are two essential causes of kyphotic deformity in adults. The first occurs with the advancing age, as a result of the degenerative process, when the lordosis of the waist is lost, and the head moves forward from the pelvis. Therefore, the SVA starts to move slowly from the sacrum into the abdomen. Another important cause is osteoporotic fractures. With each fracture, the kyphosis angle increases slightly, the projection of the head begins to protrude out of the pelvis, and the SVA progresses from the sacrum into the pelvis.

At this stage, the patients begin to straighten their spine by using their abdominal, waist, and back muscles, as described in detail above. The story is very typical. "I start walking upright, and after a while, I lean forward. My relatives warn me to walk upright." At this stage, the entire skeletal X-ray should be taken under the physician's supervision, and the patients are told to take the position they came in when they bend, and a side X-ray is taken. Then, the side radiograph is taken in straight posture. This is the posture we can achieve after surgery. There are subjective problems that we cannot resolve here. "How much is the patient leaning forward?" There is no standardization of the question, and trust is essential. In the next stage, the patient comes to the physician leaning forward, which is his/her position in which he/she continues his/her daily life. However, when we tell the patient to correct his/her posture, the patient can use muscles to straighten himself/herself as much as possible. This patient group can detect this improvement in the lateral radiographs taken while lying down and standing. These two patient groups constitute the ideal group for improvement with dynamic stabilization. There is no need for fusion in patients categorized in this group It may be necessary in cases that must be completed in the first stage. These patients may have root irritation, foraminal stenosis, or severe narrow spinal canal and may not be able to wait for 4 to 6 months. In that case, it is possible to solve the deformity with one-stage surgery, including additional iliac stabilization.[24]

Surgical Technique

The patient is operated on under general anesthesia in the prone position. Nerve roots are monitored by preoperative neuromonitoring. Then, while the table is flat, the screws are placed percutaneously using the Wiltse method described earlier. If necessary, decompression of narrowed spinal canal, foraminal decompression, and diskectomy are performed. The most important step is to make the operating table concave within the limits where the person can correct himself or herself before the operation. The C-arm is controlled and if the Dynesys system is used, the screws are tied with a thread while in this position or if Orthrus system is used, the rods are placed and tightened to the screws (**Fig. 35.16**).

This surgery can be performed in two stages depending on the bone quality. Both the operating steps can be achieved with spinal anesthesia. However, in cases where bone quality is likely to cause problems, the surgery can be performed in two stages. However, the spinal canal or foramen can be enlarged in the first stage, or diskectomy can be performed in the segment with local pathology. In addition, a temporary rod can only be placed on the screws of that distance. Then, for all remaining screws, we should wait until 4 to 6 weeks to pass and osseointegration to occur because it is not appropriate for the patient to wait this

period under the threat of painful or possible neurological damage. After confirming the osteointegration with computed tomography (CT), the second stage of the surgery is completed (**Fig. 35.17**).

If there is a loosening of the screws placed on the temporary rod or if we observe it during the surgery, we only replace these screws with larger diameter screws and complete the second stage of the surgery.

Postoperative Care

There is no extra feature in postoperative care. The patient is mobilized immediately after the surgery. If the surgery is performed in one stage, the patient is discharged after the drains placed in the muscle are removed; if it is performed in two stages, the patient can be discharged after the drains placed after the second surgery are removed. There is no chain of possible complications awaiting the patient after fusion surgery for deformity in these surgeries.

In a one-stage surgery, it is sufficient to perform the first follow-up after 4 months and the other follow-up once a year. After the two-stage surgery, the first control can be done in the 2nd month; the next controls can be done once a year.

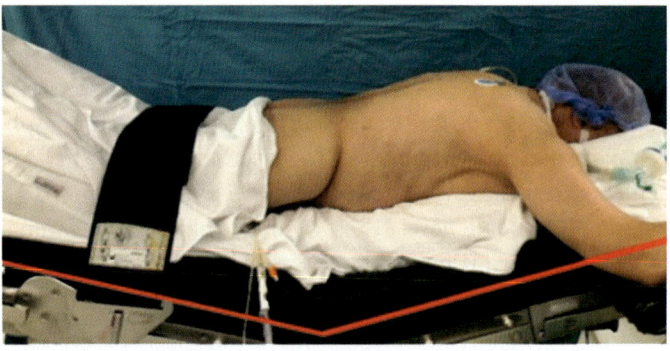

Fig. 35.16 The table is given a concave position to provide lumbar lordosis and the rods are attached to the screws in this position.

Tips and Tricks

- It is crucial to identify the adult deformity type properly for the diagnosis and further treatment of the patients
- Today, adult deformities can be easily evaluated with existing classifications. In addition, all supine and standing spine radiographs are very useful to help for diagnosis and identification.

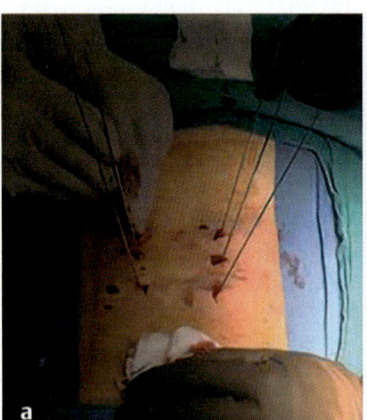
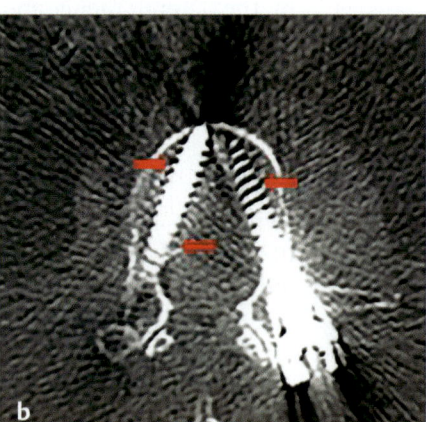
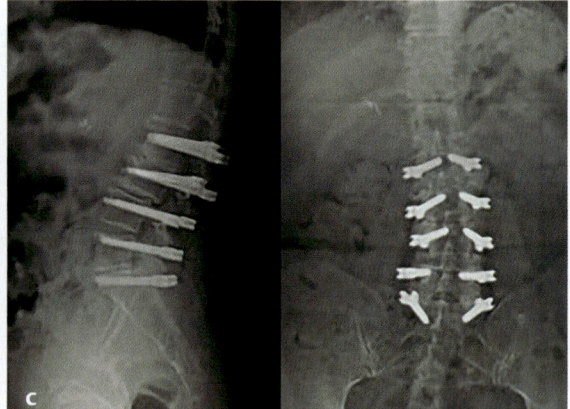

Fig. 35.17 **(a)** Placement of screws percutaneously. **(b)** After waiting for at least 4 months, computed tomography (CT) confirms that the osteointegration process of the screws is completed. **(c)** Spacers and cords are tightened to the screws and tightened in accordance with the technique.

- In all standing spine radiographs, it is very important to determine the patient's maximal level of correction. In this way, it can be predicted how much the values of spinopelvic parameters, which are abnormal in the pre-operative period, can be brought back to normal in the post-operative period.

Key Points

- Fusion surgery for deformity is a method successfully applied for many decades.

- In last two decades, the dynamic systems have been introduced, developed. The philosophy behind these systems are preserving the motion of the operated segment of the spine .

- Contrary to popular belief, dynamic stabilization systems can be successfully applied in patients with mobile deformities.

- The patients with adult deformity are mostly elderly age and osteoporotic. Therefore, two-stage surgery can be performed to prevent instrument failure in the future

Conclusion

Today, many surgeons think that "dynamic systems are dead and should be left as they are." This is not the case. Fusion surgeries are a heavy surgical method in the surgical treatment of chronic instability, and if things do not go as planned, the patient pays a hefty bill with a more severe surgery than the first one. In addition, another drawback is the mortality and morbidity rates of the elderly and patients with medical problems, especially in severe surgeries such as deformity and fusion surgery. These patients can be easily treated with the dynamic surgical techniques described above. Based on the knowledge of problems posed by fusion surgery for over hundred years, it has a solid infrastructure for solving the problem. However, they are emerging technologies and will continue to evolve. It will gradually replace unnecessary fusion surgeries with different designs and approaches. "To think that dynamic systems are dead and should be left" is a very conservative approach, and defending it is the biggest mistake against the future.

References

1. Lenke LG, Betz RR, Harms J, et al. Adolescent idiopathic scoliosis: a new classification to determine extent of spinal arthrodesis. J Bone Joint Surg Am 2001;83(8):1169–1181
2. Schwab F, Farcy J-P, Bridwell K, et al. A clinical impact classification of scoliosis in the adult. Spine 2006;31(18):2109–2114
3. Dubousset J. Three-dimensional analysis of the scoliotic deformity. In: Weinstein SL, ed. Pediatric Spine: Principles and Practice. New York, NY: Raven Press; 1994:479–496
4. Legaye J, Duval-Beaupère G, Hecquet J, Marty C. Pelvic incidence: a fundamental pelvic parameter for three-dimensional regulation of spinal sagittal curves. Eur Spine J 1998;7(2):99–103
5. Duval-Beaupère G, Schmidt C, Cosson P. A Barycentremetric study of the sagittal shape of spine and pelvis: the conditions required for an economic standing position. Ann Biomed Eng 1992;20(4):451–462
6. Schwab F, Lafage V, Patel A, Farcy J-P. Sagittal plane considerations and the pelvis in the adult patient. Spine 2009;34(17):1828–1833
7. Roussouly P, Gollogly S, Berthonnaud E, Dimnet J. Classification of the normal variation in the sagittal alignment of the human lumbar spine and pelvis in the standing position. Spine 2005;30(3):346–353
8. Barrey C, Jund J, Noseda O, Roussouly P. Sagittal balance of the pelvis-spine complex and lumbar degenerative diseases. A comparative study about 85 cases. Eur Spine J 2007;16(9):1459–1467
9. Le Huec JC, Hasegawa K. Normative values for the spine shape parameters using 3D standing analysis from a database of 268 asymptomatic Caucasian and Japanese subjects. Eur Spine J 2016;25(11):3630–3637
10. Le Huec JC, Thompson W, Mohsinaly Y, Faundez A. Sagittal balance of the spine. Eur Spine J 2019;28(9):1889–1905
11. Abrisham SMJ, Ardekani MRS, Mzarch MAB. Evaluation of the normal range of thoracic kyphosis and lumbar lordosis angles using EOS imaging. Maedica (Buchar) 2020;15(1):87–91
12. Le Huec JC, Demezon H, Aunoble S. Sagittal parameters of global cervical balance using EOS imaging: normative values from a prospective cohort of asymptomatic volunteers. Eur Spine J 2015;24(1):63–71
13. Oktenoglu T, Hekimoglu M, Aydin AL, Sasani M, Cerezci O, Ozer AF. Kyphoplasty with posterior dynamic stabilization in the surgical treatment of unstable thoracolumbar osteoporotic vertebral compression fractures. Turk Neurosurg 2021;31(6):924–930
14. Silva FE, Lenke LG. Adult degenerative scoliosis: evaluation and management. Neurosurg Focus 2010;28(3):E1
15. Berjano P, Lamartina C. Classification of degenerative segment disease in adults with deformity of the lumbar or thoracolumbar spine. Eur Spine J 2014;23(9):1815–1824
16. Schwab F, Ungar B, Blondel B, et al. Scoliosis Research Society-Schwab adult spinal deformity classification: a validation study. Spine 2012;37(12):1077–1082
17. Di Silvestre M, Lolli F, Bakaloudis G, Parisini P. Dynamic stabilization for degenerative lumbar scoliosis in elderly patients. Spine 2010;35(2):227–234
18. Di Silvestre M, Lolli F, Bakaloudis G. Degenerative lumbar scoliosis in elderly patients: dynamic stabilization without fusion versus posterior instrumented fusion. Spine J 2014;14(1):1–10
19. Di Silvestre M, Lolli F, Greggi T, Vommaro F, Baioni A. Adult's degenerative scoliosis: midterm results of dynamic stabilization without fusion in elderly patients—is it effective? Adv Orthop 2013;2013:365059
20. Lee SE, Jahng TA, Kim HJ. Decompression and nonfusion dynamic stabilization for spinal stenosis with degenerative lumbar scoliosis: clinical article. J Neurosurg Spine 2014;21(4):585–594

21. Wiltse LL, Spencer CW. New uses and refinements of the paraspinal approach to the lumbar spine. Spine 1988;13(6): 696–706

22. Wiltse LL, Bateman JG, Hutchinson RH, Nelson WE. The paraspinal sacrospinalis-splitting approach to the lumbar spine. J Bone Joint Surg Am 1968;50(5):919–926

23. Guiroy A, Sícoli A, Masanés NG, Ciancio AM, Gagliardi M, Falavigna A. How to perform the Wiltse posterolateral spinal approach: technical note. Surg Neurol Int 2018;9:38

24. Özer AF, Aydın AL, Hekimoğlu M, et al. Should iliac wing screws be included in long segment dynamic stabilization? Cureus 2021;13(2):e13543

36 Cervical Kyphosis and Arthroplasty: An Irreconcilable Relationship?

Óscar L. Alves, Rui Reinas, Leopoldina Pereira, and Margarida Luis Rios Alves

Introduction

Cervical arthroplasty (CA) offers at least equivalent clinical and cost analysis results compared to anterior cervical diskectomy and fusion (ACDF) in prospective randomized controlled trials, meta-analysis, and "real-world" data.[1-3] Not surprisingly, this effect is amplified in multilevel cervical disc disease. In addition, CA can mitigate the adverse kinematic effects of ACDF, such as loss of motion at the index level and hypermobility at adjacent levels, conferring putative protection from step-up cervical spine degeneration.

Cervical spine degeneration results not only from the natural aging process with distinctive expression in different populations, reflecting the patient's individuality, but also from sagittal malalignment. Cervical kyphosis is per se an accelerator of symptomatic cervical spondylosis and facet joint and disc degeneration. Literature on fusion shows that the development of accelerated adjacent segment degeneration (ASD) is related to segmental kyphosis at the surgical level.[4] Uchida et al demonstrated the benefit of alignment correction in maximizing the potential for clinical improvement in patients with preoperative cervical kyphosis of ≥10 degrees, confirming the importance of sagittal deformity correction.[5] A retrospective cohort study conducted by Faldini et al found that radiological ASD was present in 61% of patients fused in neutral or kyphotic alignment versus 27% of patients fused in lordotic alignment.[6] Additionally, postoperative kyphosis has proven to be related to axial pain and poor functional recovery after ACDF.

Regarding CA, evidence suggests that sagittal balance makes an essential contribution to operative and adjacent segments' longevity such as preservation of the range of motion (ROM).[7] If CA has a beneficial kinematic effect, it is also crucial to demonstrate a positive effect on cervical alignment before advocating widespread use of this technology. In this chapter, we review the relationship between CA and cervical alignment.

Real Meaning of Cervical Kyphosis

Cervical kyphosis can generally be divided into global or segmental forms. It can also be separated into reducible or irreducible types according to the results of dynamic flexion–extension lateral radiographs. Irreducible kyphosis is always associated with significant cervical degeneration or congenital bone malformation. In contrast, reducible kyphosis often relates to index level degenerative disc disease, posterior muscle weakness, or neck pain, as expressed in **Box 36.1**. Neck pain and cervical kyphosis display an intimate bidirectional link. Neck pain can be either the cause or the consequence of cervical kyphosis. Disabling neck pain is directly correlated with cervical kyphosis, as shown by Tang et al.[8]

However, it should be emphasized that up to one-third of asymptomatic volunteers may exhibit a "physiological" nonlordotic cervical spine, reflecting a degree of arbitrariness in the definition of normative values of cervical alignment.[9] Furthermore, a wide variation of normal values for cervical lordosis can be found in the literature among asymptomatic volunteers. For example, Bakoney et al reported a normal C2–C7 lordosis of 0.8 ± 13 degrees, whereas Iyer et al claimed it to be 12 ± 14 degrees.[10] Cervical kyphosis may be acceptable if a small T1 slope co-exists.[11] C2–C7 angle is driven by T1 slope and therefore by thoracolumbar alignment. Compensation in primary cervical kyphosis occurs via small T1 slope, posterior shifting of cervical sagittal vertical axis (cSVA), and significant lumbar lordosis to maintain horizontal gaze. Finally, global cervical lordosis is also a product of various demographic and pathological factors, such as patients' age, gender, body mass index, and comorbidities (e.g., obesity).

Box 36.1 Causes of cervical kyphosis

- Neck pain
- Anterior neck musculature spasm
- Weakness of posterior paraspinal muscles
- Asymmetrical loss of disc height due to disc degeneration
- Congenital bone malformation

Effects of Arthroplasty on Cervical Alignment

Regarding the effect of arthroplasty on postoperative cervical sagittal alignment, the literature reveals conflicting data, very likely related to the inclusion of different cohorts of patients, surgical techniques, and biomechanical properties of the used implants. In the early studies, CA was reported to be limited in maintaining and correcting sagittal alignment,[12] but several recent studies reported correction of cervical kyphosis in select patients.[13–16]

Sears et al found a median loss of 2 degrees in functional spinal unit (FSU) lordosis when compared with preoperative imaging ($P < 0.0001$, range: 8 degrees loss to 5 degrees gain).[17] Kim et al reported that only 36% of patients with a preoperative lordotic sagittal orientation of the index level could maintain lordosis following surgery.[18] However, the overall sagittal alignment of the cervical spine was preserved in 86% of cases at the final follow-up.[18] Using a socket–ball type of device, Barrey et al demonstrated at 24 months a significant increase in both local (from 1 ± 5 degrees to 7 ± 5 degrees, $p < 0.001$) and global lordosis (from 0.5 ± 7 degrees to 13.5 ± 10 degrees, $p < 0.01$).[19] At 2 years after surgery, the CA patients experienced a statistically significant change in lordosis of 3.0 degrees ($p < 0.001$), 0.90 degree ($p = 0.006$), and −1.9 degrees ($p < 0.001$) at the operative, cranial, and caudal adjacent levels, respectively.[14] Using a third-generation implant in 35 patients with a mean age of 48.2 years (range 37–65 years) followed up for 21.5 months (12–46 months), we reported a significant increase at index level angle of 3.4 degrees (personal communication at the 2017 Congress of the Sociedade Portuguesa de Patologia da Coluna Vertebral). The increment in global lordosis of 2.1 degrees was essentially derived from the index level lordotic increase ($r = 0.374$; $p = 0.029$). Our group also demonstrated an augmented index level (mean 1.5 ± 5.55, $p = 0.025$) and global lordosis (mean 2.1 ± 7.1, $p = 0.111$) in 32 patients subjected to multilevel CA.[20] No difference was observed if patients were stratified between two-level and three- or four-level CA. Interestingly, the increase in lordosis was coupled with a rise in global and index level ROM.

In the same way, Du et al showed that CA increased ROM of the FSU and maintained the FSU angle postoperatively.[21] However, Rabin et al, using another type of device, found that an excessively lordotic index level angle after surgery was associated with restricted segmental ROM (Pearson's $r = -0.55$; $p = 0.02$) and translation in extension (Pearson's $r = -0.58$; $p = 0.02$).[22] Lordotic configuration of prosthesis end plates is associated with restricted segmental ROM and translation from neutral to extension. The relationship between the ideal segmental alignment and ROM preservation after CA needs further research.

Published series comparing sagittal alignment between CA and fusion reflect a bias in the patient selection, with fusion groups showing a significantly less lordotic alignment than the arthroplasty group. Anakwenze et al reported that using the semiconstrained prosthesis, CA enabled a similar ability to restore sagittal alignment compared with ACDF in patients without preoperative kyphosis.[14] In both CA and ACDF, lordosis increased at the device, adjacent cranial, and total cervical levels while decreasing at the caudal adjacent level. Although ACDF facilitated a more significant increase in device level lordosis (+1.25 degrees) and less loss of lordosis at the caudal adjacent level than CA (−0.39 degrees), the clinical relevance of the slight differences remains unknown.

It is essential to underline that most published series do not include data on contemporary sagittal alignment indexes. Even after surgery, T1 slope is increasingly recognized as an essential factor that influences cervical spine sagittal balance. Kim et al noticed a significant negative correlation between preoperative T1 slope and FSU and C2–C7 angle changes. Patients with low T1 slope had more extensive changes in the FSU and C2–C7 angle, which was helpful to restore sagittal alignment in patients with kyphosis.[23] Whether regional or overall, patients with preoperative kyphosis tend to have a lower T1 slope than those without kyphosis. Patient selection based on preoperative T1 slope may add value to patients with low preoperative T1 slope as far as the device can produce lordosis by distraction.[24]

Segmental Kyphosis as a Contraindication for CA

Although the spectrum of CA indications for degenerative disc disease is increasing as more experience is gathered, segmental cervical kyphosis is still regarded as an absolute contraindication. As a significant linear relationship between preoperative and postoperative segmental angles is to be expected, proper patient selection can prevent an adverse kyphotic outcome.[25,26] Therefore, a question arises whether patients with preoperative segmental kyphosis are suitable for CA.

Interestingly, CA is more efficient in correcting global than index level lordosis. At the last follow-up after CA, Kim et al found that only 13% of preoperative kyphotic index levels became lordotic. In contrast, preoperatively kyphotic global cervical alignment resulted in lordosis in 33% of the patients.[18] Among 32 patients followed for 26.8 ± 6.4 months, Zhao et al identified 12 patients presenting with preoperative FSU kyphosis, while 9 patients had preoperative C2–C7 kyphosis. No patient had postoperative FSU or C2–C7 kyphosis. Of the 16 patients with upper adjacent segment (UAS) kyphosis, only 5 patients had postoperative UAS kyphosis. However, there was a tendency to originate lower adjacent segment (LAS) kyphosis, which increased from two to four patients after surgery.[15] CA may also restore lordosis in select cervical spondylotic myelopathy patients, as demonstrated by Park et al.[16] They described in their series of 464 patients (n = 272 CA patients versus n = 181 ACDF patients) an increase in segmental and global lordosis along with a marginal anteroinferior displacement of the center of rotation (COR). It may take several months until the implant interface is fully integrated into the end plate and the structures of the functional segmental unit (FSU) adapt to the gain in mobility offered by the CA, leading to a correction toward the physiological alignment of the patient. Similarly, we demonstrated that a physiological location of the COR is only obtained 12 months after surgery (PhD thesis, Filipe Alexandre Loureiro Pagaimo, Óscar L. Alves, PhD thesis mentor, Cervical arthroplasty characterization study? *In-vivo* biomechanical characteristics, IST, Universidade de Lisboa, September, 2019).

Focusing on isolated segmental kyphosis, we evaluated 23 patients with a mean age of 47 years (range 20–60), followed up for a mean period of 21 months (personal communication, International Society for Advancement of Spine Surgery, 2019). Among the 25 preoperative kyphotic levels identified, all showed a significant increase in segmental lordosis (+5.7 ± 6.9 degrees), as demonstrated in the case shown in **Fig. 36.1**. A slight rise in global C2–C7 lordosis (+0.8 ± 7.8 degrees) and a decrease in SVA (−2.1 ± 12.3 mm) at the expense of a slight increase in T1 slope (2.7 ± 7.64 degrees) were also observed. With increasing T1 slope, the center of gravity of the head translates more anteriorly with reinforced cervical lordotic compensation, which is compensatively associated with a decrease in the cSVA.[27] CA did not compromise nerve roots decompression and allowed reconstruction of segmental lordosis at kyphotic index levels while preserving the ROM.

We observed that in flexible cases, the correction of kyphosis enabled both pain relief and prosthesis biomechanical properties. However, in incomplete reducible kyphotic cases in extension, a posterior wedged-shaped end plate drilling was performed to reformat the disc space in a lordotic configuration-wedged osteotomy as described

in **Fig. 36.2**. In both conditions, neck strength-building exercises were crucial in the postoperative period.

Causes for Postoperative Kyphosis

It is of utmost importance to avoid segmental kyphosis because of persisting pain and symptoms of neurologic compromise, progression of adjacent degeneration, and suboptimal kinematic performance of the disc prosthesis.

Loss of anterior disc height has been identified as the most crucial indicator predicting change in the disc space angle. As expected, pre-existing straight or kyphotic segmental alignments have been implicated in the postoperative kyphotic end plate alignment, mainly due to the structural absence of lordosis incorporated into the devices. However, as Du et al described, even prosthesis with a ball and socket design that included 7 degrees of lordosis in end plates generated cases of device end plate kyphosis.[22] Because of that, in lordotic preoperative index levels, postoperative segmental kyphosis is the result of technical mistakes, often related to surgeon's experience, as shown in **Box 36.2**. **Fig. 36.3** illustrates a demonstrative case. Excessive neck positioning in extension, leading to intraoperative lordotic distraction, end plate over-drilling or asymmetric milling, and the amount of bone removed from the anterior aspect of the cephalad vertebra can all correlate with changes in FSU alignment as claimed by Sears et al.[17] Of particular relevance is the intraoperative disc space distraction that correlates with subsequent loss of disc space height. Multiple linear regression analysis confirmed that loss of disc space height and wrong angle of prosthesis insertion contributed independently. Anteriorly located implants lead to lordotic segmental angle, whereas posterior prostheses are more prone to a kyphotic segmental angle, despite the absence of effect on C2–C7 Cobb's angle.

Box 36.2   Causes of postoperative cervical kyphosis
▪ Pre-existing kyphosis
▪ Absence of disc implant structural lordosis
▪ Excessive neck positioning in extension
▪ Excessive intraoperative disc space distraction
▪ End plate over-drilling or asymmetric milling
▪ Loss of disc height
▪ Inappropriate angle of prosthesis insertion
▪ Posteriorly located implant
▪ Surgeon's experience

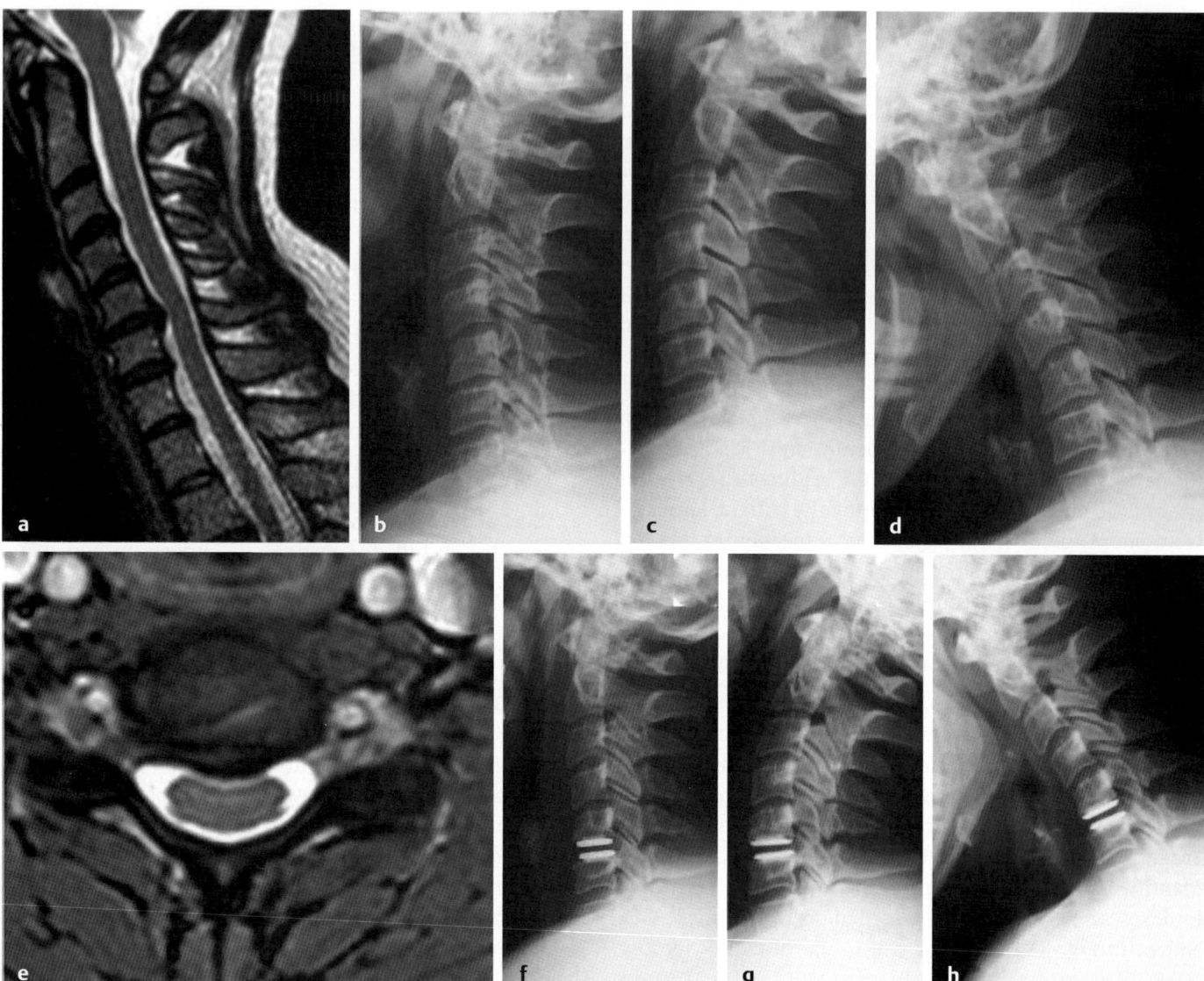

Fig. 36.1 Reversal of segmental kyphosis after cervical arthroplasty: A 43-year-old woman presented with neck pain (VAS4) and arm pain (VAS7), refractory to best medical treatment, with paresthesia but no motor deficits. On magnetic resonance imaging (MRI), she presented with a C5–C6 herniated disc causing spinal cord compression **(a, b)**, without signs of instability on dynamic lateral X-ray studies **(c–e)**. Her neutral lateral X-ray showed 4.9 degrees of global cervical lordosis and −3.5 degrees of segmental kyphosis at the C5–C6 level. In 2015, she underwent a C5–C6 diskectomy and arthroplasty with the resolution of symptoms. On 6-year follow-up lateral X-rays **(f–h)**, a minimal change of global lordosis is perceived with an increase in segmental lordosis at C5–C6 from −3.5 to 5.1 degrees. At C5–C6, in parallel to the reversal of segmental kyphosis after cervical arthroplasty, range of motion (ROM) also improved from 13.6 to 16.9 degrees. Postoperatively, both cervical sagittal vertical axis (cSVA) and T1 slope increased from 8.8 to 11.6 mm and from 23.3 to 25.9 degrees, respectively, whereas a compensatory increase in C0–C2 angle from 32.8 to 40.6 degrees to maintain horizontal gaze was observed. VAS, visual analog scale.

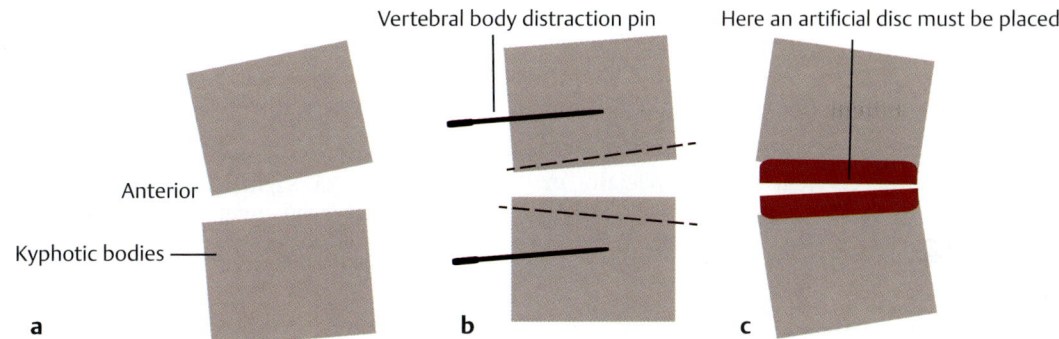

Fig. 36.2 Posterior vertebral body wedged-shaped osteotomy in segmental kyphosis is not entirely reducible in extension. The segmental kyphotic alignment of the disc space due to severe loss of anterior disc height **(a)**. Disc space distraction with divergent somatic distracters and posterior vertebral body wedged-shaped osteotomy **(b)**. Insertion of cervical disc prosthesis reformatting a lordotic-shaped disc space **(c)**.

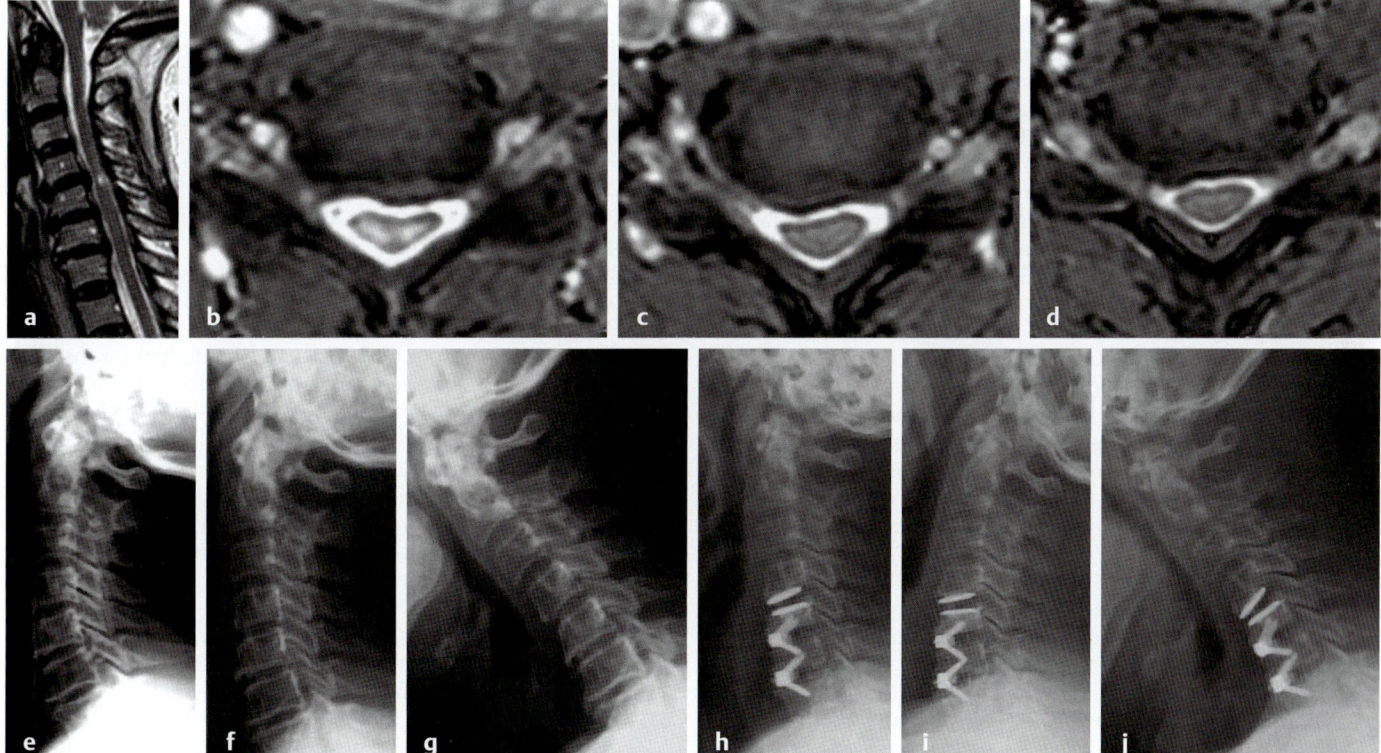

Fig. 36.3 Postoperative kyphosis as a complication after cervical arthroplasty. A 66-year-old female, previously diagnosed with rheumatoid arthritis, presented with neck pain (VAS6) and arm pain (VAS8), radiculopathy, and a modified Japanese Orthopedic Association scale for myelopathy (mJoA) of 14. Sagittal, T2-weighted magnetic imaging resonance (MRI) showing spinal cord compression at disc level C4–C7 **(a)**. Axial, T2-weighted MRI confirming spinal cord and nerve roots compression **(b–d)**. Lateral dynamic cervical radiographs exhibiting 35.8 degrees of global and 13.6 degrees of segmental C4–C5 range of motion (ROM), 14.7 degrees of C2–C7 lordosis, and 4.8 degrees of segmental lordosis at C4–C5 level **(e–g)**. The patient was pain-free and fully recovered fine motor skills after a three-level diskectomy with a hybrid construct- arthroplasty in C4–C5 and fusion at C5–C6 and C6–C7. At 1-year, postoperative lateral dynamic cervical radiographs showed proper mobility of the disc prosthesis (11.9 degrees) and absence of heterotopic calcification, but a kyphotic alignment at the index C4–C5 level (from 4.8 to 03.0 degrees) was noticed **(h–j)**. cSVA, cervical sagittal vertical axis; VAS, visual analog scale.

Conclusions

CA in degenerative disc disease can provide an optimal alignment target for surgical reconstruction of either global or segmental kyphotic cervical spine, especially in patients presenting with low T1 slope, as facet joints are not ankylosed or hypermobility is not observed.

References

1. Ament JD, Yang Z, Nunley P, Stone MB, Kim KD. Cost-effectiveness of cervical total disc replacement vs fusion for the treatment of 2-level symptomatic degenerative disc disease. JAMA Surg 2014;149(12):1231–1239

2. Radcliff K, Zigler J, Zigler J. Costs of cervical disc replacement versus anterior cervical discectomy and fusion for treatment of single-level cervical disc disease: an analysis of the Blue Health Intelligence database for acute and long-term costs and complications. Spine 2015;40(8):521–529

3. Turel MK, Kerolus MG, Adogwa O, Traynelis VC. Cervical arthroplasty: what does the labeling say? Neurosurg Focus 2017;42(2):E2

4. Katsuura A, Hukuda S, Saruhashi Y, Mori K. Kyphotic malalignment after anterior cervical fusion is one of the factors promoting the degenerative process in adjacent intervertebral levels. Eur Spine J 2001;10(4):320–324

5. Uchida K, Nakajima H, Sato R, et al. Cervical spondylotic myelopathy associated with kyphosis or sagittal sigmoid alignment: outcome after anterior or posterior decompression. J Neurosurg Spine 2009;11(5):521–528

6. Faldini C, Pagkrati S, Leonetti D, Miscione MT, Giannini S. Sagittal segmental alignment as predictor of adjacent-level degeneration after a cloward procedure. Clin Orthop Relat Res 2011;469(3):674–681

7. Fong SY, et al. Design limitations of Bryan disc arthroplasty. Spine J 2012; 233–241

8. Tang JA, Scheer JK, Smith JS, et al; ISSG. The impact of standing regional cervical sagittal alignment on outcomes in posterior cervical fusion surgery. Neurosurgery 2012;71(3): 662–669, discussion 669

9. Le Huec JC, Demezon H, Aunoble S. Sagittal parameters of global cervical balance using EOS imaging: normative values from a prospective cohort of asymptomatic volunteers. Eur Spine J 2015;24(1):63–71

10. Patel PD, Arutyunyan G, Plusch K, Vaccaro A Jr, Vaccaro AR. A review of cervical spine alignment in the normal and degenerative spine. J Spine Surg 2020;6(1):106–123

11. Staub BN, Lafage R, Kim HJ, et al; International Spine Study Group. Cervical mismatch: the normative value of T1 slope minus cervical lordosis and its ability to predict ideal cervical lordosis. J Neurosurg Spine 2018;30(1):31–37

12. Ahn P-G, Kim KN, Moon SW, Kim KS. Changes in cervical range of motion and sagittal alignment in early and late phases after total disc replacement: radiographic follow-up exceeding 2 years. J Neurosurg Spine 2009;11(6):688–695

13. Guérin P, Obeid I, Gille O, et al. Sagittal alignment after single cervical disc arthroplasty. J Spinal Disord Tech 2012;25(1): 10–16

14. Anakwenze OA, Auerbach JD, Milby AH, Lonner BS, Balderston RA. Sagittal cervical alignment after cervical disc arthroplasty and anterior cervical discectomy and fusion: results of a prospective, randomized, controlled trial. Spine 2009;34(19):2001–2007

15. Zhao J, Jiang R, Yang Y, et al. Preoperative T1 slope as a predictor of change in cervical alignment and range of motion after cervical disc arthroplasty. Med Sci Monit 2017;23:5844–5850

16. Park DK, Lin EL, Phillips FM. Index and adjacent level kinematics after cervical disc replacement and anterior fusion: in vivo quantitative radiographic analysis. Spine 2011;36(9): 721–730

17. Sears WR, Duggal N, Sekhon LH, Williamson OD. Segmental malalignment with the Bryan cervical disc prosthesis—contributing factors. J Spinal Disord Tech 2007;20(2): 111–117

18. Kim SW, Shin JH, Arbatin JJ, Park MS, Chung YK, McAfee PC. Effects of a cervical disc prosthesis on maintaining sagittal alignment of the functional spinal unit and overall sagittal balance of the cervical spine. Eur Spine J 2008; 17(1):20–29

19. Barrey C, Champain S, Campana S, Ramadan A, Perrin G, Skalli W. Sagittal alignment and kinematics at instrumented and adjacent levels after total disc replacement in the cervical spine. Eur Spine J 2012;21(8):1648–1659

20. Reinas R, Kitumba D, Pereira L, Baptista AM, Alves ÓL. Multilevel cervical arthroplasty-clinical and radiological outcomes. J Spine Surg 2020;6(1):233–242

21. Du J, Li M, Liu H, Meng H, He Q, Luo Z. Early follow-up outcomes after treatment of degenerative disc disease with the discover cervical disc prosthesis. Spine J 2011;11(4): 281–289

22. Rabin D, Bertagnoli R, Wharton N, Pickett GE, Duggal N. Sagittal balance influences range of motion: an in vivo study with the ProDisc-C. Spine J 2009;9(2):128–133

23. Kim T-H, Lee SY, Kim YC, Park MS, Kim SW. T1 slope as a predictor of kyphotic alignment change after laminoplasty in patients with cervical myelopathy. Spine 2013;38(16): E992–E997

24. Kim SW, Limson MA, Kim SB, et al. Comparison of radiographic changes after ACDF versus Bryan disc arthroplasty in single and bi-level cases. Eur Spine J 2009;18(2):218–231

25. Yoon DH, Yi S, Shin HC, Kim KN, Kim SH. Clinical and radiological results following cervical arthroplasty. Acta Neurochir (Wien) 2006;148(9):943–950

26. Walraevens JRR, Liu B, Sloten JV, Demaerel P, Goffin J. Postoperative segmental malalignment after surgery with the Bryan cervical disc prosthesis: is it related to the mechanics and design of the prosthesis? J Spinal Disord Tech 2010;23(6): 372–376

27. Park JH, Cho CB, Song JH, Kim SW, Ha Y, Oh JK. T1 slope and cervical sagittal alignment on cervical CT radiographs of asymptomatic persons. J Korean Neurosurg Soc 2013; 53(6):356–359

37 Anterior Lumbar Reconstruction and Correction for Degenerative Deformity

Bronek Boszczyk and Dileep N. Lobo

Introduction

Recent years have seen advances in the techniques available for anterior reconstruction and stabilization. There are particular advantages in restoring the shape and contour of the spine through an anterior approach as this avoids manipulation of dural structures; it is highly effective in restoring vertebral and spinal height overall and often allows the procedure to be completed with less blood loss. Advances in minimally invasive techniques have made it possible to instrument and reconstruct much of the lumbar spine from lateral minimally invasive approaches and even the lumbosacral junction. Occasionally however, these techniques are not sufficient as some patients will still require a lateral annular release, may have substantial deformities preventing the placement of minimally invasive tools, and overall, may require the preparation and dissection of the discs in a more extensive fashion to achieve the desired correction. Therefore, a technique has been described to allow surgeons an additional extensive open option for reconstruction of the entire lumbar spine to the sacrum.

Indications

This type of extensive surgery is reserved for patients with extensive degenerative scoliosis, which is considered to be unsuitable for minimally invasive reconstruction. Typically, these are performed as a staged procedure with the anterior portion of the procedure being performed a week in advance of the posterior procedure. The levels that can be reached range from the lumbosacral junction through to the thoracolumbar junction. For the access of the upper lumbar level, it is advisable to include a general surgeon for the mobilization of the visceral structure. In cases deemed to be at high risk for thrombosis and pulmonary embolism, a vena cava filter can be placed in advance of the surgery. The staged posterior procedure is often largely performed percutaneously if the anterior reconstruction is satisfactory. Sometimes, the percutaneous posterior aspect is combined with open instrumentation of the thoracic spine to the desired levels to facilitate fusion or dynamic fixation at these levels. As interbody fusion is performed at all lumbar levels, a pure percutaneous instrumentation of these levels is sufficient. If all is well with the combined procedure, total blood loss of no more than 500 mL is usual.

Definition of the Technique

The only preoperative dietary restriction is to eat light meals 2 days prior to surgery. No specific bowel preparation is necessary. The procedures are performed under general anesthesia. If required, a vena cava filter is placed preoperatively as a separate procedure. The patient is placed supine with bolsters under the knees to allow flexion of the knees and minimize tension on vascular structures. The authors' preference is to have the patient's arms extended outwards to provide easy access for two surgeons to operate. Standard prepping and draping are performed as well as antibiotic prophylaxis including coverage for Gram-negative bacteria. The incision is a standard midline incision over the desired levels as performed for laparotomy. If the access is from L3 to S1, then a standard retroperitoneal exposure is performed; if the exposure is to be performed up to the thoracolumbar junction, a transperitoneal and visceral rotation procedure is performed which extends all the way to the xiphoid. (Draping needs to include the entire abdomen in case the incision needs to be extended.) Once the posterior rectus sheath has been incised and the peritoneum has been opened, the small bowel is gently pulled to the side. Bowel can also be placed into a bowel bag temporarily, significantly reducing retractor pressure for the exposure of the spine. The dissection now involves the mobilization of the kidney, which is a primary retroperitoneal structure. It is usually fairly easy to displace medially and can be mobilized in a stepwise fashion. Particular care needs to be taken to avoid injury to the suprarenal gland. The next step is to expose the undersurface of the diaphragm. This is usually performed with the combination of manual dissection and using a harmonic scalpel. For spine surgeons new to these procedures, a visceral surgeon is highly recommended to reduce surgical time and morbidity. With a skilled visceral surgeon, the approach to the upper lumbar spine can be accomplished rapidly, often within half an hour in normal abdominal anatomy. With the mobilization of the spleen, the undersurface of the diaphragm now becomes visible (**Figs. 37.1** and **37.2**). Using the appropriate retractor frame and broad blade retractors allows the visceral structures to be gently mobilized (**Fig. 37.3**). This allows visualization of the large vessels, and entire lumbar spine up to the diaphragm. The next step is the mobilization of the vascular structures. Having a large exposure allows for a comparatively easy dissection of the segmental vessels. It is necessary to ascertain that the ureter has been mobilized medially along with the kidney. Care needs to be taken to assess the vascular supply of the distal ureter as its origin from the iliac arteries is variable. In cases where vascular supply tethers the ureter, it can also be kept lateral through gentle retroperitoneal dissection of the ureter. For the mobilization of the large vessels, it is very helpful to have reverse tip retractor blades available which can be slid under the vessels and allow these to be gently separated from the lumbar spine and retracted securely laterally (**Fig. 37.4**). Thereby the exposure achieved is very extensive. If levels need to be addressed at the thoracolumbar junction, then the lateral diaphragmatic attachments need to be lifted. This allows access up to T11 from the midline approach. It is also possible to start the exposure cranially and work toward the lower lumbar spine and sacrum according to the surgeon's preference. The authors' preference is to start crainally and work caudally as the reconstruction of the intervertebral disc space tends to restore lordosis and make access to the upper level more difficult once implants have been placed. Either will however work. Care needs to be taken when addressing the upper lumbar and thoracolumbar levels with regards to the angle of the disc space as this is compromised by the lower border of the rib cage. On occasion, the rib cage needs to be retracted separately with a second retractor to allow adequate access. The preparation of the disc space is performed as per any standard anterior lumbar interbody fusion (ALIF) procedure. This approach allows extensive access to the annulus on both sides of the vertebral disc and allows concave annular resection and height restoration in a very efficient manner. The authors use a pair of parallel intervertebral body distractors for this purpose and alternate placements in the left and right side of the discs to allow the discs to be cleared and the lateral anulus and posterior longitudinal ligament (PLL) to be resected until good height restoration can be achieved. The intervertebral devices are then placed in accordance with the surgical plan. It is also possible for less extensive pathologies to combine interbody fusion devices with motion preserving disc replacement devices whereby the use is usually off-label and needs to be considered very carefully on a case-by-case basis. Once the procedure has been completed, the visceral contents are replaced. It is prudent to inspect the bowel during the repositioning in the abdominal cavity (**Fig. 37.5**). No particular techniques are performed to fixate the abdominal contents in place. The peritoneum is usually not repaired. Mass closure of the laparotomy incision is performed with resorbable PDS sutures. In elderly patients, the use of nondissolvable sutures is acceptable as this reduces the incidence of incisional hernias.

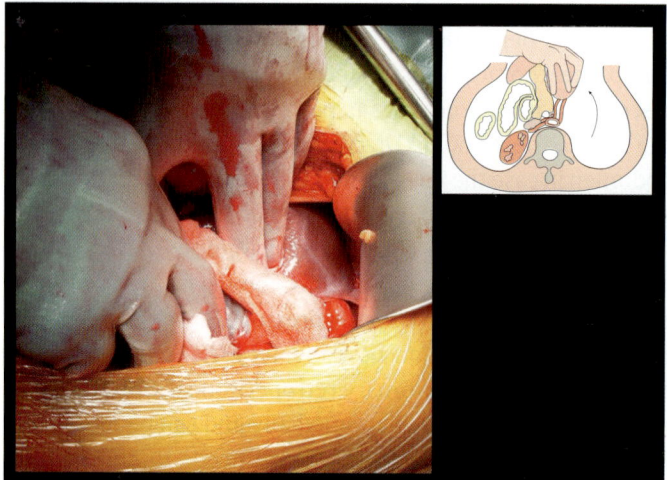

Fig. 37.1 Overview of high lumbar exposure with visceral rotation. Visceral rotation involves either mobilizing only the kidney, usually sufficient for lumbar exposure up to L2, or includes mobilizing the spleen, splenic vessels, and pancreas. The photo shows the mobilization of the spleen, still attached via the visible suspensory ligament.

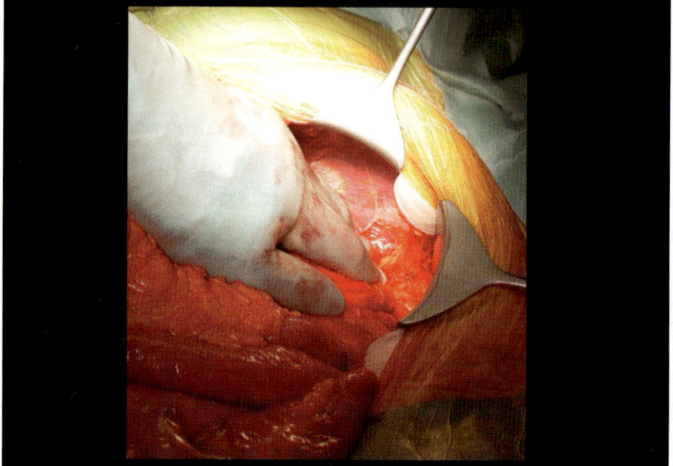

Fig. 37.2 Overview of visceral rotation with exposure of diaphragm. With the spleen mobilized, the dome of the diaphragm is visible. Note the transperitoneal approach with displacement of viscera to enable easier access.

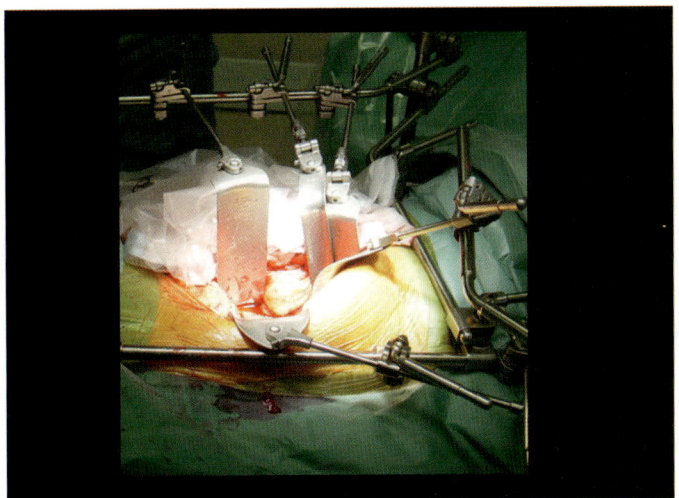

Fig. 37.3 Overview of retractor frame setup (right side is cranial). Various frame setup options are possible. The authors prefer a double layer whereby the lower layer does the "heavy lifting," retracting the rib cage and abdominal musculature. The viscera are displaced into the plastic bag. The long blades on the side of the viscera allow retraction of the abdominal wall and content while avoiding compressing the viscera. The longer narrow blade only retracts the vessels with minimal force.

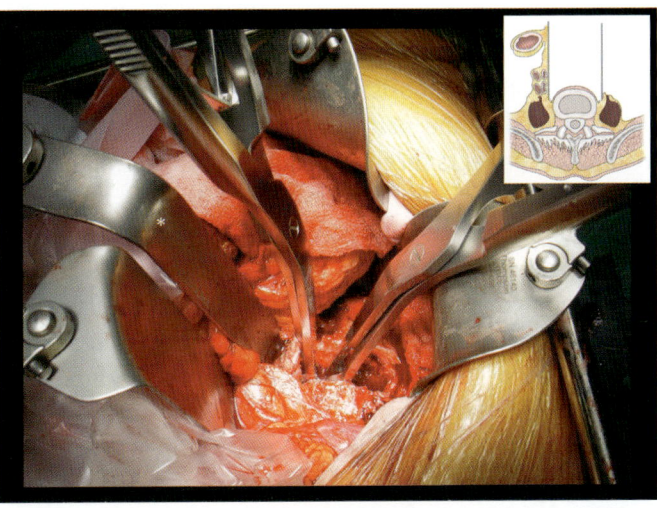

Fig. 37.4 View of the situs of exposed upper lumbar spine to thoracolumbar junction. Parallel retractors are placed in the L1/L2 disc space after release of the anulus. The reverse tip retractor (*) only holds the vessels aside while the larger blades retract the abdominal wall and content. Inset: Position of reverse tip blade.

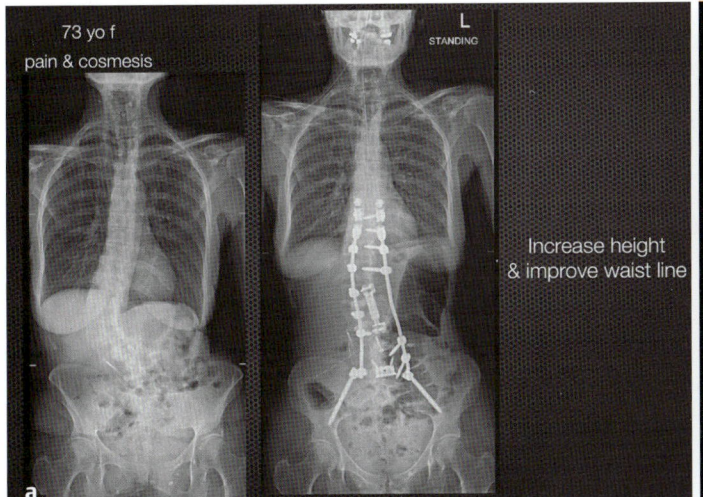

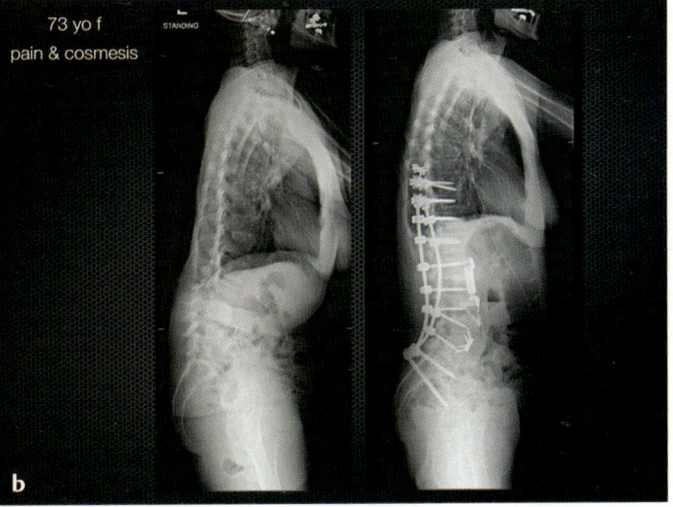

Fig. 37.5 Case example of lumbar reconstruction in degenerative scoliosis with anterior posterior reconstruction via visceral rotation. **(a)** Significant scoliotic deformity is corrected with restoration of vertebral and interbody height leading to a restored waistline and overall balance. **(b)** Anterior reconstruction facilitates restoration of lordosis with posterior instrumentation providing stability. The lower instrumentation can be inserted percutaneously or via muscle splitting approaches (as in this case) minimizing blood loss; flexible fixation at the cranial end of the construct should lessen the risk of junctional kyphosis. In the absence of complications, combined blood loss of less than 500 mL is possible.

Postoperative Management

The patient can be mobilized to a seated position within the first 1 or 2 postoperative days. For analgesic purposes, rectus sheath catheters can be placed intraoperatively. Deep drains are usually not necessary. In the event of a second posterior surgery, the mobilization of the patient depends on the structural integrity of the anterior implants; if required, a temporary brace can be useful. It is beneficial for the patient to be mobilized into a sitting position and to have brief standing periods daily. The thromboprophylaxis can be commenced on the first or second postoperative day. Patients are at risk of thrombosis due to the necessary extensive vessel retraction and particular care needs to be taken to ensure that patients receive adequate thromboprophylaxis. Intraoperative calf compression devices are very helpful to reduce thrombosis in high-risk patients, and vena cava filters may be useful too. These can be extracted once the second posterior surgery has been performed and the patient is free of complications. Typically, contrast is injected prior to extraction of the vena cava filter and if no thrombosis is found, this can be removed.

Complication Avoidance

The complications are the same as any conventional ALIF procedure. Complications range from visceral injury to splenic injury and renal injury. Including a visceral access surgeon in the team helps minimize the impact of such general surgery complications. As the access and exposure of the large vessels are substantial, any vascular repair is instantly performable by either the spine surgeon or a vascular team. The segmental vessels can be ligated securely unilaterally for the entire lumbar spine. The diaphragmatic attachments can be resutured to the spine; however, this is often technically difficult. It does not appear to be a risk factor for developing herniations. Postoperative ileus is a common complaint and regular food intake should only commence once positive bowel sounds are present and ideally once patients have opened their bowels. In the initial phase, foods with adequate fluids are recommended such as broths which are easily digestible. A urinary catheter is kept in place to assess renal output and for the comfort of the patient in the initial phase. A crush injury to the kidneys is less common with the anterior approach than a posterior approach as there is far less muscular dissection involved in the approach.

Tips and Tricks

- In elderly patients consider closing abdomen with nonresorbable sutures to avoid dehiscence and hernia.
- Consider using a retractor frame with three or four table attachments for solid retraction. This will help especially in obese patients.
- Avoid the use of Steinman pins especially in elderly patients as this can kink vessels. Rather use reverse tip retractor blades that can be slid under the vessels and securely prevent them from migrating.
- In patients susceptible to thrombosis consider a vena cava filter preoperatively. Once mobile consider removing after about a week. For this contrast is injected and if no clot is seen it can be removed, otherwise it is kept in place with anticoagulation.
- Team up with a general, hepatobiliary, or vascular surgeon for the visceral rotation.

Key Points

- Visceral rotation allows extensive midline exposure of the entire lumbar to thoracolumbar spine.
- Consider this approach in cases where annular release is required bilaterally and anteriorly.
- Reconstruction of lordosis is very effective with minimal blood loss and avoids spinal shortening and manipulation of neural structures as in pedicle subtraction osteotomy (PSO) procedures.

38 Lateral Access Surgery for Thoracolumbar Deformities

Turgut Akgül

Introduction

Norman Capener first described the lateral approach to the vertebra in 1933 for decompression surgery.[1] For several years this approach was reported with high success.[2,3] However, lateral access approaches have lost popularity due to the development of posterior instrumentation techniques and anterior approach-related morbidities for a long time. Nevertheless, lateral approaches have become popular again with minimally invasive procedures and by avoiding flank thoracoabdominal incisions.

Lateral approaches give satisfactory results in degenerative deformities because of their success in correcting them and their higher fusion rates compared to only posterior fusion surgeries. Although the lateral transpsoas approach for the lumbar spine was introduced by Pimenta in 1998, this technique was published by Ozgur et al in 2006.[4] Due to a high rate of lumbar plexus problems such as transient neuropraxia related to the transpsoas approach, another minimally invasive approach called prepsoas or antepsoas approach using a corridor between vascular structures and psoas, which has less lumbar plexus problems, was introduced by Silvestre et al in 2012.[5]

Minimally invasive lateral approaches are performed in two primary methods prepsoas–antepsoas and transpsoas, depending on where the approach is in the psoas muscle. While prepsoas approaches are used to avoid psoas irritation and are performed away from the lumbar plexus, transpsoas approaches that are far from vascular structures but close to the lumbar plexus are frequently used in lateral approaches. Attention should be paid to the lumbar plexus, main vascular structures, and ureter in the lateral approach.[6]

A minimally invasive lateral approach was described for diskectomy or short instrumentation. Also, it is possible to perform long-level vertebral body instrumentation with the lateral approach with an enlarged incision or multiple stab incisions. Posterior mobilization of the psoas muscle is required to reach the vertebral body for vertebral body instrumentation. However, correction with the lateral approach in spinal deformities was first described by Dwyer et al in 1969.[7] The rod systems providing three-plane correction with a lateral approach were popularized by

Zielke.[8] Kaneda et al reported successful results in a patient with thoracolumbar and lumbar deformities using a dual rod and screw combination.[9] They performed their surgery via a wide flank incision with approach-related morbidity due to a rigid rod system.

On the other hand, anterior surgeries for deformities give a chance to minimize instrumentation level when compared with posterior surgery. Anterior vertebral body tethering (AVBT) applications described for thoracic deformities are used in the lumbar and thoracolumbar regions for flexible deformities with satisfactory results via a minimally invasive approach such as mini-lumbotomy.[10] In particular, the use of dynamic systems and the fact that the correction maneuvers are not as rigid as other systems allow this system to be applied in a minimally invasive manner without the need for extensive openings.

Lateral Lumbar Interbody Fusion (LLIF) (Transpsoas and Antepsoas)

For the lateral retroperitoneal approach, the patient should be well-evaluated carefully before the operation to avoid complications. History of abdominal and retroperitoneal surgeries, radiotherapy, and malignancies which cause retroperitoneal adhesion related complications should be questioned. Although obesity is a huge problem for anesthesiologic complications or due to wound infection, obesity creates a large retroperitoneal space due to retroperitoneal fat tissue in the lateral decubitus position, which is better for the surgical technique.

For preoperative radiological evaluation, radiographs, computed tomography (CT), and magnetic resonance imaging (MRI) should be included. Lumbopelvic parameters and the presence and degree of spondylolisthesis should be evaluated in standard radiographs, which should be taken in anteroposterior and lateral full spine views. Vascular anatomy and position of osteophytes can be evaluated on CT sections. The position of the psoas muscle must be determined on MRI to choose the transpsoas or prepsoas approach.

Psoas morphology and position are essential due to the lumbar plexus for the transpsoas approach. Banagan et al have shown that the plexus originates partly from L1–L3 roots and partly from L4 after mapping the lumbar plexus for transpsoas approaches.[11] Nerves originating from this plexus are ilioinguinal, hypogastric, obturator, lateral femoral cutaneous, and femoral nerves. The lumbar plexus becomes more complex from the proximal to distal level, especially at the L4–L5 disc level. Although there is a wider safe area proximally, there is a more anterior safe area at the L4–L5 level.

The sympathetic chain is located approximately 8 to 13 mm anterior to the middle disc area of the psoas. Since the lumbar plexus is displaced anteriorly in the presence of anteriorly located psoas muscle on MRI, it is impossible to reach the disc distance from the safe range in these patients. However, it is possible to access the L4–L5 and L5–S1 regions with antepsoas approaches whereas it is complex and risky with the transpsoas approach.

Although there is no difference in terms of opening in antepsoas and transpsoas approaches except reaching disc space at the psoas level, anteposas approach has been described to reduce transient or permanent neurological deterioration. In this approach, the working area is located between vascular structures and the front of the psoas.

Indications

Transpsoas and antepsoas approaches are the ideal indications for degenerative scoliosis and spondylolisthesis requiring disc intervention, adjacent segment disease, cases requiring sagittal realignment, and the minimally invasive spinal deformity surgery algorithm (MISDEF) 1 and 2 cases that need to undergo minimally invasive intervention.

For the lateral transpsoas approach, patients should not have previous abdominal surgery, obesity, pelvic incidence <70 degrees and sacral slope <45 degrees, iliac crest exceeding four to five disc levels, minimal spondylolysis, lateralized vessel localization at the L5–S1 level, presence of a vein located in midline or on right at L4–L5, presence of adipose tissue between the vein and the disc, posterior location of the psoas muscle, and a problem that can be corrected with indirect compression.

Although transpsoas approaches are suitable for problems between L1 and L5, it is possible to perform surgery between L1 and S1 with antepsoas approaches.

Contraindications

Significant contraindications for the direct lateral approach are advanced spondylolisthesis, an infection that may cause adhesions in the retroperitoneal region, and previous surgery. In addition, L5–S1 pathologies, anteriorly located psoas, and high iliac crest have been shown as contraindications in transpsoas approaches.

In the presence of advanced osteoporosis, end plate fractures may occur and cage subsidence may be observed. Hence, it is not recommended for use in patients with advanced osteoporosis.

Since lateral direct approaches are performed with indirect femoral compression, patients with absolute narrow canal and foraminal osteophytes will not obtain sufficient results in terms of decompression if it is performed alone. Care should be taken in these patients.

Surgical Technique

First Step: Patient Positioning and Defining the Level

The patient's choice of anesthesia should be made in such a way that it does not interfere with the use of a neuromonitoring. Neuromonitoring should include triggered electromyography (EMG), somatosensory-evoked potential (SEP), and motor-evoked potential (MEP) modalities. Appropriate electrodes and needles for neuromonitoring must be placed after anesthesia preparation (**Fig. 38.1**).

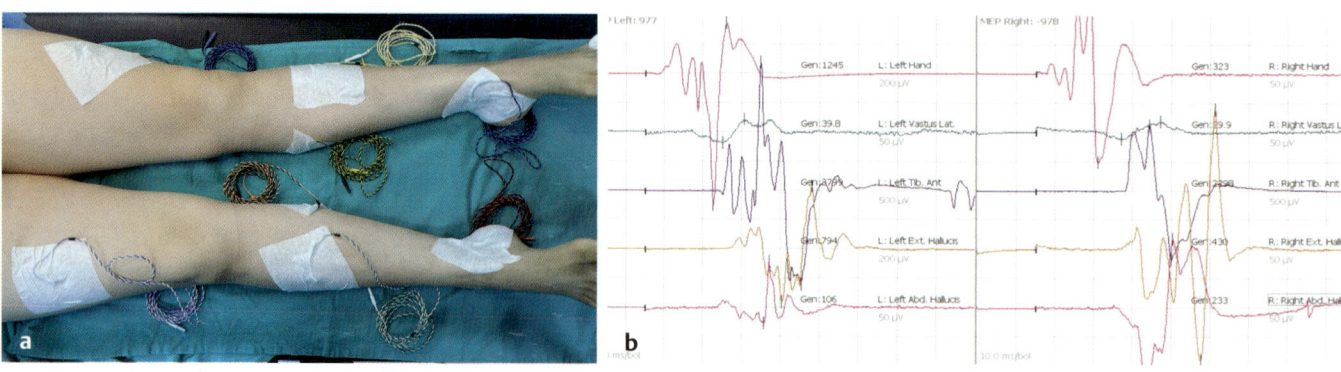

Fig. 38.1   Electrodiagnostic monitoring. Lower extremity preparation **(a)** and motor-evoked potential (MEP) value checking **(b)**.

The patient is prepared in the lateral decubitus position. Anteroposterior (AP) and lateral images can be taken with C-arm. The patient's axillary area is supported by soft pads to prevent underarm compression. Stabilization of the patient is achieved with the help of bands from the pelvic region and axillary region. In order to expand the working area, the table can be tilted so that the lateral bend or bending pads can be placed under the opposite side (**Fig. 38.2**). The patient's hip and knee should be in semiflexion position to relax the psoas, which creates a safe area to reach disc level.

The position is checked again with C-arm image intensifier to determine disc level from L1 to L5 in AP and lateral views. For the transpsoas approach, the position of the iliac crest compared to L4–L5 discs should be determined (**Fig. 38.3**). İf the iliac crest covers L4–L5 disc area, antepsoas approach is more applicable than transpsoas approach.

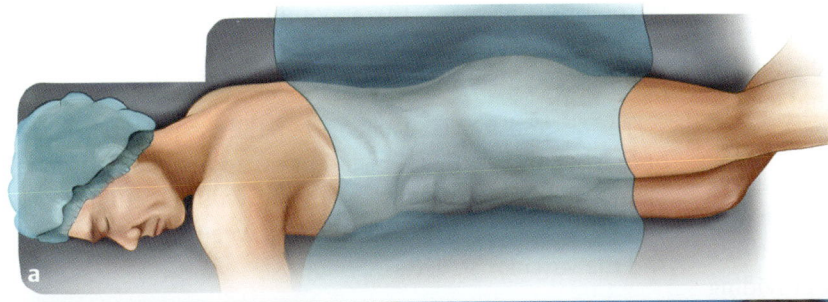

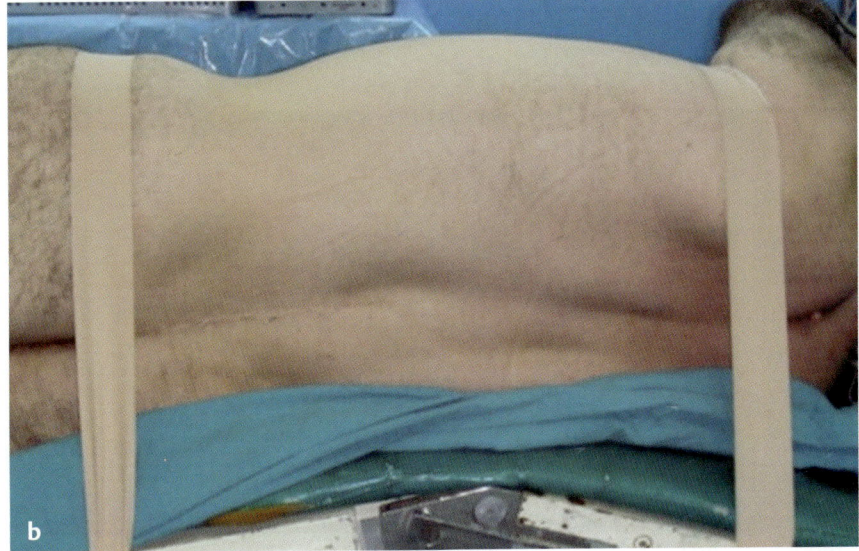

Fig. 38.2 Patient is positioned in lateral decubitus position with knee and hip in semiflexion posture **(a)**. The patient is secured with plaster at the axilla and pelvis. To create a safe working area patient's side is bent **(b)**.

Fig. 38.3 Checking iliac crest position and relationship with L4–L5 disc level is mandatory to perform the transpsoas approach.

Vertebral levels and disc distances should be determined and marked under lateral fluoroscopy control. This is important for the incision line and finding the correct level (**Fig. 38.4**).

Second Step: Incision and Deep Dissection

There are two incision techniques reported in the literature, namely, with two incisions and one incision. For the cases in which two incisions are performed, initially, the retroperitoneal region is accessed via a posterior 2 cm incision. Next, blunt finger dissection is performed to psoas muscle. Then, a second 2 cm incision is performed laterally, and the working cannula is inserted with finger guidance.

In the single-incision technique, a 3 to 4 cm long transverse or oblique incision is made just over the disc area. We suggest performing an oblique incision that gives a chance to reach more than one level safely. A clearer view of the psoas and surrounding tissues can be achieved by providing direct visualization in cases with a single incision (**Fig. 38.5**).

After the skin incision, the subcutaneous tissues are passed with the help of electrocautery. The external oblique, internal oblique, and transverse abdominus muscles are passed with the use of a dissector clamp in a line parallel to the fibers (**Fig. 38.6**). In this step, avoid harming the iliohypogastric and ilioinguinal nerves located between muscle layers. The retroperitoneal space is accessed after the transversus abdominus muscle is passed. The transverse abdominus muscle layer should be passed carefully with a hemostat not to damage the peritoneal. After reaching the retroperitoneal space, the abdominal structures are gently dissected from posterior to anterior. This dissection can be performed with a finger or tamponade (**Fig. 38.7**).

The desired area is reached when the psoas muscle is seen or touched by the finger. In antepsoas approaches, retraction of the abdominal organs anteriorly will be required. The antepsoas approach is performed between the psoas muscle and the vascular structures.

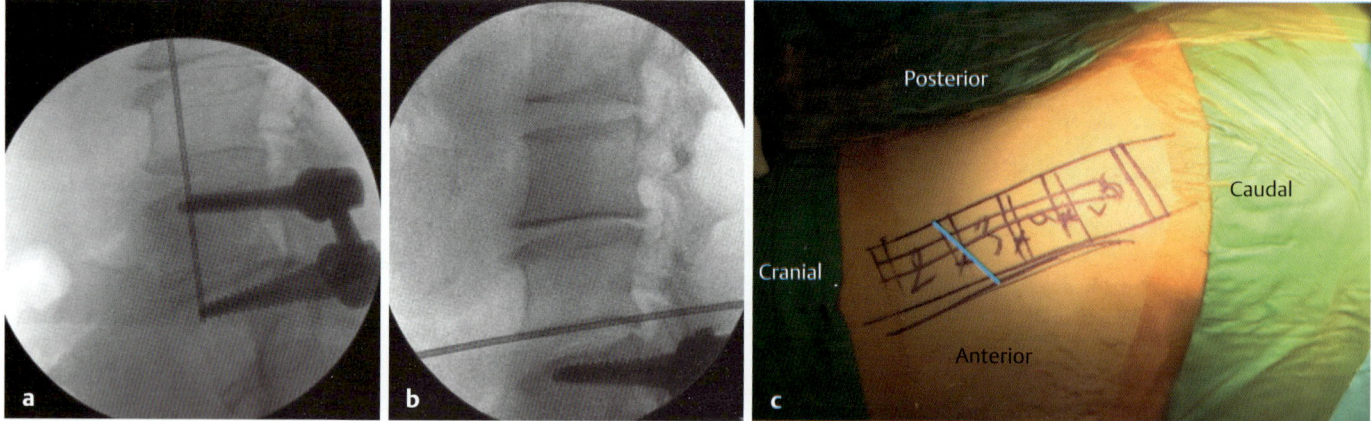

Fig. 38.4   Disc level is determined with anteroposterior (AP) and lateral views of C-arm fluoroscopy **(a, b)**. Vertebral levels and disc distances marked on the skin **(c)**.

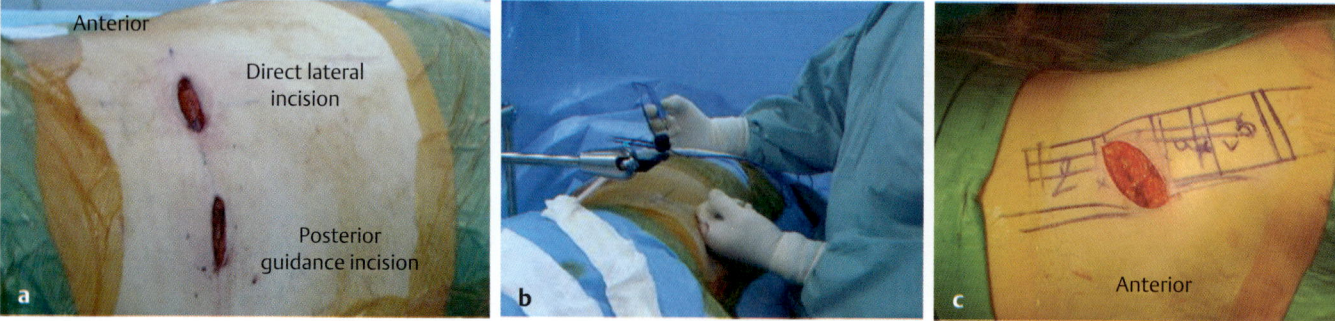

Fig. 38.5   There are two incision techniques reported in the literature, namely, with two incisions and one incision. For the cases in which two incisions are performed, initially, the retroperitoneal region is accessed via a posterior 2 cm incision. Next, blunt finger dissection is performed to psoas muscle. Then, a second 2 cm incision is performed laterally, and a working cannula is inserted with finger guidance **(a)**. In the single-incision technique, a 3 to 4 cm long transverse or oblique incision is made just over the disc area **(b)**.

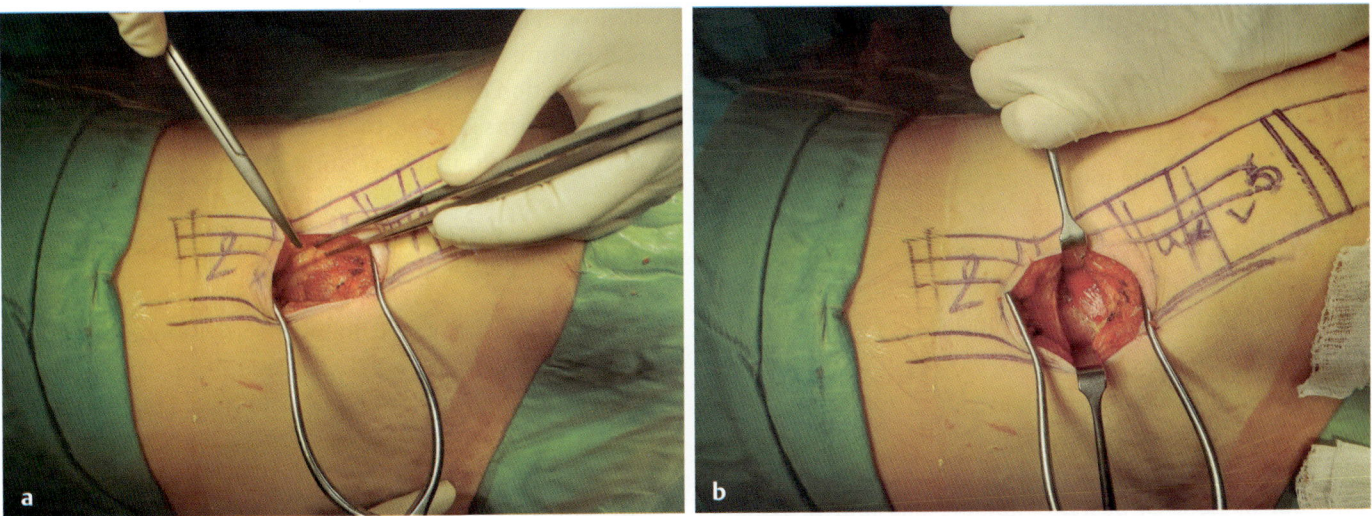

Fig. 38.6 The subcutaneous tissues are passed with the help of electrocautery, and the external oblique, internal oblique, and transverse abdominus muscles are passed with a dissector clamp in a line parallel with the fibers **(a, b)**.

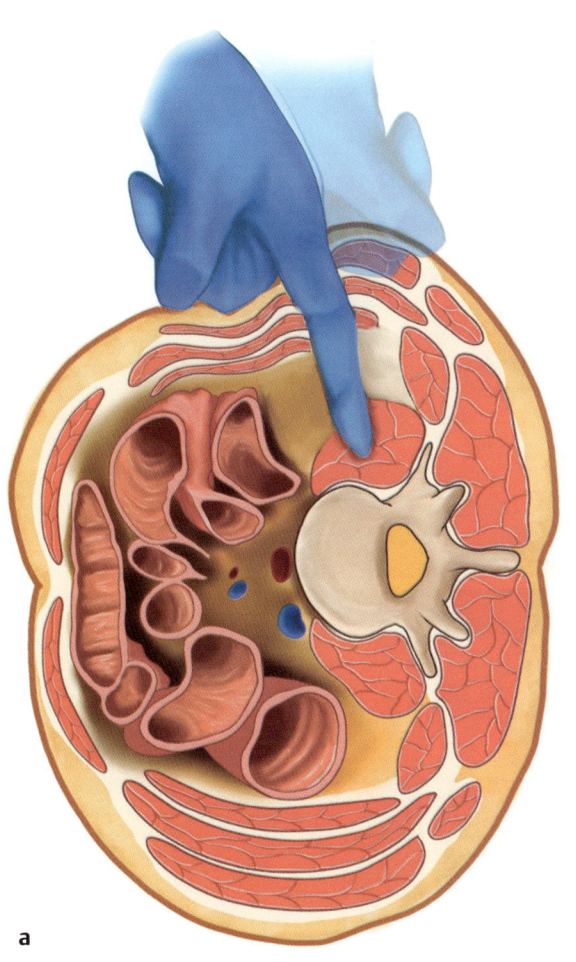

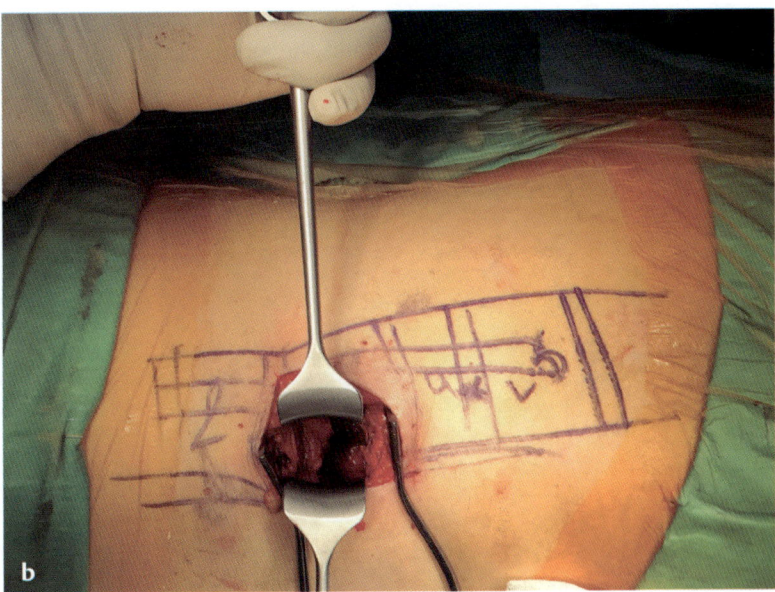

Fig. 38.7 **(a, b)** After reaching the retroperitoneal space, the abdominal structures are gently dissected from posterior to anterior. This dissection can be performed with a finger or tamponade.

Third Step: Careful Entry to Disc Space

After the psoas muscle is seen or touched by the finger, disc space is checked with the help of C-arm fluoroscopy. A triggered EMG (T-EMG) probe is inserted into the disc space to determine the safe interval at the disc space (**Fig. 38.8**). T-EMG is delivered to the distal end of the dilator as it is passed through the psoas. Direct nerve stimulation has been shown clinically to elicit average EMG responses of 2 mA. About 38,39 thresholds less than 5 mA indicate possible direct contact with the nerve.[12]

Uribe et al divided the lumbar spine disc distance into four sections according to the location of the lumbar plexus: Zone 1, anterior one-fourth; Zone 2, anterior middle one-fourth; Zone 3, posterior middle one-fourth; Zone 4, posterior one-fourth. While Zone 3 between L1 and L4 provides a safe operating range, Zone 2 between L4 and L5 offers a much safer operating range anteriorly.[13]

After the safe disc space is found, the working area is prepared with the help of dilators, and the site is secured with special retractors (**Fig. 38.9**). It has been reported in the literature that after the determination of the safe area, split retraction of the psoas can provide a safe working area without dilators (**Fig. 38.10**).[14,15] In this approach, there is no need for an additional retractor system.

Fourth Step: Diskectomy and Application of Cage

Diskectomy is performed following the annulotomy after the safe disc working area is created. While performing a diskectomy, attention should be paid to end plate fractures. It is inevitable to have cage subsidence if end plate removal is performed extensively. Taking an AP image with fluoroscopy in the end plate preparation will prevent end plate damage. The contralateral annulus should be released to create a rectangular disc area to protect end plate fracture.

After the diskectomy, the appropriate height of the disc space is determined with cage trials under the control of AP and lateral views (**Fig. 38.11**). After the proper size is selected,

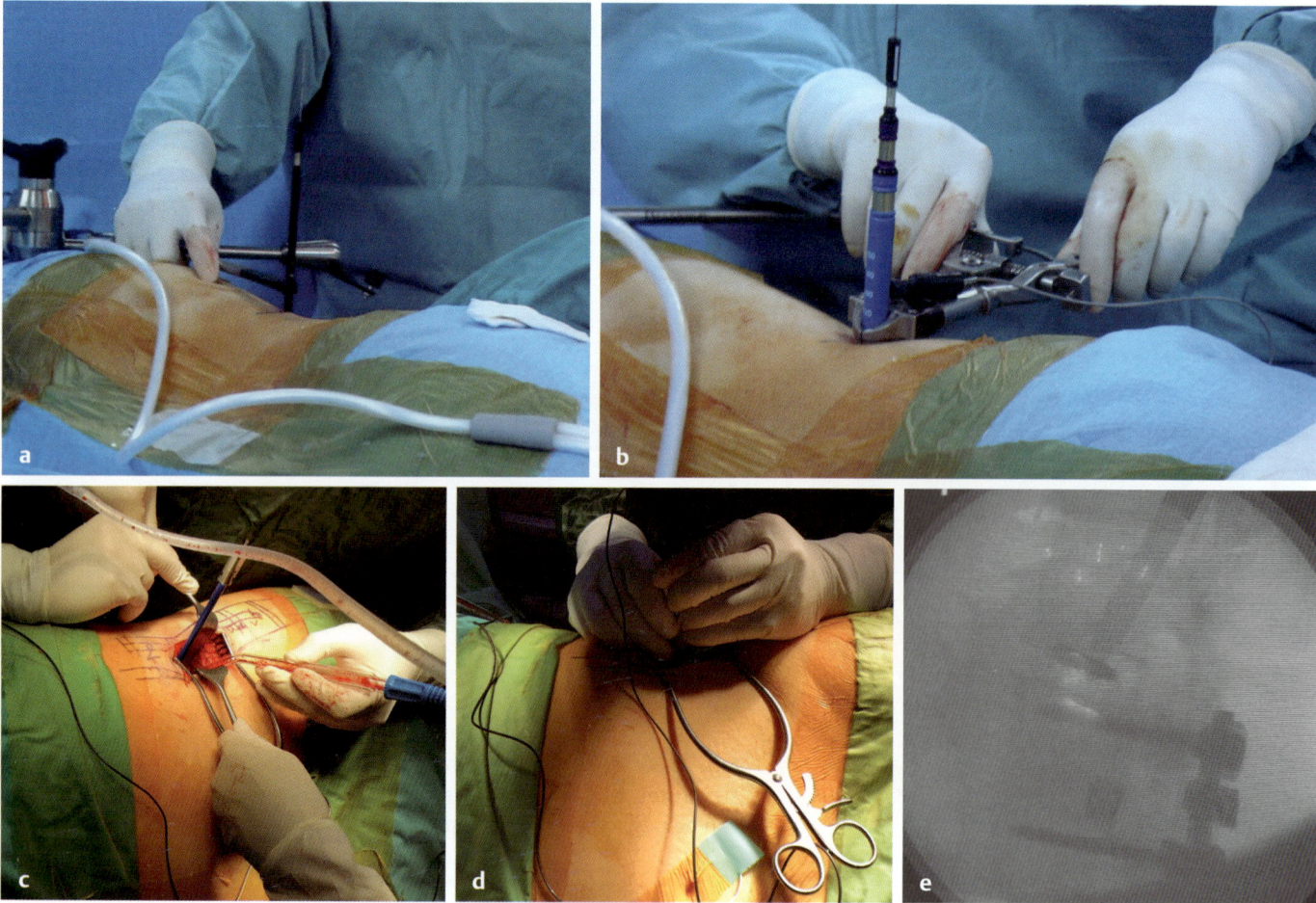

Fig. 38.8 To find a safe area for diskectomy, a triggered electromyography (EMG) probe (a different type of probe is on the market) should be used **(a–d)** and checked with C-arm fluoroscopy **(e)**.

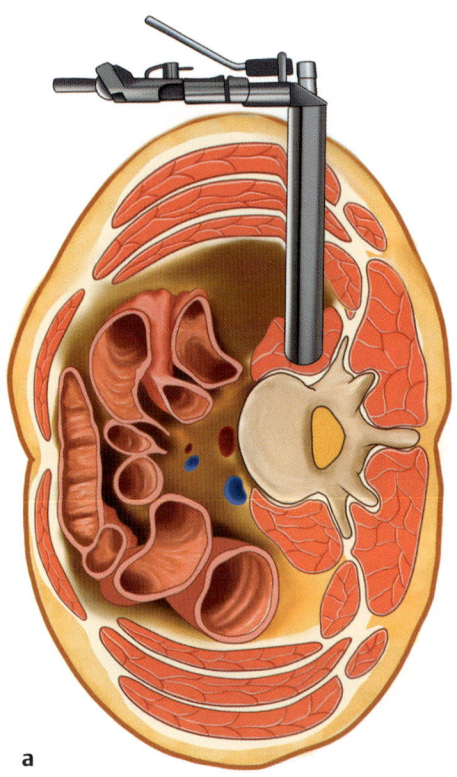

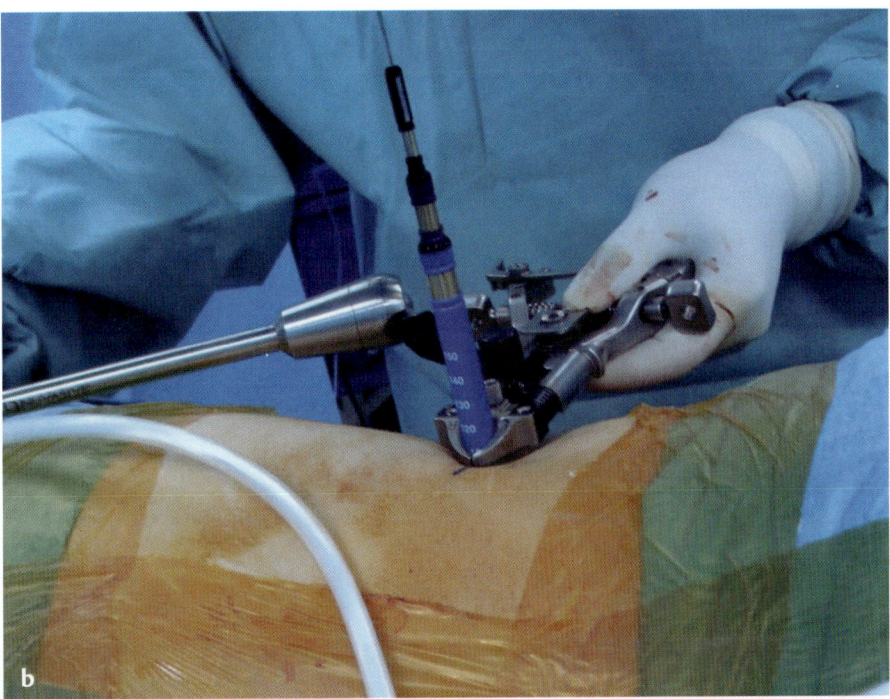

Fig. 38.9 The working area is prepared with the help of dilators and the site is secured with special retractors **(a, b)**.

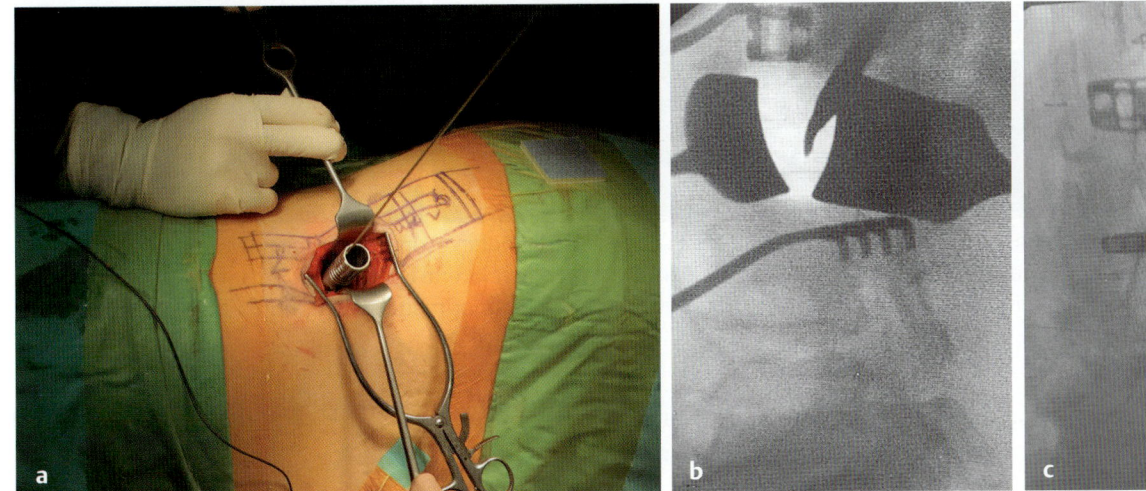

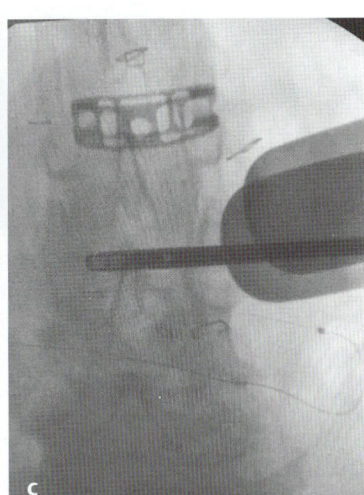

Fig. 38.10 Split retraction of the psoas can provide a safe working area without the use of dilators **(a–c)**.

the cage filled with bone graft is placed under the AP C-arm fluoroscopy. In direct lateral applications, the cage is placed perpendicular to the axial plane. In antepsoas applications, the cage is placed obliquely; then, it is positioned in its correct place with a gentle posterior maneuver (**Fig. 38.12**).

There is a difference in the choice of the cage in the transpsoas and antepsoas approaches due to the working area difference (**Fig. 38.12**). While it is possible to use longer and wider cages in the transpsoas approach, cages with less

volume are used in the antepsoas approach (**Figs. 38.13** and **38.14**).

Complications

In the lateral approach to the lumbar spine, systemic and surgery-related complications can be seen. Complications related to surgical intervention are soft tissue problems and infection, vascular injuries, injuries of abdominal structures, and temporary or permanent neurological damage.[16–18]

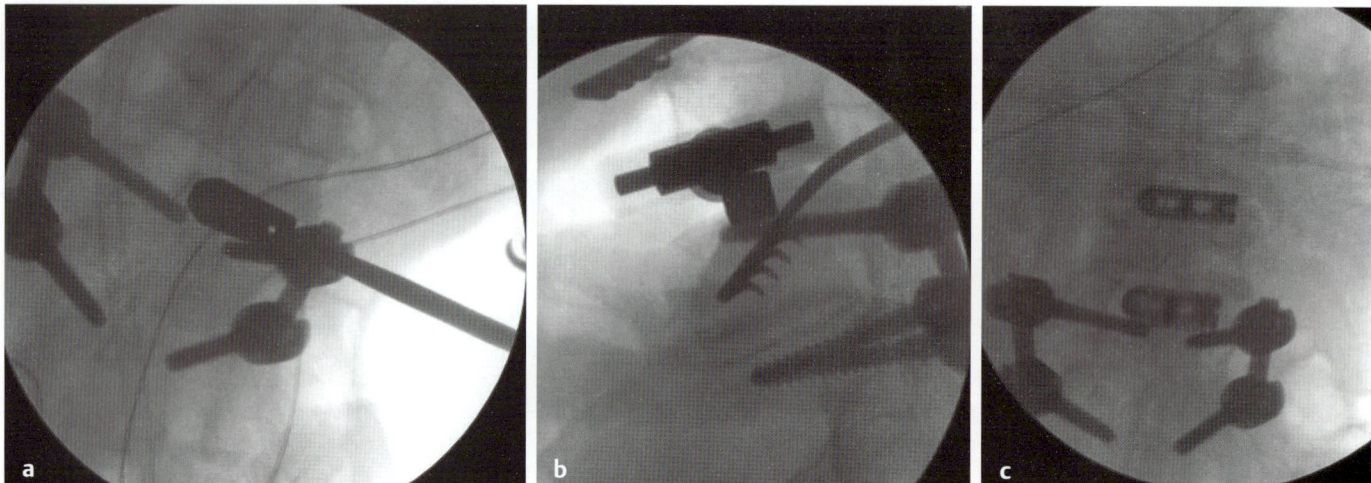

Fig. 38.11 Trial to determine appropriate cage. A trial should be controlled with C-arm fluoroscopy in anteroposterior (AP) and lateral views to avoid end plate perforation **(a–c)**.

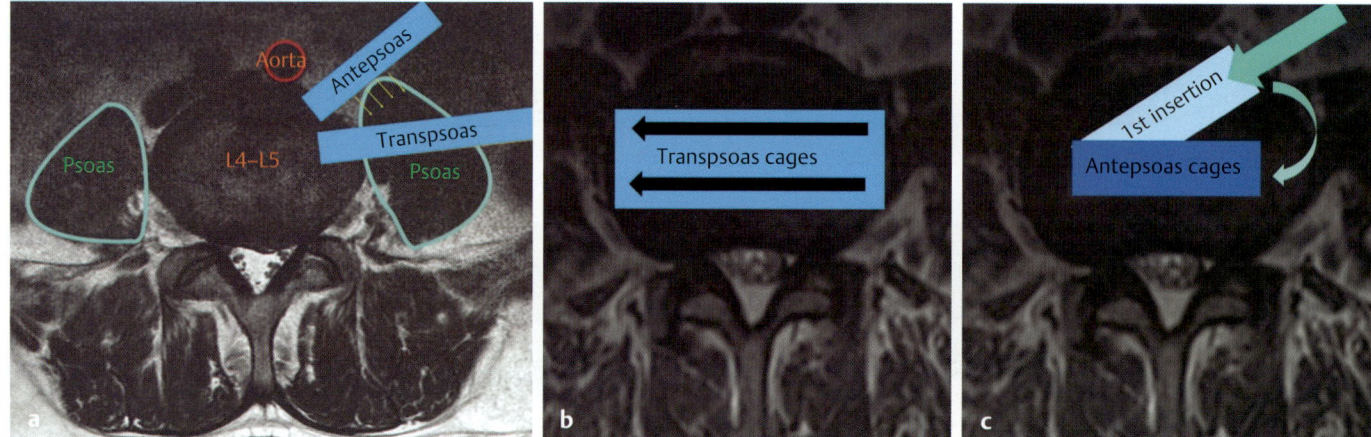

Fig. 38.12 Schematic view of transpsoas and antepsoas approaches drawn on magnetic resonance imaging (MRI) axial view to show the operative corridor **(a)**. The cage is placed perpendicular to the axial plane in direct lateral applications. In antepsoas applications, a cage is placed obliquely; then, it is positioned in its correct place with a gentle posterior maneuver **(b, c)**.

The revision rate of direct lateral approach due to nonunion, adjacent segment problems, vertebral fractures, cage malposition, or subsidence is reported to be approximately 9.2%. On the other hand, soft tissue problems, hematoma, wound problems, infection, and hernia are reported as 1.38%. There was no difference between transpsoas or antepsoas approaches regarding general complications.[16–18]

Transpsoas approaches have a higher risk of temporary and permanent neurologic injury, which is the main problem of the transpsoas approach. For the transpsoas approach, the transient neurologic injury rate is approximately 36%. Most of them resolve within 6 months. Nevertheless, 3.9% of neurological problems were reported to be permanent. With the antepsoas approach, the risk of temporary neurological injury was 14.4%, and the risk of permanent neurological injury was 1%, which is quite lower than transpsoas.[16–18]

While the risk of major vascular injury was reported as 0.4% in transpsoas approaches, it was reported as 1.8% in antepsoas approaches.[16–18] Although there is no difference between the sides in the transpsoas approach, for the antepsoas approach, the left retroperitoneal region is easier to reach since the left retroperitoneal region is wider than the right retroperitoneal area.[6] The safe place that allows working between the aorta and the psoas in the left retroperitoneal area is approximately 2.5 cm which is enough to perform disc preparation for cage insertion.[6]

The anatomy of the lumbar sympathetic chain is also essential when considering lateral approaches, as it is at

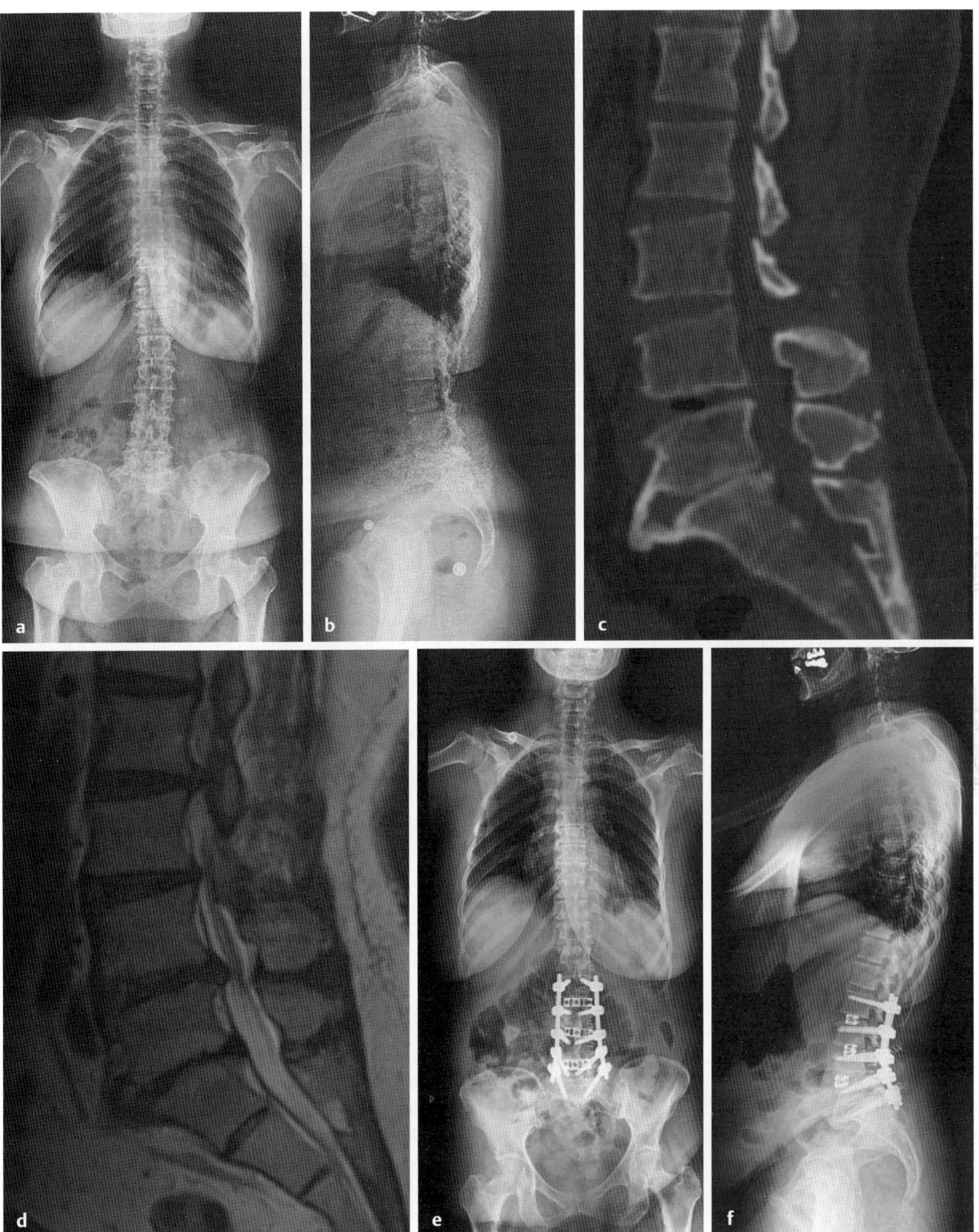

Fig. 38.13 A patient suffered from back pain and sagittal malalignment without central canal stenosis. Full spine view was taken and following measurements were obtained: pelvic incidence (PI) = 61, pelvic tilt (PT) = 30, sacral slope angle (SS) = 32, and lumbar lordosis (LL) = 44 degrees **(a, b)**. Computed tomography (CT) and magnetic resonance imaging (MRI) showed no evidence of foraminal bony osteophytes and central stenosis **(c, d)**. The patient is operated on with an anterior transpsoas approach and posterior fusion. Postoperative X-ray showed perfect sagittal alignment and corrected lumbar and pelvic mismatch **(e, f)**.

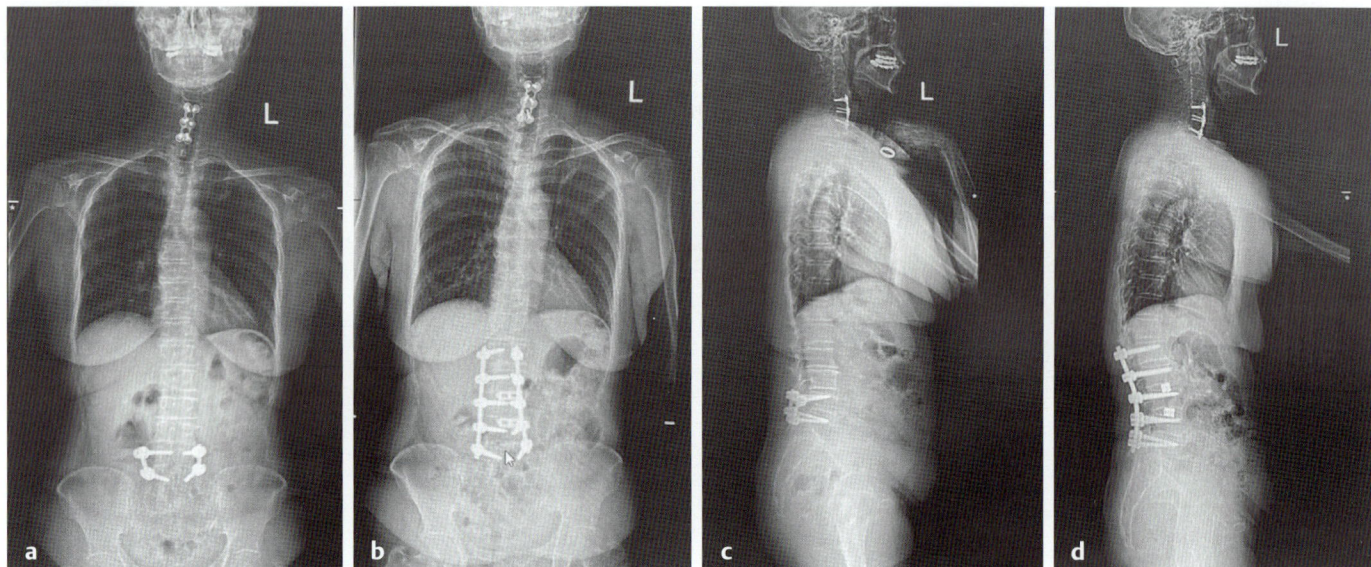

Fig. 38.14 A patient with adjacent disc disease and foraminal stenosis without central canal stenosis was operated by antepsoas approach and posterior instrumentation **(a–d)**.

risk of injury. Symptoms of injury include lower extremity temperature changes, swelling, reduced perspiration, and/or paresthesias.[16–18] Damage may be underreported due to missing this clinical diagnosis.[16–18] The incidence of antepsoas and transpsoas has been reported to be between 1.7 and 13.8%.[16–18]

In Fujibayashi et al's comparison of antepsoas and transpsoas complications, it was found that there was a significantly greater rate of ureteral injury in the antepsoas group.[18]

Mini-lumbotomy

Mini-lumbotomy can be used to reduce classical lumbotomy problems in cases that will require long-level instrumentation in the lumbar region. This technique is similar to minimally invasive lateral access, although the incision line is oblique and longer than diskectomies for this technique. This approach can be used to reach disc space, for fracture surgery, and for scoliosis surgery (**Figs. 38.15** and **38.16**). Due to the popularity of AVBT surgery recently, it is frequently used in scoliosis surgery.

Technique

First Step—Patient Positioning

The patient is positioned in the lateral decubitus position, a position that allows the surgeon to access the convex

side of the deformity. The patient is fixed with the help of supports and bands from the axillary and iliac wing parts. To provide a safer opening, the lateral bending position of the patient is obtained with the help of a table or pads similar to a minimally invasive approach.

Second Step—Incision and Deep Dissection

At the curve's apex, an oblique incision is made, extending approximately 5 to 6 cm from cranial to caudal at the convex side. After the subcutaneous fatty tissue is passed with the help of electrocautery, the external oblique, internal oblique, and transverse abdominis muscles are passed. The retroperitoneal region is accessed through the fibers of the muscles with the help of a clamp. After entering the retroperitoneal region, the abdominal structures are gently retracted from posterior to anterior. We use soft dissectors for soft tissue.

It is possible to instrument between L2 and L4 with an incision made between approximately L2 and L3. If the upper level is T10, mini-thoracotomy performed at the T12 level will enable the surgeon to access the T11–L1 region. If the level is L1, it is possible to reach it only by placing the working cannula (**Fig. 38.17**).

Third Step—Preparation of Working Space and Implant Positioning

After reaching the psoas muscle, the muscle is mobilized from anterior to posterior, providing a wide opening at the

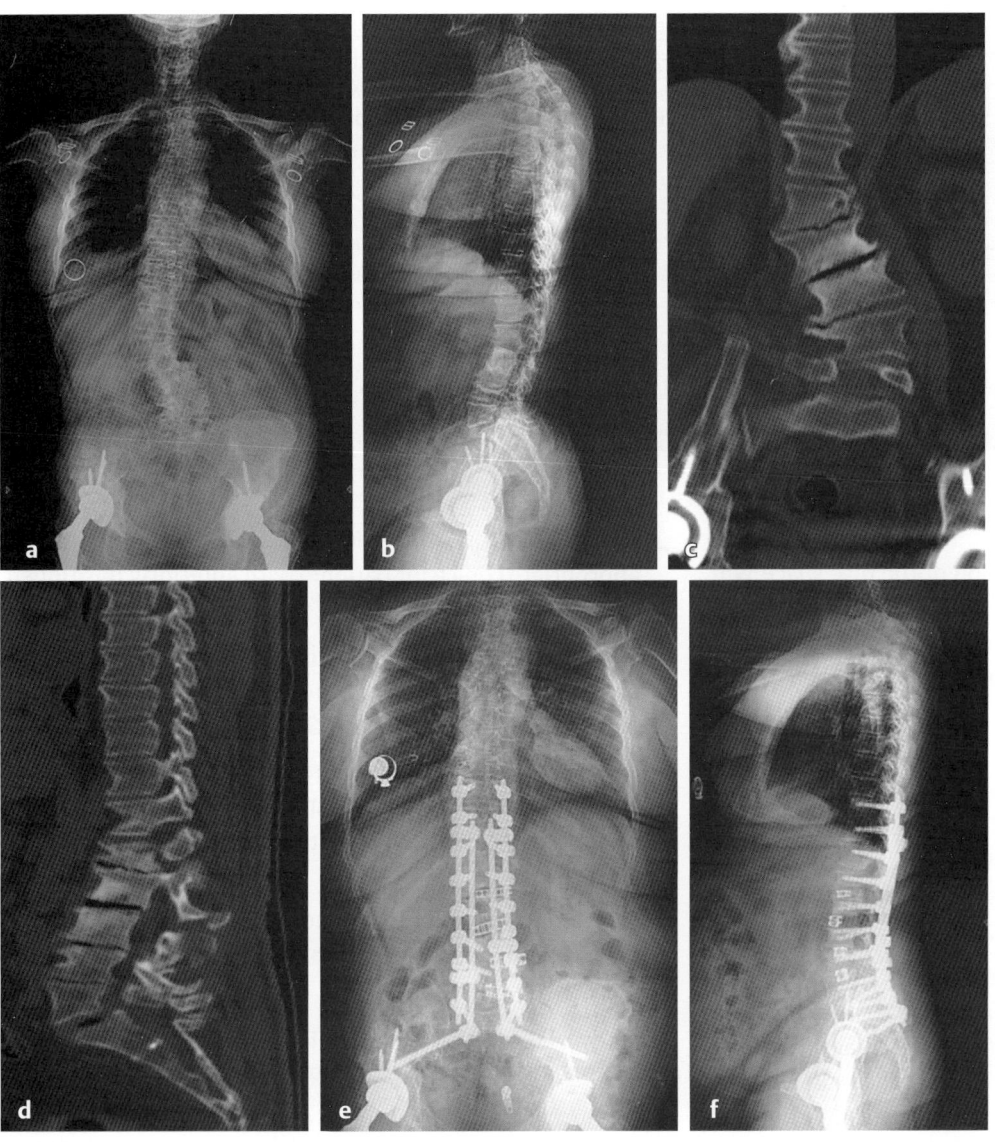

Fig. 38.15 A patient suffered from back and leg pain due to degenerative de-novo scoliosis and sagittal malalignment **(a, b)**. Computed tomography (CT) showed subchondral sclerosis and degenerative changes **(c, d)**. Mini-lumbotomy was performed to correct deformity and achieve better sagittal alignment. Antepsoas corridor was used to perform diskectomy and cage insertion. Posterior instrumentation from T10 to iliac was performed to achieve better fusion and stability **(e, f)**.

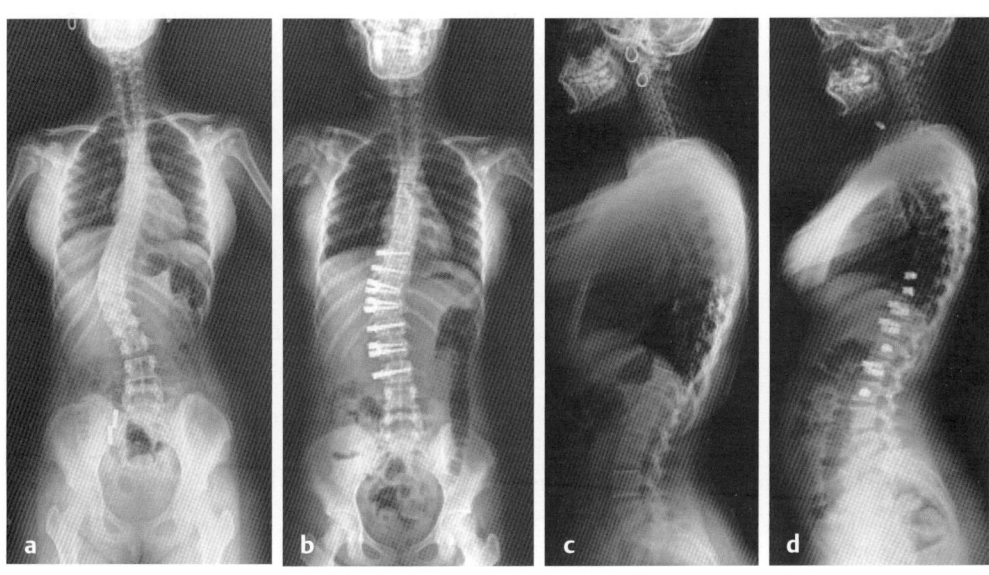

Fig. 38.16 A female patient with adolescent idiopathic scoliosis was operated on by anterior vertebral body tethering via anterior mini-lumbotomy.

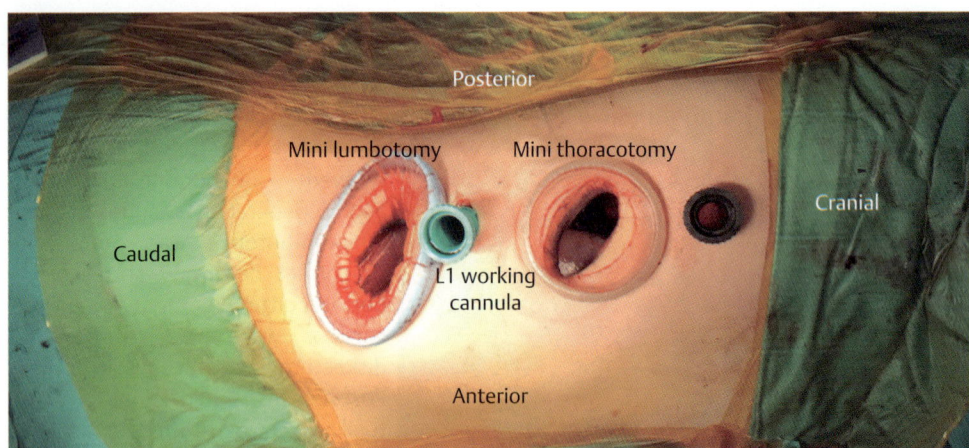

Fig. 38.17 Perioperative view of a patient operated for adolescent idiopathic scoliosis (AIS). Lumbar side surgery was performed via mini-lumbotomy, and lower thoracal surgery was performed via mini-thoracotomy. An additional working cannula was used to reach the transitional vertebra body.

disc space and lateral to the corpus. If an opening is made for isolated disc surgery, visualization of the disc space will be sufficient. In order to reach the body, segmental arteries and veins must be dissected and tied together or cauterized with electrocautery. When it is necessary to reach L4–L5 and distal, it is essential to pay attention to the external iliac artery and veins and lumbar vein.

Disc space preparation and screw placement are performed with lateral and AP images under C-arm fluoroscopy control. In screw delivery, screw placement is determined in the lateral view. Appropriate screw trajectory is controlled with AP view (**Fig. 38.18**).

Although the soft tissue incision does not differ, because screws are placed at the vertebral body, psoas retraction and scarification or retraction of segmental vascular structures will be required. Even though the complication rate of this technique is more similar to antepsoas surgery, it is also similar to the transpsoas approach in terms of psoas irritation and lumbar plexopathy. Although it is possible to place screws up to the L4 corpus with this surgical approach, it is difficult to place an implant more distally in terms of iliac crest coverage, psoas thickness, and lumbar plexus problems.

Tips and Tricks

- History of abdominal and retroperitoneal surgeries, radiotherapy, and malignancies that cause retroperitoneal adhesion related complications should be questioned.
- Psoas morphology and position are essential due to the lumbar plexus for the transpsoas approach. Anteriorly positioned psoas muscle is a contraindication for the transpsoas approach—the antepsoas approach is an appropriate choice for patients with anteriorly positioned psoas muscle.
- Transpsoas approach is used for diseases between L1 and L5. The antepsoas approach is appropriate for lumbar disc disease between L1 and S1.
- İliac crest height and coverage of the L4–S1 disc are essential for the transpsoas approach. İf the L4–L5 disc is covered by the iliac crest, antepsoas approach should be performed.
- External oblique muscle and internal oblique muscle should be dissected with a hemostat parallel to muscle fibers.
- Avoid harming iliohypogastric and ilioinguinal nerves located between external oblique and internal oblique muscle layers.
- Disc space is checked with the help of C-arm fluoroscopy after the psoas muscle is seen or touched by the finger. Triggered EMG probe is inserted into disc space to determine a safe interval at disc space. Triggered EMG is not necessary for the antepsoas approach.
- Triggered EMG, free-run EMG, MEP, and SEP should be monitored.
- The safe area for lumbar diskectomy introduced by Uribe is helpful in determining the diskectomy area.
- Contralateral annulus should be released to create a rectangular disc area to protect end plate fracture.
- There is a difference in the choice of cage between the transpsoas and antepsoas approaches. While it is possible to use longer and broader cages in the transpsoas approach, cages with less volume are used in the antepsoas approach.

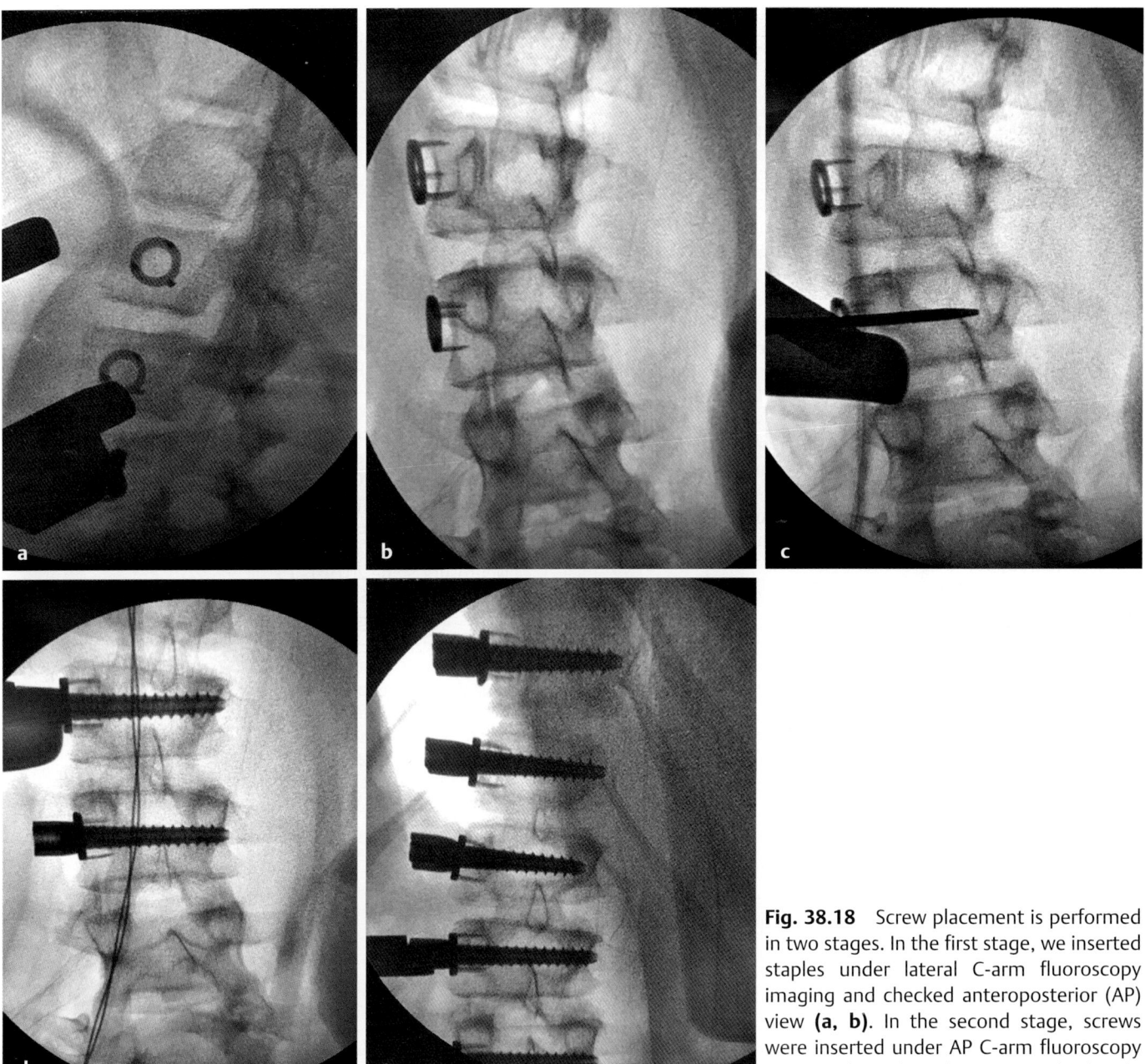

Fig. 38.18 Screw placement is performed in two stages. In the first stage, we inserted staples under lateral C-arm fluoroscopy imaging and checked anteroposterior (AP) view **(a, b)**. In the second stage, screws were inserted under AP C-arm fluoroscopy imaging through to the inner staples **(c–e)**.

Key Points

The lateral approach for spine deformity is a proper technique with a high fusion rate and acceptable complication rate. Transpsoas approach, which is performed by minimally invasive method, is the best technique for disc disease from L1 to L5. Transient or permanent neuropraxia are surgery-related complications, and the rate is higher than the other approach. İn some cases L4–L5 level disc problems cannot be treated with the transpsoas approach due to psoas muscle position and high iliac crest coverage. In such cases, the antepsoas approach can be the preferred technique. Also, the antepsoas approach has increased vascular tree, sympathetic plexus, and ureter injuries compared with transpsoas approach.

References

1. Capener N. Spondylolisthesis. Br J Surg 1932;19(75): 374–386

2. Mayer HM. A new microsurgical technique for minimally invasive anterior lumbar interbody fusion. Spine 1997;22(6): 691–699, discussion 700

3. Wolfla CE, Maiman DJ, Coufal FJ, Wallace JR. Retroperitoneal lateral lumbar interbody fusion with titanium threaded fusion cages. J Neurosurg 2002;96(1, Suppl):50–55

4. Ozgur BM, Aryan HE, Pimenta L, Taylor WR. Extreme lateral interbody fusion (XLIF): a novel surgical technique for anterior lumbar interbody fusion. Spine J 2006;6(4):435–443

5. Silvestre C, Mac-Thiong JM, Hilmi R, Roussouly P. Complications and morbidities of mini-open anterior retroperitoneal lumbar interbody fusion: oblique lumbar interbody fusion in 179 patients. Asian Spine J 2012;6(2):89–97

6. Davis TT, Hynes RA, Fung DA, et al. Retroperitoneal oblique corridor to the L2-S1 intervertebral discs in the lateral position: an anatomic study. J Neurosurg Spine 2014;21(5):785–793

7. Dwyer AF, Newton NC, Sherwood AA. An anterior approach to scoliosis. A preliminary report. Clin Orthop Relat Res 1969;62(62):192–202

8. Korovessis P, Filos KS, Zielke K. Effects of the combined VDS-Zielke and Harrington operation on the frontal rib cage deformity of double major curves in idiopathic scoliosis. Spine 1995;20(9):1061–1067

9. Kaneda K, Shono Y, Satoh S, Abumi K. New anterior instrumentation for the management of thoracolumbar and lumbar scoliosis. Application of the Kaneda two-rod system. Spine 1996;21(10):1250–1261, discussion 1261–1262

10. Lonner B, Weiner DA, Miyanji F, Hoernschemeyer DG, Eaker L, Samdani AF. Vertebral body tethering: rationale, results, and revision. Instr Course Lect 2022;71:413–425

11. Banagan K, Gelb D, Poelstra K, Ludwig S. Anatomic mapping of lumbar nerve roots during a direct lateral transpsoas approach to the spine: a cadaveric study. Spine 2011;36(11):E687–E691

12. Riley MR, Doan AT, Vogel RW, Aguirre AO, Pieri KS, Scheid EH. Use of motor evoked potentials during lateral lumbar interbody fusion reduces postoperative deficits. Spine J 2018;18(10):1763–1778

13. Uribe JS, Arredondo N, Dakwar E, Vale FL. Defining the safe working zones using the minimally invasive lateral retroperitoneal transpsoas approach: an anatomical study. J Neurosurg Spine 2010;13(2):260–266

14. Chin KR, Pencle FJR, Brown MD, Seale JA. A psoas splitting approach developed for outpatient lateral interbody fusion versus a standard transpsoas approach. J Spine Surg 2018;4(2):195–202

15. Zhengkuan X, Qixin C, Gang C, Fangcai L. The technical note and approach related complications of modified lateral lumbar interbody fusion. J Clin Neurosci 2019;66:182–186

16. Walker CT, Farber SH, Cole TS, et al. Complications for minimally invasive lateral interbody arthrodesis: a systematic review and meta-analysis comparing prepsoas and transpsoas approaches. J Neurosurg Spine 2019;1–15

17. Hijji FY, Narain AS, Bohl DD, et al. Lateral lumbar interbody fusion: a systematic review of complication rates. Spine J 2017;17(10):1412–1419

18. Fujibayashi S, Otsuki B, Kimura H, Tanida S, Masamoto K, Matsuda S. Preoperative assessment of the ureter with dual-phase contrast-enhanced computed tomography for lateral lumbar interbody fusion procedures. J Orthop Sci 2017;22(3):420–424

39 Practical Points of Intraoperative Neurophysiologic Monitoring for Spinal Deformity Surgery

Muhammad Tariq Imtiaz and Faisal R. Jahangiri

Introduction

This chapter discusses the application of various intraoperative neurophysiologic monitoring (IONM) techniques (also known as modalities) during spinal deformity surgeries. The most widely used modalities are: somatosensory-evoked potentials (SSEPs), transcranial electrical motor-evoked potentials (TCeMEPs), spontaneous electromyography (sEMG), and triggered electromyography (tEMG). Each modality is briefly discussed regarding technical and anesthetic considerations for better understanding and use during spinal deformity surgery.

The abnormal curve or alignment of the bony vertebral column is referred to as spinal deformity. There is natural curvature of some degree in the spine. However, various congenital abnormalities, age-related degeneration, neuromuscular diseases, and idiopathic reasons may also cause abnormal curves resulting in deformity. The abnormal curvature may be unnoticeable or slightly noticeable in the early stages. But over time, it can worsen and may result in pain, weakness, breathing difficulties, and other symptoms. Therefore, spinal deformities in children and adult patients should be evaluated and managed to minimize any long-term adverse outcomes.

Adult scoliosis and kyphosis can be caused by age-related wear and tear on the spinal column, trauma, or complications from past surgeries. The moderate deformity occurs when the facet joints and discs deteriorate over time and can no longer support the spine's typical posture—pain results from stressed joints and pinched nerves and mostly not from the abnormal curve. As a result, there may be loss of normal curvature resulting in flat-back syndrome. Treatment can include medications, physical therapy, injections, or surgery.

The goals of spinal deformity surgery are to alleviate symptoms and correct the existing or debilitating deformity. Spinal surgeries for major deformities are performed with standard open techniques; however, there are minimally invasive options also being applied by spinal surgeons based on disease pathology, presentation, severity, and surgeon's preference. Minimally invasive surgery (MIS) is an alternative to open deformity surgery to treat patients with adult spinal deformity. However, at this time, MIS techniques are not as versatile as open deformity techniques, and MIS techniques have been reported to result in suboptimal sagittal plane correction or pseudarthrosis when used for severe deformities. Therefore, the minimally invasive spinal deformity surgery (MISDEF) algorithm was created to provide a rational decision-making framework for surgeons considering MIS versus open spine surgery. Regardless of the surgeon's approach or preference for a spinal deformity surgery, IONM modalities generally used are the same and aim to protect the integrity of the spinal cord and nerve roots.

IONM consists of neurodiagnostic tests that allow for an early warning to minimize any injury to the nervous structures at risk during surgery. Spinal deformity surgery involves various surgical procedures that risk the spinal cord, nerve roots, and blood vessels. Therefore, over the last few decades, IONM utilization during spinal deformity surgeries has become common to evaluate spinal cord function. **IONM modalities** are neurophysiologic tests used to assess specific neurologic and functional pathways during different surgical procedures. For example, ascending somatosensory pathways (dorsal columns) and descending motor pathways (ventral columns) are monitored and protected using modalities such as SSEPs and TCeMEPs, respectively.[1] sEMG and tEMG are specific modalities that can explain nerve roots-related injuries or injuries due to incorrect positioning of screws during surgery.

Therefore, IONM is crucial in minimizing postoperative deficits during deformity surgeries with real-time feedback to the surgeons. Standard practice is to use all of the above modalities (multimodality IONM) and read the data together for better understanding and results. Multimodality IONM, in general, can prevent or lower the risk of devastating neurologic deficits in a wide variety of situations that place neural structures at risk. Although these modalities have advantages and disadvantages, they are, in combination, effective means of providing spinal cord protection resulting in the prevention of deficits postoperatively.

IONM, in other words, when applied as a multimodality tool, serves to answer various questions surgeons have in mind during surgeries. For example, questions related to the integrity of the spinal cord and its functions, medial and lateral breaches during screw placement, and questions regarding the degree of correction can be answered using multimodality IONM. In addition, IONM also provides surgeon, details about the reversibility of a change if it occurred and is identified and communicated in timely manner, also, IONM identifies data changes that are not related to direct surgical insult. For example, a data change related to suboptimal mean arterial pressure (MAP) can be identified and communicated, and correct measures are taken.

IONM Modalities

Somatosensory Evoked Potentials (SSEP)

SSEPs have been the most commonly used monitoring modality during surgical procedures since the 1960s.[2] SSEPs are used routinely during brain, spinal, and peripheral surgical procedures. SSEPs are optimal for protecting the patient's dorsal column (ascending sensory pathways) during high-risk surgical procedures.[3] These ascending dorsal column pathways mediate stereognosis, proprioception, tactile discrimination, vibration sensation, and form recognition.[4]

Upper and lower extremity SSEP monitoring is usually performed during all spinal deformity procedures. Median (C5–T1) or ulnar nerves (C7–T1) SSEP is frequently performed in the upper extremities for cervical spine pathologies, any position-related changes in thoracolumbar pathologies, or as a result, control for evaluating and identifying upper versus lower limb changes. In contrast, in the lower extremities, posterior tibial nerve (L4–L5, S1, S2) and peroneal nerve (L4–L5) SSEPs are typically performed. The SSEPs are performed by **peripheral nerves** with low-intensity electrical stimulation (20–50 mA) in the upper and lower limbs to generate SSEP signals. The **recording electrodes** are placed along the sensory pathway (brachial plexus/popliteal fossa, cervical spine, and somatosensory cortex). These multiple recording sites help identify the anatomic and functional integrity at different locations as the signal travels from the periphery to the primary sensory cortex. SSEPs are also helpful in detecting mechanical and ischemic changes in the peripheral nerves, posterior spinal cord, brainstem, and cerebral cortex.[5]

Peripheral responses, such as brachial plexus (for the upper extremities) and popliteal fossa (for the lower extremities), are monitored to confirm the adequacy of stimulation, perfusion of the peripheral limbs, and peripheral nerve compression. The peripheral and subcortical responses are less sensitive to anesthesia than the cortical responses and are frequently used to differentiate changes in SSEP resulting from anesthesia and surgical manipulation.

In response to peripheral nerve stimulation of upper limbs (ulnar and median nerves), a **negative potential (N20)** is generated in the somatosensory cortex (recorded at the scalp using electrodes after 20 milliseconds from stimulation at the wrist). Conversely, a **positive potential (P37)** is generated in the somatosensory cortex in response to posterior tibial nerve stimulation in lower limbs at the medial malleolus.

The SSEP alarm criteria used is a decrease of 50% or more in amplitude (size of the waveform, measured in microvolts) or an increase of 10% or more in the latency (duration from point A to B, measured in milliseconds). Such changes must be immediately reported to the surgeon for an intervention to reduce the risk of any postoperative neurological deficits (**Figs. 39.1** and **39.2**).

Advantages

Somatosensory (dorsal column–medial lemniscus) pathways can be monitored continuously during surgical procedures without any interference with the surgery. The SSEPs help protect the sensory fibers in the peripheral nerves, spinal cord, brainstem, or brain. Any mechanical or ischemic changes can be recorded and reported to the surgical team for immediate corrective action.

Disadvantages

SSEPs need 10 to 300 averages under general anesthesia to remove ambient noise present in electrical circuits in the operating rooms. However, if the patient is under light anesthesia, the electromyography (EMG) artifact makes it challenging to record SSEP signals leading to a longer acquisition time. It may take from a few seconds to 2 to 3 minutes to record a single SSEP trace depending upon the electrical noise and depth of anesthesia. SSEP is also limited to changes in the sensory fibers and dorsal column only. It does not detect any changes in the motor pathway. SSEP does not carry pain and temperature sensations brought by the spinothalamic tracts. Various factors affect the SSEP data, such as anesthesia, low MAP, ischemia, hypothermia, incorrect positioning of the limbs, etc.

Transcranial Electrical Motor-Evoked Potentials (TCeMEPs)

The TCeMEPs are being used to evaluate the descending corticospinal motor tracts. Since their development in the early 1980s, many studies have shown the benefits of TCeMEP monitoring to evaluate the functional integrity of descending corticospinal tracts during high-risk orthopedic and neurosurgical procedures.[6] The addition of TCeMEP

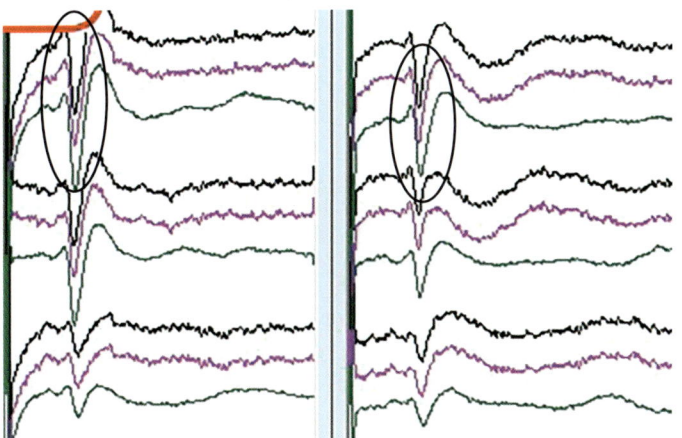

Fig. 39.1 Left and right upper (median nerves stimulated at wrist and recorded at scalp) somatosensory-evoked potentials (SSEPs) (normal data). Green-baseline data at the start of surgery; pink and black, current and previous waves.

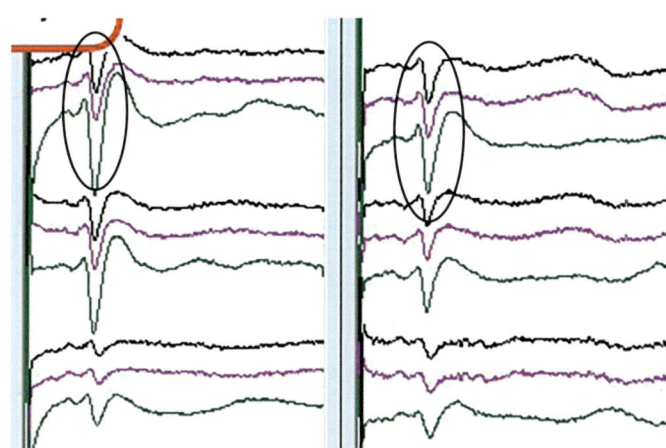

Fig. 39.2 Left and right upper (median nerves stimulated at wrist and recorded at scalp) somatosensory-evoked potentials (SSEPs) (data change and drop in amplitude recorded at scalp electrodes). Green-baseline data at the start of surgery; pink and black, current and previous waves.

to SSEP and EMG improves the patients' motor status and reduces the risk of paralysis in real-time. TCeMEP helps detect any ischemic changes in the peripheral motor nerves, spinal cord, brainstem, and motor cortex. Before introducing TCeMEP, the Stagnara wake-up test was the only way to assess the functional integrity of the motor pathways during spinal surgeries. The Stagnara wake-up test is difficult in noncompliant patients, requiring them to wake up during surgical procedures and ask them to move or wiggle their feet. The Stagnara wake-up test requires the surgeon to pause the operation and wait for the patient to wake up and comply with the commands. This technique does not give feedback in real-time and can also delay the surgical procedure.

SSEP was the only modality used for spinal cord monitoring during spine surgeries for many years. However, as we know, the ascending sensory fibers and their blood supply are different from the descending motor fibers. Therefore, if there is damage to motor pathways or ischemia to the anterior spinal artery supplying the motor pathways, it will not change SSEP signals. **Hence, the patient can wake up paralyzed with intact SSEP signals.** The TCeMEP is more sensitive to ischemic or mechanical changes than SSEP. Intraoperative loss of muscle MEPs indicates postoperative motor deficits that may be temporary or permanent. The specificity of TCeMEP is approximately 90% and has a sensitivity of 100%.[7]

TCeMEP is elicited by placing **two electrodes that serve as stimulating electrodes**—one as an anode and the other as a cathode on the patient's scalp using the EEG 10/20 electrode placement system during a spinal surgical procedure. A

high-frequency multipulse electrical stimulation activates the upper motor neurons. The signal is transmitted to the muscle fibers via lower motor neurons and neuromuscular junctions, resulting in a compound muscle action potential (CMAP) **recorded from electrodes placed in various targeted muscles in the limbs**. A pair of subdermal needles are placed in each muscle being recorded, depending on the spinal level of the surgery. The upper limb's latency is shorter than the lower limb's latencies due to the distance between the stimulation and the recording electrodes. TCeMEP responses are very sensitive to muscle relaxants and inhalational agents. Therefore, total intravenous anesthesia (TIVA) is highly recommended with propofol and narcotics with no muscle relaxants. The alarm criteria for TCeMEP include a 50 to 80% drop in the amplitude, a sudden increase in stimulation intensity by 100 volts, and/or change in the waveform morphology. Due to multiple published reading criteria about reading the TCeMEP data, at the authors' place, a combination of all standards is applied and coordinated with the step of surgery and anesthesia (**Figs. 39.3** and **39.4**).

Advantages

TCeMEPs also help the neurophysiology team detect ischemic changes in the peripheral motor nerves, spinal cord, brainstem, and primary motor cortex. TCeMEP is used to assess the functional integrity of the descending corticospinal pathways. It minimizes postoperative motor deficits in patients undergoing spinal surgeries. Recent literature has shown that TCeMEP is more sensitive to nerve root injuries than SSEP.[8]

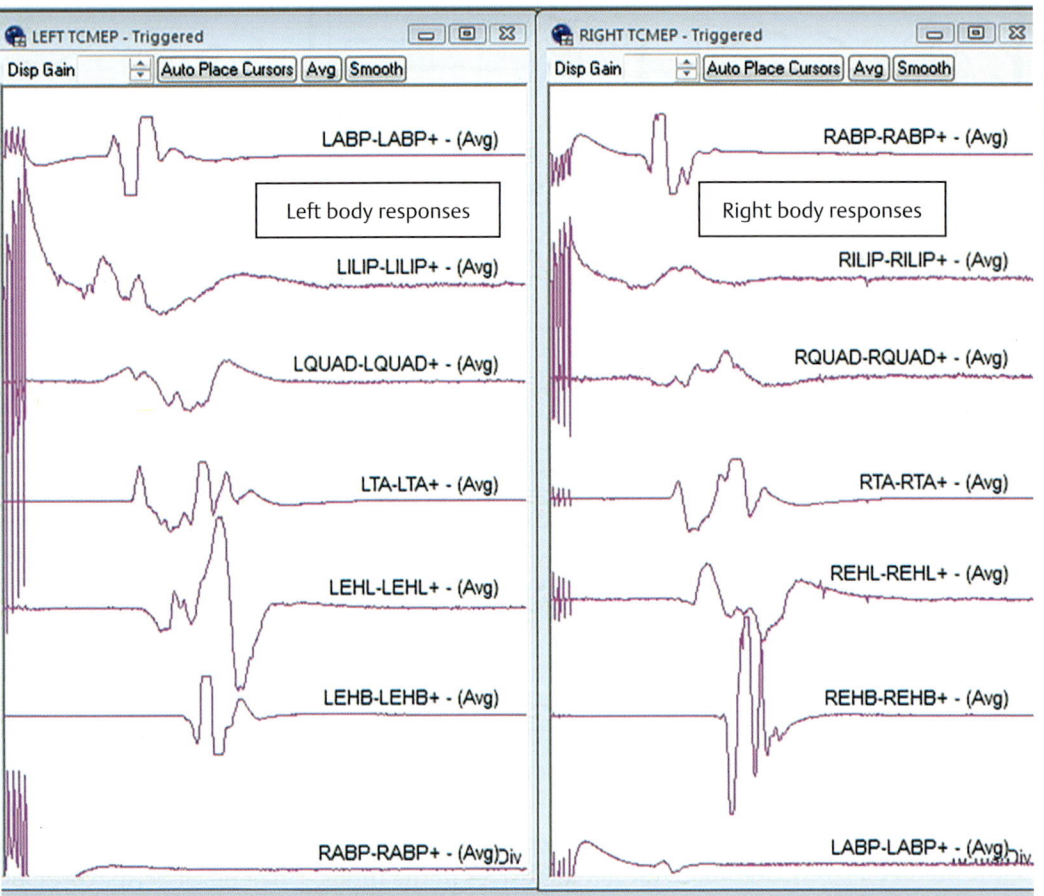

Fig. 39.3 Left and right transcranial electrical motor-evoked potentials (TCeMEP) recorded from left and right body muscles; stimulation at the scalp (normal data).

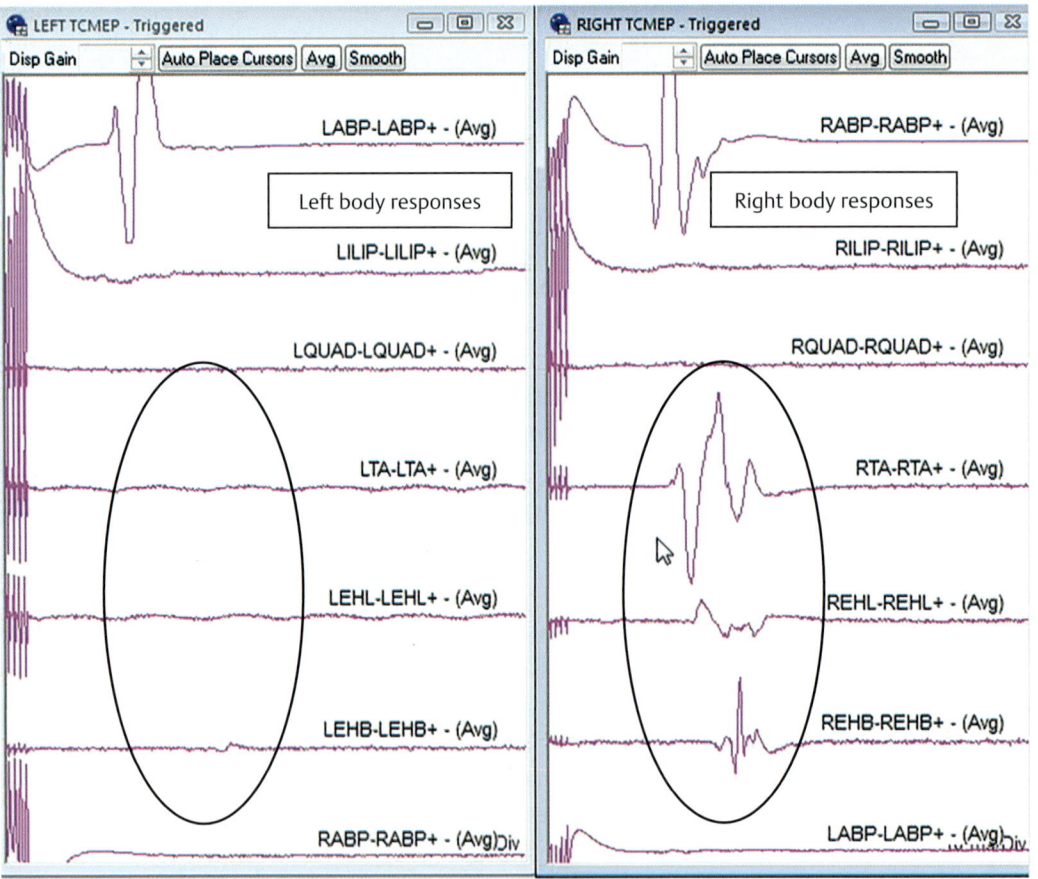

Fig. 39.4 Left and right transcranial electrical motor-evoked potentials (TCeMEP) recorded from left and right body muscles; stimulation at the scalp (data drop on left and right side lower limb muscles). Notice the left and right upper limb muscle (control) is stable.

Disadvantages

TCeMEP monitoring requires a strict anesthesia regimen with TIVA. Muscle relaxants cannot be used to block the responses by paralyzing the muscles. TCeMEP is also sensitive to dexmedetomidine if given at or higher than 0.3 to 0.5 μg/kg/hr. There is no contraindication for monitoring TCeMEP, and special considerations must be given to patients with a history of seizure, pacemakers, deep brain stimulation, and cochlear implants. The benefit of TCeMEP monitoring must be weighed against a limitation in these patients. The technique is considered safe, but surgery may be paused to run TCeMEP because of patient movement. Tongue lacerations can also be avoided by placing appropriate protection using a bite block.

Spontaneous Electromyography (sEMG)

EMG records muscle activity produced by nerve root irritation during surgical procedures. In addition, the muscles supplied by the nerve roots at risk during spinal surgeries are monitored by sEMG. Recording subdermal paired needle electrodes are bilaterally placed in upper and lower extremity muscles during spinal deformity surgeries. The sEMG is very sensitive to any nerve injury and will produce abnormal sEMG activity due to stretching, compression, retraction, or heating of the nerve roots. The abnormal sEMG firing seen are spikes, bursts, trains, and neurotonic discharges due to mechanical, electrical, or thermal irritation. A preoperative nerve root irritation or compression may be identified by the presence of a baseline EMG activity, such as fasciculations or fibrillations.

Intraoperative EMG monitoring focuses on identifying abnormal activity in any muscle supplied by the nerve roots at risk. Prolonged or sustained neurotonic (high amplitude and high frequency) discharges are considered to represent a more severe nerve injury. The muscles monitored during spinal deformity surgery may include the adductor magnus, quadriceps femoris, tibialis anterior, gastrocnemius, abductor hallucis, and anal sphincter depending on the nerve root at risk. In addition, the urethral sphincter muscle monitoring has recently been reported in spinal surgeries.[8] In cervical spine surgeries, the muscles mainly used are deltoids, biceps, triceps, brachioradialis, abductor pollicis brevis, and adductor digiti minimi (**Figs. 39.5–39.7**).

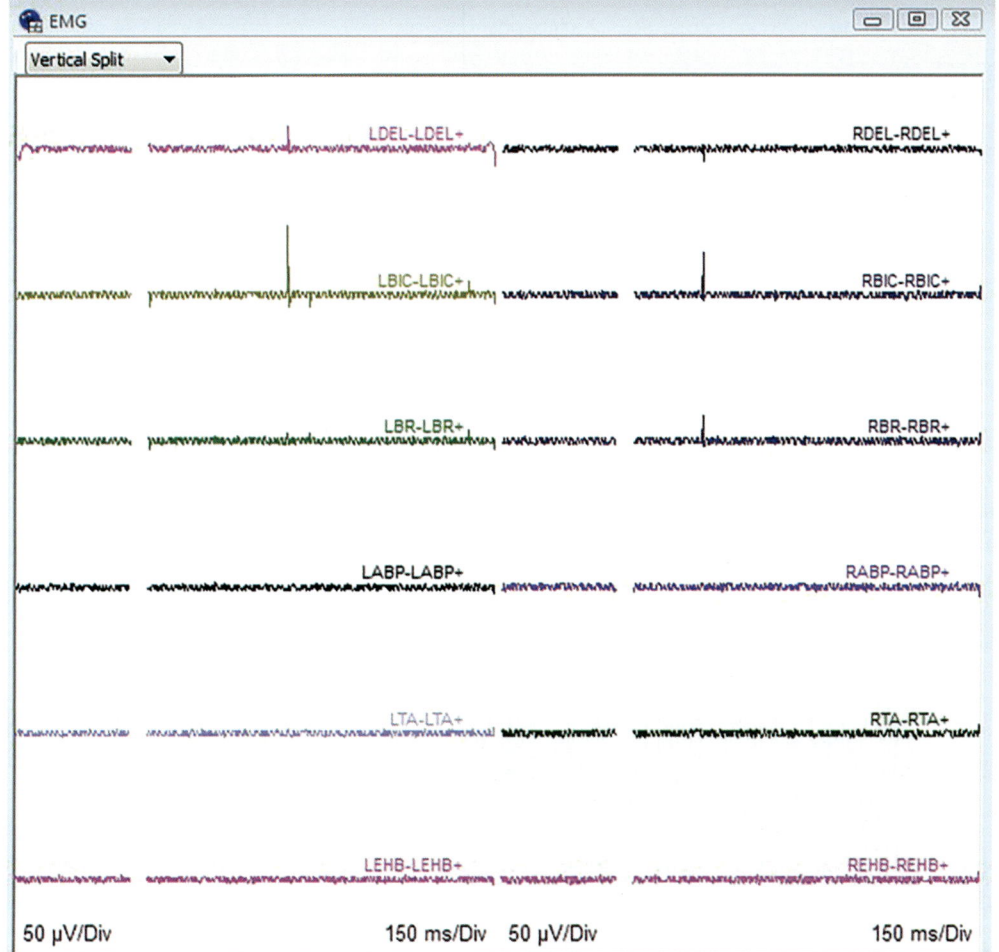

Fig. 39.5 Left and right electromyography (EMG) recorded from left and right upper and lower limb muscles (normal EMG, no alarm is needed).

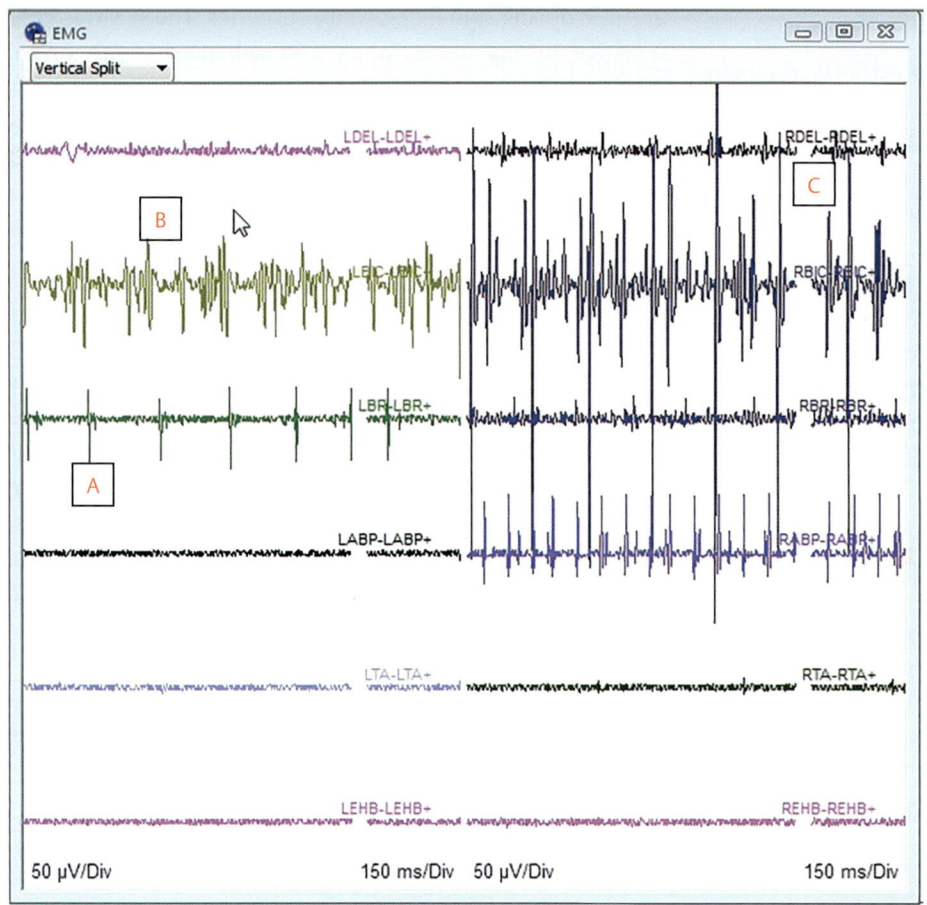

Fig. 39.6 Left and right electromyography (EMG) recorded from left and right upper and lower limb muscles (alarm is needed). A, mild fasciculations; B, bursts (surgeon needs to be notified); C, trains of discharges (red alert to surgeon).

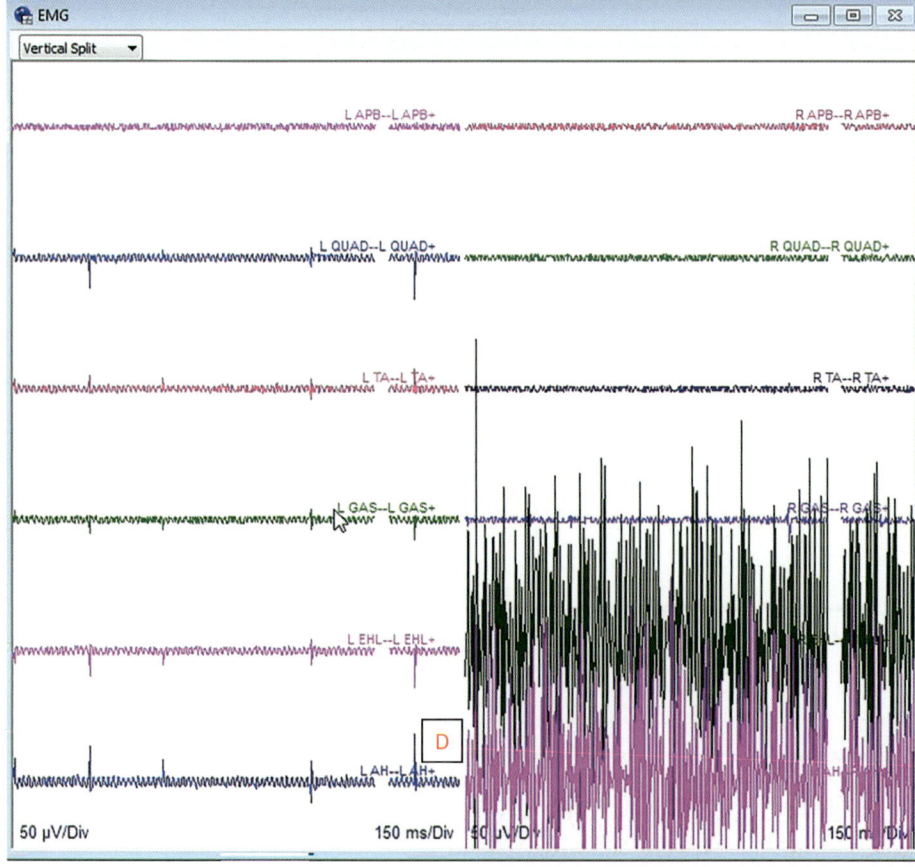

Fig. 39.7 Left and right electromyography (EMG) recorded from left and right upper and lower limb muscles. Right side muscles showing abnormal discharges (red alert and alarm is needed). D, neurotonic discharges (worse form of EMG irritation; if goes unchecked may result in postoperative motor deficit of that muscle group).

Advantages

Free-run or sEMG gives real-time and immediate feedback to the surgeon. This immediate feedback and alert allow the surgeon to act immediately and remove any nerve traction causing abnormal EMG activity.

Disadvantages

Any use of muscle relaxants will interfere with sEMG monitoring. Therefore, the muscle relaxant should only be used for intubation for optimal sEMG monitoring during the surgical procedure. In addition, various biological and electrical artifacts also interfere with the sEMG monitoring, such as electrocautery devices, X-ray machines, C-arm, microscope, electrocardiogram (EKG), etc. Therefore, surgeons should be notified that no EMG data is available while electrical appliances such as electrocautery are in use.

Triggered Electromyography (Direct Nerve and Pedicle Screw Stimulation)

Intraoperative tEMG modality for identifying the nerve root or testing the pedicle screw is utilized routinely during spinal deformity surgeries.[9,10] The tEMG with a monopolar handheld probe gives immediate feedback about any pedicle wall breach. If the breached pedicle screw is not identified correctly, it may cause damage to the spinal cord or the nerve root at that level immediately or during correction

maneuvers. The subdermal needle electrodes placed in the corresponding limb muscles for sEMG are used for recording tEMG responses. Any malpositioned screw will show a threshold of 10 mA or a lower value for screw testing at lumbar levels. The positive predictive value may be 99% if the threshold exceeds 15 mA. The most common reasons for the false-negative responses include muscle relations, chronically irritated nerves, current shunting due to fluid in the exposed area, coated screws, etc. Therefore, the train of four (TOF) testing is intermittently performed during the surgery to confirm the level of muscle relaxation in centers where muscle relaxants are routinely used. At the authors' place, muscle relaxants are totally avoided (**Figs. 39.8** and **39.9**).

Advantages

There is widely published data regarding tEMG stimulation intensity numbers for lumbar screws. Stimulating a lumbar screw using a monopolar stimulator and recording from relevant myotome or relevant muscle for that level at 10 mA or higher is considered a safe screw.

Disadvantages

This test is highly sensitive, and the chances of false positives are high in minor screw breaches. Current will exit at the smallest breach, reach the relevant muscle, and produce a CMAP at lower intensity numbers, creating a false alarm.

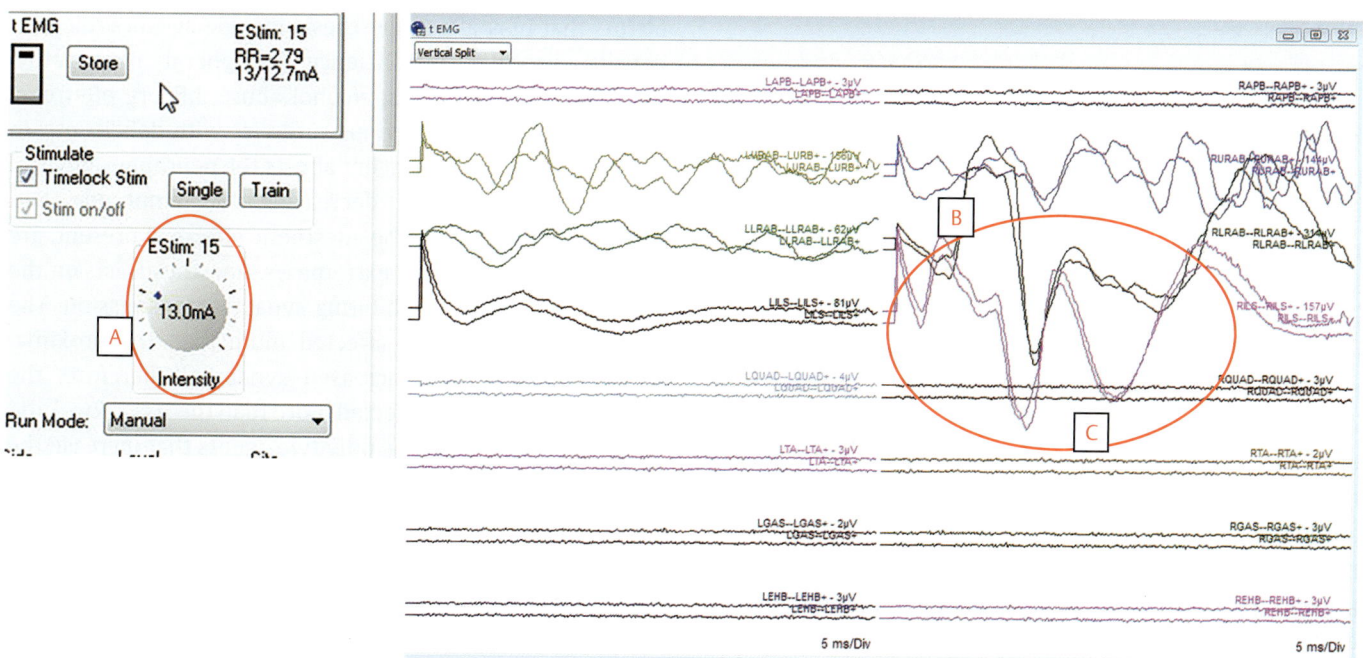

Fig. 39.8 Stimulation intensity (A), artifact (B) that needs to be carefully excluded from true data at the time of interpretation, and true response (C) recorded from right iliopsoas muscle after stimulation of right L1 screw using a monopolar ball tip stimulator at 13 mA. Intensity of response higher than 10 mA for lumbar level screws can be considered safe screws.

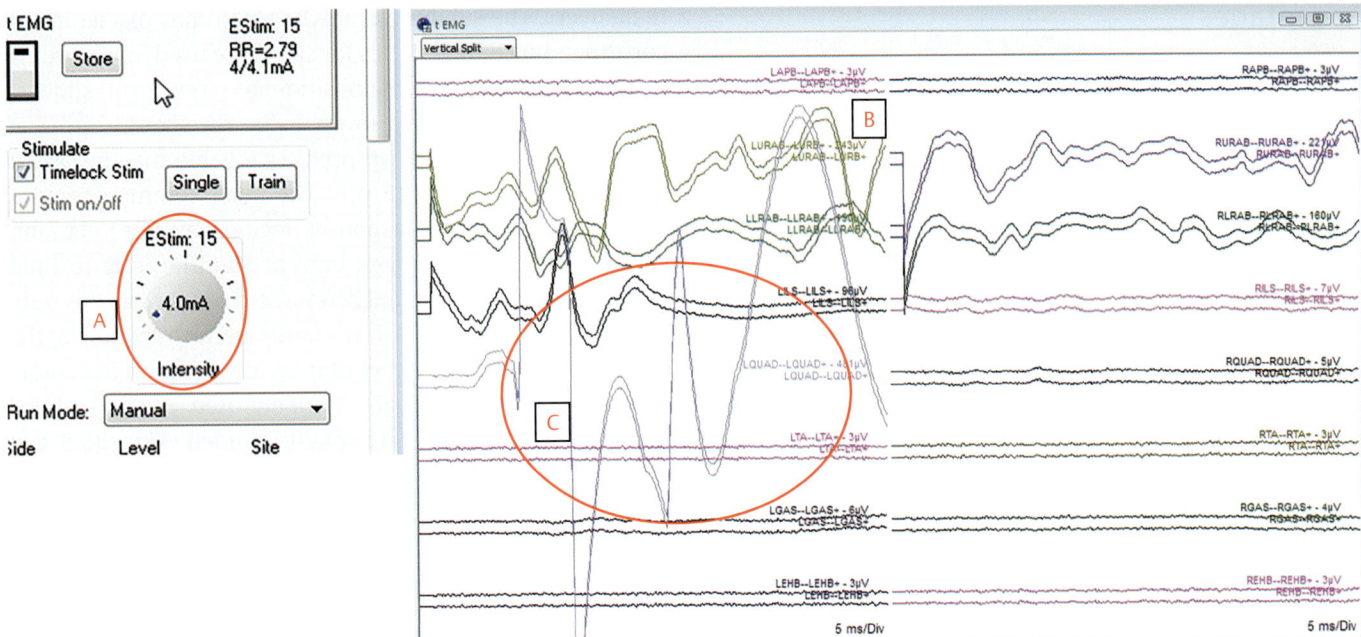

Fig. 39.9 Stimulation ntensity (A), artifact (B) that needs to be carefully excluded from true data at the time of interpretation, and true response (C) recorded from left quadriceps muscle after stimulation of left L3 screw using a monopolar ball tip stimulator at 4 mA. This screw needs to be repositioned. Intensity of response higher than 10 mA for lumbar level screws can be considered safe screws.

Hence, this test is always communicated clearly, and a change must be looked at in TCeMEPs data for that muscle group. Most surgeons would not change screws if they felt good purchase during screw placement. Also, there is insufficient data demonstrating good numbers for thoracic and cervical spine screws.

Train of Four

The level of the neuromuscular blocking agent is monitored by the TOF modality. TOF monitoring is performed from the most distal muscle for optimal TCeMEP and EMG recordings.[11] For example, the posterior tibial nerve is stimulated at the medial malleolus, and responses are recorded in the foot's abductor hallucis and extensor hallucis brevis muscles. The TOF stimulation is performed at the rate of 2.0 Hz for 2 seconds, with four stimuli. The presence of 4/4 twitches corresponds to a 0 to 65% blockade, 3/4 to a 75% blockade, 2/4 twitches corresponds to an 85% blockade, 1/4 twitch corresponds to a 95% blockade, and 0/4 twitches (or absence of any visible twitch) corresponds to a 100% muscle blockade. Therefore, at least 4/4 or 3/4 twitches must be present to perform appropriate intraoperative monitoring, especially TCeMEP, sEMG, and tEMG.

Effects of Anesthesia on Neurophysiologic Monitoring

Anesthetic agents significantly affect neurophysiological signals and vary from one patient to another. Various factors that may affect anesthesia include age, neurological deficits, vascular insufficiency, peripheral neuropathy, neuromuscular disorders, alcohol abuse, history of stroke, metabolic disorders, previous surgeries with deficits etc. In addition, the anesthetic agent affects the neurophysiological monitoring signals by decreasing the amplitude and increasing the latency. The anesthetic effects, if present, are primarily observed in all extremities. Anesthesia acts on the evoked potentials by inhibiting synaptic transmission. The later cortical peaks are affected more than the proximal ones because of the increased synapses. Therefore, the cortical responses are affected more than the subcortical and peripheral responses. The only two agents that increase the amplitude of the SSEP and TCeMEP responses are ketamine and etomidate at low to moderate doses.[12]

All the inhalational agents, including isoflurane, sevoflurane, desflurane, and nitrous oxide (N_2O), significantly suppress SSEP and TCeMEP responses. On the other hand, intravenous agents have minimal effect on SSEP and TCeMEP responses if given as continuous steady-state infusion. Therefore, TIVA with a combination of propofol with a narcotic agent, such as fentanyl, or remifentanil, without any muscle relaxant is recommended for optimal recordings during procedures with multimodality neuromonitoring.[13] In addition, neuromuscular blocking agents have minimal SSEP changes but should be avoided and used only for intubation when monitoring TCeMEP and EMG during spinal deformity surgeries. Dexmedetomidine is increasingly being used in conjunction with TIVA. Dexmedetomidine causes a significant decrease in MEP amplitude when used at infusion rates of 0.3 to 0.5 µg/kg/hr during spinal surgeries and deterioration can be profound in pediatric age groups especially in case of congenital and neuromuscular etiologies[14] (**Figs. 39.10** and **39.11**).

Positioning and Traction Related Data Change

The proper positioning of the patient during the surgery is essential to avoid any peripheral nerve injury. An improper patient positioning may cause compression, stretching, or peripheral nerve ischemia. In addition, the upper limbs are more at risk of postoperative position-related neuropathy. A multimodality IONM with SSEP and TCeMEP can help identify any position-related changes during spine surgeries.[15] The literature supports this view, indicating that brachial plexopathy can occur from improper arm or shoulder positioning during prone position surgeries. When the arms are tucked and pulled down, additional pressure to the brachial plexus stretches the brachial plexus (**Fig. 39.12**).

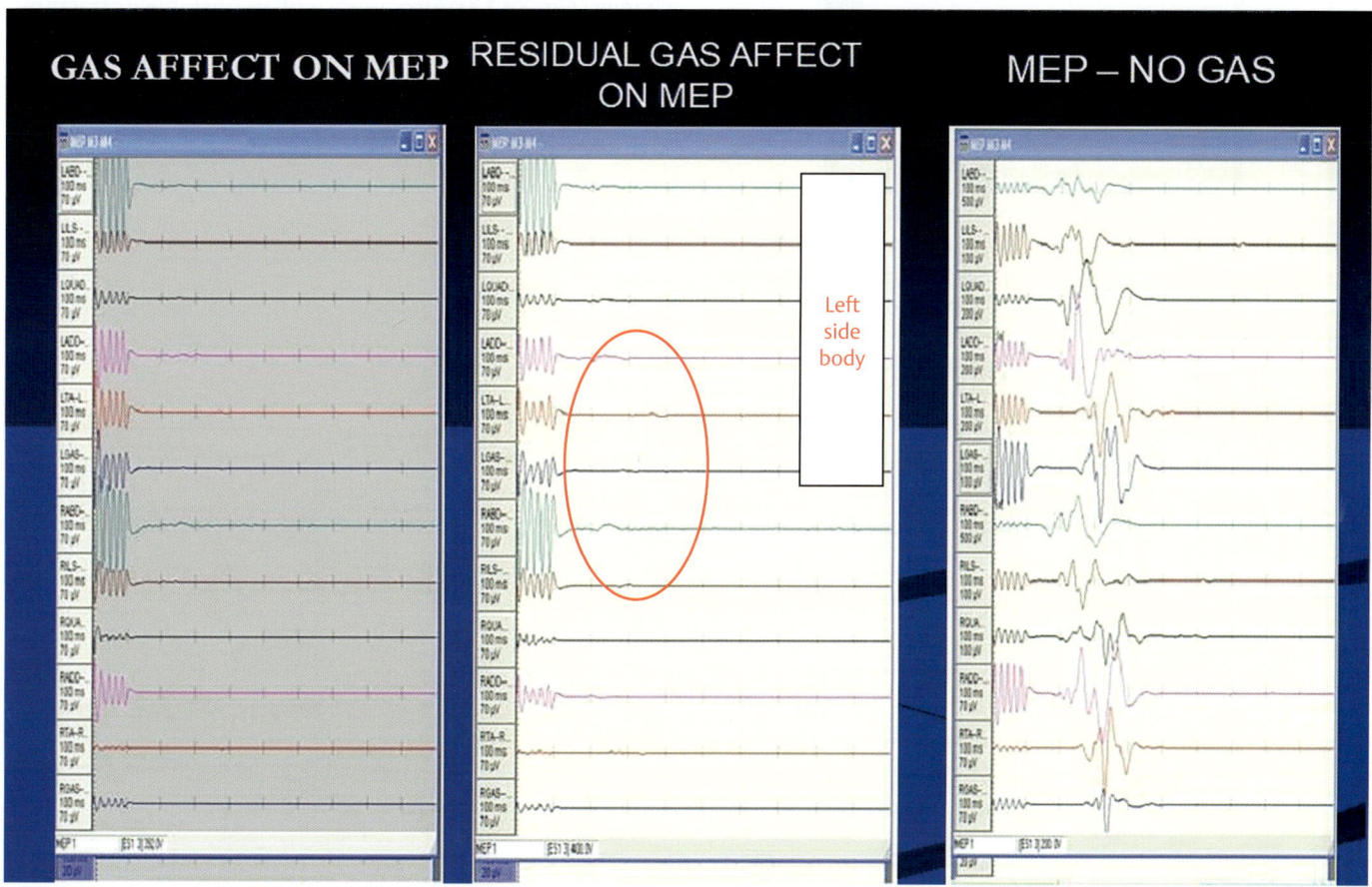

Fig. 39.10 Effect of residual inhalational anesthetics on transcranial electrical motor-evoked potentials (TCeMEP) data. Circle shows small amplitude compound muscle action potentials (CMAPs) starting to show up with sevoflorine at 1.2% approximately (0.5 minimum alveolar concentration (MAC), showing the effects of inhalational anesthetics on TCeMEP data.

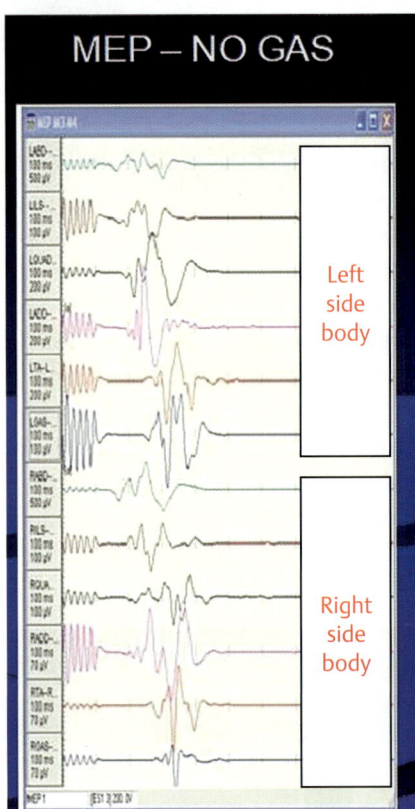

Fig. 39.11 Effect of no inhalational anesthetic Transcranial electrical motor-evoked potentials (TCeMEP) data with total intravenous anesthesia regimen of propofol and remifentanil. Both right and left side showing healthy compound muscle action potentials (CMAPs) at lesser intensity from upper and lower limb muscles compared with **Fig. 39.10**.

According to the American Society of Anesthesiology report, male patients are at higher risk for position-related nerve injuries.[16] The other factors that may increase position-related injuries may include diabetes mellitus, obesity, vascular compromise, and preexisting spinal cord diseases. Therefore, ulnar and median nerve SSEP and upper limb TCeMEP monitoring is recommended for any position-related injuries in spinal surgeries. The neuromonitoring team should immediately inform the anesthesiologist and the surgeon of any change in ulnar SSEP or upper limb TCeMEP responses. The affected limb should be repositioned until the signals return to the baselines to minimize long-term sequelae.[17]

In addition, surgeons sometimes prefer to apply traction at the head and/or body with weights from 5 pounds to 20 to 30 pounds. Therefore, it is imperative that data need to be carefully evaluated in case of traction-related data change (**Fig. 39.13**). Also, in case of an unstable or fractured spine, preposition data needs to be compared with post-position data, and any change needs to be evaluated and communicated to the surgeon with immediate corrective measures applied.

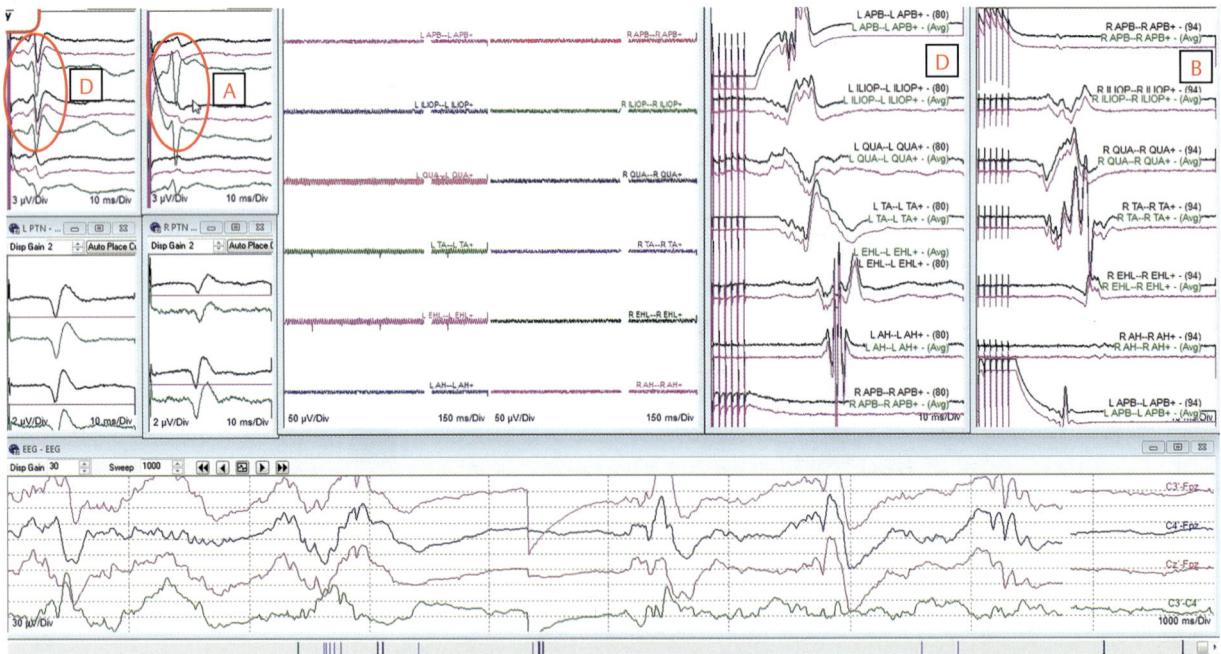

Fig. 39.12 Positioning effect with changes on right side ulnar nerve somatosensory-evoked potentials (SSEPs) showing data change (drop in amplitude shown with red circle) as well as right side motor change in upper limb muscle. A, right ulnar nerve data change (compare green baselines with pink, compare with left ulnar nerve SSEPs in D); B, right upper limb transcranial electrical motor-evoked potentials (TCeMEP) drop (compare right side with left hand D).

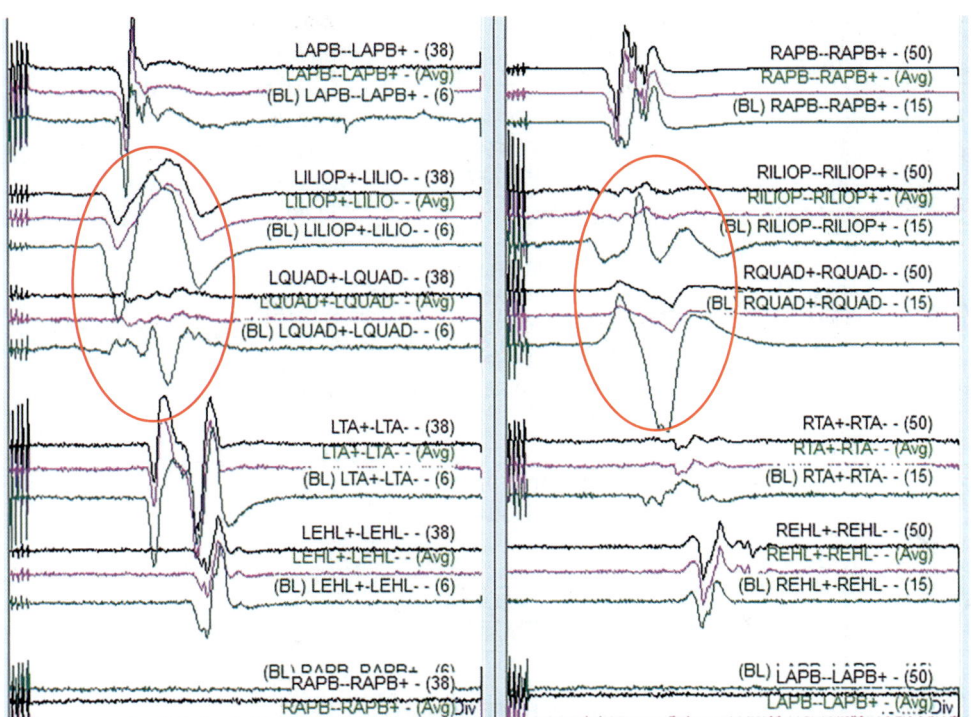

Fig. 39.13 Post-traction data change selectively noticed in more than one muscle groups on both left and right side lower limb muscle transcranial electrical motor-evoked potentials (TCeMEP). Green-baselines; Pink-current wave form after traction.

Effect of Hypotension

Both SSEP and TCeMP responses are affected by hypotension resulting in either decreased, delayed, or lost responses due to ischemia. The gray matter within the spinal cord is most sensitive to ischemia.[18] The loss of synaptic activity in the gray matter occurs within 1 to 2 minutes. On the other hand, the changes are observed between 11 and 20 minutes due to ischemia of the white matter tracts. In addition, poor patient positioning, blood pressure cuff-pressure, tourniquets, and vascular compromise result in peripheral response changes due to limb hypoperfusion. A decrease in the cerebral blood from the average of 50 mL/minute/100 g to less than 20 mL/minute/100 g significantly affects the cortical SSEP responses. The SSEP signals are lost when cerebral blood is between 13 and 18 mL/minute/100g. A loss of SSEP and/or TCeMEP responses may result from a significant decrease in the MAP. Therefore, the MAP should be frequently monitored and documented during spinal deformity surgeries, especially in hypertensive patients. The neuromonitoring team must immediately alert the surgeon and the anesthesiologist to elevate the MAP above the baseline level to avoid ischemic injury of the nervous system. It is the authors' practice to maximize normotensive exposure, especially in more extensive deformity correction surgeries (**Fig. 39.14**). Consideration also needs to be given to blood loss, and correction of hemoglobin may be warranted if data shows a global change in both upper and lower extremities in a thoracolumbar deformity surgery.

Effect of Hypothermia

Neurophysiological signals are affected by hypothermia due to reduced neuronal synaptic functions. The changes in the data are noted by a decrease in the amplitude and an increase in the latency of the evoked responses. A delay in the peripheral limb responses with average interpeak latencies results from limb hypothermia. These changes are significant in the cortical responses due to multiple synapses along the pathway.[19] Cold intravenous fluids can cause whole-body hypothermia, and cold irrigation fluids can cause local hypothermia. In general, these changes can be easily avoided by communicating with anesthesia team and noting body temperature.

Real-Time Monitoring with Trained and Experienced Staff

Utilizing a highly trained IONM team will improve patient outcomes.[20] Intraoperative neurophysiological monitoring by a certified technologist (Certification in Intraoperative Neurophysiological Monitoring [CNIM][21] in the operative room, with onsite or remote real-time, regardless of location, oversight by a board-certified neurophysiologist [DABNM, FASNM]),[22] and/or an IONM fellowship-trained neurologist[23] will have a better patient outcome than less or nontrained teams.

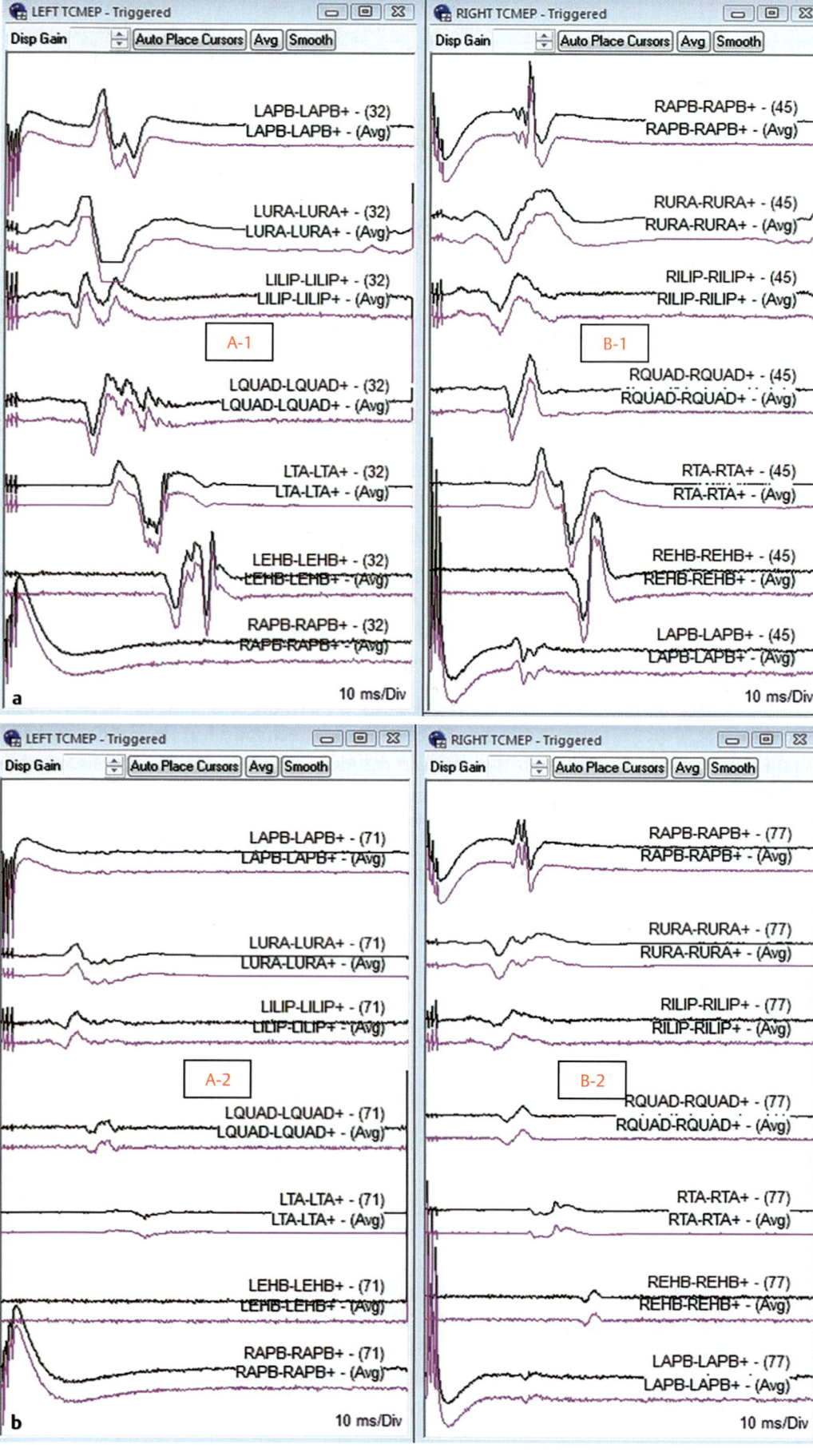

Fig. 39.14 Mean arterial pressure (MAP) drop at 60 mm Hg showing a global change in transcranial electrical motor-evoked potentials (TCeMEP) data on both right and left sides including upper and lower limbs. Most such data changes can easily be corrected by keeping a healthy MAP of 75 mm Hg. Left side A1 at MAP of 75 mm Hg; right side B1 at MAP of 75 mm Hg ; left side A2 at MAP of 60 mm Hg; right side B2 at MAP of 60 mm Hg.

Conclusion

It is highly recommended to utilize a multimodality neurophysiologic monitoring approach during spinal deformity surgeries. Multimodality monitoring approach with SSEP, TCeMEP, sEMG, and tEMG can reduce the risk of neurologic injury during spinal deformity surgeries.[24] There are advantages and disadvantages of each modality. Still, when used in combination, the increase in sensitivity and specificity helps in preventing and minimizing any devastating postoperative neurologic deficits.

References

1. Eager M, Shimer A, Jahangiri FR, Shen F, Arlet V. Intraoperative neurophysiological monitoring (IONM): lessons learned from 32 case events in 2069 spine cases. Am J Electroneurodiagn Technol 2011;51(4):247–263
2. Larson SJ, Sances A Jr. Evoked potentials in man. Neurosurgical applications. Am J Surg 1966;111(6):857–861
3. Nuwer MR, Dawson EG, Carlson LG, Kanim LE, Sherman JE. Somatosensory evoked potential spinal cord monitoring reduces neurologic deficits after scoliosis surgery: results of a large multicenter survey. Electroencephalogr Clin Neurophysiol 1995;96(1):6–11
4. Khan MH, Smith PN, Balzer JR, et al. Intraoperative somatosensory evoked potential monitoring during cervical spine corpectomy surgery: experience with 508 cases. Spine 2006;31(4):E105–E113
5. Jahangiri FR. Surgical Neurophysiology: A Reference Guide to Intraoperative Neurophysiological Monitoring (IONM). 2nd ed. Lexington, KY: 2012
6. Deletis V, Sala F. Intraoperative neurophysiological monitoring of the spinal cord during spinal cord and spine surgery: a review focus on the corticospinal tracts. Clin Neurophysiol 2008;119(2):248–264
7. Jahangiri FR, Silverstein JW, Trausch C, et al. Motor evoked potential recordings from the urethral sphincter muscles (USMEPs) during spine surgeries. Neurodiagn J 2019;59(1):34–44
8. Wilent WB, Tesdahl EA, Harrop JS, et al. Utility of motor evoked potentials to diagnose and reduce lower extremity motor nerve root injuries during 4,386 extradural posterior lumbosacral spine procedures. Spine J 2020;20(2):191–198
9. Jahangiri FR, Asdi RA, Tarasiewicz I, Azzubi M. Intraoperative triggered electromyography recordings from the external urethral sphincter muscles during spine surgeries. Cureus 2019;11(6):e4867
10. Jahangiri FR, Sheryar M, Al Behairy Y. Early detection of pedicle screw-related spinal cord injury by continuous intraoperative neurophysiological monitoring (IONM). Neurodiagn J 2014;54(4):323–337
11. Ali HH, Utting JE, Gray C. Stimulus frequency in the detection of neuromuscular block in humans. Br J Anaesth 1970;42(11):967–978
12. Hasan MS, Tan JK, Chan CYW, Kwan MK, Karim FSA, Goh KJ. Comparison between effect of desflurane/remifentanil and propofol/remifentanil anesthesia on somatosensory evoked potential monitoring during scoliosis surgery—a randomized controlled trial. J Orthop Surg (Hong Kong) 2018;26(3):2309499018789529
13. Tamkus AA, Rice KS, Kim HL. Differential rates of false-positive findings in transcranial electric motor evoked potential monitoring when using inhalational anesthesia versus total intravenous anesthesia during spine surgeries. Spine J 2014;14(8):1440–1446
14. Holt F, Strantzas S, Zaarour C, et al. The effect of dexmedetomidine on motor-evoked potentials during pediatric posterior spinal fusion surgery: a retrospective case-control study. Can J Anaesth 2020;67(10):1341–1348
15. Overzet K, Wang C, Jahangiri FR. The incidence of positioning-related intraoperative neurophysiological monitoring (IONM) changes: a review of 5894 surgeries. EC Neurology 2019;11(1):46–54
16. Schwartz DM, Sestokas AK, Hilibrand AS, et al. Neurophysiological identification of position-induced neurologic injury during anterior cervical spine surgery. J Clin Monit Comput 2006;20(6):437–444
17. Pajewski TN, Arlet V, Phillips LH. Current approach on spinal cord monitoring: the point of view of the neurologist, the anesthesiologist and the spine surgeon. Eur Spine J 2007;16(Suppl 2):S115–S129
18. Shlobin NA, Raz E, Shapiro M, et al. Spinal neurovascular complications with anterior thoracolumbar spine surgery: a systematic review and review of thoracolumbar vascular anatomy. Neurosurg Focus 2020;49(3):E9
19. Markand ON, Warren C, Mallik GS, King RD, Brown JW, Mahomed Y. Effects of hypothermia on short latency somatosensory evoked potentials in humans. Electroencephalogr Clin Neurophysiol 1990;77(6):416–424
20. Kim SM, Kim SH, Seo DW, Lee KW. Intraoperative neurophysiologic monitoring: basic principles and recent update. J Korean Med Sci 2013;28(9):1261–1269
21. ABRET: Neurodiagnostic Credentialing and Accreditation - CNIM exam eligibility requirements. (2021). Accessed August 24, 2021 at: https://www.abret.org/candidates/credentials/cnim/
22. ABNM: American Board of Neurophysiologic Monitoring. Accessed December 26, 2021: http://www.abnm.info/
23. Gertsch JH, Moreira JJ, Lee GR, et al; membership of the ASNM. Practice guidelines for the supervising professional: intraoperative neurophysiological monitoring. J Clin Monit Comput 2019;33(2):175–183
24. Thirumala PD, Huang J, Thiagarajan K, Cheng H, Balzer J, Crammond DJ. Diagnostic accuracy of combined multimodality somatosensory evoked potential and transcranial motor evoked potential intraoperative monitoring in patients with idiopathic scoliosis. Spine 2016;41(19):E1177–E1184

40 Complication Avoidance for Adult Degenerative Deformity Surgery

Mehmet Zileli and Nevhis Akıntürk

Introduction

Adult degenerative deformity incidence increases in the elderly population as life expectancy increases. The presentation of the disease is usually with intolerable pain, neurological deficits, and disability of the patient.[1-3] Therefore, the mainstay of the surgery is to correct the deformity, decrease the pain and improve the neurological deficits. To achieve these goals, open, minimally invasive, and hybrid surgeries might be performed.[4]

However, adult degenerative deformity surgery may have a high rate of complications and reoperations due to medical comorbidities, osteoporosis, and severe deformity.[5-9] The complication rates after deformity surgery may vary from 37 to 71% in recent series.[2,8,10-12] Complications may affect patient outcomes and the quality of life.[2] Prevention of complications decreases costs, especially for high-risk patients.[5]

The complications are primarily associated with patients' age > 70, osteoporosis, posterior surgery, obesity, more than seven fusion levels, hospital length of stay of >7 days, nutrition, and sagittal balance.[5,13] It is found that obese patients have an 80% increase of risk of readmission.[5,14] Due to infection and instrumentation failure, a reoperation rate of 10.1% is also reported.[15] The most common factors for short-term reoperations are wound infection, screw malposition, and proximal junctional failure.[9] Osteoporotic patients have a 98% reoperation rate in 5 years.[16]

Selection of the patient and the type of surgery in adult degenerative deformity is quite challenging. Hence, preventing complications, the impact on quality of life, and the overall cost will be improved.

Definition

Adult degenerative deformity surgery is seen widely in the aging population. With the development of the fusion techniques, the deformities are treatable. However, the complications also become more compelling.[13,17,18]

The risk factors for deformity surgery are age, gender, comorbidities, obesity, duration of symptoms, and number of fused levels.[11,17-19] Neurological impairment, dural tears, excessive blood loss, and other systemic complications are mostly encountered while correcting the deformity. In addition, implant failure, pseudoarthrosis, and proximal junctional kyphosis are seen frequently as long-term complications.

The intraoperative, perioperative, and postoperative complication rates are reported at 30.5, 48.5, and 58.7%, respectively.[20] The total complication rates were similar between the open and hybrid groups; however, the intraoperative complication rate was higher in the open group.[19] Recent studies show that minimally invasive surgery reduces complication rates.[21,22]

Glassman et al's system and Clavien-Dindo classification system are mostly used for complications of adult generative deformity surgery.[2,23,24] This chapter will classify complications as systemic, neurologic, instrumentation, wound problems, and infection.

Systemic Complications

Pulmonary complications are often seen after degenerative spine surgery, and the incidence is 7.6%.[14] Atelectasis and pneumonia are the other major pulmonary problems postoperatively.[25] The risk of pulmonary embolism increases with age and longer operation time. To avoid this complication, pneumatic stockings and low molecular weight heparin usage should be used accordingly.

Excessive blood loss was the most common operative complication, leading to massive blood transfusion and myocardial infarction.[8,20] Also, low hemoglobin levels after blood loss can lead to a delay in wound healing.[18]

Minimally invasive surgery is found to be related to less blood loss, shorter operation time, and minor muscle damage.[26] Also, it has a shorter duration of hospital stay and leads to early mobilization.

Significant frailty was associated with a worse outcome for the patient.[27] Preoperative assessment of the patient must be done carefully to decrease the complications.

Neurologic Complications

During the correction of the malalignment, decompression, osteotomy, and placing of the instruments, there is always a potential risk of spinal cord injury. The quality of life decreases with the new onset of neurological deficits during the surgery. The overall complication rate was reported as 10.8%.[28,29] Retraction of the spinal cord, malposition of the instruments, and pressure applied by Kerrison are the primary factor of spinal cord injury.[30] Using high-speed drills may solve the problem of pressure application with the Kerrison rongeur, and intraoperative neuromonitoring, fluoroscopy, and navigation systems could be the other solutions for decreasing spinal cord injury.

During degenerative deformity surgery, spinal cord injury could be observed before decompression during positioning, during decompression because of direct damage, and after/during osteotomy.

Neurological complication incidence is approximately 20%. To clarify the cause, magnetic resonance imaging (MRI) and computed tomography (CT) scans should be done.[31] Spinal cord injury, insufficient decompression, hematoma/ischemia, and instrumentation placement must be assessed with the scans. Hematoma evacuation, decompression, or screw revision must be performed without wasting time.

The mean arterial pressure must be monitored and kept at approximately 90 to 95 mm Hg.[32] Corticosteroid administration is still controversial. The application of methylprednisolone is still favored for the improvement of neurological deficits.[33]

Wound Problems and Infection

The risk factors for wound infection are diabetes, obesity, and prolonged operation time.[34] The overall infection rate was found to be between 1.2 and 4%.[35] To decrease infection rates, prophylactic antibiotics are commonly used. On the other hand, vancomycin powder, rifampicin, and gentamicin are used topically to prevent wound infections.[36] Anterior approaches are associated with less blood loss and shorter operation times, leading to fewer infections.[37]

After the operation, wound management is also essential to avoid pressure, to regulate blood sugar levels, and for early mobilization. Cerebrospinal fluid leakage is a challenging complication; surgical sites and systemic infection reduce wound healing. The primary treatment regimens are bed rest, patient hydration, and antibiotic prophylaxis. However, epidural blood patch, lumbar drainage, and revision surgery must be considered.

Instrumentation Complications

Pedicle screw fixation is used commonly in adult degenerative deformity surgery. Due to vertebral rotation, screw placement is always challenging in these patients. Malposition of the screws may cause root irritation or spinal cord injury resulting in severe pain and deficits.[38] CT-based navigation systems have better accuracy in screw insertion than freehand techniques.[38] Using electromyography (EMG) intraoperatively to detect malposition of the instrumentation is another technique.[39]

Even though it is a rare complication, great vessel injury is one of the problems in instrumentation, as the aorta lies on the left side and vena cava and azygous vein on the right side. Therefore, preoperative measurement of the vertebral bodies and anteroposterior fluoroscopy controls should be done.

Wrong-level surgery is also one of the most devastating complications of spine surgery. Even if the incidence is low at 0.13%, this complication is avoidable with the appropriate counting of vertebral bodies with fluoroscopy intraoperatively. Transitional vertebras should be kept in mind according to preoperative images and intraoperatively counting should be done from the top or bottom of the spine.

Mechanical implant failure after degenerative deformity surgery is one of the challenging and devastating complications. The most common reasons for mechanical implant failure are proximal junctional kyphosis and rod breakage.[40]

Elderly patients, osteoporosis, obesity, excessive correction of the deformity, and postoperative sagittal imbalance are the risk factors for proximal junctional kyphosis (PKJ).[41] PJK is often present with a fracture of the adjacent vertebra or screw loosening at the upper level of the construct.[40,41] To avoid this complication, treatment of osteoporosis should be considered before the surgery. Vertebroplasty is used as a prophylactic technique to prevent the fracture of the vertebra.[40]

In some series, the most common complication of implant failure is rod breakage.[8] It is seen mainly in elderly and obese patients and long-segment fusions.[6] Multi-rod construct systems were developed to encounter this complication.

The risk factors for pseudoarthrosis are smoking, older age, and suboptimal spinal balance.[40] Revision surgery must be considered if the patient is symptomatic and using auto-allograft, and the construct should be augmented. To avoid adjacent segment implant failure and pseudoarthrosis, pelvic fixation and multi-rod systems are preferred.[42] The mechanical complications increase the risk of reoperation rate by 32 to 72%.[20]

Tips and Tricks

- Avoidance of systemic complications
  - Cardiopulmonary complications
    - Preoperative medical treatment
    - Intraoperative monitoring, prevention of excessive blood loss
    - Early mobilization
  - Thromboembolic complications
    - Medical treatment, both pre- and postoperatively
    - Early mobilization
    - Using compression stockings intra- and postoperatively
  - Renal complications
    - Avoiding excessive blood loss
  - Excessive blood loss prevention
    - Positioning of the patient
    - Careful hemostasis during surgery
    - Autologous blood transfusion
    - Intraoperative antifibrinolytic treatment
- Avoidance of neurological complications
  - High-speed drill instead of Kerrison rongeur, operation microscope for laminectomy
  - Less retraction of the neural tissues
  - Using intraoperative neuromonitoring
  - Fluoroscopy, neuronavigation
- Avoidance of wound problems and infection
  - Antibiotic prophylaxis
  - Skin preparation
  - Less blood loss and short operation time
  - Regulation of blood sugar levels
  - Minimally invasive surgery
  - Irrigation with topical antibiotics
- Avoidance of implant complications
  - Intraoperative fluoroscopy, neuromonitoring, navigation
  - Osteoporosis treatment
  - Adequate bone grafts
  - Achieving good sagittal balance and avoiding excessive sagittal vertical axis (SVA) corrections
  - Hybrid constructs
  - Good selection of end vertebra, both cranial and caudal levels
  - Interbody fusions if necessary

Key Points

- Adult degenerative deformity surgery is challenging in every aspect.
- Careful evaluation of the patient and preoperative assessment of the comorbidities are mandatory to avoid complications.
- Minimally invasive surgery should be the first-line treatment of choice in selected patients to avoid excessive blood loss, proximal junctional kyphosis, and vertebra fracture.

References

1. Yen CP, Mosley YI, Uribe JS. Role of minimally invasive surgery for adult spinal deformity in preventing complications. Curr Rev Musculoskelet Med 2016;9(3):309–315
2. Wick JB, Le HV, Lafage R, et al; International Spine Study Group. Assessment of adult spinal deformity complication timing and impact on 2-year outcomes using a comprehensive adult spinal deformity classification system. Spine 2022;47(6):445–454
3. Schwab F, Dubey A, Gamez L, et al. Adult scoliosis: prevalence, SF-36, and nutritional parameters in an elderly volunteer population. Spine (Phila Pa 1976) 2005;30(9):1082–5
4. Koller H, Pfanz C, Meier O, et al. Factors influencing radiographic and clinical outcomes in adult scoliosis surgery: a study of 448 European patients. Eur Spine J 2016;25(2):532–548
5. Taliaferro K, Rao A, Theologis AA, Cummins D, Callahan M, Berven SH. Rates and risk factors associated with 30- and 90-day readmissions and reoperations after spinal fusions for adult lumbar degenerative pathology and spinal deformity. Spine Deform. 2022;10(3):625–637
6. Soroceanu A, Burton DC, Oren JH, et al; International Spine Study Group. Medical complications after adult spinal deformity surgery: incidence, risk factors, and clinical impact. Spine 2016;41(22):1718–1723
7. Zanirato A, Damilano M, Formica M, et al. Complications in adult spine deformity surgery: a systematic review of the recent literature with reporting of aggregated incidences. Eur Spine J 2018;27(9):2272–2284
8. Smith JS, Klineberg E, Lafage V, et al; International Spine Study Group. Prospective multicenter assessment of perioperative and minimum 2-year postoperative complication rates associated with adult spinal deformity surgery. J Neurosurg Spine 2016;25(1):1–14
9. Crawford CH III, Glassman SD, Carreon LY, et al. Prevalence and indications for unplanned reoperations following index surgery in the adult symptomatic lumbar scoliosis NIH-sponsored clinical trial. Spine Deform 2018;6(6):741–744
10. Jain A, Hassanzadeh H, Puvanesarajah V, et al; International Spine Study Group. Incidence of perioperative medical complications and mortality among elderly patients

undergoing surgery for spinal deformity: analysis of 3519 patients. J Neurosurg Spine 2017;27(5):534–539

11. Acosta FL Jr, McClendon J Jr, O'Shaughnessy BA, et al. Morbidity and mortality after spinal deformity surgery in patients 75 years and older: complications and predictive factors. J Neurosurg Spine 2011;15(6):667–674

12. Kwan KYH, Bow C, Samartzis D, et al. Non-neurologic adverse events after complex adult spinal deformity surgery: results from the prospective, multicenter Scoli-RISK-1 study. Eur Spine J 2019;28(1):170–179

13. Barbanti Bròdano G, Terzi S, Gasbarrini A, Bandiera S, Simoes C, Boriani S. Do benefits overcome the risks related to surgery for adult scoliosis? A detailed analysis of a consecutive case series. Eur Spine J 2013;22(Suppl 6):S795–S802

14. Manoharan SR, Baker DK, Pasara SM, Ponce B, Deinlein D, Theiss SM. Thirty-day readmissions following adult spinal deformity surgery: an analysis of the National Surgical Quality Improvement Program (NSQIP) database. Spine J 2016;16(7):862–866

15. Mok JM, Cloyd JM, Bradford DS, et al. Reoperation after primary fusion for adult spinal deformity: rate, reason, and timing. Spine 2009;34(8):832–839

16. Puvanesarajah V, Shen FH, Cancienne JM, et al. Risk factors for revision surgery following primary adult spinal deformity surgery in patients 65 years and older. J Neurosurg Spine 2016;25(4):486–493

17. De la Garza Ramos R, Nakhla J, Echt M, et al. Risk factors for 30-day readmissions and reoperations after 3-column osteotomy for spinal deformity. Global Spine J 2018;8(5):483–489

18. Camino-Willhuber G, Guiroy A, Servidio M, et al. Unplanned Readmission Following Early Postoperative Complications After Fusion Surgery in Adult Spine Deformity: A Multicentric Study. Global Spine J. 2023;13(1):74–80

19. Uribe JS, Deukmedjian AR, Mummaneni PV, et al; International Spine Study Group. Complications in adult spinal deformity surgery: an analysis of minimally invasive, hybrid, and open surgical techniques. Neurosurg Focus 2014;36(5):E15

20. Klineberg EO, Passias PG, Poorman GW, et al. Classifying complications: assessing adult spinal deformity 2-year surgical outcomes. Global Spine J 2020;10(7):896–907

21. Anand N, Baron EM, Khandehroo B, Kahwaty S. Long-term 2- to 5-year clinical and functional outcomes of minimally invasive surgery for adult scoliosis. Spine 2013;38(18):1566–1575

22. Khajavi K, Shen AY. Two-year radiographic and clinical outcomes of a minimally invasive, lateral, transpsoas approach for anterior lumbar interbody fusion in the treatment of adult degenerative scoliosis. Eur Spine J 2014;23(6):1215–1223

23. Glassman SD, Hamill CL, Bridwell KH, Schwab FJ, Dimar JR, Lowe TG. The impact of perioperative complications on clinical outcome in adult deformity surgery. Spine 2007;32(24):2764–2770

24. Dindo D, Demartines N, Clavien PA. Classification of surgical complications: a new proposal with evaluation in a cohort of 6336 patients and results of a survey. Ann Surg. 2004;240(2):205–13

25. Imposti F, Cizik A, Bransford R, Bellabarba C, Lee MJ. Risk factors for pulmonary complications after spine surgery. Evid Based Spine Care J 2010;1(2):26–33

26. Than KD, Mummaneni PV, Bridges KJ, et al. Complication rates associated with open versus percutaneous pedicle screw instrumentation among patients undergoing minimally invasive interbody fusion for adult spinal deformity. Neurosurg Focus 2017;43(6):E7

27. Zileli M, Dursun E. How to improve outcomes of spine surgery in geriatric patients. World Neurosurg 2020;140:519–526

28. Bhagat S, Vozar V, Lutchman L, Crawford RJ, Rai AS. Morbidity and mortality in adult spinal deformity surgery: Norwich Spinal Unit experience. Eur Spine J 2013;22(Suppl 1):S42–S46

29. Zeng Y, Chen Z, Guo Z, Qi Q, Li W, Sun C. Complications of correction for focal kyphosis after posterior osteotomy and the corresponding management. J Spinal Disord Tech 2013;26(7):367–374

30. He B, Yan L, Xu Z, Guo H, Liu T, Hao D. Treatment strategies for the surgical complications of thoracic spinal stenosis: a retrospective analysis of two hundred and eighty three cases. Int Orthop 2014;38(1):117–122

31. Lenke LG, Fehlings MG, Shaffrey CI, et al. Neurologic outcomes of complex adult spinal deformity surgery: results of the prospective, multicenter scoli-RISK-1 study. Spine 2016;41(3):204–212

32. Walters BC, Hadley MN, Hurlbert RJ, et al. American Association of Neurological Surgeons; Congress of Neurological Surgeons. Guidelines for the management of acute cervical spine and spinal cord injuries: 2013 update. Neurosurgery. 2013;60(CN_suppl_1):82–91

33. Bracken MB. Steroids for acute spinal cord injury. Cochrane Database Syst Rev 2012;1(1):CD001046

34. Farah K, Lubiato A, Meyer M, et al. Surgical site infection following surgery for spinal deformity: about 102 patients. Neurochirurgie 2021;67(2):152–156

35. Charosky S, Guigui P, Blamoutier A, Roussouly P, Chopin D; Study Group on Scoliosis. Complications and risk factors of primary adult scoliosis surgery: a multicenter study of 306 patients. Spine 2012;37(8):693–700

36. Bakhsheshian J, Dahdaleh NS, Lam SK, Savage JW, Smith ZA. The use of vancomycin powder in modern spine surgery: systematic review and meta-analysis of the clinical evidence. World Neurosurg 2015;83(5):816–823

37. Lee NJ, Kothari P, Kim JS, et al. Early complications and outcomes in adult spinal deformity surgery: an NSQIP study based on 5803 patients. Global Spine J 2017;7(5):432–440

38. Gelalis ID, Paschos NK, Pakos EE, et al. Accuracy of pedicle screw placement: a systematic review of prospective in vivo studies comparing free hand, fluoroscopy guidance and navigation techniques. Eur Spine J 2012;21(2):247–255

39. Samdani AF, Tantorski M, Cahill PJ, et al. Triggered electromyography for placement of thoracic pedicle screws: is it reliable? Eur Spine J 2011;20(6):869–874

40. Yagi M, Akilah KB, Boachie-Adjei O. Incidence, risk factors and classification of proximal junctional kyphosis: surgical outcomes review of adult idiopathic scoliosis. Spine 2011;36(1):E60–E68

41. Nguyen NL, Kong CY, Hart RA. Proximal junctional kyphosis and failure-diagnosis, prevention, and treatment. Curr Rev Musculoskelet Med 2016;9(3):299–308

42. Guevara-Villazón F, Boissiere L, Hayashi K, et al. Multiple-rod constructs in adult spinal deformity surgery for pelvic-fixated long instrumentations: an integral matched cohort analysis. Eur Spine J 2020;29(4):886–895

Index